PUBLIC HEALTH PERSPECTIVES ON DEPRESSIVE DISORDERS

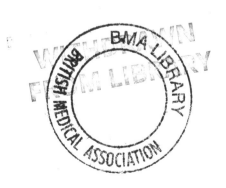

Public Health Perspectives on Depressive Disorders

EDITED BY

NEAL L. COHEN, MD

Clinical Professor, Department of Psychiatry,
    Icahn School of Medicine at Mount Sinai
Adjunct Professor, Department of Population Health,
    New York University School of Medicine
Senior Medical Advisor, New York State Office of Mental Health
Former Commissioner, New York City Departments
    of Health and Mental Health

JOHNS HOPKINS UNIVERSITY PRESS
BALTIMORE

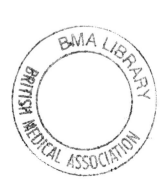

© 2017 Johns Hopkins University Press
All rights reserved. Published 2017
Printed in the United States of America on acid-free paper
9 8 7 6 5 4 3 2 1

Johns Hopkins University Press
2715 North Charles Street
Baltimore, Maryland 21218-4363
www.press.jhu.edu

Library of Congress Cataloging-in-Publication Data

Names: Cohen, Neal L., editor.
Title: Public health perspectives on depressive disorders / edited by Neal L. Cohen.
Description: Baltimore : Johns Hopkins University Press, 2017. | Includes bibliographical
    references and index.
Identifiers: LCCN 2016046992 | ISBN 9781421422794 (hardcover : alk. paper) | ISBN 1421422794
    (hardcover : alk. paper) | ISBN 9781421422800 (pbk. : alk. paper) | ISBN 1421422808
    (pbk. : alk. paper) | ISBN 9781421422817 (electronic) | ISBN 1421422816 (electronic)
Subjects: | MESH: Depressive Disorder—prevention & control | Depressive Disorder—therapy |
    Public Health Practice | Cost of Illness
Classification: LCC RC537 | NLM WM 171.5 | DDC 616.85/27—dc23
    LC record available at https://lccn.loc.gov/2016046992

A catalog record for this book is available from the British Library.

*Special discounts are available for bulk purchases of this book. For more information, please contact
Special Sales at 410-516-6936 or specialsales@press.jhu.edu.*

Johns Hopkins University Press uses environmentally friendly book materials, including recycled
text paper that is composed of at least 30 percent post-consumer waste, whenever possible.

CONTENTS

CONTRIBUTORS

SERGIO AGUILAR-GAXIOLA, MD, PhD Center for Reducing Health Disparities, School of Medicine, University of California, Davis, Sacramento, California

JOAN ROSENBAUM ASARNOW, PhD Semel Institute for Neuroscience and Human Behavior, David Geffen School of Medicine, University of California, Los Angeles, California

ALFIEE M. BRELAND-NOBLE, PhD, MHSc Department of Psychiatry, Georgetown University Medical Center, Washington, DC

EVELYN J. BROMET, PhD Departments of Psychiatry and Preventive Medicine, The State University of New York at Stony Brook, Stony Brook, New York

HELEN CERIGO, MSc Department of Epidemiology, Biostatistics and Occupational Health, McGill University, Montreal, Canada

TRINA CHANG, MD, MPH Depression Clinical and Research Program, Massachusetts General Hospital, Harvard Medical School, Boston, Massachusetts

NEAL L. COHEN, MD Department of Psychiatry, Icahn School of Medicine at Mount Sinai, New York; New York State Office of Mental Health, Albany, New York

WILSON M. COMPTON, MD, MPE National Institute on Drug Abuse, the National Institutes of Health, Bethesda, Maryland

PATRICK W. CORRIGAN, PsyD Department of Psychology, Illinois Institute of Technology, Chicago, Illinois

PIM CUIJPERS, PhD Department of Clinical Psychology, VU University, Amsterdam, The Netherlands

APRIL JOY DAMIAN, MSc Johns Hopkins Bloomberg School of Public Health, Baltimore, Maryland

PETER DE JONGE, PhD Department of Developmental Psychology, Interdisciplinary Center Psychopathology and Emotion Regulation, University of Groningen, Groningen, The Netherlands

J. KONADU FOKUO Department of Psychology, Illinois Institute of Technology, Chicago, Illinois

AMELIA R. GAVIN, PhD University of Washington School of Social Work, Seattle, Washington

CONSTANCE L. HAMMEN, PhD Department of Psychiatry and Biobehavioral Sciences, Semel Institute for Neuroscience and Human Behavior, David Geffen School of Medicine, University of California, Los Angeles, California

Beth Han, MD, PhD, MPH Substance Abuse and Mental Health Services Administration, Rockville, Maryland

Deborah Hasin, PhD Department of Psychiatry, College of Physicians and Surgeons, Columbia University, New York; New York State Psychiatric Institute, New York, New York

Jennifer L. Hughes, PhD Department of Psychiatry, University of Texas Southwestern Medical Center, Dallas, Texas

Ronald C. Kessler, PhD Department of Health Care Policy, Harvard Medical School, Boston, Massachusetts

Daniel N. Klein, PhD Department of Psychology, The State University of New York at Stony Brook, Stony Brook, New York

Daniel C. Kopala-Sibley, PhD Department of Psychology, The State University of New York at Stony Brook, Stony Brook, New York

Amy Kwan, MPH The Graduate Center, City University of New York, New York

Alissa R. Link, MPH New York University Langone Medical Center, New York, New York

Gustavo Loera, EdD Center for Reducing Health Disparities, School of Medicine, University of California, Davis, Sacramento, California

Richard McKeon, PhD, MPH Substance Abuse and Mental Health Services Administration, Rockville, Maryland

Tamar Mendelson, PhD Johns Hopkins Bloomberg School of Public Health, Baltimore, Maryland

Jacquelyn L. Meyers, PhD Department of Psychiatry and Behavioral Sciences, The State University of New York, Downstate Medical Center, Brooklyn, New York

Jeanne Miranda, PhD Center for Health Services and Society, Department of Psychiatry and Biobehavioral Sciences, David Geffen School of Medicine, University of California, Los Angeles, California

Regina Miranda, PhD Hunter College and The Graduate Center, City University of New York, New York

Ana Ortin, PhD New York State Psychiatric Institute, Columbia University Medical Center, New York, New York

Charles Platkin, PhD, MPH New York City Food Policy Center at Hunter College, City University of New York, New York

Lillian Polanco-Roman, MA, MPhil The Graduate Center, City University of New York, New York

Amélie Quesnel-Vallée, PhD Department of Epidemiology, Biostatistics and Occupational Health, Department of Sociology, McGill University, Montreal, Canada

Rebecca Rebbe, MSW University of Washington School of Social Work, Seattle, Washington

KATE SCOTT, PhD, MA Department of Psychological Medicine, University of Otago, Dunedin, New Zealand

VICTORIA SHAHLY, PhD Department of Health Care Policy, Harvard Medical School, Boston, Massachusetts

EFRAIN TALAMANTES, MD, MS Center for Reducing Health Disparities, School of Medicine, University of California, Davis, Sacramento, California

JORGE VALDERRAMA, PhD The Graduate Center, City University of New York, New York

DANIEL VIGO, MD Harvard T. H. Chan School of Public Health, Boston, Massachusetts

MARSHA WILCOX, EdD, ScD Janssen Pharmaceutical Research and Development, Titusville, New Jersey

ALBERT YEUNG, MD, ScD Depression Clinical and Research Program, Massachusetts General Hospital, Harvard Medical School, Boston, Massachusetts

ACKNOWLEDGMENTS

I am grateful to all the authors who have contributed chapters to this book. I have learned a great deal from them throughout the process of creating the volume.

I am also grateful to my colleagues, past and present, at the New York City Department of Health and Mental Hygiene and the New York State Office of Mental Health for helping to advance a vision of a truly integrated health and mental health care system that recognizes the important contribution of mental health to overall health.

The book is dedicated, as always, to Ilene, Alex, Becca, and Jake.

PUBLIC HEALTH PERSPECTIVES ON DEPRESSIVE DISORDERS

CHAPTER 1

The Path to the Public Health Recognition of Depressive Disorders

Neal L. Cohen, MD

Depression has long been known to be one of the most common manifestations of psychological distress in Western societies. Consequently, the training of mental health practitioners has routinely addressed depression as a target of intervention, most frequently as an individual treatment approach. This volume, however, builds on a body of knowledge largely advanced over the past two decades that recognizes depression as a major public health issue worldwide, one that is amenable to public health approaches to disease prevention (McLaughlin, 2011). Research data that underscore the importance of bringing public mental health systems into much closer alignment with mainstream public health practice to benefit both mental health and overall population health are presented.

Over the past 150 years, public health systems have made dramatic and ongoing improvements in health and life expectancy. The containment of infectious diseases, largely through systematic improvements in air, water, and food safety, and advances in population-level health education and promotion have largely contributed to the increase in life expectancy of greater than three decades (Greene, 2001). The seminal work of McGinnis and Foege (1993) described the modifiable factors contributing to poor health outcomes, which have helped bring about greater public health focus on lifestyle and behavioral patterns contributing to the increasing burden of chronic diseases. These efforts, at either individual or population-level behavioral changes, to improve health outcomes are often stymied by the social and environmental realities of people's lives. As public health practice examines the disparities in health outcomes across communities, attention to the social determinants of health, such as the stresses associated with urban living (Freudenberg, Galea, & Vlahov, 2006) and the consequences of poverty for overall health (Andrulis, 2006), has helped raise awareness of mental health as a major component of public health. This century's increased public health focus on the burden of chronic diseases will require far greater attention to the interface of health and behavioral health, particularly the contributions that mental well-being can make to overall population health.

The Emergence and Contributions of Psychiatric Epidemiology

Psychiatric epidemiology as a distinct discipline began to emerge in the mid-twentieth century, stimulated by the efforts made by military screening for psychological symptoms and impairments during World War II (Tohen, Bromet, Murphy, & Tsuang, 2000). Larger community surveys of mental well-being during the second half of the twentieth century, such as the Midtown Manhattan Study (Srole et al., 1962) and the Stirling County Study (Leighton, 1959), were the beginning of a new era of descriptive psychiatry and assessment of psychopathology prevalence in the general population. But it was the publication of the third edition of the *Diagnostic and Statistical Manual of Mental Disorders* (*DSM-III*; American Psychiatric Association, 1980) that provided empirical data to allow for a clearer and more standardized classification of mental illness. Consequently, a series of survey instruments were developed to assess mental disorders in the general population consistent with *DSM* criteria that were used in a number of large, national, population-based studies, such as the Epidemiologic Catchment Area study (Regier et al., 1984) and the National Comorbidity Surveys (Kessler et al., 1994), which provided estimates of the prevalence of psychopathology nationwide. With these surveys estimating approximately 16%–17% of US adults and 11%–12% of adolescents experiencing a major depressive episode at least once in their lifetime (Kessler et al., 2003; Merikangas et al., 2010), major depression is one of the most common mental disorders (Kessler, Chiu, Demier, Merikangas, & Walters, 2005). Moving beyond counting the number of affected individuals, significant advances in mental health epidemiology in the first decade of the twenty-first century have also allowed for new models and approaches to quantify the prevalence and burden of mental disorders, the adequacy of service delivery models, and the risk factors that contribute to morbidity and premature mortality (Susser, Schwartz, Morabia, & Bromet, 2006).

The past two decades have seen major advances toward a population approach to mental health that has underscored the significance of mental health to population health. The Global Burden of Disease Study (Murray & Lopez, 1996) developed a new metric, disability-adjusted life years, which combines information on both mortality and disability to quantify the contribution of chronic diseases to human suffering and population health. In a comparative analysis examining the impact of more than two hundred disease conditions worldwide, the researchers were able to use disability-adjusted life years to quantify the global burden attributable to depressive disorders, calculated by adding years lived with a disability to years of lost life because of disease-specific premature death.

When disability was accounted for and mortality was no longer the sole indicator of disease burden, the follow-up Global Burden of Disease Study (Üstün, Ayuso-Mateos, Chatterji, Mathers, & Murray, 2004), conducted in 2000, found that depressive disorders were the fourth leading cause of disease burden worldwide, after lower respiratory infections, diarrheal diseases, and conditions arising during the perinatal period. According to the 2010 GBD study (Ferrari et al. 2013), when compared with other diseases and injuries, major depressive disorder (MDD) accounted for 8.2% of global YLDs in 2010, making it the second leading cause of global disability. The global burden of depressive disorders had increased by 37.5% between 1990 and 2010 because of population growth and aging, with projections of even greater burden for depressive disorders by 2020.

Further underscoring the public health significance of mental health, the release of a series of reports on mental health (US Public Health Service, 1999a; 1999b; 2000; 2001) by then–US Surgeon General David Satcher brought new awareness of the high prevalence of mental disorders worldwide and an established therapeutic armamentarium for their treatment. As a former head of the Centers for Disease Control and Prevention and leading public health authority, Dr. Satcher's advocacy for the inclusion of mental health into the mainstream of the nation's public health agenda was greatly influential in drawing both professional and public attention to the importance of mental health to overall health.

Incorporating mental health into the mainstream public health agenda requires the application of tools and strategies of public health practice, such as surveillance, screening and early identification, preventive interventions, health promotion, and community action (Cohen & Galea, 2011). The adoption of a population-level focus on mental health, along with the training needed to apply public health tools and strategies to the work, is now progressing, fueled by the growing body of research evidence that has established the interrelationship of health and mental health in chronic health conditions (Kessler et al., 2011). With one-quarter of the US population afflicted with a mental disorder in any one year, and half of the adult population with one or more chronic medical conditions, the rate of comorbidity is high (Kessler et al., 2005), and importantly, comorbidity is associated with significantly elevated health risks and negative outcomes.

Most closely studied has been the prevalent comorbidity of depressive disorders with chronic health conditions (e.g., Benton, Staab, & Evans, 2007). Evidence has mounted over the past few decades for a bidirectional link between depression and medical illness that derives from a complex interaction between physiological and environmental factors (Gleason, Pierce, Walker, & Warnock, 2013). In a controlled study of patients hospitalized for acute coronary syndrome who screened positive for MDD, Glassman, Bigger, and Gaffney (2009) found that mortality more than doubled over 6.7 years of follow-up for those with greater MDD severity or failure to significantly improve over the first six months of treatment. Importantly, effective and persistent treatment of depression among those with comorbid chronic health conditions appears to mitigate the likelihood of increased morbidity and mortality (Bogner, Morales, Post, & Bruce, 2007). Furthermore, a systematic literature review by Huffman and colleagues (2014) found that those integrated care interventions that targeted both mental health and chronic medical illness may have superior outcomes over treatments that separate the domains of health and mental health.

As the evidence of the need for integrating behavioral health and medical care has mounted, models of intervention are being developed, tested, and implemented. The treatment of depression in primary care has gained significant traction over the past decade, with numerous community-based programs and interventions, and hospital-based collaborations that have emphasized the screening and treatment for depression in general adult medical practice. Moreover, the evidence for a bidirectional link between major depression with poor health outcomes associated with huge medical costs and lessened quality of life challenges the traditional model of bifurcated health and mental health care.

Organization and Content of the Book

This volume has been organized into three parts. In the first part, "Impact," four chapters underscore the public health significance of depressive illness by focusing on the evidence provided by recent approaches to nosology, epidemiology, illness burden, and impact on overall health. In the first chapter, Kopala-Sibley and Klein describe the phenomenology of depressive disorders and provide a clear framework for the study of community-level depression that informs efforts at early detection and preventive interventions. Next, Kessler and colleagues describe how the World Mental Health Surveys have extended our understanding of the public health impact of depressive illness worldwide through measurement of the impairment and disability that accompanies these disorders. Building on their review of the data for the descriptive epidemiology of depressive illness, Kessler and colleagues underscore the high prevalence, early age of onset, chronicity, associated impairments in role functioning, and comorbidity with many physical disorders as confirming depression's worldwide impact. Next, Aguilar-Gaxiola and colleagues report on a growing body of literature that links depression with multiple chronic health conditions. Given the evidence for the association of major depression with poor health outcomes, the data strongly suggest that failing to address population-level depressive illness may hinder public health efforts to improve population-level physical health. Meyers and Hasin examine the well-documented comorbidity of major depression with alcohol and drug disorders as well as the challenge to service delivery programs to provide integrated models of treatment. Importantly, Meyers and Hasin highlight the finding that persons with comorbid major depression and substance use disorder will likely have greater depressive symptomatology and functional impairment, and be at greater risk of dying by suicide than those without the comorbidity.

In the second part, "Influences," three chapters examine the social and environmental influences on depressive disorders that are critical to future efforts to prevent illness and promote mentally healthy communities. Cerigo and Quesnel-Vallée observe the epidemiology of social inequalities in depression and the pathways by which these inequalities are manifested. Their findings lead to the authors' support for those policies that may disrupt the cycle of poor social and economic circumstances with human suffering due to depressive illness. In the next chapter, Hammen reviews evidence for the influence of maternal depression on the intergenerational transmission and continuity of depression and stress in children. With nearly half of all children with depressed mothers experiencing some diagnosable mental disorder, Hammen cites the need for more research that addresses the mechanisms of depression transmission and the treatments and preventive interventions for families with parental depression. Fokuo and Corrigan conclude this section by examining the ways that mental health stigma can impede recovery from depression and the research needed to identify and change the social structures that maintain stigma.

The third part, "Risk, Strategies, and Interventions," comprises 10 chapters that address the challenges to a number of population-level groups that are found to be at elevated risk for depressive disorders. Addressing the vulnerability of diverse groups to depressive illness, chapter authors discuss best practices to mitigate risk and improve both the preventive and therapeutic armamentarium.

In the first chapter, Hughes and Asarnow describe the unique challenges of recognizing and addressing the clinical care needs of children and adolescents presenting with stress, suicide, or symptoms of mood disturbance. They highlight the opportunity for school-based interventions to both identify those at greatest risk for depressive disorders and create ways in which schools can promote well-being in children and adolescents.

Miranda and colleagues address the public health significance of adolescent suicidality, as it is among the leading three causes of death in adolescence, with suicidal thoughts and behaviors at highest prevalence during the adolescent years. With greater than half of adolescent deaths by suicide occurring in first-time attempts, the authors underscore the need for research efforts to improve suicide risk assessment and the treatment of those adolescents most at risk. Han and colleagues examine the interrelationship of suicidality and depressive disorders, including the implications for suicide prevention strategies at the population and individual levels. Using a public health lens, they highlight the importance of research needed to focus suicide prevention strategies during high-risk time periods and to promote help-seeking and mental health treatment among individuals with depressive disorders and suicidal ideation or behavior.

Mendelson and Damian review mindfulness-based interventions, both school- and community-based, which train capacities for attention, awareness, compassion, and self-regulation of thoughts and emotions for chronically stressed and disadvantaged urban youth. The authors see many challenges and opportunities for the implementation of mindfulness to enhance social-emotional learning among adolescents, including depression management for significant public health impact.

As the leading cause of disease-related disability among women worldwide (Lopez & Mathers, 2006), major depression assumes an especially impactful role during pregnancy and in the early child-rearing years. Gavin and Rebbe report on the prevalence and risk factors associated with depressive disorders during pregnancy, concluding with the recommendation for universal screening for depression during the prenatal period and the availability of effective treatment options.

Breland-Noble and Miranda describe the underutilization of adequate mental health services for depressive disorders among racial and ethnic minorities. Despite generally having better mental health than white Americans, minorities suffer from disparities in mental health care, with elevated rates of more severe illness resulting in greater need for emergency room care and hospital admission. Next, Chang and Yeung examine promising interventions to identify and address depressive illness in primary care settings. Pioneered by Katon and colleagues (1995), the collaborative care model has expanded to many diverse primary care populations. The authors review the potential for the collaborative care model to address the needs of depressed minority patients who are more likely to present in primary care than in mental health settings.

Cohen examines the public health challenge of addressing late-life depressive illness worldwide with the population of people aged 65 or older, which is projected to triple from an estimated 524 million in 2010 to nearly 1.5 billion in 2050 (National Institute on Aging, 2011). In the United States, "late-life depression" is associated with very significant increases in health care costs, even after adjusting for chronic medical illness and mental health treatment. With the accumulation of chronic health conditions among the aging population, there is a uniquely important public health opportunity to address the underdiagnosis and undertreatment of depressive illness in older adults with models of integrated mental health and physical health care.

Platkin and colleagues describe the many ways in which advances in health technology and the wide utilization of social media can reach, inform, and support various diverse populations that are less likely to access office-based mental health care until depression symptoms evolve into more seriously disabling levels of major depression. The digital revolution is creating new tools with internet-based applications to health care that can enhance mental health surveillance and deliver both preventive and therapeutic interventions to many.

In the final chapter, Cuijpers reports on those efforts that address key challenges in preventing depressive illness and promoting mental health in a population-based framework. Going forward, prevention may become an important way, in addition to treatment, to reduce the enormous public health burden of depression in the coming years.

With its focus on depressive illness within a broader public health framework, this volume aims to highlight the centrality of mental health to public health, underscoring the universality of the challenge to recognize and promote improved care for depressive illness. I hope this book serves as an invaluable resource for researchers and practitioners to develop and facilitate the conduct of pilot and feasibility studies of promising treatment and preventive interventions that might mitigate the progression toward major depression and other mental disorders among populations at risk.

The past 25 years have seen mental health advance with greater application of the tools and strategies of the public health field (e.g., surveillance, screening and early identification, preventive interventions, health promotion, and community action) toward a twenty-first-century public mental health policy and practice. With legislative changes now bringing parity in health and behavioral health insurance coverage, health and mental health professionals can better move beyond their traditional professional silos to advance collaborative care models that deliver holistic and integrated care, and remove the long-standing marginalization of mental health from other efforts to improve population health. As World Health Organization scientists stated nearly a decade ago, "there is no health without mental health" (Prince et al., 2007).

References

American Psychiatric Association. (1980). *Diagnostic and statistical manual of mental disorders* (3rd ed.). Washington, DC: American Psychiatric Association.

Andrulis, D. (2006). Access to high-quality health care in US cities: Balancing community need and service system survival. In N. Freudenberg, S. Galea, & D. Vlahov (Eds.), *Cities and the health of the public* (pp. 85–105). Nashville, TN: Vanderbilt University Press.

Benton, T., Staab, J., & Evans, D. L. (2007). Medical co-morbidity in depressive disorders. *Annals of Clinical Psychiatry, 19*(4), 289–303.

Bogner, H. R., Morales, K. H., Post, E. P., & Bruce, M. L. (2007). Diabetes, depression, and death: A randomized controlled trial of a depression treatment program for older adults based in primary care (PROSPECT). *Diabetes Care, 30*(12), 3005–3010.

Cohen, N., & Galea, S. (Eds.). (2011). *Population mental health: Evidence, policy, and public health practice.* New York, NY: Routledge Press.

Ferrari, A. J., Charlson, F. J., Norman, R. E., Patten, S. B., Freedman, G., Murray, C. J., . . . Whiteford, H. A. (2013). Burden of depressive disorders by country, sex, age, and year: Findings from the Global Burden of Disease Study 2010. *PLoS Med 10*(11): e1001547. doi:10.1371/journal.pmed.1001547

Freudenberg, N., Galea, S., & Vlahov, D. (Eds.). (2006). *Cities and the health of the public.* Nashville, TN: Vanderbilt University Press.

Glassman, A. H., Bigger, J. T., & Gaffney, M. (2009). Psychiatric characteristics associated with long-term mortality among 361 patients having an acute coronary syndrome and major depression: Seven-year follow-up of SADHART participants. *Archives of General Psychiatry, 66*(9), 1022–1029.

Gleason, O. C., Pierce, A. M., Walker, A. E., & Warnock, J. K. (2013). The two-way relationship between medical illness and late-life depression. *Psychiatric Clinics of North America, 36*(4), 533–544.

Greene, V. W. (2001). Personal hygiene and life expectancy improvements since 1850: Historic and epidemiologic associations. *American Journal of Infection Control, 29*(4), 203–206.

Huffman, J. C., Niazi, S. K., Rundell, J. R., Sharpe, M., & Katon, W. J. (2014). Essential articles on collaborative care models for the treatment of psychiatric disorders in medical settings: A publication by the Academy of Psychosomatic Medicine Research and Evidence-Based Practice Committee. *Psychosomatics, 55*(2), 109–122.

Katon, W., Von Korff, M., Lin, E., Walker, E., Simon, G. E., Bush, T., . . . Russo, J. (1995). Collaborative management to achieve treatment guidelines: Impact on depression in primary care. *JAMA, 273*(13), 1026–1031.

Kessler, R. C., Aguilar-Gaxiola, S., Alonso, J., Chatterji, S., Lee, S., Levinson, D., . . . Wang, P. S. (2011). The burden of mental disorders worldwide: Results from the World Mental Health Surveys. In N. Cohen & S. Galea (Eds.), *Population mental health: Evidence, policy, and public health practice* (pp. 9–37). New York, NY: Routledge.

Kessler, R. C., Berglund, P., Demler, O., Jin, R., Koretz, D., Merikangas, K. R., . . . Walters, E. D. (2003). The epidemiology of major depressive disorder: Results from the National Comorbidity Survey Replication (NCS-R). *Journal of the American Medical Association, 289*(23), 3095–3105.

Kessler, R. C., Chiu, W. T., Demier, O., Merikangas, K. R., & Walters, E. E. (2005). Prevalence, severity, and comorbidity of 12-month *DSM-IV* disorders in the National Comorbidity Survey Replication. *Archives of General Psychiatry, 62*(6), 617–627.

Kessler, R. C., McGonagle, K. A., Zhao, S., Nelson, C. B., Hughes, M., Eshleman, S., . . . Kendler, K. S. (1994). Lifetime and 12-month prevalence of *DSM-III-R* psychiatric disorders in the United States: Results from the National Comorbidity Survey. *Archives of General Psychiatry, 51*(1), 8–19.

Leighton, A. H. (1959). *My name is legion: Foundations for a theory of man in relation to culture* (Vol. 1.). New York, NY: Basic Books.

Lopez, A. D., & Mathers, C. D. (2006). Measuring the global burden of disease and epidemiological transitions: 2002–2030. *Annals of Tropical Medicine & Parasitology, 100*(5–6), 481–499.

McGinnis, J. M., & Foege, W. H. (1993). Actual causes of death in the United States. *JAMA, 270*, 2207–2212.

McLaughlin, K. A. (2011). The public health impact of major depression: A call for interdisciplinary prevention efforts. *Prevention Science, 12*, 361–371.

Merikangas, K. R., He, J., Burstein, M., Swanson, S. A., Avenevoli, S., Cui, L., . . . Swendsen, J. (2010). Lifetime prevalence of mental disorders in US adolescents: Results from the National Comorbidity Survey Replication-Adolescent Supplement (NCS-A). *Journal of the American Academy of Child and Adolescent Psychiatry, 49*, 980–989.

Murray, C. J., & Lopez, A. D. (Eds.). (1996). *The global burden of disease: A comprehensive assessment of mortality and disability from diseases, injuries and risk factors in 1990 and projected to 2020*. Boston, MA: Harvard School of Public Health, World Health Organization, and World Bank.

National Institute on Aging. (2011). *Global health and aging*. Rockville, MD: US Government Printing Office.

Prince, M., Patel, V., Sexena, S., Maj, M., Maselko, J., Phillips, M. R., & Rahman, A. (2007). Global mental health 1: No health without mental health. *Lancet, 370*(9590), 859–877.

Regier, D. A., Myers, J. K., Kramer, M., Robins, L. N., Blazer, D. G., Hough, R. L., . . . Locke, B. Z. (1984). The NIMH Epidemiologic Catchment Area program: Historical context, major objectives, and study population characteristics. *Archives of General Psychiatry, 41*(10), 934–941.

Srole, L., Langer, T. S., Michael, S. T., Kirkpatrick, P., Opler, M., & Rennie, T. A. (1962). *Mental health in the metropolis*. New York, NY: Harper & Row.

Susser, E., Schwartz, S., Morabia, A., & Bromet, E. J. (2006). *Psychiatric epidemiology*. New York, NY: Oxford University Press.

Tohen, M., Bromet, E., Murphy, J. M., & Tsuang, M. T. (2000). Psychiatric epidemiology. *Harvard Review of Psychiatry, 8*(3), 111–125.

US Public Health Service. (1999a). *Mental health: A report of the Surgeon General*. Washington, DC: US Department of Health and Human Services.

US Public Health Service. (1999b). *The Surgeon General's call to action to prevent suicide*. Washington, DC: US Department of Health and Human Services.

US Public Health Service. (2000). *Report of the Surgeon General's conference on children's mental health: A national action agenda*. Washington, DC: US Department of Health and Human Services.

US Public Health Service. (2001). *Mental health: Culture, race and ethnicity. Supplement to Mental health: A report of the Surgeon General*. Washington, DC: US Department of Health and Human Services.

Ustün, T. B., Ayuso-Mateos, J. L., Chatterji, S., Mathers, C., & Murray, C. J. (2004). Global burden of depressive disorders in the year 2000. *British Journal of Psychiatry, 184*(5), 386–392.

PART I **IMPACT**

CHAPTER 2

Depressive Disorders
Presentation, Classification, Developmental Trajectories, and Course

Daniel C. Kopala-Sibley, PhD
Daniel N. Klein, PhD

Depression is a pervasive, highly disabling mental disorder that carries substantial costs to the individual suffering from it, to those around them, and to society at large. It often has its onset early in life and is frequently chronic or likely to recur, even with treatment. As such, understanding the nature, etiology, prevalence, and course of depressive disorders is highly important from a public health perspective, as this serves to inform public health policy regarding early detection, prevention, and intervention. At the same time, the etiology of depression is complex. It appears to be a multifactorial and etiologically heterogeneous condition—the outcome of multiple developmental pathways (equifinality). Moreover, few risk factors are specific to depression (multifinality), and overlapping etiological factors may contribute to its rates of comorbidity with other psychiatric and general medical disorders. As a result, understanding depression continues to be a formidable challenge.

The goal of this chapter is to provide an overview of depressive disorders for health professionals and other researchers who are concerned about the public health implications of depression. We selectively review the literature pertaining to the diagnosis and classification of different forms of depressive disorders, the developmental epidemiology and clinical course of depression and its genetics, key environmental risk factors, as well as personality and cognitive vulnerabilities with which it is associated. It is beyond the scope of this chapter to summarize the rapidly growing literature on the cognitive affective neuroscience of depression, but we conclude by offering an outline for an integrative model of the biopsychosocial causes of depression.

Individual and Societal Costs Associated with Depressive Disorders

Before reviewing the nature, prevalence, and course of depression, it is important to recognize the substantial physical, psychological, social, and financial costs associated with this disorder. According to the World Health Organization (Ustün et al., 2004), depressive disorders are the second leading cause of years lived with disability and account for almost 12% of all total years lived with disability worldwide. Moreover, depressed outpatients across the United States show levels of functional impairment that are comparable to patients with a wide variety of chronic general medical conditions (Papakostas et al., 2004) and display poor functioning in an array of social and vocational roles (Donohue & Pincus, 2007; Leader & Klein, 1996).

Finally, depression imposes a substantial financial burden on employers and society in general. Between 1.8% and 3.6% of workers in the US labor force suffer from depression at any given time. While 17%–21% of the workforce in general experiences short-term disability during any given year, 37%–48% of workers with depression experience short-term disability at some point (Goldberg & Steury, 2001). In one review of the economic costs associated with depression, across 24 studies (Luppa, Heinrich, Angermeyer, König, & Riedel-Heller, 2007), estimates for the average annual cost per case of depression ranged from $1,000 to $2,500 for direct costs, from $2,000 to $3,700 for morbidity costs, and from $200 to $400 for mortality costs. In sum, depression imposes substantial costs to society at numerous different levels.

Classification and Diagnosis of Depressive Disorders
Major Depressive Disorder

The most commonly diagnosed form of depression is major depressive disorder (MDD). Although the recent update of the *Diagnostic and Statistical Manual for Mental Disorders* (*DSM-5*; 2013), published by the American Psychiatric Association, contained many changes to the classification of disorders, the criteria for MDD were unchanged with the exception that the bereavement exclusion criterion for MDD was removed. The *DSM-5* criteria for a diagnosis of MDD are summarized in Table 2.1.

To receive a diagnosis of MDD, symptoms also must not be better explained by the presence of general medical conditions (e.g., anemia, which can mimic many of the symptoms of MDD) or by medication/substance use. These criteria are consistent with those used by the International Classification of Diseases (World Health Organization, 2012).

It is useful to understand how MDD can appear in someone suffering from it, as it may not always be clear how these symptoms manifest in day-to-day life. In terms of their family relationships and vocational or academic performance, a mild-to-moderately depressed person may appear quiet, disengaged, or somewhat oppositional or disagreeable, and show decreasing effort and performance at work. A more severely

Table 2.1. DSM-5 *criteria for major depressive disorder (MDD)*

Core criteria
  1. Depressed mood or a loss of interest or pleasure in daily activities for more than two weeks.
  2. Mood represents a change from the person's baseline.
  3. Impaired functioning (social, occupational, educational) or significant distress.

Specific symptoms: Five of these nine present nearly every day for the same two-week period
  1. Depressed or irritable mood most of the day, nearly every day, as indicated by subjective report (e.g., feels sad or empty) or observations made by others (e.g., appears tearful)
  2. Decreased interest or pleasure in most activities, most of each day
  3. Significant weight change or change in appetite
  4. Change in sleep: insomnia or hypersomnia
  5. Change in activity: psychomotor agitation or retardation
  6. Fatigue or loss of energy
  7. Feelings of worthlessness or excessive or inappropriate guilt
  8. Diminished ability to think or concentrate, or indecisiveness
  9. Thoughts of death and/or suicidal ideation

depressed individual may isolate themselves and hardly engage with family members or work colleagues at all. They may lack nearly all motivation or be aggressive, fail in terms of work performance, or be absent frequently. Moderate depression may be accompanied by periodic thoughts of self-harm or suicide, whereas a more severely depressed individual may have frequent thoughts of self- harm or suicide, have plans of self-harm, or may have made attempts to do so. In sum, depression, both at mild-moderate and severe levels, may manifest in observable and highly impairing behaviors across several domains of psychosocial functioning.

Persistent Depressive Disorder, or Dysthymia/Chronic Depression

Previous editions of the *DSM* included the category of dysthymic disorder, a mild, chronic condition defined by many of the same symptoms as MDD but with less severe symptoms that lasted at least two years. In recognition of the fact that there are relatively few differences between various forms of chronic depression, including dysthymia, double depression (i.e., an episode of MDD on top of a preexisting dysthymia), and chronic MDD (Klein, 2010), the *DSM-5* replaced dysthymic disorder with the diagnosis of persistent depressive disorder (PDD). Whereas MDD requires symptoms to be present for at least two weeks, a diagnosis of PDD requires that the depressive symptoms are present for at least two years. Differentiating these two categories is important for several reasons. First, those with PDD, relative to MDD, are more likely to have other comorbid disorders, a family history of chronic depression, and early developmental adversity, such as childhood maltreatment (Klein & Allmann, 2014). Furthermore, whether individuals experience MDD or PDD tends to predict whether future episodes will be acute or chronic (Klein, Shankman, & Rose, 2006).

Continuous versus Categorical Models of Depression and Subthreshold/Minor Depression

Numerous theorists and researchers have argued for a continuous or dimensional classification of depression, rather than the currently used categorical approach. Categorical diagnoses imply that individuals with symptoms exceeding the diagnostic threshold are qualitatively distinct from those with fewer symptoms, whereas the dimensional perspective proposes that they differ only in degree. From a continuity perspective, depression ranges in severity from nonexistent to mild, moderate, or severe and occurs, to some degree, in nearly all individuals at some point in their lives (Blatt, 2004). Studies using taxometric methods to formally test the latent structure of depression have generally found greater support for a continuous model of depression than for qualitatively distinct boundaries (e.g., Hankin, Fraley, Lahey, & Waldman, 2005). Klein (2008) proposed classifying depression along two dimensions, one reflecting severity and the other chronicity, in recognition of the fact that depression can vary along each of these axes, and that both dimensions convey important information relevant to prognosis, treatment, and etiology.

The number and duration of symptoms required to meet criteria for a diagnosis of MDD or PDD are somewhat arbitrary, and individuals with depressive symptoms that fall below the diagnostic threshold often experience substantial impairment. For instance, Judd, Paulus, Wells, and Rapaport (1996) found that individuals with subthreshold depression showed equally high levels of household strain, interpersonal irritability, and financial strain as well as limitations in physical or job functioning, restricted activity days, days spent in bed, and poor health status compared to individuals who met full criteria for MDD. Moreover, Kessler, Zhao, Blazer, and Swartz (1997) reported that there is a linear increase in number and length of depressive episodes, impairment, and comorbidity as one goes from subthreshold, or minor depression, to MDD with five to six symptoms, to MDD with seven to nine symptoms.

Perhaps more importantly, subthreshold depression is one of the most powerful predictors of later episodes of MDD (Cuijpers & Smit, 2004). For instance, elevated but subclinical levels of depressive symptoms predict a two- to threefold greater risk for a major depressive episode (Pine, Cohen, Cohen, & Brook, 1999). The risk is particularly high in individuals with persistent or recurrent subthreshold symptoms (Klein, Shankman, Lewinsohn, & Seeley, 2009).

Comorbidity

In addition to questions about the boundary between depression and nondepression, the boundaries between depression and other psychiatric disorders, particularly anxiety, bipolar disorder, and the psychotic disorders, are also unclear (Klein, Shankman, & McFarland, 2006a). Indeed, there is substantial overlap between depression and other psychiatric disorders, and the majority of individuals with depressive disorders also meet criteria for other diagnoses (Richards & O'Hara, 2014). The causes of comorbidity are complex and poorly understood, but they may include one disorder predisposing the other, the two comorbid conditions sharing etiological factors, both diagnoses reflecting aspects of a single disorder that has been erroneously split into two separate categories, and overlapping diagnostic criteria for depression and other disorders that increases the chances that an individual will meet criteria for both diagnoses (Klein & Riso, 1993).

Explanations of comorbidity may not be mutually exclusive, as multiple processes are likely to be involved. For example, in a longitudinal twin study, Eaves, Silberg, and Erkanli (2003) reported that childhood anxiety influences the development of depression in adolescence through three distinct pathways: (1) the same genes influence early anxiety and later depression (i.e., heterotypic continuity); (2) the genes that affect early anxiety increase sensitivity to adverse life events, indirectly increasing risk for depression (an example of passive gene-environment interaction, as discussed later); and (3) genes that increase risk for early anxiety increase exposure to depressogenic environmental influences (an example of gene-environment correlation, also discussed later).

Bereavement and Depression

There has been recent controversy over the removal of the bereavement exclusionary criteria from the diagnosis of MDD in *DSM-5* (Shear et al., 2011). In *DSM-IV*, clinicians were advised not to diagnose MDD if it followed the loss of a loved one, even if the individual otherwise met full criteria for the diagnosis. In part, the rationale behind this was that depression following bereavement, as long as it lasted less than two months, was a normative reaction to the loss of a loved one. In contrast, the *DSM-5* takes the position that such an event may indeed precipitate an episode of MDD, and when MDD occurs in the context of bereavement, it adds an additional risk for suffering, feelings of worthlessness, suicidal ideation, poorer somatic health, and worse interpersonal and work functioning. This decision was based on several lines of argument. Many, but not all, studies indicate that depressive episodes in the context of bereavement are not fundamentally different from depressive episodes in other contexts (Mojtabai, 2011; Zisook et al., 2012). For example, bereavement-related major depression is also most likely to occur in individuals with past personal and family histories of major depressive episodes, and is associated with similar personality characteristics, patterns of comorbidity, and risks of chronicity or recurrence as non-bereavement-related major depressive episodes. Moreover, the depressive symptoms associated with bereavement-related depression respond to the same psychosocial and medication treatments as non-bereavement-related depression (Zisook et al., 2012). The *DSM-5* also recognizes that bereavement does not typically resolve within two months but, rather, may last years.

Finally, it appears arbitrary to single out bereavement over other severe life events, such as divorce or physical disability, which may also contribute to the onset of MDD. The bereavement exclusion also results in untenable exclusions; for instance, one may be diagnosed with MDD following the news of a loved one's terminal illness, but the diagnosis is no longer applicable after the loved one dies. In *DSM-5*, clinicians are not compelled to diagnose MDD simply because a person is experiencing a recent bereavement, allowing clinicians more flexibility in assigning the diagnosis. Alternatively, critics argue that suspension of the bereavement exclusion criterion risks "pathologizing" normal reactions to bereavement (Frances & Widiger, 2012).

Subtypes of Depression

Depression shows substantial heterogeneity as a disorder. Researchers have sought to understand this heterogeneity by delineating ostensibly discrete subtypes of depression, including recurrent, psychotic, melancholic, atypical, and seasonal. Here, we briefly review the characteristics of these proposed subtypes as well as evidence regarding their validity as diagnostic categories and their utility as clinical diagnoses.

There is substantial debate over whether discrete subtypes of depression represent valid categories and whether these distinctions show clinical utility. For instance, Baumeister and Parker (2012), in their metareview, identified a range of subtypes that they argue will help delineate the etiology and response to treatment of depression. However, Van Loo, De Jonge, Romeijn, Kessler, and Schoevers (2012), in their review of data-driven approaches (e.g., factor, principal component, and latent class analyses) to delineating subtypes of depression, argued that the current evidence does not support the existence of specific depressive dimensions or symptomatic subtypes.

Recurrent Depression

MDD may be classified as either a single episode or recurrent episodes. Indeed, if an individual experiences a single episode of depression, then there is roughly a 50% likelihood of recurrence (Klein & Allmann, 2014; Monroe & Harkness, 2012). Individuals who will experience a recurrence typically show more severe symptoms and more comorbidity (Burcusa & Iacono, 2007; Hardeveld, Spijker, De Graaf, Nolen, & Beekman, 2010). The recurrent subtype is also associated with a greater likelihood of a family history of depression (Burcusa & Iacono, 2007; Klein, Lewinsohn, Rohde, Seeley, & Durbin, 2002; Sullivan, Neale, & Kendler, 2000) as well as experiences of maltreatment in childhood (Burcusa & Iacono, 2007; Nanni, Uher, & Danese, 2012). It is worth noting that there is overlap between PDD and recurrent depression, as they are predicted by many of the same variables. This has led researchers to propose that chronic and recurrent depressions lie along a continuum (Klein, 2008; Klein & Allmann, 2014). For instance, someone with a first episode in adolescence who was then free of depression until a recurrence in middle age would be on one end of this spectrum, whereas someone who experiences episodes every few years and is dysthymic in between episodes would be further along the spectrum, while a third person with chronic, unremitting MDD for decades would be yet further along the spectrum.

Psychotic Depression

Early studies found that about 14% of those with depression also experience psychotic symptoms such as delusions and hallucinations (Johnson, Horwath, & Weissman, 1991). Depressed individuals with and without psychosis differ in a number of significant respects (Klein et al., 2006a). For example, depressed individuals with psychosis experience a more severe course in terms of persistence over one year, risk for relapse, suicide attempts, hospitalization, and financial dependency (Johnson, Horwath, & Weissman, 1991). In addition, when patients with psychotic depression experience a recurrence, it is more likely to be psychotic (Coryell, 1997). Patients with psychotic depression also exhibit more severe levels of a variety of neurocognitive and neurobiological abnormalities (Gomez et al., 2006), and have higher rates of bipolar disorder, psychotic depression, and MDD in their relatives (Coryell, 1997; Østergaard, Waltoft, Mortensen, & Mors, 2013). Finally, psychotic depression does not respond to antidepressant medications alone but must be treated with the combination of an antidepressant and an antipsychotic medication or with electroconvulsive therapy (Klein et al., 2006a). However, it is still unclear whether psychotic depression represents a discrete subtype of depression or if it should be considered quantitatively more severe than depression without psychosis (Coryell, 1997; Klein et al., 2006a).

Melancholic Depression

Melancholic depression is a subtype of depression that is characterized by severe anhedonia, lack of reactivity to positive events, and vegetative symptoms such as severe loss of appetite. It was a specifier of major depression under *DSM-IV*; however, the diagnostic criteria were not specific enough to distinguish it from other subtypes of depression, or even from major depression (Parker et al., 2013; Taylor & Fink, 2008). Some evidence suggests that melancholia is associated with some distinct behavioral and biological features compared to major depression, including psychomotor retardation, hypercortisolemia, and specific sleep abnormalities, such as reduced rapid eye movement latency, increased rapid eye movement time, and reduced delta sleep, although many studies have failed to corroborate these differences (Klein et al., 2006a). Some studies also report that melancholic individuals experience fewer negative life events preceding their depression and have a higher likelihood of completed suicide and a lower likelihood of a comorbid personality disorder, but again these findings are inconsistent (Coryell, 2007; Leventhal & Rehm, 2005). Despite long-standing claims that melancholia is associated with a favorable response to electroconvulsive therapy and antidepressant medication, and does not respond to psychotherapy (Baumeister & Parker, 2012), the evidence for this is weak at best (Klein et al., 2006a). Finally, melancholia does not appear to have a qualitatively distinct symptom profile compared to other forms of depression (Van Loo et al., 2012). In sum, there is only marginal support for the validity of melancholia as a subtype of depression.

Atypical Depression

In *DSM-IV*, the atypical subtype is defined by mood reactivity in combination with two or more of the following symptoms: weight gain or increased appetite, hypersomnia, leaden paralysis, and long-standing vulnerability to rejection. It is estimated that 15%–50% of all depressed patients meet these criteria (Thase, 2006). The initial support for the "atypical" subtype was based on reports of a poor response to tricyclic antidepressant medications and a superior response to monoamine oxidase inhibitors (Davidson, 2006), although subsequent evidence has been equivocal (Pae, Tharwani, Marks, Masand, & Patkar, 2009; Stewart & Thase, 2007). Moreover, it has been debated whether the criteria for atypical depression are able to distinguish it from melancholia and other depressive conditions (Baumeister & Parker, 2012). Generally, there are few biological or psychosocial correlates that distinguish atypical depression from other forms of depression, apart from some evidence of hypo-, rather than hyper-, cortisolemia and abnormally increased posterior right hemisphere electrocortical activity compared to melancholia and other depressive subtypes (Posternak, 2003; Thase, 2009). Overall, there does not appear to be strong support for atypical depression as a distinct subtype.

Seasonal Depression / Seasonal Affective Disorder

The criteria for seasonal affective disorder are the same as those for major depression with the exception that the onset of symptoms must show a seasonal pattern, with depression in the winter and remissions (or occasionally hypomania) during the summer. Currently, there is debate over whether seasonal affective disorder (SAD) is a distinct subtype or rather just reflects a more extreme variant of a mood-sensitive seasonality trait that characterizes much of the population (Hansen, Skre, & Lund, 2008; Rosenthal, 2009; Westrin & Lam, 2007). SAD is hypothesized to stem from the shorter winter photoperiod or from circadian rhythms that are phase delayed relative to the external time (Levitan, 2007; Rohan, Roecklein, & Haaga, 2009; Sohn & Lam, 2005). This suggests that the prevalence of SAD should be associated with distance from the equator, as seasons get more extreme. However, there is only a weak association between the likelihood of seasonal depression and latitude (Sohn & Lam, 2005). The hallmark of SAD is a rapid response to light therapy. However, SAD is also responsive to exercise and antidepressant medication (Howland, 2009; Westrin

& Lam, 2007), and there is some evidence that light therapy may be effective in the treatment of nonseasonal depressions (Even, Schröder, Friedman, & Rouillon, 2008; Golden et al., 2005). Thus, there continue to be significant questions about the validity of the distinction between SAD and nonseasonal depression.

Prevalence, Development, and Course of Depression

Although depression affects individuals of both genders across the life span, prevalence rates vary considerably as a function of age and sex. Thus, it is important to understand the periods of life during which risk increases and gender differences appear. In the following section, we also describe the normative trajectories for an episode of MDD, factors that mitigate or exacerbate risk for MDD, and risk for recurrent or chronic episodes of depression.

Prevalence across the Life Span

Globally, the reported prevalence throughout the world of depressive episodes is 16 per 100,000 per year for males and 25 per 100,000 per year for females (Ustün et al., 2004). A number of large-scale epidemiological surveys have examined the lifetime and point prevalence of depression (Kessler & Bromet, 2013). For example, the National Comorbidity Survey reported a 12-month prevalence of 8.6% and a lifetime prevalence of 14.9% for MDD in the population (Kessler, 1994). In the National Comorbidity Survey-Replication (NCS-R), the 12-month prevalence was 6.6% and the lifetime prevalence was 16.2% (Kessler et al., 2003). In virtually all epidemiological studies of adults and adolescents, rates of depression are approximately twice as high in females compared to males (Kessler & Bromet, 2013).

Age of Onset of Risk

While depression occurs in children, it is not until adolescence that rates of depression increase substantially and the increased risk for women emerges. Using developmentally modified *DSM-IV* criteria for preschool depression in children aged 3–5 (Luby et al., 2002), studies have estimated prevalence rates that range from 0.5% (Keren & Tyano, 2006) to 3% (Bufferd, Dougherty, Carlson, & Klein, 2011; Costello, Erkanli, & Angold, 2006; Egger & Angold, 2006). Thus, while depression exists in very young children, it is relatively rare. In later childhood, prevalence rates remain fairly low; one study reported rates of depressive disorders of 1.4% for six-year-olds and 3.0% for prepubertal children (Fleming & Offord, 1990), while Merikangas and colleagues (2010) found a 2.5% 12-month prevalence rate in children aged 8–11 years.

In adolescence, we see a sharp increase in the prevalence of depression, as well as the emergence of gender differences in rates of depression. For example, Hankin and colleagues (1998) followed a large cohort of children from preadolescence to age 18.

At age 13, approximately 1%–2% of both boys and girls experienced a depressive episode in the previous year. However, by age 15, 4% of females and 1% of males had experienced an episode in the past year. By age 18, 23% of females and 11% of males had experienced an episode in the past year. Moreover, by age 21, 40% of females and 21% of males had experienced at least one episode of depression in their lifetime. Similarly, in a longitudinal study from adolescence through adulthood, Rohde, Lewinsohn, Klein, Seeley, and Gau (2013) found that 5% of participants reported experiencing an episode of MDD in childhood (aged 5–13) compared to 20% in adolescence (aged 13–17), 28% in emerging adulthood (aged 18–23), and 26% in young adulthood (aged 24–30). Consistent with Hankin and colleagues (1998), the appearance of gender difference in rates was first evident around age 13 (Rohde et al., 2013). This suggests that early adolescence (aged 13–15) represents a key period for the emergence of gender differences in depression, while emerging adulthood represents the period of maximal risk for MDD.

These findings have been broadly corroborated by many other studies. For example, in a prospective study, Hamdi and Iacono (2014) reported that lifetime prevalence rates of depression more than doubled in both men and women between the ages of 18 and 27, while other epidemiological research (Kessler & Bromet, 2013) has found that the gender difference in rates of depression emerges in late adolescence and continues through middle age. It should also be noted that MDD remains a common problem in individuals in later life; in one meta-analysis of rates of MDD in individuals older than 75, Luppa et al. (2007) reported that point prevalence rates in those over 75 ranged from 4% to 9%, with a pooled estimate of 7.2%.

There is considerable continuity in depression from adolescence through adulthood. Kessler (1994) found that nearly three-quarters of all cases of adult depression had an onset prior to the age of 18. Moreover, studies that have followed individuals from adolescence to adulthood report that approximately 40%–70% of adolescents who experience MDD will have a recurrence in adulthood (Fergusson & Woodward, 2002; Lewinsohn, Rohde, Klein, & Seeley, 1999; Pine, Cohen, Gurley, Brook, & Ma, 1998; Weissman et al., 1999a). Findings of continuity of depression from childhood to adolescence or to adulthood are less consistent, as some studies find that children with MDD are more likely to experience depression in adolescence or adulthood, while other studies do not (Copeland, Shanahan, Costello, & Angold, 2009; Geller, Zimerman, Williams, Bolhofner, & Craney, 2001; Harrington, Fudge, Rutter, Pickles, & Hill, 1990; Weissman et al., 1999b).

Gender Differences in Rates of Depression

Numerous theories have been posited to explain why, from adolescence onward, depression is twice as common in women compared to men, and include a range of both biological and psychosocial models. Some have suggested that women are genetically more predisposed to depression. Results generally suggest a higher heritability in women compared to men (Kendler, Gardner, Neale, & Prescott, 2001). The genetic correlation between the sexes is approximately .60 (Flint & Kendler, 2014), highlighting the somewhat different effects genes may play in the etiology of depression in males compared to females.

Others have suggested that changes in hormone levels at various points in development may account for gender differences. For instance, Angold, Costello, and Worthman (1998) found that pubertal status predicted the differential sex ratio better than age did, suggesting that hormonal, rather than social, changes played a bigger role. Angold, Costello, Erkanli, and Worthman (1999) also found that, after controlling for morphological status, estrogen and androgen levels in early adolescence predicted depression.

Other researchers have emphasized the role of social, cultural, and personality factors over biological effects. Crick (1997) showed that parents accept more anger or assertiveness from boys and more submissive behaviors from girls, while Aubé, Fichman, Saltaris, and Koestner (2000) showed that irrespective of gender, these more "feminine" traits were related to increased levels of depression. According to the gender identification hypothesis (Wichstrøm, 1999), around puberty women begin to identify more strongly with the stereotypical ideal female body image. However, pubertal development moves females further away from this female ideal body image, whereas males move closer to their ideal. This often leads to body dissatisfaction, which is associated with depression in females but not males (Wichstrøm, 1999). Importantly, in a high school sample, Allgood-Merten, Lewinsohn, and Hops (1990) found that the gender difference in depression was eliminated when body image and self-esteem were controlled. Similarly, Rudolph and Conley (2005) reported that social-evaluative concerns accounted fully for the gender difference in depression.

A ruminative response style, or the tendency to engage in repetitive and passive negative thinking while focusing on their symptoms and the meaning of their distress, has also been widely studied as a factor underlying the gender difference in depression (Nolen-Hoeksema, 1987, 2000). Individuals who tend to engage in ruminative responses to stress experiences manifest increases in depressive symptoms over time, are more likely to experience depressive episodes, and are more vulnerable to stress than nonruminators (Nolen-Hoeksema, 2000; Nolen-Hoeksema, Wisco, & Lyubormirsky, 2008). Women, relative to men, tend to ruminate about their depressed mood, causing their depressed mood to continue (Nolen-Hoeksema, 1987), whereas men tend to distract themselves, thereby dampening their depressed mood.

In addition, gender differences in exposure to stress and increased reactivity to stress (diathesis-stress) may contribute to the increased prevalence of depression in females. For example, Shih, Eberhart, Hammen, and Brennan (2006) found that adolescent girls experienced more interpersonal stress than boys. In addition, after controlling for maternal depression and number of stressors, gender partially mediated the relationship between stress and depression, indicating that girls were more reactive to interpersonal stress than boys. Hankin, Mermelstein, and Roesch (2007) also reported that adolescent girls experienced a greater number of stressors than boys and that these stressors partially mediated the relationship between gender and depression. These investigators also found that even when the number of stressors was equal, women reacted with greater increases in depression.

The Clinical Course of Depressive Disorders

It is useful for researchers, clinicians, patients, and families to understand the typical course of depressive disorders, including the duration of episodes, probabilities of recovery and relapse, and factors that might predict persistence and relapse. Estimates of the duration of depressive episodes range from a few months to a year. In a nationally representative community sample, the NCS-R reported an average episode duration of 5.5 months (Kessler et al., 2003). Similarly, a 12-year follow-up of a community sample from the Baltimore site of the Epidemiological Catchment Area (ECA) study found a mean episode duration of 6.75 months (Eaton et al., 2008).

A longer time to recovery is predicted by multiple factors, including living alone, having a more severe episode, comorbid dysthymia (Keitner, Ryan, Miller, Kohn, & Epstein, 1991; Mueller et al., 1996), being unemployed, having experienced a recent bereavement, or having other comorbid psychiatric disorders (Ohayon, Priest, Guilleminault, & Caulet, 1999). Experiencing a more severe depressive episode or having had experienced previous depressive episodes can double the length of a current depressive episode (Spijker et al., 2002). A minority of episodes are chronic (i.e., persist for two years or more); in the Baltimore ECA study, 15% of individuals with an MDD episode experienced an unremitting chronic course lasting at least two years (Eaton et al., 2008). In the National Institute of Mental Health (NIMH) Collaborative Depression Study (CDS), although 70% of depressed patients recovered within 1 year (Keller, Shapiro, Lavori, & Wolfe, 1982), by 2 years 20% had not recovered, by 5 years 12% (Keller et al., 1992), by 10 years 7% (Mueller et al., 1996), and by 15 years 6% of depressed individuals still had not recovered (Keller & Boland, 1998).

Of those who recover from a depressive episode, many will experience a recurrence in the future. In a long-term follow-up of the Baltimore ECA sample, about 50% of individuals with MDD recovered from their first episode with no future episodes, but 35% went on to experience recurrent episodes (Eaton et al., 2008).

Recurrence rates are higher in clinical samples. The NIMH CDS reported an initial recurrence rate of 25%–40% after 2 years. This rate increased over time, up to 60% after 5 years, 75% after 10 years, and 85% after 15 years (Keller & Boland, 1998). Being female, having never married, and having had prior episodes of depression, a longer current episode, comorbid dysthymia, or other comorbid psychiatric disorders all predicted an increased likelihood of relapse. The Group for Longitudinal Affective

Disorders Study in Japan reported somewhat similar rates of relapse: 21% for a 12-month period, 30% by 2 years, and 42% by 5 years (Kanai et al., 2003). The risk of future recurrence appears to increase by about 16% with each successive recurrence but decreases as the length of time spent recovered increases (Solomon et al., 2000).

An important factor in the rate and timing of recurrence is the extent of recovery. Individuals in the CDS who fully recovered (i.e., were asymptomatic at follow-up) had much lower rates (66%) of recurrence than did those with some symptoms (87%) during follow-up (Mueller et al., 1996). Residual symptoms at time of recovery is arguably the most powerful predictor of recurrence (Klein & Small, 2014).

Etiological Factors in the Development of Risk for Depression

A comprehensive review of factors that mitigate or exacerbate risk for depression is beyond the scope of this chapter. However, in the following sections we briefly review the role of genetic, environmental, and trait-like personality or cognitive factors.

Genetics

The role of genetics in depression has been investigated using a number of approaches, including twin, adoption, candidate-gene, and genome-wide association studies (Flint & Kendler, 2014). Twin studies indicate that MDD has a heritability of approximately 37% (Sullivan et al., 2000), and heritability appears to be higher for women (40%–42%) than men (29%–30%) (Kendler et al., 2001). Researchers have also conducted genome-wide association studies in order to examine if common variants of specific genes are related to risk for MDD. A large majority of these studies have failed to find significant associations; however, if depression is highly polygenic (many genes, each with very small effects), statistical power may not have been sufficient to detect associations (Flint & Kendler, 2014).

The failure to identify genes associated with MDD raises the question of how to reconcile the results of twin studies and genome-wide association studies (i.e., the problem of missing heritability). Genome-wide complex trait analysis, in which the heritability of MDD is estimated by comparing the degree of sharing of common genetic variants and risk for MDD, attempts to resolve this issue. In these studies, the heritability estimates for MDD range from 21% (Lee et al., 2013) to 30% (Lubke et al., 2012). These results confirm that many common genetic variants each make a small contribution to the genetic susceptibility to depression (Flint & Kendler, 2014).

Longitudinal studies of large samples of twins provide information about how the roles of genes and environment change over the course of development. These studies suggest that environmental influences play a larger role in early life, while genes account for an increasing amount of variance in depression as children develop into adolescence, and from adolescence into young adulthood and adulthood (Bergen,

Gardner, & Kendler, 2007; Kendler, Gardner, & Lichtenstein, 2008; Waszczuk, Zavos, Gregory, & Eley, 2014). Moreover, these studies also indicate that there is genetic innovation and attenuation; that is, the influence of particular genes on depression emerge and dissipate at different points in development.

Evidence from twin studies that genes account for less than half the variance in depression suggests the importance of environmental influences. However, other designs provide firmer evidence for environmental effects on depression. For instance, depression in adoptive parents predicts the likelihood of depression in their adopted children, just as it does in their biological offspring (Tully, Iacono, & McGue, 2008). Children of twin studies have also confirmed the effects of parental depression as an environmental predictor of child depression, over and above shared genes (Singh et al., 2011), while studies of children conceived through in vitro fertilization have found that parenting behaviors predict child depression whether the child is biologically related to the parent or not, over and above the effects of parental history of depression (Harold et al., 2011).

Finally, a number of studies have examined whether specific genetic variants (candidate genes) confer vulnerability to depression, especially following negative events, adversity, or other forms of stress. The gene X environment literature is currently the source of considerable controversy (Munafo, Zammit, & Flint, 2014; Rutter, 2014); however, some meta-analyses have supported initial findings indicating that the serotonin transporter 5-HTTLPR variant is associated with greater risk for depression following adversity, particularly when it occurs in childhood (Karg, Burmeister, Shedden, & Sen, 2011).

Environmental Influences

Twin and adoption studies provide indirect approaches to testing the role of environmental influences on depression. Numerous studies have also directly examined associations between measured environmental factors and depression. For instance, there is considerable evidence that negative experiences with parents, including emotional or physical abuse, neglect, rejection, or high levels of physical or psychological control, appear to confer risk for later depression (McLeod, Weisz, & Wood, 2007; Widom, DuMont, & Czaja, 2007). These studies cannot rule out the possibility that gene-environment correlations (i.e., the same parents who provide the poor family environment also provide the child's genes) account for these effects. However, studies of identical twins who are discordant for a traumatic event have shown that the twin who experienced the trauma has the greater risk for depression (e.g., Nelson et al., 2002), indicating that the effect of the stressor must operate via an environmental mechanism.

What mechanisms mediate the association of early adversity with the subsequent development of depression? These effects appear, at least partially, to reflect the effects of parenting and early adversity on the development of personality or cognitive traits that are more proximal risk factors for depression (Hankin et al., 2009; Kopala-Sibley & Zuroff, 2014) or confer an increased likelihood of exposure to stress (Hammen, 1991; Liu & Alloy, 2010). In addition, early adversity appears to contribute to dysregulation of the hypothalamic-pituitary-adrenal axis (Ali & Pruessner, 2012; Heim, Plotsky, & Nemeroff, 2004; Penza, Heim, & Nemeroff, 2003), one of the major biological stress response systems that has been strongly implicated in depression (Stetler & Miller, 2011).

Other more proximal environmental influences on depression include poor-quality relationships with siblings and peers. For instance, peer victimization or bullying predicts the development of depressive symptoms in adolescents (Hawker & Boulton, 2000; La Greca & Harrison, 2005; Prinstein, Boergers, Spirito, Little, & Grapentine, 2000), while the quality of relationships with siblings in adolescence predicts depressive symptoms 30 years later (Waldinger, Vaillant, & Orav, 2007).

The effects of negative life events have also received much attention as an etiological factor in the onset of depression. A large body of literature over the past 35 years has confirmed the role of life events or stressors in depression (Monroe, Slavich, & Georgiades, 2014). For instance, depressed patients experience a greater number of stressful events in the several months preceding the onset of their disorder compared to healthy controls, and this holds true for events over which the individual had no control (Brown & Harris, 1978). Kessler and colleagues (1997) noted that both cumulative stress over a long period of time as well as the occurrence of specific, more severe events contribute to increases in depressive symptoms, the occurrence of a first episode of depression, and recurrence of major depression.

Trait Vulnerabilities to Depression

Children may also show early trait-like risk factors for later depression. For instance, child temperament has received much attention in the literature as an early risk factor for later depression (Klein, Dyson, Kujawa, & Kotov, 2012). Child negative and positive emotionality at age 3, for instance, predict depressive symptoms at age 10 (Dougherty, Klein, Durbin, Hayden, & Olino, 2010). Caspi, Moffitt, Newman, and Silva (1996) reported that children who were rated as socially reticent, inhibited, and easily upset at age 3 had elevated rates of depressive (but not anxiety or substance use) disorders at age 21. There is also a robust association between temperamental or personality traits and depressive disorders in adults (Kotov, Gamez, Schmidt, & Watson, 2010). Indeed, several prospective studies have found that neuroticism predicts the first onset of depression in adults (Kendler, Kessler, Neale, Heath, & Eaves, 1993; Kendler, Kuhn, & Prescott, 2004).

A number of other trait-like personality or cognitive variables have been proposed to confer vulnerability to depression in adolescents and adults by exacerbating the effects of stress on depression. Some of the most widely studied include self-criticism and dependency (Blatt, 1974; Blatt, D'Afflitti, & Quinian, 1976; Blatt & Zuroff, 1992), sociotropy and autonomy (Beck, Epstein, Harrison, & Emery, 1983), perfectionism (Hewitt & Flett, 1991), and hopelessness (Abramson, Metalsky, & Alloy, 1989). High levels of self-criticism, autonomy, and perfectionism are associated with excessive fears of failure, concerns about social status, and feelings of guilt and low self-worth (Beck et al., 1983; Blatt, 2004, 2007; Blatt & Luyten, 2009; Dunkley, Zuroff, & Blankstein, 2006), while the personality traits of dependency and sociotropy are characterized by excessive dependence on close others and fears of abandonment and interpersonal loss (Beck et al., 1983; Blatt & Luyten, 2009). A hopeless cognitive style is characterized by a pervasive pattern in which the person tends to make stable, global attributions for the causes of events and to infer negative consequences about the events as well as negative characteristics about him- or herself (Abramson et al., 1989). Evidence generally suggests that these personality factors, both in isolation and in interaction with negative events, do confer vulnerability to depression (Abramson et al., 1998; Alloy et al., 2004; Blatt & Zuroff, 1992; Hankin, Abramson, Miller, & Haeffel, 2004; Kopala-Sibley & Zuroff, 2014; Zuroff, Mongrain, & Santor, 2004).

Outline of an Integrative Perspective

The field is still far from being able to formulate a comprehensive model of depression. For heuristic purposes, however, we briefly outline one plausible, but undoubtedly oversimplified, model of the etiopathogenesis of depression (Klein, Kujawa, Black, & Pennock, 2013; Kopala-Sibley & Zuroff, 2014).

We can begin by positing two key sets of distal etiological factors: genetic susceptibilities and early environmental adversity, including poor parenting. The nature of the genetic effects is only beginning to be elucidated. There are multiple common gene variants, each with small effects, and there may also be some rare mutations with large effects on only a small number of cases. In addition, due to developmentally mediated changes in gene expression, the relation between genotype and phenotype may vary over time, with the same set of genetic influences producing different phenotypes at various points in development and different genetic factors producing similar phenotypes at different ages.

The nature and specificity of the environmental influences also remain to be fully elucidated; however, experiences that convey to the child a sense of being worthless or unlovable appear to be central (Kopala-Sibley & Zuroff, 2014). The overall strength of the genetic influences appears to increase with age; conversely, environmental influences may play a greater role at younger ages, although they can have effects that persist throughout adulthood. These two sets of distal causes often co-occur (i.e., passive gene-environment correlation), and they may have additive or interactive effects (Klein et al., 2013).

Genetic susceptibilities may be expressed in the form of temperamental vulnerabilities that, at the behavioral level, are reflected by low positive or high negative emotionality, and are accompanied by dysregulation in key neurobiological systems (Klein et al., 2012). Key neural systems include reward (e.g., a dopaminergically mediated circuit that includes the prefrontal cortex and nucleus accumbens in the ventral striatum), threat (a circuit that includes the prefrontal cortex, anterior cingulate, amygdala, and hippocampus), and stress response (e.g., the hypothalamic-pituitary-adrenal axis), all of which appear to be dysregulated in depressed individuals, often prior to the onset of the disorder (Disner, Beevers, Haigh, & Beck, 2011; Gotlib, Joormann, & Foland-Ross, 2014; Pizzagalli & Treadway, 2014). These temperamental vulnerabilities and dysregulation of reward, threat, and stress response systems are also influenced by environmental adversity. At the same time, uncaring or overly controlling parenting can result in traits characterized by poor self-worth and high self-criticism or by insecure attachment and dependency on others, which can also have persisting effects on later interpersonal functioning (Kopala-Sibley & Zuroff, 2014).

As the child enters the early school-age years, temperamental vulnerabilities may be elaborated cognitively, leading to the emergence of depressotypic personality or cognitive styles/biases, which include attentional and memory biases oriented toward negative self-relevant material and trait-like schemas revolving around low self-worth (Gotlib & Joormann, 2010; Kopala-Sibley & Zuroff, 2014). At the same time, temperamental and cognitive vulnerabilities and insecure attachment can lead to interpersonal deficits that, in turn, reinforce cognitive styles/biases and generate stressors that may further sensitize neurobiological threat and stress response systems and dampen reward systems (Kopala-Sibley & Zuroff, 2014; Pizzagalli & Treadway, 2014; Uliaszek et al., 2012). These various vulnerabilities and environmental stressors combine, either additively or interactively, to produce depressive symptoms and may escalate to a full depressive episode.

This process can occur at virtually any point during the life span. However, because of developmental effects on gene expression, the development of critical neurobiological and cognitive systems, and the developmental challenges and transitions associated with adolescence and early adulthood, this escalation is particularly likely to occur during this period. Moreover, it is much more likely to occur in females and is probably related to sex differences in preexisting vulnerability factors and a greater increase in depression-relevant (e.g., interpersonal) stressors in adolescence.

Conclusion

Depression is a highly prevalent, disabling disorder that affects individuals of all ages across the globe. It has substantial personal, social, and economic costs both to the individual and society at large. As such, from a public health perspective, understanding the prevalence, course, and etiology of depression will serve to inform public health policy regarding early detection, prevention, and intervention. Adolescence and emerging adulthood appear to be a particularly important time for the first onset of depression, although it is by no means limited to this period. While many individuals who experience a depressive episode will recover from it, a substantial number go on to develop chronic depression or to experience multiple episodes. Even with treatment, the risk for relapse is still substantial. Although there has been progress in understanding depression, much more work is needed before we have a full picture of its complex, multifactorial causes.

References

Abramson, L. Y., Alloy, L. B., Hogan, M. E., Whitehouse, W. G., Cornette, M., Akhavan, S., & Chiara, A. (1998). Suicidality and cognitive vulnerability to depression among college students: A prospective study. *Journal of Adolescence, 21*(4), 473–487.

Abramson, L. Y., Metalsky, G. I., & Alloy, L. B. (1989). Hopelessness depression: A theory-based subtype of depression. *Psychological Review, 96*(2), 358–372.

Ali, N., & Pruessner, J. C. (2012). The salivary alpha amylase over cortisol ratio as a marker to assess dysregulations of the stress systems. *Physiology & Behavior, 106*(1), 65–72.

Allgood-Merten, B., Lewinsohn, P. M., & Hops, H. (1990). Sex differences and adolescent depression. *Journal of Abnormal Psychology, 99*(1), 55–63.

Alloy, L. B., Abramson, L. Y., Gibb, B. E., Crossfield, A. G., Pieracci, A. M., Spasojevic, J., & Steinberg, J. A. (2004). Developmental antecedents of cognitive vulnerability to depression: Review of findings from the cognitive vulnerability to depression project. *Journal of Cognitive Psychotherapy, 18*(2), 115–133.

American Psychiatric Association. (2013). *Diagnostic and statistical manual of mental disorders (DSM-5)*. Arlington, VA: American Psychiatric Publishing.

Angold, A., Costello, E. J., Erkanli, A., & Worthman, C. M. (1999). Pubertal changes in hormone levels and depression in girls. *Psychological Medicine, 29*(5), 1043–1053.

Angold, A., Costello, E. J., & Worthman, C. M. (1998). Puberty and depression: The roles of age, pubertal status and pubertal timing. *Psychological Medicine, 28*(1), 51–61.

Aubé, J., Fichman, L., Saltaris, C., & Koestner, R. (2000). Gender differences in adolescent depressive symptomatology: Towards an integrated social-developmental model. *Journal of Social and Clinical Psychology, 19*(3), 297–313.

Baumeister, H., & Parker, G. (2012). Meta-review of depressive subtyping models. *Journal of Affective Disorders, 139*(2), 126–140.

Beck, A. T., Epstein, N., Harrison, R. P., & Emery, G. (1983). *Development of the Sociotropy-Autonomy Scale: A measure of personality factors in psychopathology*. Unpublished manuscript, University of Pennsylvania, Philadelphia, PA.

Bergen, S. E., Gardner, C. O., & Kendler, K. S. (2007). Age-related changes in heritability of behavioral phenotypes over adolescence and young adulthood: A meta-analysis. *Twin Research and Human Genetics, 10*(3), 423–433.

Blatt, S. J. (1974). Levels of object representation in anaclitic and introjective depression. *The Psychoanalytic Study of the Child, 29*, 107–157.

Blatt, S. J. (2004). *Experiences of depression: Theoretical, clinical, and research perspectives.* Washington, DC: American Psychological Association.

Blatt, S. J. (2007). A fundamental polarity in psychoanalysis: Implications for personality development, psychopathology, and the therapeutic process. *Psychoanalytic Inquiry, 26*(4), 494–520.

Blatt, S. J., D'Afflitti, J. P., & Quinian, D. M. (1976). Experiences of depression in normal young adults. *Journal of Abnormal Psychology, 85*(4), 383–389.

Blatt, S. J., & Luyten, P. (2009). A structural–developmental psychodynamic approach to psychopathology: Two polarities of experience across the life span. *Development and Psychopathology, 21*(3), 793–814.

Blatt, S. J., & Zuroff, D. C. (1992). Interpersonal relatedness and self-definition: Two prototypes for depression. *Clinical Psychology Review, 12*(5), 527–562.

Brown, G. W., & Harris, T. (1978). *Social origins of depression: A study of psychiatric disorder in women.* New York, NY: Free Press.

Bufferd, S. J., Dougherty, L. R., Carlson, G. A., & Klein, D. N. (2011). Parent-reported mental health in preschoolers: Findings using a diagnostic interview. *Comprehensive Psychiatry, 52*(4), 359–369.

Burcusa, S. L., & Iacono, W. G. (2007). Risk for recurrence in depression. *Clinical Psychology Review, 27*(8), 959–985.

Caspi, A., Moffitt, T. E., Newman, D. L., & Silva, P. A. (1996). Behavioral observations at age 3 years predict adult psychiatric disorders: Longitudinal evidence from a birth cohort. *Archives of General Psychiatry, 53*(11), 1033–1039.

Copeland, W. E., Shanahan, L., Costello, E. J., & Angold, A. (2009). Childhood and adolescent psychiatric disorders as predictors of young adult disorders. *Archives of General Psychiatry, 66*(7), 764–772.

Coryell, W. (1997). Do psychotic, minor, and intermittent depressive disorders exist on a continuum? *Journal of Affective Disorders, 45*(1–2), 75–83.

Coryell, W. (2007). The facets of melancholia. *Acta Psychiatrica Scandinavica, 115*(s433), 31–36.

Costello, J. E., Erkanli, A., & Angold, A. (2006). Is there an epidemic of child or adolescent depression? *Journal of Child Psychology and Psychiatry, 47*(12), 1263–1271.

Crick, N. R. (1997). Engagement in gender normative versus nonnormative forms of aggression: Links to social–psychological adjustment. *Developmental Psychology, 33*(4), 610.

Cuijpers, P., & Smit, F. (2004). Subthreshold depression as a risk indicator for major depressive disorder: A systematic review of prospective studies. *Acta Psychiatrica Scandinavica, 109*(5), 325–331.

Davidson, J. R. (2006). A history of the concept of atypical depression. *Journal of Clinical Psychiatry, 68*(2), 10–15.

Disner, S. G., Beevers, C. G., Haigh, E. A. P., & Beck, A. T. (2011). Neural mechanisms of the cognitive model of depression. *Nature Reviews Neuroscience, 12*, 467–477.

Donohue, J. M., & Pincus, H. A. (2007). Reducing the societal burden of depression. *Pharmacoeconomics, 25*(1), 7–24.

Dougherty, L. R., Klein, D. N., Durbin, C. E., Hayden, E. P., & Olino, T. M. (2010). Temperamental positive and negative emotionality and children's depressive symptoms: A longitudinal prospective study from age three to age ten. *Journal of Social and Clinical Psychology, 29*(4), 462–488.

Dunkley, D. M., Zuroff, D. C., & Blankstein, K. R. (2006). Specific perfectionism components versus self-criticism in predicting maladjustment. *Personality and Individual Differences, 40*(4), 665–676.

Eaton, W. W., Martins, S. S., Nestadt, G., Bienvenu, O. J., Clarke, D., & Alexandre, P. (2008). The burden of mental disorders. *Epidemiologic Reviews, 30*(1), 1–14.

Eaves, L., Silberg, J., & Erkanli, A. (2003). Resolving multiple epigenetic pathways to adolescent depression. *Journal of Child Psychology and Psychiatry, 44*(7), 1006–1014.

Egger, H. L., & Angold, A. (2006). Common emotional and behavioral disorders in preschool children: Presentation, nosology, and epidemiology. *Journal of Child Psychology and Psychiatry, 47*(3–4), 313–337.

Even, C., Schröder, C. M., Friedman, S., & Rouillon, F. (2008). Efficacy of light therapy in nonseasonal depression: A systematic review. *Journal of Affective Disorders, 108*(1), 11–23.

Fergusson, D. M., & Woodward, L. J. (2002). Mental health, educational, and social role outcomes of adolescents with depression. *Archives of General Psychiatry, 59*(3), 225–231.

Fleming, J. E., & Offord, D. R. (1990). Epidemiology of childhood depressive disorders: A critical review. *Journal of the American Academy of Child and Adolescent Psychiatry, 29*(4), 571–580.

Flint, J., & Kendler, K. S. (2014). The genetics of major depression. *Neuron, 81*(3), 484–503.

Frances, A. J., & Widiger, T. (2012). Psychiatric diagnosis: Lessons from the *DSM-IV* past and cautions for the *DSM-5* future. *Annual Review of Psychology, 8*, 109–130.

Geller, B., Zimerman, B., Williams, M., Bolhofner, K., & Craney, J. L. (2001). Bipolar disorder at prospective follow-up of adults who had prepubertal major depressive disorder. *American Journal of Psychiatry, 158*(1), 125–127.

Goldberg, R. J., & Steury, S. (2001). Depression in the workplace: Costs and barriers to treatment. *Depression, 52*(12), 1639–1643.

Golden, R. N., Gaynes, B. N., Ekstrom, R. D., Hamer, R. M., Jacobsen, F. M., Suppes, T., . . . Nemeroff, C. B. (2005). The efficacy of light therapy in the treatment of mood disorders: A review and meta-analysis of the evidence. *American Journal of Psychiatry, 162*(4), 656–662.

Gomez, R. G., Fleming, S. H., Keller, J., Flores, B., Kenna, H., DeBattista, C., . . . Schatzberg, A. F. (2006). The neuropsychological profile of psychotic major depression and its relation to cortisol. *Biological Psychiatry, 60*(5), 472–478.

Gotlib, I. H., & Joormann, J. (2010). Cognition and depression: Current status and future directions. *Annual Review of Clinical Psychology, 6*, 285–312.

Gotlib, I. H., Joormann, J., & Foland-Ross, L. C. (2014). Understanding familial risk for depression: A 25-year perspective. *Perspectives on Psychological Science, 9*(1), 94–108.

Hamdi, N. R., & Iacono, W. G. (2014). Lifetime prevalence and co-morbidity of externalizing disorders and depression in prospective assessment. *Psychological Medicine, 44*(2), 315–324.

Hammen, C. (1991). Generation of stress in the course of unipolar depression. *Journal of Abnormal Psychology, 100*(4), 555–561.

Hankin, B. L., Abramson, L. Y., Miller, N., & Haeffel, G. J. (2004). Cognitive vulnerability-stress theories of depression: Examining affective specificity in the prediction of depression versus anxiety in three prospective studies. *Cognitive Therapy and Research, 28*(3), 309–345.

Hankin, B. L., Abramson, L. Y., Moffitt, T. E., Silva, P. A., McGee, R., & Angell, K. E. (1998). Development of depression from preadolescence to young adulthood: Emerging gender differences in a 10-year longitudinal study. *Journal of Abnormal Psychology, 107*(1), 128.

Hankin, B. L., Fraley, R. C., Lahey, B. B., & Waldman, I. D. (2005). Is depression best viewed as a continuum or discrete category? A taxometric analysis of childhood and adolescent depression in a population-based sample. *Journal of Abnormal Psychology, 114*(1), 96–110.

Hankin, B. L., Mermelstein, R., & Roesch, L. (2007). Sex differences in adolescent depression: Stress exposure and reactivity models. *Child Development, 78*(1), 279–295.

Hankin, B. L., Oppenheimer, C., Jenness, J., Barrocas, A., Shapero, B. G., & Goldband, J. (2009). Developmental origins of cognitive vulnerabilities to depression: Review of processes contributing to stability and change across time. *Journal of Clinical Psychology, 65*(12), 1327–1338.

Hansen, V., Skre, I., & Lund, E. (2008). What is this thing called "SAD"? A critique of the concept of seasonal affective disorder. *Epidemiologia e Psichiatria Sociale, 17*(2), 120–127.

Hardeveld, F., Spijker, J., De Graaf, R., Nolen, W. A., & Beekman, A. T. F. (2010). Prevalence and predictors of recurrence of major depressive disorder in the adult population. *Acta Psychiatrica Scandinavica, 122*(3), 184–191.

Harold, G. T., Rice, F., Hay, D. F., Boivin, J., Van Den Bree, M., & Thapar, A. (2011). Familial transmission of depression and antisocial behavior symptoms: Disentangling the contribution of inherited and environmental factors and testing the mediating role of parenting. *Psychological Medicine, 41*(6), 1175–1185.

Harrington, R., Fudge, H., Rutter, M., Pickles, A., & Hill, J. (1990). Adult outcomes of childhood and adolescent depression: I. Psychiatric status. *Archives of General Psychiatry, 47*(5), 465–473.

Hawker, D. S., & Boulton, M. J. (2000). Twenty years' research on peer victimization and psychosocial maladjustment: A meta-analytic review of cross-sectional studies. *Journal of Child Psychology and Psychiatry, 41*(4), 441–455.

Heim, C., Plotsky, P. M., & Nemeroff, C. B. (2004). Importance of studying the contributions of early adverse experience to neurobiological findings in depression. *Neuropsychopharmacology, 29*(4), 641–648.

Hewitt, P. L., & Flett, G. L. (1991). Perfectionism in the self and social contexts: Conceptualization, assessment, and association with psychopathology. *Journal of Personality and Social Psychology, 60*(3), 456–470.

Howland, R. H. (2009). An overview of seasonal affective disorder and its treatment options. *The Physician and Sports Medicine, 37*(4), 104–115.

Johnson, J., Horwath, E., & Weissman, M. M. (1991). The validity of major depression with psychotic features based on a community study. *Archives of General Psychiatry, 48*(12), 1075–1081.

Judd, L. L., Paulus, M. P., Wells, K. B., & Rapaport, M. H. (1996). Socioeconomic burden of subsyndromal depressive symptoms and major depression in a sample of the general population. *American Journal of Psychiatry, 153*(11), 1411–1417.

Kanai, T., Takeuchi, H., Furukawa, T. A., Yoshimura, R., Imaizumi, T., Kitamura, T., & Takahashi, K. (2003). Time to recurrence after recovery from major depressive episodes and its predictors. *Psychological Medicine, 33*(5), 839–845.

Karg, K., Burmeister, M., Shedden, K., & Sen, S. (2011). The serotonin transporter promoter variant (5-HTTLPR), stress, and depression meta-analysis revisited: Evidence of genetic moderation. *Archives of General Psychiatry, 68*(5), 444–454.

Keitner, G. I., Ryan, C. E., Miller, I. W., Kohn, R., & Epstein, N. B. (1991). 12-month outcome of patients with major depression and comorbid psychiatric or medical illness (compound depression). *American Journal of Psychiatry, 148*(3), 345–350.

Keller, M. B., & Boland, R. J. (1998). Implications of failing to achieve successful long-term maintenance treatment of recurrent unipolar major depression. *Biological Psychiatry, 44*(5), 348–360.

Keller, M. B., Lavori, P. W., Mueller, T. I., Endicott, J., Coryell, W., Hirschfeld, R. M. A., & Shea, T. (1992). Time to recovery, chronicity, and levels of psychopathology in major depression: A 5-year prospective follow-up of 431 subjects. *Archives of General Psychiatry, 49*(10), 809–816.

Keller, M. B., Shapiro, R. W., Lavori, P. W., & Wolfe, N. (1982). Relapse in major depressive disorder: Analysis with the life table. *Archives of General Psychiatry, 39*(8), 911–915.

Kendler, K. S., Gardner, C. O., & Lichtenstein, P. (2008). A developmental twin study of symptoms of anxiety and depression: Evidence for genetic innovation and attenuation. *Psychological Medicine, 38*(11), 1567–1575.

Kendler, K. S., Gardner, C. O., Neale, M. C., & Prescott, C. A. (2001). Genetic risk factors for major depression in men and women: Similar or different heritabilities and same or partly distinct genes? *Psychological Medicine, 31*(4), 605–616.

Kendler, K. S., Kessler, R. C., Neale, M. C., Heath, A. C., & Eaves, L. J. (1993). The prediction of major depression in women: Toward an integrated etiologic model. *American Journal of Psychiatry, 150*(8), 1139–1148.

Kendler, K. S., Kuhn, J., & Prescott, C. A. (2004). The interrelationship of neuroticism, sex, and stressful life events in the prediction of episodes of major depression. *American Journal of Psychiatry, 161*(4), 631–636.

Keren, M., & Tyano, S. (2006). Depression in infancy. *Child and Adolescent Psychiatric Clinics of North America, 15*(4), 883–897.

Kessler, R. C. (1994). The National Comorbidity Survey of the United States. *International Review of Psychiatry, 6*(4), 365–376.

Kessler, R. C., Berglund, P., Demler, O., Jin, R., Koretz, D., Merikangas, K. R., . . . Wang, P. S. (2003). The epidemiology of major depressive disorder: Results from the National Comorbidity Survey-Replication (NCS-R). *JAMA, 289*(23), 3095–3105.

Kessler, R.C., & Bromet, E. (2013). The epidemiology of depression across cultures. *Annual Review of Public Health, 34*, 119–138.

Kessler, R. C., Zhao, S., Blazer, D. G., & Swartz, M. (1997). Prevalence, correlates, and course of minor depression and major depression in the National Comorbidity Survey. *Journal of Affective Disorders, 45*(1), 19–30.

Klein, D. N. (2008). Classification of depressive disorders in the *DSM-V*: Proposal for a two-dimension system. *Journal of Abnormal Psychology, 117*(3), 552.

Klein, D. N. (2010). Chronic depression: Diagnosis and classification. *Current Directions in Psychological Science, 19*(2), 96–100.

Klein, D. N., & Allmann, A. E. S. (2014). Course of depression: Persistence and recurrence. In I. H. Gotlib & C. L. Hammen (Eds.), *Handbook of depression and its treatment* (3rd ed.) (pp. 64–83). New York, NY: Guilford Press.

Klein, D. N., Dyson, M. W., Kujawa, A. J., & Kotov, R. (2012). Temperament and internalizing disorders. In M. Zentner and R. Shiner (Eds.), *Handbook of temperament* (pp. 541–561). New York, NY: Guilford Press.

Klein, D. N., Kujawa, A. J., Black, S. R., & Pennock, A. T. (2013). Depressive disorders. In T. P. Beauchaine and S. P. Hinshaw (Eds.), *Child and adolescent psychopathology* (2nd ed.) (pp. 543–576). Hoboken, NJ: John Wiley & Sons.

Klein, D. N., Lewinsohn, P. M., Rohde, P., Seeley, J. R., & Durbin, E. C. (2002). Clinical features of major depressive disorder in adolescents and their relatives: Impact on familial aggregation, implications for phenotype definition, and specificity of transmission. *Journal of Abnormal Psychology, 111*(1), 98–106.

Klein, D. N., & Riso, L. P. (1993). Psychiatric diagnoses: Problems of boundaries and co-occurrences. In C. G. Costello (Ed.), *Basic issues in psychopathology* (pp. 19–66). New York, NY: Guilford Press.

Klein, D. N., Shankman, S. A., Lewinsohn, P. M., & Seeley, J. R. (2009). Subthreshold depressive disorder in adolescents: Predictors of escalation to full syndrome depressive disorders. *Journal of the American Academy of Child and Adolescent Psychiatry, 48*(7), 703–710.

Klein, D. N., Shankman, S. A., & McFarland, B. (2006a). Classification of mood disorders. In D. J. Stein, D. J. Kupfer, and A. F. Schatzberg (Eds.), *The American Psychiatric Publishing textbook of mood disorders* (pp. 17–32). Washington, DC: American Psychiatric Publishing, Inc.

Klein, D. N., Shankman, S. A., & Rose, S. (2006b). Ten-year prospective follow-up study of the naturalistic course of dysthymic disorder and double depression. *American Journal of Psychiatry, 163*(5), 872–880.

Klein, D. N., & Small, A. E. (2014). Course of depression: Persistence and recurrence. In I. H. Gotlib & C. L. Hammen (Eds.), *Handbook of depression: Third edition* (pp. 64–83). New York, NY: Guilford Press.

Kopala-Sibley, D. C., & Zuroff, D. C. (2014). The developmental origins of personality factors from the self-definitional and relatedness domains: A review of theory and research. *Review of General Psychology, 18*(3), 137.

Kotov, R., Gamez, W., Schmidt, F., & Watson, D. (2010). Linking "big" personality traits to anxiety, depressive, and substance use disorders: A meta-analysis. *Psychological Bulletin, 136*(5), 768.

La Greca, A. M., & Harrison, H. M. (2005). Adolescent peer relations, friendships, and romantic relationships: Do they predict social anxiety and depression? *Journal of Clinical Child and Adolescent Psychology, 34*(1), 49–61.

Leader, J. B., & Klein, D. N. (1996). Social adjustment in dysthymia, double depression, and episodic major depression. *Journal of Affective Disorders, 37*(2–3), 91–101.

Lee, S. H., Ripke, S., Neale, B. M., Faraone, S. V., Purcell, S. M., Perlis, R. H., . . . Witte, J. S. (2013). Genetic relationship between five psychiatric disorders estimated from genome-wide SNPs. *Nature Genetics, 45*(9), 984–994.

Leventhal, A. M., & Rehm, L. P. (2005). The empirical status of melancholia: Implications for psychology. *Clinical Psychology Review, 25*(1), 25–44.

Levitan, R. D. (2007). The chronobiology and neurobiology of winter seasonal affective disorder. *Dialogues in Clinical Neuroscience, 9*(3), 315.

Lewinsohn, P. M., Rohde, P., Klein, D. N., & Seeley, J. R. (1999). Natural course of adolescent major depressive disorder: I. Continuity into young adulthood. *Journal of the American Academy of Child and Adolescent Psychiatry, 38*(1), 56–63.

Liu, R. T., & Alloy, L. B. (2010). Stress generation in depression: A systematic review of the empirical literature and recommendations for future study. *Clinical Psychology Review, 30*(5), 582–593.

Lubke, G. H., Hottenga, J. J., Walters, R., Laurin, C., De Geus, E. J., Willemsen, G., . . . Boomsma, D. I. (2012). Estimating the genetic variance of major depressive disorder due to all single nucleotide polymorphisms. *Biological Psychiatry, 72*(8), 707–709.

Luby, J. L., Heffelfinger, A. K., Mrakotsky, C., Hessler, M. J., Brown, K. M., & Hildebrand, T. (2002). Preschool major depressive disorder: Preliminary validation for developmentally modified *DSM-IV* criteria. *Journal of the American Academy of Child and Adolescent Psychiatry, 41*(8), 928–937.

Luppa, M., Heinrich, S., Angermeyer, M. C., König, H. H., & Riedel-Heller, S. G. (2007). Cost-of-illness studies of depression: A systematic review. *Journal of Affective Disorders, 98*(1), 29–43.

McLeod, B. D., Weisz, J. R., & Wood, J. J. (2007). Examining the association between parenting and childhood depression: A meta-analysis. *Clinical Psychology Review, 27*(8), 986–1003.

Merikangas, K. R., He, J. P., Brody, D., Fisher, P. W., Bourdon, K., & Koretz, D. S. (2010). Prevalence and treatment of mental disorders among US children in the 2001–2004 NHANES. *Pediatrics, 125*(1), 75–81.

Mojtabai, R. (2011). Bereavement-related depressive episodes: Characteristics, 3-year course, and implications for *DSM-5*. *Archives of General Psychiatry, 68*(9), 920–928.

Monroe, S. M., & Harkness, K. L. (2012). Is depression a chronic mental illness? *Psychological Medicine, 42*(5), 899–902.

Monroe, S. M., Slavich, G. M., & Georgiades, K. (2014). The social environment and depression: The roles of life stress. In I. H. Gotlib and C. L. Hammen (Eds.), *Handbook of depression and its treatment* (3rd ed.) (pp. 296–314). New York, NY: Guilford Press.

Mueller, T. I., Keller, M. B., Leon, A. C., Solomon, D. A., Shea, M. T., Coryell, W., & Endicott, J. (1996). Recovery after 5 years of unremitting major depressive disorder. *Archives of General Psychiatry, 53*(9), 794–799.

Munafo, M. R., Zammit, S., & Flint, J. (2014). Practitioner review: A critical perspective on gene-environment interaction models—what impact should they have on clinical perceptions and practice? *Journal of Child Psychology and Psychiatry, 55*(10), 1092–1101.

Nanni, V., Uher, R., & Danese, A. (2012). Childhood maltreatment predicts unfavorable course of illness and treatment outcome in depression: A meta-analysis. *American Journal of Psychiatry, 169*(2), 141–151.

Nelson, E. C., Heath, A. C., Madden, P. A., Cooper, M. L., Dinwiddie, S. H., Bucholz, K. K., . . . Martin, N. G. (2002). Association between self-reported childhood sexual abuse and adverse psychosocial outcomes: Results from a twin study. *Archives of General Psychiatry, 59*(2), 139–145.

Nolen-Hoeksema, S. (1987). Sex differences in unipolar depression: Evidence and theory. *Psychological Bulletin, 101*(2), 259.

Nolen-Hoeksema, S. (2000). The role of rumination in depressive disorders and mixed anxiety/depressive symptoms. *Journal of Abnormal Psychology, 109*(3), 504–511.

Nolen-Hoeksema, S., Wisco, B. E., & Lyubomirsky, S. (2008). Rethinking rumination. *Perspectives on Psychological Science, 3*(5), 400–424.

Ohayon, M. M., Priest, R. G., Guilleminault, C., & Caulet, M. (1999). The prevalence of depressive disorders in the United Kingdom. *Biological Psychiatry, 45*(3), 300–307.

Østergaard, S. D., Waltoft, B. L., Mortensen, P. B., & Mors, O. (2013). Environmental and familial risk factors for psychotic and non-psychotic severe depression. *Journal of Affective Disorders, 147*(1), 232–240.

Pae, C. U., Tharwani, H., Marks, D. M., Masand, P. S., & Patkar, A. A. (2009). Atypical depression. *CNS Drugs, 23*(12), 1023–1037.

Papakostas, G. I., Petersen, T., Mahal, Y., Mischoulon, D., Nierenberg, A. A., & Fava, M. (2004). Quality of life assessments in major depressive disorder: A review of the literature. *General Hospital Psychiatry, 26*(1), 13–17.

Parker, G., McCraw, S., Blanch, B., Hadzi-Pavlovic, D., Synnott, H., & Rees, A. M. (2013). Discriminating melancholic and non-melancholic depression by prototypic clinical features. *Journal of Affective Disorders, 144*(3), 199–207.

Penza, K. M., Heim, C., & Nemeroff, C. B. (2003). Neurobiological effects of childhood abuse: Implications for the pathophysiology of depression and anxiety. *Archives of Women's Mental Health, 6*(1), 15–22.

Pine, D. S., Cohen, E., Cohen, P., & Brook, J. (1999). Adolescent depressive symptoms as predictors of adult depression: Moodiness or mood disorder? *American Journal of Psychiatry, 156*(1), 133–135.

Pine, D. S., Cohen, P., Gurley, D., Brook, J., & Ma, Y. (1998). The risk for early-adulthood anxiety and depressive disorders in adolescents with anxiety and depressive disorders. *Archives of General Psychiatry, 55*(1), 56–64.

Pizzagalli, D. A., & Treadway, M. T. (2014). Neuroimaging approaches to the study of major depressive disorder: From regions to circuits. In I.H. Gotlib and C.L. Hammen (Eds.), *Handbook of depression and its treatment* (3rd ed.) (pp. 202–219). New York, NY: Guilford Press.

Posternak, M. A. (2003). Biological markers of atypical depression. *Harvard Review of Psychiatry, 11*(1), 1–7.

Prinstein, M. J., Boergers, J., Spirito, A., Little, T. D., & Grapentine, W. L. (2000). Peer functioning, family dysfunction, and psychological symptoms in a risk factor model for adolescent inpatients' suicidal ideation severity. *Journal of Clinical Child Psychology, 29*(3), 392–405.

Richards, C. S., & O'Hara, M. W. (2014). *Oxford handbook of depression and comorbidity.* New York, NY: Oxford University Press.

Rohan, K. J., Roecklein, K. A., & Haaga, D. A. (2009). Biological and psychological mechanisms of seasonal affective disorder: A review and integration. *Current Psychiatry Reviews, 5*(1), 37–47.

Rohde, P., Lewinsohn, P. M., Klein, D. N., Seeley, J. R., & Gau, J. M. (2013). Key characteristics of major depressive disorder occurring in childhood, adolescence, emerging adulthood, and adulthood. *Clinical Psychological Science, 1*(1), 41–53.

Rosenthal, N. E. (2009). Issues for *DSM-V*: Seasonal affective disorder and seasonality. *American Journal of Psychiatry, 166*(8), 852–853.

Rudolph, K. D., & Conley, C. S. (2005). The socioemotional costs and benefits of social-evaluative concerns: Do girls care too much? *Journal of Personality, 73*(1), 115–138.

Rutter, M. (2014). Commentary: G x E in child psychiatry and psychology: A broadening of the scope of enquiry as prompted by Munafo et al. (2014). *Journal of Child Psychology and Psychiatry, 55*(10), 1102–1104.

Shear, M. K., Simon, N., Wall, M., Zisook, S., Neimeyer, R., Duan, N., . . . Keshaviah, A. (2011). Complicated grief and related bereavement issues for *DSM-5*. *Depression and Anxiety, 28*(2), 103–117.

Shih, J. H., Eberhart, N. K., Hammen, C. L., & Brennan, P. A. (2006). Differential exposure and reactivity to interpersonal stress predict sex differences in adolescent depression. *Journal of Clinical Child and Adolescent Psychology, 35*(1), 103–115.

Singh, A. L., D'Onofrio, B. M., Slutske, W. S., Turkheimer, E., Emery, R. E., Harden, K. P., . . . Martin, N. G. (2011). Parental depression and offspring psychopathology: A children of twins study. *Psychological Medicine, 41*(7), 1385–1395.

Sohn, C. H., & Lam, R. W. (2005). Update on the biology of seasonal affective disorder. *CNS Spectrums, 10*(8), 635–646.

Solomon, D. A., Keller, M. B., Leon, A. C., Mueller, T. I., Lavori, P. W., Shea, M. T., . . . Endicott, J. (2000). Multiple recurrences of major depressive disorder. *American Journal of Psychiatry, 157*(2), 229–233.

Spijker, J., De Graaf, R., Bijl, R. V., Beekman, A. T., Ormel, J., & Nolen, W. A. (2002). Duration of major depressive episodes in the general population: Results from the Netherlands Mental Health Survey and Incidence Study (NEMESIS). *British Journal of Psychiatry, 181*(3), 208–213.

Stetler, C., & Miller, G. E. (2011). Depression and hypothalamic-pituitary-adrenal activation: A quantitative summary of four decades of research. *Psychosomatic Medicine, 73*(2), 114–126.

Stewart, J. W., & Thase, M. E. (2007). Treating *DSM-IV* depression with atypical features. *Journal of Clinical Psychiatry, 68*(4), e10.

Sullivan, P. F., Neale, M. C., & Kendler, K. S. (2000). Genetic epidemiology of major depression: Review and meta-analysis. *Genetic Epidemiology, 157*(10), 1552–1562.

Taylor, M. A., & Fink, M. (2008). Restoring melancholia in the classification of mood disorders. *Journal of Affective Disorders, 105*(1), 1–14.

Thase, M. E. (2006). Recognition and diagnosis of atypical depression. *Journal of Clinical Psychiatry, 68*(Suppl. 8), 11–16.

Thase, M. E. (2009). Atypical depression: Useful concept, but it's time to revise the *DSM-IV* criteria. *Neuropsychopharmacology, 34*(13), 2633–2641.

Tully, E. C., Iacono, W. G., & McGue, M. (2008). An adoption study of parental depression as an environmental liability for adolescent depression and childhood disruptive disorders. *American Journal of Psychiatry, 165*(9), 1148–1154.

Uliaszek, A. A., Zinbarg, R. E., Mineka, S., Craske, M. G., Griffith, J. W., Sutton, J.M., . . . Hammen, C. (2012). A longitudinal examination of stress generation in depressive and anxiety disorders. *Journal of Abnormal Psychology, 121*(1), 4–15.

Ustün, T. B., Ayuso-Mateos, J. L., Chatterji, S., Mathers, C., & Murray, C. J. (2004). Global burden of depressive disorders in the year 2000. *British Journal of Psychiatry, 184*(5), 386–392.

Van Loo, H. M., De Jonge, P., Romeijn, J. W., Kessler, R. C., & Schoevers, R. A. (2012). Data-driven subtypes of major depressive disorder: A systematic review. *BMC Medicine, 10*(1), 156.

Waldinger, R. J., Vaillant, G. E., & Orav, E. J. (2007). Childhood sibling relationships as a predictor of major depression in adulthood: A 30-year prospective study. *American Journal of Psychiatry, 164*(6), 949–954.

Waszczuk, M. A., Zavos, H. M., Gregory, A. M., & Eley, T. C. (2014). The phenotypic and genetic structure of depression and anxiety disorder symptoms in childhood, adolescence, and young adulthood. *JAMA Psychiatry, 71*(8), 905–916.

Weissman, M. M., Wolk, S., Goldstein, R. B., Moreau, D., Adams, P., Greenwald, S., . . . Wickramaratne, P. (1999a). Depressed adolescents grown up. *JAMA, 281*(18), 1707–1713.

Weissman, M. M., Wolk, S., Wickramaratne, P., Goldstein, R. B., Adams, P., Greenwald, S., . . . Steinberg, D. (1999b). Children with prepubertal-onset major depressive disorder and anxiety grown up. *Archives of General Psychiatry, 56*(9), 794–801.

Westrin, Å., & Lam, R. W. (2007). Seasonal affective disorder: A clinical update. *Annals of Clinical Psychiatry, 19*(4), 239–246.

Wichstrøm, L. (1999). The emergence of gender difference in depressed mood during adolescence: The role of intensified gender socialization. *Developmental Psychology, 35*(1), 232.

Widom, C. S., DuMont, K., & Czaja, S. J. (2007). A prospective investigation of major depressive disorder and comorbidity in abused and neglected children grown up. *Archives of General Psychiatry, 64*(1), 49–56.

World Health Organization. (2012). *International classification of diseases (ICD)*. Geneva: World Health Organization.

Zisook, S., Corruble, E., Duan, N., Iglewicz, A., Karam, E. G., Lanuoette, N., . . . Young, I. T. (2012). The bereavement exclusion and *DSM-V*. *Depression and Anxiety, 29*(5), 425–443.

Zuroff, D. C., Mongrain, M., & Santor, D. A. (2004). Conceptualizing and measuring personality vulnerability to depression: Comment on Coyne and Whiffen (1995). *Psychological Bulletin, 130*(3), 489–511.

CHAPTER 3

The Burden of Depressive Illness

Ronald C. Kessler, PhD
Evelyn J. Bromet, PhD
Peter de Jonge, PhD
Victoria Shahly, PhD
Marsha Wilcox, EdD, ScD

The initial report of the World Health Organization (WHO) Global Burden of Disease (GBD) Study first called widespread attention to the enormous burden of depressive illness. That study concluded, based on a selective review of the world epidemiological literature on comparative disease prevalence combined with a rating exercise using an international panel of experts on comparative disease severity, that unipolar depressive disorder was the fourth leading cause of disease burden in the world as of 1990 (Murray & Lopez, 1996). An update of the GBD estimates for 2000, based on a series of epidemiological surveys carried out in selected countries, concluded that unipolar depressive disorder was at that time the third leading cause of disease burden in the world (Üstün, Ayuso-Mateos, Chatterji, Mathers, & Murray, 2004). The subsequent GBD update, which was based on a much more exhaustive review of the world epidemiological literature along with an expansion of the definition to include not only major depressive disorder (MDD) but also dysthymic disorder and improved statistical estimation methods, concluded that unipolar MDD was the second leading cause of years lived with disability in the world (exceeded only by low back pain) and the first to fourth leading cause (out of nearly 300 considered) in each region of the world. Dysthymic disorder was the 19th leading cause (Vos et al., 2012).

These high estimates are due to depressive disorders having both high prevalence (e.g., MDD was estimated by GBD investigators to be the 19th most common of the 50 most burdensome diseases in the world) and high severity (indicated by MDD being rated as having the second-highest ranking as a cause of disability). But an argument could be made that GBD nonetheless underestimated the total burden of depression because the GBD methodology precluded any lost years of life being attributed to depression due to the fact that early mortality was attributed to direct causes (e.g., suicide, ischemic heart disease), even though those direct causes might have been influenced by depression. Subsequent reanalysis of the GBD data suggests that the global disease burden of MDD would increase by about 25% (from 3.0% to 3.8% of all disability-adjusted life years) if the indirect effects on early mortality due to suicide and ischemic heart disease were taken into consideration (Ferrari et al., 2013).

Even when these indirect effects of MDD on early mortality are taken into consideration, a good case could be made that the overall human costs of depression are substantially underestimated by GBD due to the fact that the GBD methodology focused on the effects of current disorders on productive functioning and mortality risk. Three other important types of burdens were excluded. The first are the burdens associated with the fact that early onset depression has adverse effects on life course role incumbency. The second are the burdens associated with the fact that both lifetime and current depressive illness influence role functioning in ways that go well beyond the effects on productive functioning that were the focus of GBD. The third are the burdens associated with the fact that lifetime history of depression influences risk of onset, persistence, and severity of a wide range of other disorders not captured in the GBD analysis of indirect effects through suicide and ischemic heart disease. We present an overview of the literature on all three of these additional burdens of depressive illness in this chapter. In addition, we explore the argument that at least some of the putative burden of depression is actually due to comorbid disorders, especially comorbid anxiety disorders. But before turning to any of these topics, we present a brief overview of the basic descriptive epidemiology of depressive illness, as a background in this literature is important for understanding the processes underlying the burden of depressive illness.

Basic Descriptive Epidemiology of Depressive Illness
Point Prevalence

Up to 20% of adults and up to 50% of children and adolescents report depressive symptoms in community epidemiological surveys over recall periods between one week and six months (Kessler & Bromet, 2013). Point prevalence estimates for MDD in community epidemiological surveys that use structured diagnostic interviews are considerably lower, with rates of current MDD typically less than 1% among children (reviewed by Merikangas & Angst, 1995), up to 6% among adolescents (reviewed by Kessler, Avenevoli, & Ries Merikangas, 2001), and 2%–4% among adults (reviewed by Kessler & Bromet, 2013).

The discrepancy between the high symptom prevalence and lower MDD prevalence means many people have subthreshold depressive symptoms. Epidemiological studies investigating these symptoms have been hampered by inconsistent definitions of subthreshold depression (Rodriguez, Nuevo, Chatterji, & Ayuso-Mateos, 2012) but have documented rates among both adolescents (Kessler & Walters, 1998) and adults (Judd, Akiskal, & Paulus, 1997) as high as, if not higher than, rates of MDD, with especially high relative rates among the elderly (Meeks, Vahia, Lavretsky, Kulkarni, & Jeste, 2011). Longitudinal research shows that subthreshold depression is a powerful predictor of subsequent MDD (Klein et al., 2013). The WHO's World Mental Health (WMH) Survey found that subthreshold depression is quite common throughout the world, is associated with similar risk factors to major depressive episodes, and is associated with substantial decrements in health (Ayuso-Mateos, Nuevo, Verdes, Naidoo, & Chatterji, 2010).

Twelve-Month Prevalence

Many community surveys focus on 12-month prevalence of depressive illness (i.e., the percentage of people with depression at some time in the 12 months before the interview) based on the fact that public health planning is typically made on an annual basis. The most recent such data came from the WHO WMH surveys, which are large household surveys in 18 countries with a combined sample of 89,037 respondents (Bromet et al., 2011). The average 12-month prevalence estimate of *DSM-IV* major depressive episodes (which includes MDD and depressive episodes due to bipolar disorder) was 5.5% in the 10 WMH surveys in high-income countries and 5.9% in the 8 surveys in low-middle-income countries. These estimates are somewhat higher than the 3.2% 12-month prevalence of major depressive episodes *alone* found among 245,404 respondents in 60 countries in the World Health Surveys (Moussavi et al., 2007), but the World Health Surveys also showed that 9.3%–23.0% of respondents with chronic physical conditions had *comorbid* major depressive episodes.

Lifetime Prevalence

Epidemiological surveys generally use retrospective reports to assess lifetime prevalence and age of onset (AOO) of major depressive episodes. Lifetime prevalence estimates in US surveys have ranged widely, from as low as 6% (Weissman, Livingston, Leaf, Florio, & Holzer, 1991) to as high as 25% (Lewinsohn, Rohde, Seeley, & Fischer, 1991). The WMH surveys estimated that lifetime prevalence of major depressive episodes was 14.6% in the 10 high-income countries assessed and 11.1% in the 8 low-middle-income countries assessed (Bromet et al., 2011).

Age of Onset

Lifetime prevalence estimates represent cumulative prevalence to date. Some survey respondents who never had a depressive illness will have one later in life. Lifetime *risk* (as opposed to lifetime *prevalence*) can be estimated with actuarial methods that use retrospective AOO reports to predict subsequent risk for respondents who have not yet passed through the risk period. This type of analysis was carried out in the WMH surveys (Kessler et al., 2007). Median AOO of depressive illness across countries was in the range 29–43 years, with the AOO distributions across countries showing consistently low risk through the early teens, a roughly linear increase thereafter through late-middle age, and a more gradual increase later in life. Projected lifetime risk by age 75 was 40%–170% greater than the proportion of respondents with lifetime-to-date depressive illness at the time of the interview.

In considering these results, it is important to recognize that the WMH lifetime risk projections assumed that conditional risk is constant across cohorts. This assumption is clearly incorrect, as shown by the fact that AOO curves differ substantially by cohort, with estimated risk successively higher in each younger cohort. This pattern of intercohort variation could be due to the risk of depression increasing in successively more recent cohorts, to various methodological possibilities involving cohort-related differences in willingness to admit depression or to recall past episodes of depression (Giuffra & Risch, 1994), or to some combination of substantive and methodological influences.

There is no way to adjudicate among these contending interpretations definitively with cross-sectional data of the sort available in the WMH surveys. Longitudinal data are needed. Longitudinal studies in the United States (Kessler et al., 2005) and Netherlands (de Graaf, ten Have, van Gool, & van Dorsselaer, 2012) failed to find evidence of significant time trends in prevalence. Although one other study suggested that depression prevalence increased dramatically in the United States between 1991–1992 and 2001–2002 (Compton, Conway, Stinson, & Grant, 2006), that report was in error due to an implausibly low estimate in the baseline assessment created by a methodological error that was corrected in the second survey, leading to the false impression of an increase in prevalence.

Course

Little longitudinal research has been carried out to study the course of major depressive episodes in general population samples (but for important exceptions, see Gamma, Angst, Ajdacic, Eich, & Rossler, 2007; Yaroslavsky, Pettit, Lewinsohn, Seeley, & Roberts, 2013). However, cross-sectional surveys consistently find the ratio of 12-month to lifetime major depressive episodes to be in the range of .5 to .6 (Bromet et al., 2011), suggesting that between one-half and two-thirds of people with these lifetime episodes will be in episode in any given year for the remainder of their lives. At least three separate processes contribute to the size of this ratio: (1) probability of first episode chronicity, (2) probability of episode recurrence among people with a history of nonchronic episodes, and (3) speed of episode recovery.

Epidemiological studies show that the first of these three processes is quite small, with only a small fraction of people reporting a single lifetime depressive episode persisting for many years. Prevalence of dysthymia and chronic minor depression are somewhat higher but still only in the range of 3%–4% of the population (Kessler &

Bromet, 2013). Episode recurrence, in contrast, is very common, with the vast majority of people with lifetime major depression having recurrent episodes (Hardeveld, Spijker, de Graaf, Nolen, & Beekman, 2013; Pettit, Hartley, Lewinsohn, Seeley, & Klein, 2013). Finally, the speed of episode recovery appears to be highly variable, although the epidemiological evidence on this issue is lacking (Kendler, Walters, & Kessler, 1997; McLeod, Kessler, & Landis, 1992).

Comorbidity

An issue we return to in the last substantive section of this chapter is that studies of diagnostic patterns in community surveys consistently find high comorbidity between depressive illness and other mental disorders (Kessler, Ormel, et al., 2011). Indeed, lifetime comorbidity is the norm among people with major depressive episodes. In the US National Comorbidity Survey Replication (NCS-R), for example, nearly three-quarters of respondents with lifetime major depressive episodes also had at least one other lifetime *DSM-IV* disorder (Kessler et al., 2003), including 59% with an anxiety disorder, 31.9% with an impulse control disorder, and 24.0% with a substance disorder. Lifetime comorbidity was even higher among respondents with 12-month major depressive episodes, implying importantly that comorbid major depression is more persistent. Comparison of retrospective AOO reports in the NCS-R showed that major depression was reported to have started at an earlier age than all other comorbid disorders in only 12.4% of lifetime cases, although temporal priority was much more common in cases of comorbidity with substance use disorders (41.3%–49.2%) than with either anxiety disorders (13.7%–14.6%) or impulse control disorders (17.9%–20.9%).

Controversy exists about the extent to which this high comorbidity is an artifact of changes in the diagnostic systems used in almost all recent studies of comorbidity (Frances et al., 1992). Beginning with *DSM-III*, these systems dramatically increased the number of diagnostic categories and reduced the number of exclusion criteria so that many people who would have received only a single diagnosis in previous systems now receive multiple diagnoses. The intention was to retain potentially important differentiating information that could be useful in refining understanding of etiology, course, and likely treatment response (First, Spitzer, & Williams, 1990). However, it can also be argued that this had the unintended negative consequence of artificially inflating estimates of comorbidity. This uncertainty might be resolved in future attempts to determine the validity of diagnostic distinctions, based on the new National Institute of Mental Health Research Domain Criteria initiative. The Research Domain Criteria initiative is designed to go beyond *DSM* diagnoses to focus on the underlying domains and constructs that account for psychopathology. Identifying the common domains and constructs in which dysfunction is occurring may ultimately help explain the high diagnostic overlap and comorbidity between depression and other *DSM* disorders. Until that time, we are left with a situation in which major depression appears to be highly comorbid with a number of other disorders.

As noted previously, the majority of comorbid major depression is temporally secondary in the sense that first onset of major depression occurs subsequent to first onset of other comorbid disorders. Survival analysis of cross-sectional data in the WMH surveys using retrospective AOO reports to determine temporal priority shows that a wide range of temporally primary disorders predict subsequent major depression onset (Kessler, Ormel, et al., 2011). Importantly, most of these associations are confined to associations with active, as opposed to remitted, primary disorders, which suggests indirectly that earlier disorders are (variable) risk factors rather than (fixed) risk markers (Kraemer et al., 1997). We discuss the implications of this finding later in this chapter.

Effects of Depressive Illness on Life Course Role Incumbency

Given its typically early AOO, depressive illness might be expected to have adverse effects on critical developmental transitions, such as educational attainment and timing of marriage. A number of epidemiological studies have examined these effects, with a focus on four domains: education, marital timing and stability, childbearing, and employment status.

Education

Several studies show that early onset mental disorders are associated with premature termination of education (Breslau, Lane, Sampson, & Kessler, 2008; Breslau, Miller, Chung, & Schweitzer, 2011; Kessler, Foster, Saunders, & Stang, 1995; Lee et al., 2009; McLeod & Kaiser, 2004; Porche, Fortuna, Lin, & Alegria, 2011; Vaughn et al., 2011; Woodward & Fergusson, 2001). While disruptive behavior disorders and bipolar disorder tend to have the strongest associations in these studies, major depression is also significantly associated with a roughly 60% elevated odds of failure to complete secondary school than otherwise comparable youth in high-income countries. Low educational attainment, in turn, is associated with reduced income and increased occupational instability throughout the life course.

Marital Timing and Stability

Several studies have examined associations of premarital mental disorders with subsequent marriage (Breslau et al., 2011; Forthofer, Kessler, Story, & Gotlib, 1996; Whisman, Tolejko, & Chatav, 2007). Early onset mental disorders predict low probability of ever marrying but are either positively associated (Forthofer et al., 1996) or unrelated (Breslau, Miller, Jin, et al., 2011) with early marriage (before age 18), which is known to be associated with a number of adverse outcomes, and negatively associated with on-time and late marriage, which are known to be associated with a number of benefits (e.g., financial security, social support). These associations are largely the same for men and women and across countries. Major depression is one of the most important of these premarital mental disorders. A separate set of studies has shown that premarital history of mental disorders predicts divorce (Butterworth & Rodgers, 2008; Kessler, Walters, & Forthofer, 1998), again with associations quite similar for husbands and wives across all countries, and major depression among the most important disorders in this regard (Breslau, Miller, Jin, et al., 2011).

Teen Childbearing

Although not a topic of sustained research, we are aware of one study that examined the association between child-adolescent mental disorder and subsequent teen childbearing (Kessler et al., 1997). Major depression and a number of other early onset mental disorders were significant predictors of increased teen childbearing. Disaggregation found that the overall associations were due to disorders predicting increased sexual activity but not decreased use of contraception.

Employment Status

We noted earlier that early onset depression is associated with reduced educational attainment, which, in turn, is associated with unstable employment throughout the life course. However, this effect is not generally appreciated in the epidemiological literature. Instead, although a good deal of research in samples of adults has documented significant associations of depression with unemployment, most of this research has emphasized the impact of job loss on depression rather than depression as a risk factor for job loss (Dooley, Fielding, & Levi, 1996). However, a recent analysis of data from the WMH surveys documented the latter association by showing that history of mental disorders as of the age of completing schooling, depression being among the most important of these disorders, predicted current (at the time of the interview) unemployment and work disability (Kawakami et al., 2012). Interestingly, though, this association was significant only in high-income countries, raising the possibility that depression becomes more detrimental to work performance as the substantive complexity of work increases.

Effects of Depressive Illness on Role Performance

A considerably larger amount of research has been carried out on the associations of depressive illness with various aspects of role performance, with a special focus on *productive* role performance. As noted in the introduction, the GBD Study focused on the effects of health problems on productive role performance, but depressive illness has additional effects on affiliative role performance (friendship, marriage, parenting), which also warrant consideration.

Days Out of Role

Considerable research has examined days out of role associated with various physical and mental disorders in an effort to produce data on comparative disease burden for health policy planning purposes (Alonso et al., 2004; Merikangas et al., 2007). These studies typically find that major depression is associated with among the highest number of days out of role at the societal level of any physical or mental disorder due to its combination of comparatively high prevalence and comparatively strong individual-level association (Collins et al., 2005; Munce, Stansfeld, Blackmore, & Stewart, 2007; Wang et al., 2003). In the WMH surveys, for example, 62,971 respondents across 24 countries were assessed for a wide range of common physical and mental disorders as well as for days out of role in the 30 days before the interview (Alonso et al., 2011). MDD was associated with 5.1% of all days out of role, the fourth highest population attributable risk proportion of all the disorders considered (exceeded only by headache or migraine, other chronic pain conditions, and cardiovascular disorders) and by far the largest among the mental disorders. A number of epidemiological surveys in the United States have estimated the workplace costs of major depression on absenteeism and low work performance (often referred to as *presenteeism*) (Greenberg et al., 2003; Kessler et al., 2006; Stewart, Ricci, Chee, Hahn, & Morganstein, 2003a; Wang, Simon, & Kessler, 2003). All these studies found that depression significantly predicts overall lost work performance. Several studies attempted to estimate the annual salary-equivalent human capital value of these losses. These estimates were in the range of $30.1 billion (Stewart, Ricci, Chee, Hahn, & Morganstein, 2003a) to $51.5 billion (Greenberg et al., 2003).

Financial Success

One of the most striking aspects of the impairment associated with major depression is that the personal earnings and household income of people with depression are substantially lower than those of people without depression (Ford et al., 2010; Insel, 2008; Kessler et al., 2008; Levinson et al., 2010; Marcotte & Wilcox-Gok, 2001; McMillan, Enns, Asmundson, & Sareen, 2010). However, it is unclear whether depression is primarily a cause, consequence, or both in these associations due to the possibility of reciprocal causation between income-earnings and depression (Muntaner, Eaton, Miech, & O'Campo, 2004). Causal effects of low income on depression have been documented in quasi-experimental studies of job loss (Dooley et al., 1996). Time series analyses have also documented aggregate associations between unemployment rates and suicide rates (Jones, 1991). Previous studies of the effects of mental disorders on reductions in income have not controlled for these reciprocal effects, making the size of the adverse effects of depression on income-earnings uncertain. One way to sort out this temporal order would be to take advantage of the fact that depression often starts in childhood or adolescence and use prospective epidemiological data to study long-term associations between early onset disorders and subsequent income-earnings. Several such studies exist, all of them suggesting that depression in childhood-adolescence predicts reduced income-earnings in adulthood (Goodman, Joyce, & Smith, 2011; Smith & Smith, 2010).

Marital Functioning

It has long been known that marital dissatisfaction and discord are strongly related to depressive symptoms (e.g., Culp & Beach, 1998; Whisman, 1999), with an average Pearson correlation between marital dissatisfaction and depressive symptoms of approximately 0.4 across studies and very similar patterns for men and women (Whisman, 2001). Longitudinal studies show that the association is bidirectional (Mamun et al., 2009; Whisman & Uebelacker, 2009), but with a stronger time-lagged association of marital discord predicting depressive symptoms than vice versa (Proulx, Helms, & Buehler, 2007). Fewer studies have considered the effects of depressive illness on marital functioning (Coyne, Thompson, & Palmer, 2002; Kronmuller et al., 2011; Pearson, Watkins, Kuyken, & Mullan, 2010), but those studies consistently document significant adverse effects.

Considerable research documents that both perpetration of and victimization by physical violence in marital relationships are significantly associated with depression (Stith, Smith, Penn, Ward, & Tritt, 2004). While these studies have generally focused on presumed mental health *consequences* of relationship violence (Afifi et al., 2009; Kim, Laurent, Capaldi, & Feingold, 2008; Renner, 2009), a growing body of research has more recently suggested that preexisting mental disorders are also important *causes* of marital violence (Kessler, Molnar, Feurer, & Appelbaum, 2001; Lorber & O'Leary, 2004; O'Leary, Tintle, Bromet, & Gluzman, 2008; Riggs, Caulfield, & Street, 2000). Indeed, longitudinal studies consistently find that premarital history of mental disorders, including depression, predicts subsequent marital violence perpetration (Fang, Massetti, Ouyang, Grosse, & Mercy, 2010; Lorber & O'Leary, 2004) and victimization (Lehrer, Buka, Gortmaker, & Shrier, 2006; O'Leary et al., 2008; Riggs et al., 2000; Stith et al., 2004). However, few of these studies adjusted for comorbidity. A recent study in the WMH surveys (Miller et al., 2011) found that the association between premarital history of MDD and subsequent marital violence disappears after controls are introduced for disruptive behavior disorders and substance use disorders, suggesting that depression might be a risk marker rather than a causal risk factor.

Parental Functioning

A number of studies have documented significant associations of both maternal (Lovejoy, Graczyk, O'Hare, & Neuman, 2000) and paternal (Wilson & Durbin, 2010) depression with negative parenting behaviors. These associations are found throughout the age range of children, but are most pronounced for the parents of young children. Although only an incomplete understanding exists of pathways, both laboratory and naturalistic studies of parent-infant microinteractions have documented subtle ways in which parent depression leads to maladaptive interactions that impede infant affect regulation and later child development (Tronick & Reck, 2009).

Comparative Role Impairments

A number of community surveys, most of them carried out in the United States, have examined the comparative effects of diverse diseases on various aspects of role functioning (Kessler, Greenberg, Mickelson, Meneades, & Wang, 2001; Lerner, Allaire, & Reisine, 2005; Merikangas et al., 2007; Stewart, Ricci, Chee, & Morganstein, 2003b; Verbrugge & Patrick, 1995; Wang, Beck, et al., 2003). MDD was included in a number of these studies, and the results typically showed that musculoskeletal disorders and major depression were associated with the highest levels of disability at the individual level among all commonly occurring disorders assessed. The most compelling study of this sort outside the United States was based on 15 national surveys carried out as part of the WMH surveys in which disorder-specific disability scores were compared across people who experienced each of 10 chronic physical disorders and 10 mental disorders in the year before the interview (Ormel et al., 2008). This study is of special importance because role impairment was disaggregated to distinguish impairments in productive roles (employment, housework) from impairments in affiliative roles (close intimate relationships, social relationships).

MDD and bipolar disorder were the mental disorders most often rated severely impairing across all these areas of role functioning. None of the physical disorders considered had impairment levels as high as those for these mood disorders, despite the fact that the physical disorders included such severe conditions as cancer, diabetes, and heart disease. Nearly all the higher mental-than-physical ratings were statistically significant at the .05 level. It is noteworthy that comparable results were obtained when analyses focused exclusively on subsamples of respondents who were in treatment and when comparisons were restricted to respondents who had both disorders in a given mental-physical pair (e.g., respondents who had both MDD and cancer or both MDD and heart disease). Importantly, these significant greater effects of mood disorders than physical disorders on role functioning were most pronounced for impairments in intimate relationships and social relationships, both of which were ignored in the GBD ratings.

Effects of Depressive Illness on Secondary Disorders

We noted previously that the majority of lifetime comorbid depressive illness is temporally secondary to the other mental disorders with which it is comorbid. That is, first onset of depressive illness typically occurs subsequent to first onset of comorbid mental disorders. As a result, there is little evidence that temporally primary depressive illness is associated with elevated risk of the subsequent first onset of other common mental disorders. The one exception is that temporally primary MDD is significantly associated with elevated risk of subsequent generalized anxiety disorder (Kessler, Ormel, et al., 2011), although this might be due to symptom overlap between MDD and generalized anxiety disorder (Cramer, Waldorp, van der Maas, & Borsboom, 2010). However, it is also possible that depressive illness influences the persistence and severity of comorbid mental disorders. While this is, as of yet, not an active area of research, we are aware of a number of epidemiological studies documenting associations between initial major depressive episodes and the subsequent persistence and severity of comorbid mental disorders (Roy-Byrne et al., 2000; Wardenaar, Giltay, van Veen, Zitman, & Penninx, 2012), although other studies show that change in comorbid symptoms over time is unrelated to baseline levels of depression (Fineberg et al., 2013; Leadbeater, Thompson, & Gruppuso, 2012).

More compelling evidence exists for associations of temporally primary major depression with subsequent onset and persistence of numerous chronic physical disorders, including arthritis, asthma, cancer, cardiovascular disease, diabetes, hypertension, chronic respiratory disorders, and a variety of chronic pain conditions (Baxter, Charlson, Somerville, & Whiteford, 2011). Although most data documenting these associations come from clinical samples, similar data exist in community epidemiological surveys. These associations have considerable individual and public health significance and can be thought of as representing costs of depressive illness in at least two ways. First, to the extent that depression is a causal risk factor, it leads to increased prevalence of physical disorders. Evidence about depression as a cause is spotty, though we know from meta-analyses of longitudinal studies that depression is a consistent predictor of subsequent first onset of coronary artery disease, stroke, diabetes, heart attacks, and certain types of cancer. A number of biologically plausible mechanisms have been proposed to explain these prospective associations (de Jonge et al., 2010). Second, even if depression is a consequence rather than cause of chronic physical disorders, comorbid depression is often associated with a worse course of the physical disorder (Gillen, Tennen, McKee, Gernert-Dott, & Affleck, 2001), possibly through nonadherence to treatment regimens (Ziegelstein et al., 2000). Based on these considerations, it is not surprising that depression is associated with elevated risk of early death (Carney, Freedland, Miller, & Jaffe, 2002). This is true not only because people with depression have high risks of suicide and heart disease, as taken into consideration in the GBD Study, but also because depression is associated with elevated risk of many types of disorders and with elevated mortality risk among people with a number of disorders. These associations are reviewed in more detail in chapter 4.

Effects of Anxiety Disorders on Secondary Depressive Illness

The severity of depressive illness is highly variable (Birnbaum et al., 2010; Li et al., 2014). Indeed, severity is the most consistent discriminating characteristic in empirical studies of depression symptom subtypes (van Loo, de Jonge, Romeijn, Kessler, & Schoevers, 2012). One of the strongest predictors of depression severity is comorbid anxiety disorder (Mineka & Vrshek-Shallhorn, 2014; Wu & Fang, 2014). As noted earlier, in the subsection on comorbidity, epidemiological studies consistently show that depressive illness is highly comorbid with numerous anxiety disorders (Andrade et al., 2003; Kessler, Petukhova, & Zaslavsky, 2011; Lamers et al., 2011), and that comorbid anxiety disorders typically have earlier AOO than depression in cross-sectional surveys that assess AOO retrospectively (Kessler, 1995; Kessler, Ormel, et al., 2011) and in prospective studies that examine unfolding of comorbidity over time (Bittner et al., 2004; Copeland, Shanahan, Costello, & Angold, 2009; Klein et al., 2013; Murphy, Olivier, Sobol, Monson, & Leighton, 1986). Depression is also more severe and persistent when accompanied by comorbid anxiety disorders (Fichter, Quadflieg, Fischer, & Kohlboeck, 2010; McLaughlin, Khandker, Kruzikas, & Tummala, 2006; Ormel et al., 1994; Roy-Byrne et al., 2000). Furthermore, people with anxious depression are also significantly more likely to seek treatment (Jacobi et al., 2004; Kessler, Keller, & Wittchen, 2001) but are significantly less likely to respond to treatment (Jakubovski & Bloch, 2014; Saveanu et al., 2015) than those with nonanxious depression.

Although most epidemiological studies of comorbid anxiety-depression use a narrow definition of comorbid anxiety or examine only one anxiety disorder (typically generalized anxiety disorder or panic disorder), a recent analysis of the WMH survey data corrected this problem by creating a composite measure that included a wide range of anxiety disorders in an analysis of comorbidity, AOO priority, and severity persistence (Kessler et al., 2015). Close to half (45.7%) of respondents with lifetime major depression also had a lifetime anxiety disorder. A somewhat higher proportion (51.7%) of respondents with 12-month depression had a lifetime anxiety disorder. Perhaps most striking, though, was that only a slightly lower proportion of respondents with 12-month depression had a 12-month anxiety disorder (41.6%). Only 13.5% of respondents with lifetime comorbid anxiety-depression reported that the depression was temporally primary. Significantly higher proportions of respondents with 12-month anxious depression than nonanxious depression reported severe role impairment (64.4% vs. 46.0%) and suicide ideation (19.5% vs. 8.9%). All these results were quite consistent across countries.

These WMH results argue quite strongly that the major burden of depressive illness on role functioning and impairment is associated not so much with depression per se as with anxious depression. This specification was not taken into consideration in the GBD Study. However, based on an increasing awareness of the importance of comorbid anxiety (Das-Munshi et al., 2008), a new diagnosis of mixed anxiety-depression is being proposed for the upcoming revision of the *ICD* diagnostic system (Lam et al., 2013), while the recently revised *DSM-5* system includes a new major depression specifier of "with anxious distress" (American Psychiatric Association, 2013).

But even more broadly, recent research on comorbidity suggests that both anxiety and depression might be most accurately conceptualized as indicators of an underlying predisposition to internalizing disorders that has a more fundamental effect than either of the component disorders. This line of thinking can be traced to an influential paper by Krueger (1999) that documented, using factor analysis, associations among hierarchy-free anxiety, mood, behavior, and substance disorders consistent with the existence of two latent internalizing and externalizing disorders. The internalizing dimension was further divided into secondary dimensions of fear (e.g., panic, phobia) and distress (e.g., major depressive episode, generalized anxiety disorder) in the original paper as well as a number of replications and extensions (Beesdo-Baum et al., 2009; Cox & Swinson, 2002; Krueger & Markon, 2006a; Lahey et al., 2008; Slade & Watson, 2006; Vollebergh et al., 2001). While initially used to argue for a reorganization of the classification of mental disorders in the *DSM* and *ICD* diagnostic systems (Andrews et al., 2009; Goldberg, Krueger, Andrews, & Hobbs, 2009; Krueger & Markon, 2006b; Watson, 2005; Wittchen, Beesdo, & Gloster, 2009), subsequent analysis showed that the theoretical structure was insufficiently robust to serve as the basis for such a reorganization (Beesdo-Baum et al., 2009; Wittchen et al., 2009), although it has been used to support the creation of an anxious depression disorder in *ICD-11*.

The general finding of strong comorbidity within the internalizing domain has raised the question whether common risk factors exist for disorders in these domains and, if so, whether risk factors for and consequences of individual disorders in previous studies are actually risk factors for and consequences of the broader predispositions. This issue of specificity versus generality of risk factors is of considerable importance, as a number of hypotheses about causal pathways posit very specific associations between particular risk factors and particular outcomes that would be called into question if empirical research showed that risk factors have less specific predictive effects (Green et al., 2010). In addition, evidence that a risk factor has a broad effect on a wide range of disorders would increase interest in that risk factor as an intervention target (Mrazek & Haggerty, 1994). It is noteworthy that not only environmental risk factors but also genes might be generalized risk targets of this sort, as recent studies suggest that some genes have pleiotropic effects that confer risk for a range of psychiatric disorders (Smoller et al., 2013).

Although use of latent variable models to study risk factor specificity is only in its infancy, research has already shown considerable value. For example, Kramer, Krueger, and Hicks (2008) found that the widely observed association of gender with MDD became insignificant when controls were included for latent internalizing and externalizing dimensions, arguing that gender is more directly associated with these overall latent dimensions than with MDD or any other disorder within these dimensions. In another example, Kessler and colleagues (2010) found that the effects of childhood adversities on onset of major depression and other individual mental disorders were largely mediated by more direct effects on predispositions for internalizing and externalizing disorders. More recent studies have examined the extent to which a latent internalizing predisposition might account for the development of lifetime comorbidity between depression and other disorders based on analysis of the WMH survey data (Kessler, Cox, et al., 2011; Kessler, Ormel, et al., 2011; Kessler, Petukhova, et al., 2011). These analyses found good fit of a latent variable model, suggesting that common causal pathways account for most comorbidities of major depression with anxiety disorders. However, those analyses focused on predicting lifetime first onset of these disorders using retrospective analyses. Large-scale, multiwave longitudinal data are needed to determine whether these retrospective results can be replicated and extended to study onset and persistence of disorders over time. Such data exist (Beesdo, Pine, Lieb, & Wittchen, 2010; Beesdo-Baum et al., 2009), and analyses of this sort are under way, but results are not yet available.

Discussion

Depressive illness is commonly occurring and burdensome. The high prevalence, early AOO, high persistence, and strong associations of depression with impairments in role functioning as well as with secondary physical disorders in the many different countries where epidemiological surveys have been administered confirm the high worldwide importance of the illness. Evidence is not definitive that depression plays a causal role in its associations with the many adverse outcomes reviewed here. And questions remain about the specifying role of comorbid anxiety disorders and about the extent to which the causes and consequences of depression parallel those of a broader class of internalizing disorders. Nonetheless, clear evidence exists that depression has causal effects on a number of important biological mediators, making it difficult to assume anything other than that depression has strong causal effects on many dimensions of burden.

These results have been used to argue for the likely cost-effectiveness of expanded depression treatment from a societal perspective (Wang et al., 2006). Two separate large-scale, randomized workplace depression treatment effectiveness trials have been carried out in the United States to evaluate the cost-effectiveness of expanded treatment from an employer perspective (Rost, Smith, & Dickinson, 2004; Wang, Simon, et al., 2007). Both trials had positive returns on investment to employers. A substantial expansion of worksite depression care management programs has occurred in the United States subsequent to the publication of these trials (Rost, Marshall, Shearer,

& Dietrich, 2011). Yet the proportion of people with depressive illness who receive treatment remains low in the United States and even lower in other parts of the world. A recent US study found that only about half of workers with major depression received treatment in the year of the interview and that fewer than half of treated workers received treatment consistent with published treatment guidelines (Kessler, Merikangas, & Wang, 2008). Although the treatment rate was higher for more severe cases, even those with severe major depression often failed to receive treatment (Birnbaum et al., 2010). The WMH surveys show that treatment rates are even lower in many other developed countries and consistently much lower in developing countries (Wang, Aguilar-Gaxiola, et al., 2007). Less information is available on rates of depression treatment among patients with chronic physical disorders, but available evidence suggests that expanded treatment could be of considerable value (Katon, Lin, & Kroenke, 2007). Randomized controlled trials are needed to expand our understanding of the effects of detection and treatment of depression among people in treatment for chronic physical disorders. In addition, controlled effectiveness trials with long-term follow-ups are needed to increase our understanding of the effects of early depression treatment interventions on changes in life course role trajectories, role performance, and onset of secondary physical disorders. Only in the basis of such experimental analyses will we be able to obtain definitive data on the full scope of the burdens of depressive illness.

Acknowledgments

The WHO World Mental Health (WMH) Survey Initiative is supported by the National Institute of Mental Health (NIMH; R01 MH070884), the John D. and Catherine T. MacArthur Foundation, the Pfizer Foundation, the US Public Health Service (R13-MH066849, R01-MH069864, and R01 DA016558), the Fogarty International Center (FIRCA R03-TW006481), the Pan American Health Organization (PAHO), Eli Lilly & Company Foundation, Ortho-McNeil Pharmaceutical, Inc., GlaxoSmithKline, Sanofi-Aventis, and Bristol-Myers Squibb. Peter de Jonge is supported by a VICI grant (no: 91812607) from the Netherlands Research Foundation (NWO-ZonMW). We thank the WMH staff for assistance with instrumentation, fieldwork, and data analysis. A complete list of WMH publications can be found at https://www.hcp.med.harvard.edu/wmh/.

Each WMH country obtained funding for its own survey. The São Paulo Megacity Mental Health Survey is supported by the State of São Paulo Research Foundation (FAPESP) Thematic Project Grant 03/00204-3. The Bulgarian Epidemiological Study of common mental disorders EPIBUL is supported by the Ministry of Health and the National Center for Public Health Protection. The Beijing, People's Republic of China World Mental Health Survey Initiative is supported by the Pfizer Foundation. The Shenzhen, People's Republic of China Mental Health Survey is supported by the Shenzhen Bureau of Health and the Shenzhen Bureau of Science, Technology, and Information. The Colombian National Study of Mental Health (NSMH) is supported by the Ministry of Social Protection. Implementation of the Iraq Mental Health Survey (IMHS), and data entry were carried out by the staff of the Iraqi Ministry of Health and Ministry of Planning with direct support from the Iraqi IMHS team and funding from both the Japanese and European Funds through United Nations Development Group Iraq Trust Fund (UNDG ITF). The Israel National Health Survey is funded by the Ministry of Health with support from the Israel National Institute for Health Policy and Health Services Research and the National Insurance Institute of Israel. The World Mental Health Japan (WMHJ) Survey is supported by the Grant for Research on Psychiatric and Neurological Diseases and Mental Health (H13-SHOGAI-023, H14-TOKUBETSU-026, H16-KOKORO-013) from the Japan Ministry of Health, Labour and Welfare. The Lebanese National Mental Health Survey (L.E.B.A.N.O.N.) is supported by the Lebanese Ministry of Public Health, the World Health Organization (WHO; Lebanon), National Institute of Health / Fogarty International Center (R03 TW006481-01), Sheikh Hamdan Bin Rashid Al Maktoum Award for Medical Sciences, anonymous private donations to the Institute for Development, Research, Advocacy and Applied Care (IDRAAC), Lebanon, and unrestricted grants from AstraZeneca, Eli Lilly, GlaxoSmithKline, Hikma Pharm, Pfizer, Roche, Sanofi-Aventis, Servier, and Novartis. The Mexican National Comorbidity Survey (MNCS) is supported by the National Institute of Psychiatry Ramon de la Fuente (INPRFMDIES 4280) and by the National Council on Science and Technology (CONACyT-G30544-H), with supplemental support from PAHO. Te Rau Hinengaro: The New Zealand Mental Health Survey (NZMHS) is supported by the New Zealand Ministry of Health, Alcohol Advisory Council, and the Health Research Council. The Nigerian Survey of Mental Health and Well-Being (NSMHW) is supported by the WHO (Geneva), the WHO (Nigeria), and the Federal Ministry of Health, Abuja, Nigeria. The Northern Ireland Study of Mental Health was funded by the Health & Social Care Research & Development Division of the Public Health Agency. The Portuguese Mental Health Study was carried out by the Department of Mental Health, Faculty of Medical Sciences, NOVA University of Lisbon, with collaboration with the Portuguese Catholic University, and was funded by Champalimaud Foundation, Gulbenkian Foundation, Foundation for Science and Technology (FCT) and the Ministry of Health. The Romania WMH study projects "Policies in Mental Health Area" and "National Study regarding Mental Health and Services Use" were carried out by National School of Public Health & Health Services Management (former National Institute for Research & Development in Health, present National School of Public Health Management & Professional Development, Bucharest), with technical support of Metro Media Transilvania, the National Institute of Statistics—National Centre for Training in Statistics, SC Cheyenne Services SRL, Statistics Netherlands, and were funded by the Ministry of Public Health (former Ministry of Health) with supplemental support of Eli Lilly Romania SRL. The Ukraine Comorbid

Mental Disorders during Periods of Social Disruption (CMDPSD) study is funded by the US National Institute of Mental Health (RO1-MH61905). The US National Comorbidity Survey Replication (NCS-R) is supported by the National Institute of Mental Health (NIMH; U01-MH60220) with supplemental support from the National Institute of Drug Abuse (NIDA), the Substance Abuse and Mental Health Services Administration (SAMHSA), the Robert Wood Johnson Foundation (RWJF; Grant 044708), and the John W. Alden Trust. Additional support for preparation of this report was provided by Janssen Pharmaceuticals.

Portions of this chapter have appeared in R. C. Kessler, N. A. Sampson, P. Berglund, et al. (2015). Anxious and non-anxious major depressive disorder in the World Health Organization World Mental Health surveys, *Epidemiology and Psychiatry Sciences, 24*(3), 210–26; R. C. Kessler (2012). The costs of depression, *Psychiatric Clinics of North America, 35*(1), 1–14; R. C. Kessler, P. de Jonge, V. Shahly, et al. (2014). Epidemiology of depression, in I. H. Gotlib & C. L. Hammen (Eds.), *Handbook of depression: Third edition* (pp. 7–24). New York, NY: The Guilford Press. All used with permission.

References

Afifi, T. O., MacMillan, H., Cox, B. J., Asmundson, G. J., Stein, M. B., & Sareen, J. (2009). Mental health correlates of intimate partner violence in marital relationships in a nationally representative sample of males and females. *Journal of Interpersonal Violence, 24*(8), 1398–1417.

Alonso, J., Angermeyer, M. C., Bernert, S., Bruffaerts, R., Brugha, T. S., Bryson, H., . . . Vollebergh, W. A. (2004). Disability and quality of life impact of mental disorders in Europe: Results from the European Study of the Epidemiology of Mental Disorders (ESEMeD) project. *Acta Psychiatrica Scandinavica, Supplementum* (420), 38–46.

Alonso, J., Petukhova, M., Vilagut, G., Chatterji, S., Heeringa, S., Üstün, T. B., . . . Kessler, R. C. (2011). Days out of role due to common physical and mental conditions: Results from the WHO World Mental Health surveys. *Molecular Psychiatry, 16*(12), 1234–1246.

American Psychiatric Association. (2013). *Diagnostic and statistical manual of mental disorders (DSM-5)*. Arlington, VA: American Psychiatric Association.

Andrade, L., Caraveo-Anduaga, J. J., Berglund, P., Bijl, R. V., de Graaf, R., Vollebergh, W., . . . Wittchen, H. U. (2003). The epidemiology of major depressive episodes: Results from the International Consortium of Psychiatric Epidemiology (ICPE) Surveys. *International Journal of Methods in Psychiatric Research, 12*(1), 3–21.

Andrews, G., Goldberg, D. P., Krueger, R. F., Carpenter, W. T., Hyman, S. E., Sachdev, P., & Pine, D. S. (2009). Exploring the feasibility of a meta-structure for *DSM-V* and *ICD-11*: Could it improve utility and validity? *Psychological Medicine, 39*(12), 1993–2000.

Ayuso-Mateos, J. L., Nuevo, R., Verdes, E., Naidoo, N., & Chatterji, S. (2010). From depressive symptoms to depressive disorders: The relevance of thresholds. *The British Journal of Psychiatry: The Journal of Mental Science, 196*(5), 365–371.

Baxter, A. J., Charlson, F. J., Somerville, A. J., & Whiteford, H. A. (2011). Mental disorders as risk factors: Assessing the evidence for the Global Burden of Disease Study. *BMC Medicine, 9*(1), 134.

Beesdo, K., Pine, D. S., Lieb, R., & Wittchen, H. U. (2010). Incidence and risk patterns of anxiety and depressive disorders and categorization of generalized anxiety disorder. *Archives of General Psychiatry, 67*(1), 47–57.

Beesdo-Baum, K., Hofler, M., Gloster, A. T., Klotsche, J., Lieb, R., Beauducel, A., . . . Wittchen, H. U. (2009). The structure of common mental disorders: A replication study in a community sample of adolescents and young adults. *International Journal of Methods in Psychiatric Research, 18*(4), 204–220.

Birnbaum, H. G., Kessler, R. C., Kelley, D., Ben-Hamadi, R., Joish, V. N., & Greenberg, P. E. (2010). Employer burden of mild, moderate, and severe major depressive disorder: Mental health services utilization and costs, and work performance. *Depression and Anxiety, 27*(1), 78–89.

Bittner, A., Goodwin, R. D., Wittchen, H. U., Beesdo, K., Hofler, M., & Lieb, R. (2004). What characteristics of primary anxiety disorders predict subsequent major depressive disorder? *Journal of Clinical Psychiatry, 65*(5), 618–626, quiz 730.

Breslau, J., Lane, M., Sampson, N., & Kessler, R. C. (2008). Mental disorders and subsequent educational attainment in a US national sample. *Journal of Psychiatric Research, 42*(9), 708–716.

Breslau, J., Miller, E., Chung, W. J. J., & Schweitzer, J. B. (2011). Childhood and adolescent onset psychiatric disorders, substance use, and failure to graduate high school on time. *Journal of Psychiatric Research, 45*(3), 295–301.

Breslau, J., Miller, E., Jin, R., Sampson, N. A., Alonso, J., Andrade, L. H., . . . Kessler, R. C. (2011). A multinational study of mental disorders, marriage, and divorce. *Acta Psychiatrica Scandinavica, 124*(6), 474–486.

Bromet, E., Andrade, L. H., Hwang, I., Sampson, N. A., Alonso, J., de Girolamo, G., . . . Kessler, R. C. (2011). Cross-national epidemiology of *DSM-IV* major depressive episode. *BMC Medicine, 9*(1), 90.

Butterworth, P., & Rodgers, B. (2008). Mental health problems and marital disruption: Is it the combination of husbands and wives' mental health problems that predicts later divorce? *Social Psychiatry and Psychiatric Epidemiology, 43*(9), 758–763.

Carney, R. M., Freedland, K. E., Miller, G. E., & Jaffe, A. S. (2002). Depression as a risk factor for cardiac mortality and morbidity: A review of potential mechanisms. *Journal of Psychosomatic Research, 53*(4), 897–902.

Collins, J. J., Baase, C. M., Sharda, C. E., Ozminkowski, R. J., Nicholson, S., Billotti, G. M., . . . Berger, M. L. (2005). The assessment of chronic health conditions on work performance, absence, and total economic impact for employers. *Journal of Occupational and Environmental Medicine / American College of Occupational and Environmental Medicine, 47*(6), 547–557.

Compton, W. M., Conway, K. P., Stinson, F. S., & Grant, B. F. (2006). Changes in the prevalence of major depression and comorbid substance use disorders in the United States between 1991–1992 and 2001–2002. *American Journal of Psychiatry, 163*(12), 2141–2147.

Copeland, W. E., Shanahan, L., Costello, E. J., & Angold, A. (2009). Childhood and adolescent psychiatric disorders as predictors of young adult disorders. *Archives of General Psychiatry, 66*(7), 764–772.

Cox, B. J., & Swinson, R. P. (2002). Instrument to assess depersonalization-derealization in panic disorder. *Depression and Anxiety, 15*(4), 172–175.

Coyne, J. C., Thompson, R., & Palmer, S. C. (2002). Marital quality, coping with conflict, marital complaints, and affection in couples with a depressed wife. *Journal of Family Psychology, 16*(1), 26–37.

Cramer, A. O., Waldorp, L. J., van der Maas, H. L., & Borsboom, D. (2010). Comorbidity: A network perspective. *The Behavioral and Brain Sciences, 33*(2–3), 137–150; discussion 150–193.

Culp, L. N., & Beach, S. R. H. (1998). Marriage and depressive system: The role and bases of self-esteem differ by gender. *Psychology of Women Quarterly, 22*(4), 647–663.

Das-Munshi, J., Goldberg, D., Bebbington, P. E., Bhugra, D. K., Brugha, T. S., Dewey, M. E., . . . Prince, M. (2008). Public health significance of mixed anxiety and depression: Beyond current classification. *The British Journal of Psychiatry: The Journal of Mental Science, 192*(3), 171–177.

de Graaf, R., ten Have, M., van Gool, C., & van Dorsselaer, S. (2012). Prevalence of mental disorders and trends from 1996 to 2009. Results from the Netherlands Mental Health Survey and Incidence Study-2. *Social Psychiatry and Psychiatric Epidemiology, 47*(2), 203–213.

de Jonge, P., Rosmalen, J. G., Kema, I. P., Doornbos, B., van Melle, J. P., Pouwer, F., & Kupper, N. (2010). Psychophysiological biomarkers explaining the association between depression and prognosis in coronary artery patients: A critical review of the literature. *Neuroscience and Biobehavioral Reviews, 35*(1), 84–90.

Dooley, D., Fielding, J., & Levi, L. (1996). Health and unemployment. *Annual Review of Public Health, 17*(1), 449–465.

Fang, X., Massetti, G. M., Ouyang, L., Grosse, S. D., & Mercy, J. A. (2010). Attention-deficit / hyperactivity disorder, conduct disorder, and young adult intimate partner violence. *Archives of General Psychiatry, 67*(11), 1179–1186.

Ferrari, A. J., Charlson, F. J., Norman, R. E., Patten, S. B., Freedman, G., Murray, C. J., . . . Whiteford, H. A. (2013). Burden of depressive disorders by country, sex, age, and year: Findings from the Global Burden of Disease Study 2010. *PLoS Medicine, 10*(11), e1001547.

Fichter, M. M., Quadflieg, N., Fischer, U. C., & Kohlboeck, G. (2010). Twenty-five-year course and outcome in anxiety and depression in the Upper Bavarian Longitudinal Community Study. *Acta Psychiatrica Scandinavica, 122*(1), 75–85.

Fineberg, N. A., Hengartner, M. P., Bergbaum, C., Gale, T., Rossler, W., & Angst, J. (2013). Lifetime comorbidity of obsessive-compulsive disorder and sub-threshold obsessive-compulsive symptomatology in the community: Impact, prevalence, socio-demographic and clinical characteristics. *International Journal of Psychiatry in Clinical Practice, 17*(3), 188–196.

First, M. B., Spitzer, R. L., & Williams, J. B. W. (1990). Exclusionary principles and the comorbidity of psychiatric diagnoses: A historical review and implications for the future. In J. D. Maser & C. R. Cloninger (Eds.), *Comorbidity of mood and anxiety disorders* (pp. 83–109). Washington, DC: American Psychiatric Press.

Ford, E., Clark, C., McManus, S., Harris, J., Jenkins, R., Bebbington, P., . . . Stansfeld, S. A. (2010). Common mental disorders, unemployment and welfare benefits in England. *Public Health, 124*(12), 675–681.

Forthofer, M. S., Kessler, R. C., Story, A. L., & Gotlib, I. H. (1996). The effects of psychiatric disorders on the probability and timing of first marriage. *Journal of Health and Social Behavior, 37*(2), 121–132.

Frances, A., Manning, D., Marin, D., Kocsis, J., McKinney, K., Hall, W., & Kline, M. (1992). Relationship of anxiety and depression. *Psychopharmacology, 106 Suppl*(1), S82–86.

Gamma, A., Angst, J., Ajdacic, V., Eich, D., & Rossler, W. (2007). The spectra of neurasthenia and depression: Course, stability and transitions. *European Archives of Psychiatry and Clinical Neuroscience, 257*(2), 120–127.

Gillen, R., Tennen, H., McKee, T. E., Gernert-Dott, P., & Affleck, G. (2001). Depressive symptoms and history of depression predict rehabilitation efficiency in stroke patients. *Archives of Physical Medicine and Rehabilitation, 82*(12), 1645–1649.

Giuffra, L. A., & Risch, N. (1994). Diminished recall and the cohort effect of major depression: A simulation study. *Psychological Medicine, 24*(2), 375–383.

Goldberg, D. P., Krueger, R. F., Andrews, G., & Hobbs, M. J. (2009). Emotional disorders: Cluster 4 of the proposed meta-structure for *DSM-V* and *ICD-11*. *Psychological Medicine, 39*(12), 2043–2059.

Goodman, A., Joyce, R., & Smith, J. P. (2011). The long shadow cast by childhood physical and mental problems on adult life. *Proceedings of the National Academy of Sciences of the United States of America, 108*(15), 6032–6037.

Green, J. G., McLaughlin, K. A., Berglund, P. A., Gruber, M. J., Sampson, N. A., Zaslavsky, A. M., & Kessler, R. C. (2010). Childhood adversities and adult psychiatric disorders in the National Comorbidity Survey Replication I: Associations with first onset of *DSM-IV* disorders. *Archives of General Psychiatry, 67*(2), 113–123.

Greenberg, P. E., Kessler, R. C., Birnbaum, H. G., Leong, S. A., Lowe, S. W., Berglund, P. A., & Corey-Lisle, P. K. (2003). The economic burden of depression in the United States: How did it change between 1990 and 2000? *Journal of Clinical Psychiatry, 64*(12), 1465–1475.

Hardeveld, F., Spijker, J., de Graaf, R., Nolen, W. A., & Beekman, A. T. (2013). Recurrence of major depressive disorder and its predictors in the general population: Results from the Netherlands Mental Health Survey and Incidence Study (NEMESIS). *Psychological Medicine, 43*(1), 39–48.

Insel, T. R. (2008). Assessing the economic costs of serious mental illness. *American Journal of Psychiatry, 165*(6), 663–665.

Jacobi, F., Wittchen, H. U., Holting, C., Hofler, M., Pfister, H., Muller, N., & Lieb, R. (2004). Prevalence, co-morbidity and correlates of mental disorders in the general population: Results from the German Health Interview and Examination Survey (GHS). *Psychological Medicine, 34*(4), 597–611.

Jakubovski, E., & Bloch, M. H. (2014). Prognostic subgroups for citalopram response in the STAR*D trial. *Journal of Clinical Psychiatry, 75*(7), 738–747.

Jones, L. (1991). The health consequences of economic recessions. *Journal of Health & Social Policy, 3*(2), 1–14.

Judd, L. L., Akiskal, H. S., & Paulus, M. P. (1997). The role and clinical significance of subsyndromal depressive symptoms (SSD) in unipolar major depressive disorder. *Journal of Affective Disorders, 45*(1–2), 5–17; discussion 17–18.

Katon, W., Lin, E. H., & Kroenke, K. (2007). The association of depression and anxiety with medical symptom burden in patients with chronic medical illness. *General Hospital Psychiatry, 29*(2), 147–155.

Kawakami, N., Abdulghani, E. A., Alonso, J., Bromet, E. J., Bruffaerts, R., Caldas-de-Almeida, J. M., . . . Kessler, R. C. (2012). Early-life mental disorders and adult household income in the World Mental Health surveys. *Biological Psychiatry, 72*(3), 228–237.

Kendler, K. S., Walters, E. E., & Kessler, R. C. (1997). The prediction of length of major depressive episodes: Results from an epidemiological sample of female twins. *Psychological Medicine, 27*(1), 107–117.

Kessler, R. C. (1995). Epidemiology of psychiatric comorbidity. In M. T. Tsuang & G. E. P. Zahner (Eds.), *Textbook in psychiatric epidemiology* (Vol. 18, pp. 179–197). New York, NY: John Wiley & Sons, Inc.

Kessler, R. C., Akiskal, H. S., Ames, M., Birnbaum, H., Greenberg, P., Hirschfeld, R. M., . . . Wang, P. S. (2006). Prevalence and effects of mood disorders on work performance in a nationally representative sample of US workers. *American Journal of Psychiatry, 163*(9), 1561–1568.

Kessler, R. C., Angermeyer, M., Anthony, J. C., de Graaf, R., Demyttenaere, K., Gasquet, I., . . . Ustün, T. B. (2007). Lifetime prevalence and age-of-onset distributions of mental disorders in the World Health Organization's World Mental Health Survey Initiative. *World Psychiatry: Official Journal of the World Psychiatric Association, 6*(3), 168–176.

Kessler, R. C., Avenevoli, S., & Ries Merikangas, K. (2001). Mood disorders in children and adolescents: An epidemiologic perspective. *Biological Psychiatry, 49*(12), 1002–1014.

Kessler, R. C., Berglund, P., Demler, O., Jin, R., Koretz, D., Merikangas, K. R., . . . Wang, P. S. (2003). The epidemiology of major depressive disorder: Results from the National Comorbidity Survey Replication (NCS-R). *JAMA, 289*(23), 3095–3105.

Kessler, R. C., Berglund, P. A., Foster, C. L., Saunders, W. B., Stang, P. E., & Walters, E. E. (1997). Social consequences of psychiatric disorders, II: Teenage parenthood. *American Journal of Psychiatry, 154*(10), 1405–1411.

Kessler, R. C., & Bromet, E. J. (2013). The epidemiology of depression across cultures. *Annual Review of Public Health, 34*(1), 119–138.

Kessler, R. C., Cox, B. J., Green, J. G., Ormel, J., McLaughlin, K. A., Merikangas, K. R., . . . Zaslavsky, A. M. (2011). The effects of latent variables in the development of comorbidity among common mental disorders. *Depression and Anxiety, 28*(1), 29–39.

Kessler, R. C., Demler, O., Frank, R. G., Olfson, M., Pincus, H. A., Walters, E. E., . . . Zaslavsky, A. M. (2005). Prevalence and treatment of mental disorders, 1990 to 2003. *The New England Journal of Medicine, 352*(24), 2515–2523.

Kessler, R. C., Foster, C. L., Saunders, W. B., & Stang, P. E. (1995). Social consequences of psychiatric disorders, I: Educational attainment. *American Journal of Psychiatry, 152*(7), 1026–1032.

Kessler, R. C., Greenberg, P. E., Mickelson, K. D., Meneades, L. M., & Wang, P. S. (2001). The effects of chronic medical conditions on work loss and work cutback. *Journal of Occupational and Environmental Medicine / American College of Occupational and Environmental Medicine, 43*(3), 218–225.

Kessler, R. C., Heeringa, S., Lakoma, M. D., Petukhova, M., Rupp, A. E., Schoenbaum, M., . . . Zaslavsky, A. M. (2008). Individual and societal effects of mental disorders on earnings in the United States: Results from the National Comorbidity Survey Replication. *American Journal of Psychiatry, 165*(6), 703–711.

Kessler, R. C., Keller, M. B., & Wittchen, H. U. (2001). The epidemiology of generalized anxiety disorder. *Psychiatric Clinics of North America, 24*(1), 19–39.

Kessler, R. C., McLaughlin, K. A., Green, J. G., Gruber, M. J., Sampson, N. A., Zaslavsky, A. M., . . . Williams, D. R. (2010). Childhood adversities and adult psychopathology in the WHO World Mental Health surveys. *The British Journal of Psychiatry: The Journal of Mental Science, 197*(5), 378–385.

Kessler, R. C., Merikangas, K. R., & Wang, P. S. (2008). The prevalence and correlates of workplace depression in the National Comorbidity Survey Replication. *Journal of Occupa-*

tional and Environmental Medicine / American College of Occupational and Environmental Medicine, 50(4), 381–390.

Kessler, R. C., Molnar, B. E., Feurer, I. D., & Appelbaum, M. (2001). Patterns and mental health predictors of domestic violence in the United States: Results from the National Comorbidity Survey. *International Journal of Law and Psychiatry, 24*(4–5), 487–508.

Kessler, R. C., Ormel, J., Petukhova, M., McLaughlin, K. A., Green, J. G., Russo, L. J., . . . Ustün, T. B. (2011). Development of lifetime comorbidity in the World Health Organization World Mental Health surveys. *Archives of General Psychiatry, 68*(1), 90–100.

Kessler, R. C., Petukhova, M., & Zaslavsky, A. M. (2011). The role of latent internalizing and externalizing predispositions in accounting for the development of comorbidity among common mental disorders. *Current Opinion in Psychiatry, 24*(4), 307–312.

Kessler, R. C., Sampson, N. A., Berglund, P., Gruber, M. J., Al-Hamzawi, A., Andrade, L., . . . Wilcox, M. A. (2015). Anxious and non-anxious major depressive disorder in the World Health Organization World Mental Health surveys. *Epidemiology and Psychiatric Sciences, 24*(3), 210–226.

Kessler, R. C., & Walters, E. E. (1998). Epidemiology of *DSM-III-R* major depression and minor depression among adolescents and young adults in the National Comorbidity Survey. *Depression and Anxiety, 7*(1), 3–14.

Kessler, R. C., Walters, E. E., & Forthofer, M. S. (1998). The social consequences of psychiatric disorders, III: Probability of marital stability. *American Journal of Psychiatry, 155*(8), 1092–1096.

Kim, H. K., Laurent, H. K., Capaldi, D. M., & Feingold, A. (2008). Men's aggression toward women: A 10-year panel study. *Journal of Marriage and the Family, 70*(5), 1169–1187.

Klein, D. N., Glenn, C. R., Kosty, D. B., Seeley, J. R., Rohde, P., & Lewinsohn, P. M. (2013). Predictors of first lifetime onset of major depressive disorder in young adulthood. *Journal of Abnormal Psychology, 122*(1), 1–6.

Kraemer, H. C., Kazdin, A. E., Offord, D. R., Kessler, R. C., Jensen, P. S., & Kupfer, D. J. (1997). Coming to terms with the terms of risk. *Archives of General Psychiatry, 54*(4), 337–343.

Kramer, M. D., Krueger, R. F., & Hicks, B. M. (2008). The role of internalizing and external-izing liability factors in accounting for gender differences in the prevalence of common psychopathological syndromes. *Psychological Medicine, 38*(1), 51–61.

Kronmuller, K. T., Backenstrass, M., Victor, D., Postelnicu, I., Schenkenbach, C., Joest, K., . . . Mundt, C. (2011). Quality of marital relationship and depression: Results of a 10-year prospective follow-up study. *Journal of Affective Disorders, 128*(1–2), 64–71.

Krueger, R. F. (1999). The structure of common mental disorders. *Archives of General Psychiatry, 56*(10), 921–926.

Krueger, R. F., & Markon, K. E. (2006a). Reinterpreting comorbidity: A model-based approach to understanding and classifying psychopathology. *Annual Review of Clinical Psychology, 2*(1), 111–133.

Krueger, R. F., & Markon, K. E. (2006b). Understanding psychopathology: Melding behavior genetics, personality, and quantitative psychology to develop an empirically based model. *Current Directions in Psychological Science, 15*(3), 113–117.

Lahey, B. B., Rathouz, P. J., Van Hulle, C., Urbano, R. C., Krueger, R. F., Applegate, B., . . . Waldman, I. D. (2008). Testing structural models of *DSM-IV* symptoms of common forms of child and adolescent psychopathology. *Journal of Abnormal Child Psychology, 36*(2), 187–206.

Lam, T. P., Goldberg, D. P., Dowell, A. C., Fortes, S., Mbatia, J. K., Minhas, F. A., & Klinkman, M. S. (2013). Proposed new diagnoses of anxious depression and bodily stress syndrome in ICD-11-PHC: An international focus group study. *Family Practice, 30*(1), 76–87.

Lamers, F., van Oppen, P., Comijs, H. C., Smit, J. H., Spinhoven, P., van Balkom, A. J., . . . Penninx, B. W. (2011). Comorbidity patterns of anxiety and depressive disorders in a large cohort study: The Netherlands Study of Depression and Anxiety (NESDA). *Journal of Clinical Psychiatry, 72*(3), 341–348.

Leadbeater, B., Thompson, K., & Gruppuso, V. (2012). Co-occurring trajectories of symptoms of anxiety, depression, and oppositional defiance from adolescence to young adulthood. *Journal of Clinical Child and Adolescent Psychology, American Psychological Association, Division 53, 41*(6), 719–730.

Lee, S., Tsang, A., Breslau, J., Aguilar-Gaxiola, S., Angermeyer, M., Borges, G., . . . Kessler, R. C. (2009). Mental disorders and termination of education in high-income and low- and middle-income countries: Epidemiological study. *The British Journal of Psychiatry: The Journal of Mental Science, 194*(5), 411–417.

Lehrer, J. A., Buka, S., Gortmaker, S., & Shrier, L. A. (2006). Depressive symptomatology as a predictor of exposure to intimate partner violence among US female adolescents and young adults. *Archives of Pediatrics & Adolescent Medicine, 160*(3), 270–276.

Lerner, D., Allaire, S. H., & Reisine, S. T. (2005). Work disability resulting from chronic health conditions. *Journal of Occupational and Environmental Medicine / American College of Occupational and Environmental Medicine, 47*(3), 253–264.

Levinson, D., Lakoma, M. D., Petukhova, M., Schoenbaum, M., Zaslavsky, A. M., Angermeyer, M., . . . Kessler, R. C. (2010). Associations of serious mental illness with earnings: Results from the WHO World Mental Health surveys. *The British Journal of Psychiatry: The Journal of Mental Science, 197*(2), 114–121.

Lewinsohn, P. M., Rohde, P., Seeley, J. R., & Fischer, S. A. (1991). Age and depression: Unique and shared effects. *Psychology and Aging, 6*(2), 247–260.

Li, Y., Aggen, S., Shi, S., Gao, J., Tao, M., Zhang, K., . . . Kendler, K. S. (2014). Subtypes of major depression: Latent class analysis in depressed Han Chinese women. *Psychological Medicine, 44*(15), 3275–3288.

Lorber, M. F., & O'Leary, K. D. (2004). Predictors of the persistence of male aggression in early marriage. *Journal of Family Violence, 19*(6), 329–338.

Lovejoy, M. C., Graczyk, P. A., O'Hare, E., & Neuman, G. (2000). Maternal depression and parenting behavior: A meta-analytic review. *Clinical Psychology Review, 20*(5), 561–592.

Mamun, A. A., Clavarino, A. M., Najman, J. M., Williams, G. M., O'Callaghan, M. J., & Bor, W. (2009). Maternal depression and the quality of marital relationship: A 14-year prospective study. *Journal of Women's Health, 18*(12), 2023–2031.

Marcotte, D. E., & Wilcox-Gok, V. (2001). Estimating the employment and earnings costs of mental illness: Recent developments in the United States. *Social Science & Medicine, 53*(1), 21–27.

McLaughlin, T. P., Khandker, R. K., Kruzikas, D. T., & Tummala, R. (2006). Overlap of anxiety and depression in a managed care population: Prevalence and association with resource utilization. *Journal of Clinical Psychiatry, 67*(8), 1187–1193.

McLeod, J. D., & Kaiser, K. (2004). Childhood emotional and behavioral problems and educational attainment. *American Sociological Review, 69*(5), 636–658.

McLeod, J. D., Kessler, R. C., & Landis, K. R. (1992). Speed of recovery from major depressive episodes in a community sample of married men and women. *Journal of Abnormal Psychology, 101*(2), 277–286.

McMillan, K. A., Enns, M. W., Asmundson, G. J., & Sareen, J. (2010). The association between income and distress, mental disorders, and suicidal ideation and attempts: Findings from the Collaborative Psychiatric Epidemiology Surveys. *The Journal of Clinical Psychiatry, 71*(9), 1168–1175.

Meeks, T. W., Vahia, I. V., Lavretsky, H., Kulkarni, G., & Jeste, D. V. (2011). A tune in "a minor" can "b major": A review of epidemiology, illness course, and public health implications of subthreshold depression in older adults. *Journal of Affective Disorders, 129*(1–3), 126–142.

Merikangas, K. R., Ames, M., Cui, L., Stang, P. E., Ustün, T. B., Von Korff, M., & Kessler, R. C. (2007). The impact of comorbidity of mental and physical conditions on role disability in the US adult household population. *Archives of General Psychiatry, 64*(10), 1180–1188.

Merikangas, K. R., & Angst, J. (1995). Comorbidity and social phobia: Evidence from clinical, epidemiologic, and genetic studies. *European Archives of Psychiatry and Clinical Neuroscience, 244*(6), 297–303.

Miller, E., Breslau, J., Petukhova, M., Fayyad, J., Green, J. G., Kola, L., . . . Kessler, R. C. (2011). Premarital mental disorders and physical violence in marriage: Cross-national study of married couples. *The British Journal of Psychiatry: The Journal of Mental Science, 199*(4), 330–337.

Mineka, S., & Vrshek-Shallhorn, S. (2014). Comorbidity of unipolar depressive and anxiety disorders. In I. H. Gotlib & C. L. Hammen (Eds.), *Handbook of depression* (pp. 94–102). New York, NY: Guilford Press.

Moussavi, S., Chatterji, S., Verdes, E., Tandon, A., Patel, V., & Ustün, B. (2007). Depression, chronic diseases, and decrements in health: Results from the World Health Surveys. *Lancet, 370*(9590), 851–858.

Mrazek, P. J., & Haggerty, R. J. (1994). *Reducing risks for mental disorders: Frontiers for preventive intervention research.* Washington, DC: National Academy Press.

Munce, S. E., Stansfeld, S. A., Blackmore, E. R., & Stewart, D. E. (2007). The role of depression and chronic pain conditions in absenteeism: Results from a national epidemiologic survey. *Journal of Occupational and Environmental Medicine / American College of Occupational and Environmental Medicine, 49*(11), 1206–1211.

Muntaner, C., Eaton, W. W., Miech, R., & O'Campo, P. (2004). Socioeconomic position and major mental disorders. *Epidemiologic Reviews, 26*(1), 53–62.

Murphy, J. M., Olivier, D. C., Sobol, A. M., Monson, R. R., & Leighton, A. H. (1986). Diagnosis and outcome: Depression and anxiety in a general population. *Psychological Medicine, 16*(1), 117–126.

Murray, C. J. L., & Lopez, A. D. (1996). *The global burden of disease: A comprehensive assessment of mortality and disability from diseases, injuries, and risk factors in 1990 and projected to 2020.* Boston, MA: Harvard School of Public Health, World Health Organization, and World Bank.

National Institute of Mental Health. *Research Domain Criteria (RDoC).* Retrieved from http://www.nimh.nih.gov/research-priorities/rdoc/index.shtml

O'Leary, K. D., Tintle, N., Bromet, E. J., & Gluzman, S. F. (2008). Descriptive epidemiology of intimate partner aggression in Ukraine. *Social Psychiatry and Psychiatric Epidemiology, 43*(8), 619–626.

Ormel, J., Petukhova, M., Chatterji, S., Aguilar-Gaxiola, S., Alonso, J., Angermeyer, M. C., . . . Kessler, R. C. (2008). Disability and treatment of specific mental and physical disorders across the world. *The British Journal of Psychiatry: The Journal of Mental Science, 192*(5), 368–375.

Ormel, J., VonKorff, M., Ustün, T. B., Pini, S., Korten, A., & Oldehinkel, T. (1994). Common mental disorders and disability across cultures. Results from the WHO Collaborative Study on Psychological Problems in General Health Care. *JAMA, 272*(22), 1741–1748.

Pearson, K. A., Watkins, E. R., Kuyken, W., & Mullan, E. G. (2010). The psychosocial context of depressive rumination: Ruminative brooding predicts diminished relationship satisfaction in individuals with a history of past major depression. *The British Journal of Clinical Psychology/The British Psychological Society, 49*(Pt 2), 275–280.

Pettit, J. W., Hartley, C., Lewinsohn, P. M., Seeley, J. R., & Klein, D. N. (2013). Is liability to recurrent major depressive disorder present before first episode onset in adolescence or acquired after the initial episode? *Journal of Abnormal Psychology, 122*(2), 353–358.

Porche, M. V., Fortuna, L. R., Lin, J., & Alegria, M. (2011). Childhood trauma and psychiatric disorders as correlates of school dropout in a national sample of young adults. *Child Development, 82*(3), 982–998.

Proulx, C. M., Helms, H. M., & Buehler, C. (2007). Marital quality and personal well-being: A meta-analysis. *Journal of Marriage and Family, 69*(3), 576–593.

Renner, L. M. (2009). Intimate partner violence victimization and parenting stress: Assessing the mediating role of depressive symptoms. *Violence Against Women, 15*(11), 1380–1401.

Riggs, D. S., Caulfield, M. B., & Street, A. E. (2000). Risk for domestic violence: Factors associated with perpetration and victimization. *Journal of Clinical Psychology, 56*(10), 1289–1316.

Rodriguez, M. R., Nuevo, R., Chatterji, S., & Ayuso-Mateos, J. L. (2012). Definitions and factors associated with subthreshold depressive conditions: A systematic review. *BMC Psychiatry, 12*(1), 181.

Rost, K., Marshall, D., Shearer, B., & Dietrich, A. J. (2011). Depression care management: Can employers purchase improved outcomes? *Depression Research and Treatment, 2011*, 942519.

Rost, K., Smith, J. L., & Dickinson, M. (2004). The effect of improving primary care depression management on employee absenteeism and productivity: A randomized trial. *Medical Care, 42*(12), 1202–1210.

Roy-Byrne, P. P., Stang, P., Wittchen, H. U., Ustün, B., Walters, E. E., & Kessler, R. C. (2000). Lifetime panic-depression comorbidity in the National Comorbidity Survey: Association with symptoms, impairment, course and help-seeking. *The British Journal of Psychiatry: The Journal of Mental Science, 176*(3), 229–235.

Saveanu, R., Etkin, A., Duchemin, A. M., Goldstein-Piekarski, A., Gyurak, A., Debattista, C., . . . Williams, L. M. (2015). The International Study to Predict Optimized Treatment in Depression (iSPOT-D): Outcomes from the acute phase of antidepressant treatment. *Journal of Psychiatric Research, 61*, 1–12.

Slade, T., & Watson, D. (2006). The structure of common *DSM-IV* and ICD-10 mental disorders in the Australian general population. *Psychological Medicine, 36*(11), 1593–1600.

Smith, J. P., & Smith, G. C. (2010). Long-term economic costs of psychological problems during childhood. *Social Science & Medicine, 71*(1), 110–115.

Smoller, J. W., Ripke S., Lee P. H., Neale B., Nurnberger J. I., Santangelo S., Sullivan P. F., . . . Kendler, K. S. (2013). Identification of risk loci with shared effects on five major psychiatric disorders: A genome-wide analysis. *Lancet, 381*(9875), 1371–1379.

Stewart, W. F., Ricci, J. A., Chee, E., Hahn, S. R., & Morganstein, D. (2003a). Cost of lost productive work time among US workers with depression. *JAMA, 289*(23), 3135–3144.

Stewart, W. F., Ricci, J. A., Chee, E., & Morganstein, D. (2003b). Lost productive work time costs from health conditions in the United States: Results from the American Productivity Audit. *Journal of Occupational and Environmental Medicine / American College of Occupational and Environmental Medicine, 45*(12), 1234–1246.

Stith, S. M., Smith, D. B., Penn, C. E., Ward, D. B., & Tritt, D. (2004). Intimate partner physical abuse perpetration and victimization risk factors: A meta-analytic review. *Aggression and Violent Behavior, 10*(1), 65–98.

Tronick, E., & Reck, C. (2009). Infants of depressed mothers. *Harvard Review of Psychiatry, 17*(2), 147–156.

Ustün, T. B., Ayuso-Mateos, J. L., Chatterji, S., Mathers, C., & Murray, C. J. (2004). Global burden of depressive disorders in the year 2000. *The British Journal of Psychiatry: The Journal of Mental Science, 184*(5), 386–392.

van Loo, H. M., de Jonge, P., Romeijn, J. W., Kessler, R. C., & Schoevers, R. A. (2012). Data-driven subtypes of major depressive disorder: A systematic review. *BMC Medicine, 10*(1), 156.

Vaughn, M. G., Wexler, J., Beaver, K. M., Perron, B. E., Roberts, G., & Fu, Q. (2011). Psychiatric correlates of behavioral indicators of school disengagement in the United States. *Psychiatric Quarterly, 82*(3), 191–206.

Verbrugge, L. M., & Patrick, D. L. (1995). Seven chronic conditions: Their impact on US adults' activity levels and use of medical services. *American Journal of Public Health, 85*(2), 173–182.

Vollebergh, W. A., Iedema, J., Bijl, R. V., de Graaf, R., Smit, F., & Ormel, J. (2001). The structure and stability of common mental disorders: The NEMESIS study. *Archives of General Psychiatry, 58*(6), 597–603.

Vos, T., Flaxman, A. D., Naghavi, M., Lozano, R., Michaud, C., Ezzati, M., . . . Memish, Z. A. (2012). Years lived with disability (YLDs) for 1160 sequelae of 289 diseases and injuries 1990–2010: A systematic analysis for the Global Burden of Disease Study 2010. *Lancet, 380*(9859), 2163–2196.

Wang, P. S., Aguilar-Gaxiola, S., Alonso, J., Angermeyer, M. C., Borges, G., Bromet, E. J., . . . Wells, J. E. (2007). Use of mental health services for anxiety, mood, and substance disorders in 17 countries in the WHO World Mental Health surveys. *Lancet, 370*(9590), 841–850.

Wang, P. S., Beck, A., Berglund, P., Leutzinger, J. A., Pronk, N., Richling, D., . . . Kessler, R. C. (2003). Chronic medical conditions and work performance in the Health and Work Performance Questionnaire calibration surveys. *Journal of Occupational and Environmental Medicine / American College of Occupational and Environmental Medicine, 45*(12), 1303–1311.

Wang, P. S., Patrick, A., Avorn, J., Azocar, F., Ludman, E., McCulloch, J., . . . Kessler, R. (2006). The costs and benefits of enhanced depression care to employers. *Archives of General Psychiatry, 63*(12), 1345–1353.

Wang, P. S., Simon, G. E., Avorn, J., Azocar, F., Ludman, E. J., McCulloch, J., . . . Kessler, R. C. (2007). Telephone screening, outreach, and care management for depressed workers and impact on clinical and work productivity outcomes: A randomized controlled trial. *JAMA, 298*(12), 1401–1411.

Wang, P. S., Simon, G., & Kessler, R. C. (2003). The economic burden of depression and the cost-effectiveness of treatment. *International Journal of Methods in Psychiatric Research, 12*(1), 22–33.

Wardenaar, K. J., Giltay, E. J., van Veen, T., Zitman, F. G., & Penninx, B. W. (2012). Symptom dimensions as predictors of the two-year course of depressive and anxiety disorders. *Journal of Affective Disorders, 136*(3), 1198–1203.

Watson, D. (2005). Rethinking the mood and anxiety disorders: A quantitative hierarchical model for *DSM-V. Journal of Abnormal Psychology, 114*(4), 522–536.

Weissman, M. M., Livingston, B. M., Leaf, P. J., Florio, L. P., & Holzer, C. I. (1991). Affective disorders. In L. N. Robins & D. A. Regier (Eds.), *Psychiatric disorders in America: The Epidemiologic Catchment Area Study* (pp. 53–80). New York, NY: The Free Press.

Whisman, M. A. (1999). Marital dissatisfaction and psychiatric disorders: Results from the National Comorbidity Survey. *Journal of Abnormal Psychology, 108*(4), 701–706.

Whisman, M. A. (2001). The association between depression and marital dissatisfaction. In S. R. H. Beach (Ed.), *Marital and family processes in depression: A scientific foundation for clinical practice* (pp. 3–24). Washington, DC: American Psychological Association.

Whisman, M. A., Tolejko, N., & Chatav, Y. (2007). Social consequences of personality disorders: Probability and timing of marriage and probability of marital disruption. *Journal of Personality Disorders, 21*(6), 690–695.

Whisman, M. A., & Uebelacker, L. A. (2009). Prospective associations between marital discord and depressive symptoms in middle-aged and older adults. *Psychology and Aging, 24*(1), 184–189.

Wilson, S., & Durbin, C. E. (2010). Effects of paternal depression on fathers' parenting behaviors: A meta-analytic review. *Clinical Psychology Review, 30*(2), 167–180.

Wittchen, H. U., Beesdo, K., & Gloster, A. T. (2009). A new meta-structure of mental disorders: A helpful step into the future or a harmful step back to the past? *Psychological Medicine, 39*(12), 2083–2089.

Wittchen, H. U., Beesdo-Baum, K., Gloster, A. T., Hofler, M., Klotsche, J., Lieb, R., . . . Kessler, R. C. (2009). The structure of mental disorders re-examined: Is it developmentally stable and robust against additions? *International Journal of Methods in Psychiatric Research, 18*(4), 189–203.

Woodward, L. J., & Fergusson, D. M. (2001). Life course outcomes of young people with anxiety disorders in adolescence. *Journal of the American Academy of Child and Adolescent Psychiatry, 40*(9), 1086–1093.

Wu, Z., & Fang, Y. (2014). Comorbidity of depressive and anxiety disorders: Challenges in diagnosis and assessment. *Shanghai Archives of Psychiatry, 26*(4), 227–231.

Yaroslavsky, I., Pettit, J. W., Lewinsohn, P. M., Seeley, J. R., & Roberts, R. E. (2013). Heterogeneous trajectories of depressive symptoms: Adolescent predictors and adult outcomes. *Journal of Affective Disorders, 148*(2–3), 391–399.

Ziegelstein, R. C., Fauerbach, J. A., Stevens, S. S., Romanelli, J., Richter, D. P., & Bush, D. E. (2000). Patients with depression are less likely to follow recommendations to reduce cardiac risk during recovery from a myocardial infarction. *Archives of Internal Medicine, 160*(12), 1818–1823.

CHAPTER 4

The Burden of Comorbidity
Depressive and Physical Disorders

Sergio Aguilar-Gaxiola, MD, PhD
Gustavo Loera, EdD
Daniel Vigo, MD
Efrain Talamantes, MD, MS
Kate Scott, PhD

Depression is a highly prevalent disease that has been forecasted to reach number one in the ranking of global burden of disease (GBD) in terms of years lived with disability (YLDs) by 2030 (Lépine & Briley, 2011). Indeed, it has advanced from third to the second leading cause of YLDs in the last GBD revision (Institute for Health Metrics and Evaluation, 2013; Vos et al., 2015), and its impact on people's lives and on communities' well-being is gaining increased attention.

Depression diminishes people's interest in and enjoyment of activities that were once considered pleasurable, and increases a sense of worthlessness and suicidal thinking; it leads to worse physical health outcomes, social isolation, and decreased productivity. Depressive disorders currently account for 61.6 million YLDs, which represent 8% of global disability due to all causes (Vos et al., 2015). Recent epidemiological surveys conducted in general populations worldwide have found the lifetime prevalence of depression to be between 10% and 15% (Lépine & Briley, 2011). Clearly, depression is a significant contributor to the global burden of disease that diminishes role functioning and quality of life in populations worldwide (Bromet et al., 2011; Kessler et al., 2003; Kessler & Wang, 2009; Spijker et al., 2004; Ustün, Ayuso-Mateos, Chatterji, Mathers, & Murray, 2004).

The enormous public health impact of depression is evidenced by the World Health Organization's (WHO) projection that it will have affected 350 million people over the course of the first three decades of the twenty-first century—making it the leading cause of disease burden among developed and developing countries (WHO, 2008; 2012). Mathers and Loncar (2006) estimated that by 2030, depression will be the second leading cause of disability-adjusted life years (DALYs) worldwide and first among high-income countries. By 2030, depression is expected to be the leading chronic and recurrent illness with highly detrimental effects on mental and physical functioning, further underscoring the urgency of establishing depression as a core domain of the public health framework (Cohen & Galea, 2011).

Comorbidity

Comorbidity refers to the co-occurrence of two or more disorders in the same person, either at the same time or over the life span, regardless of the chronological order in which they occurred (Valderas, Starfield, Sibbald, Salisbury, & Roland, 2009). Numerous epidemiological studies have shown that people who suffer from physical and comorbid mental disorders more likely were exposed to multiple risk factors early in life and less likely to have received adequate treatment and resources (e.g., Kessler et al., 2003; Kohn, Saxena, Levav, & Saraceno, 2004). People at greater risk of comorbidity disproportionally live in communities that have historically been un- or underserved and inappropriately served due to limited or lack of access to services and resources. Consequently, the twenty-first-century public health practice will require a more systemic approach to understanding and addressing depression comorbidity.

The epidemiologic transition has led to a landscape of multimorbidity, in which 22 of the leading 25 causes of disability are noncommunicable diseases (NCDs). The percentage of working-age adults living with five or more chronic health conditions ranges from 32% of working-age adults in high-income countries to 62% in Sub-Saharan Africa, highlighting the challenge of building and adapting health systems able to manage multimorbidity across the life span (Atun, 2015; Vos et al., 2015). Comorbidity should not be seen as an isolated clinical condition but as a social and economic phenomenon that contributes to burden of disease worldwide. Systemic transformations in public health practices—improving access, availability, appropriateness, affordability, and advocacy—must be a public health priority to reduce disease burden and disability.

A number of key points are raised in the research literature relevant to an examination of depression from a population-based approach and its integration into twenty-first-century public health practice: (1) without adequate treatment, depression will most likely become more chronic, recurrent, and associated with increasing disability over time (Kohn et al., 2004); (2) depression is commonly associated with chronic physical disorders (Kang et al., 2015; Kessler & Bromet, 2013; Scott et al., 2007a); and (3) there is an urgency to take action in curbing depression by addressing it as a public health priority in order to reduce burden and disability, and improving the overall health of populations (Cohen & Galea, 2011).

Use of Epidemiology in Public Health

Epidemiological studies are concerned with the extent and types of illnesses in populations and with the risk factors that influence their distribution (Merikangas, Nakamura, & Kessler, 2009). The aim of epidemiological studies is to identify the etiology of a disease in order to prevent or intervene on the progression of the disorder (Kessler & Bromet, 2013). As research advocates of this approach, we argue that mental health is complex and multifaceted, requiring a comprehensive understanding of the etiology of mental disorders (i.e., depression) and their burden on individuals and populations. That is, understanding and addressing depression and its interaction with physical conditions from a multidimensional, systemic, and population-based approach is critical to the prospect of changing its course and severity through adequate prevention, intervention, and treatment.

Most researchers agree that the causes of mental disorders are multidirectional across psychobiological processes (e.g., Kendler, 2005). In Kendler's efforts to apply the philosophy of science to psychiatry, he advocates that psychiatry needs to be more diverse and creative with the goal of piecemeal integration to explain complex pathways to illness incrementally. Put another way, Kendler contends that the complex etiological pathways that lead to mental disorders cannot be understood through simple linear causations or sophisticated explanations that rarely translate into meaningful practices. Other researchers have also advocated for the broadening of psychiatric epidemiology through innovative discoveries that are directly relevant to genetic and biological research (Schwartz & Susser, 2010; Susser & Smith, 2011). Again, this further illustrates the utility of epidemiological research not only in understanding the underpinnings of disease but also the treatment gaps and population-based practices needed to improve the overall health of populations.

Epidemiological Perspectives on Comorbid Depression and Physical Conditions
The WHO World Mental Health Survey Initiative

The World Mental Health (WMH) surveys provide more than two decades of cross-national data about the prevalence and correlates of mental and physical disorders (e.g., Costello, He, Sampson, Kessler, & Merikangas, 2014; Demyttenaere et al., 2007; Gureje et al., 2008; He et al., 2008; Nock, Hwang, Sampson, & Kessler, 2010; Scott et al., 2007a, 2007b, 2008a; Von Korff, Scott, & Gureje, 2009). To date, the WMH Survey data is the most comprehensive and cited populations survey approach to epidemiological research and diagnosis in the area of mental disorders, and has provided foundation population data on mental-physical comorbidity. In all WMH Survey studies, depression and other mental disorders were defined according to the diagnostic criteria of the *Diagnostic and Statistical Manual of Mental Disorders, Fourth Edition* (*DSM-IV*; American Psychiatric Association, 1994), using the Composite International Diagnostic Interview (CIDI; Kessler & Üstün, 2004) when collecting data. The CIDI was designed for use by trained lay nonclinical interviewers to gather self-report data from community-dwelling individuals with and without a history of a mental disorder.

The WMH Surveys provide data from developed and developing countries about common mental disorders and their association with physical health conditions, although the data collected on physical conditions is much less comprehensive and detailed than the data collected on mental disorders. For these associations, the WMH Surveys estimated odd ratios (ORs) to determine the strength of a relationship between mental disorders including depression and physical conditions—in other words, the odds of developing a mental disorder (e.g., depression) among people with a specific chronic physical condition compared to those without that physical condition (or conversely, the odds of developing a physical condition among people with depression compared to those without a depressive disorder).

Some 20 years ago, the concept of GBD was brought to the forefront by a landmark study (Murray & Lopez, 1996) recognizing depression as a major contributor to human suffering and disability across the globe. Currently, depression is among the most prevalent of all mental disorders and the single most burdensome illness in the world in terms of human suffering and economic hardship (Gotlib & Joormann, 2010). Furthermore, a strong body of evidence from the WMH Surveys has highlighted depression as a common, disabling, and highly prevalent disorder among patients with multiple physical disorders (e.g., Kessler et al., 2010; Kessler, Merikangas, & Wang, 2008; Kovess-Masfety et al., 2013; Scott et al., 2007b; Scott et al., 2013a; Stein et al., 2010a; Wardenaar et al., 2014). For example, a one-year WMH Survey study of 9,090 adults in the United States found the prevalence of major depression to be common, widely distributed, and associated with symptom severity and role impairment (Kessler et al., 2003). Specifically, these authors found the prevalence for one year to be 6.6% (confidence interval [CI], 5.9–7.3) (13.1–14.2 million US adults) and 16.2% (CI, 15.1–17.3) (32.6–35.1 million US adults) for lifetime. Naylor and colleagues (2012) found that people with physical health conditions are more likely to experience depression and other mental disorders.

WMH Surveys researchers contend that early life experiences of stress and adverse social conditions may also influence comorbid outcomes. Additional results from the WMH Surveys documented in the 2009 *Global Perspectives on Mental-Physical Comorbidity in the WHO World Mental Health Surveys* found that the prevalence of mood disorders, such as major depression, was higher among persons with chronic physical conditions in both developed and developing countries (see Figure 4.1; Von Korff et al., 2009).

It is also important to note that depression worsens the prognosis for people with comorbid physical health problems, such as heart disease (Frasure-Smith & Lespérance, 2008), and increases the risks for other physical or medical disorders (Evans et al., 2005). This is consistent with the findings from Scott and colleagues (2008b) that older persons with mental disorders tend to show chronic physical/pain comorbidity. Epidemiologic researchers (e.g., Huffman, Celano, Beach, Motiwala, & Januzzi, 2013; Katon, 2011) have found comorbid depression to be associated with increased chronic

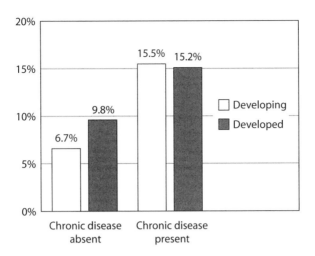

FIGURE 4.1 The prevalence of depressive disorders comorbid with chronic diseases in developed and developing countries

Source: M. Von Korff, K. M. Scott, & O. Gureje (Eds.). (2009). *Global perspectives on mental-physical comorbidity in the WHO World Mental Health Surveys.* Cambridge: Cambridge University Press.

physical health symptom burden, functional impairment, medical costs, and increased risk of mortality in patients with a chronic health condition (e.g., heart disease).

Case History

The following case history illustrates a common presentation. A 34-year-old married, working mother of six children (four sons aged 15, 11, 10, and 3, and 3-month-old twin daughters) lives in a two-bedroom apartment in a low-income community. She works at home as a seamstress to help support her family. For 15–20 hours per day, she sews *and* completes other activities such as caring for her newborn daughters and keeping up with housework. Consequently, she is very sleep deprived. One evening, starting with a persistent headache and high fever, she suffers a heart attack and is in a coma for eight days and in the hospital for two months. During the time she was in the hospital, her husband had to place their twin daughters with two different relatives during the day so he could continue working. Additionally, the 15-year-old son dropped out of school to help care for his three younger siblings. Upon awakening from her coma, the doctor tells her that due to her heart attack, she should no longer work as a seamstress, work that she always loved doing, in order to reduce her stress. Having to manage her medical condition and no longer being able to work, she becomes increasingly worried and preoccupied with how her family will be able to survive financially. The worries evolve into increasing depression, feeling incompetent and useless to her family, and eating and sleeping poorly. Her husband, concerned about the stress in her life and the fear of her having another heart attack and dying, sold her sewing machine, causing her to become even more depressed. Now, at 48 years of age, a physical examination reveals that she has mild arthritis. Living with chronic pain has begun to contribute to her depression, and as a result of her depression, she is not eating properly. She is also mostly sedentary due to her arthritis and has gained a lot of weight. Two years later, during another visit to her doctor, she is diagnosed with hypertension, worsening her depression.

This case history suggests that mental and physical disorders are associated via bi-directional links (Evans et al., 2005). In this particular case, a middle-age person was exposed to stressful conditions that interacted with lifestyle, genetic, and biological factors, resulting in a chronic physical condition. Heart disease increased her risk of depression, and her depression increased her risk of developing other chronic physical conditions. In addition, depression in earlier life may have contributed to the psychobiological pathways leading to heart disease.

Heart Disease and Depression

Many studies have suggested that heart disease and depression can each act as an independent predictor of comorbidity (e.g., Goldston & Baillie, 2008; Thomas, Kalaria, & O'Brien, 2004), so that heart disease and depression can each act as an independent predictor of comorbidity.

A recent WMH Survey study of 52,095 adults from 19 countries found that depression was associated with the subsequent diagnosis of heart disease and that this association was stronger for those whose heart disease diagnosis occurred earlier rather than later in life (Scott et al., 2013a). Multiple studies have shown that depression and other mental disorders are most prevalent early in life, and treatable when detected early, so early detection and treatment of depression could be very helpful in preventing later comorbidity with chronic health conditions such as heart disease.

Returning to the prior case history, the seamstress mother was diagnosed with heart disease at the age of 34, and the burden of the disease diminished her ability to work and help support her family. We know that those who develop depression following medical diagnoses such as heart disease have usually had prior episodes of depression, so a prior history of depression may have been instrumental in accelerating the heart disease in this case. Furthermore, the depressive episode that followed her heart attack could have become a risk factor for her arthritis later in life.

Arthritis and Depression

Another prevalence study of depression and other DSM-IV and CIDI mental disorders and subsequent onset of arthritis among 52,095 adults from 19 WMH studies conducted by the WMH Survey Initiative (Aguilar-Gaxiola et al., 2015) found depression to be associated with the onset of arthritis. The odds ratio for the association of depression with onset of arthritis was (OR = 1.7), and the overall odds ratios for other mental disorders (e.g., anxiety, impulse-control, and substance) ranged from 1.5 to 2.8, indicating that individuals with these disorders had a 50% to 180% greater likelihood of developing arthritis than those without these mental disorders. Aguilar-Gaxiola and colleagues (2015) also found the association between depression and arthritis to be stronger among women with regard to burden of disease and diminished abilities to participate in life activities. Additionally, 17 WMH Survey studies that examined the prevalence of specific mental disorders among persons with arthritis (He et al., 2008) found arthritis to be significantly associated with depression.

Our current knowledge, although incomplete, strongly suggests that the link between depression and arthritis is bidirectional. Just as with depression and heart disease, a causal relationship between depression and arthritis is still inconclusive. Returning to our case history, based on the current literature, it is difficult to conclude that the seamstress mother's depression was causally linked to her mild arthritis. Kendler (2005) suggested that we can find, at best, small explanations from a variety of explanatory perspectives with careful examination of multiple risk factors that can help us better understand the etiological processes that led to these disorders.

Hypertension and Depression

WMH Survey researchers examining the association between mental disorders and subsequent hypertension among 52,095 adults from 19 countries found depression and other mental disorders to be significantly associated with the subsequent diagnosis of hypertension (Stein et al., 2014). Furthermore, adults with late onset depression (OR = 1.3, 95% CI 1.2–1.4) had a stronger association with hypertension than did early onset depression. Stein and colleagues (2014) suggested that the effects of depression on subsequent hypertension may be too subtle compared to the impact of aging. Early life adversities may also explain the association between depression and hypertension (Stein et al., 2010b). Returning to our case profile, the woman's history of heart disease combined with arthritis and bouts of depression may be contributing to her hypertension, along with aging. Becoming aware of her functional impairments appears to have triggered a worsening of her depression.

In summary, depression and other mental disorders often have been viewed as the consequence of life stressors or stressful life experiences (Scott et al., 2013b). Another path is that depression and other mental disorders are experienced as stressors that can further exacerbate another mental disorder or trigger a physical disorder. McEwen (2003) referred to this overexposure to stress that eventually leads to chronic disorders as "allostatic load." Allostatic load can be viewed as the wear and tear due to repeated exposure to stress. Again, this helps to shed some light on our case history in that intensive stress exposure may have contributed to the woman's heart condition and triggered a chronic depression that influenced other aspects of her life and led to other chronic physical disorders.

The Burden of Comorbid Depression and Physical Conditions

In 2013, the WMH Surveys Initiative published a volume titled *The Burdens of Mental Disorders: Global Perspectives from the WHO World Mental Health Surveys* (Alonso, Chatterji, & He, 2013), compiling a set of analyses using WMH Survey data from more than 150,000 respondents across 28 countries worldwide. Results from this volume found that lifetime prevalence estimates of *DSM-IV* mental disorders range from 18.1% to 36.1%, with depression emerging as the most prevalent and disabling illness worldwide (Alonso, 2012). Depression and heart disease continue to be two of the leading causes of disability and disease burden worldwide (Perez-Prada, 2011). They have continued to increase both from 1990 to 2005 and from 2005 to 2013 (Murray et al., 2015), and are projected to further increase in women by 2020 (Meyer, 2000; Reddy, 2010; Ustün et al., 2004).

Overall findings from Alonso and colleagues (2013) recognized depression as the most impacting condition on physical health, further emphasizing the burden associated with depression and physical condition comorbidity. Depression's impact on public health was perceived to be most harmful in social, personal, and productive role functioning.

The presence of depression intersecting with specific physical disorders has a particularly significant impact on families with dire consequences to their overall quality of life, including social, educational, marital, and occupational functioning (Kessler, Walters, & Forthofer, 1998; Olfson et al., 1997; Scott et al., 2013b). With one in four families having at least one member suffering from a mental disorder (WHO, 2003), family members become the primary caregivers and shoulder the vast majority of long-term care responsibilities of a loved one with a mental disorder (Carter, 2008; Keitner et al., 1995). The burdens associated with serious mental and physical health conditions are significant, making family members more vulnerable to additional stressors. Viana and colleagues (2013) found that among the WMH Survey respondents with an ill relative, 23%–27% reported experiencing psychological distress, 22%–31% reported burden of time caring for a relative, and 11%–19% reported financial burden.

The consequence of this burden for family members leads to the loss of workdays and productivity, the inability to participate in community activities or contribute to the economy and feel like a productive member of society, and, ultimately, poor quality of life. This is true for the spouse or parent caring for the ill relative. As illustrated in our case history, the patient's chronic physical condition became a burden to the spouse and older son in regard to financial burden and time devoted in caring for spouse and siblings, which may have worsened with her ongoing depression. It may also have had a negative impact on the proper care of her twins, placing them at higher risk of suffering from major depression themselves later in life. In addition to these devastating consequences of depression at the personal and family level, the micro- and macro-economic impact is also staggering; the disease burden is accompanied by economic burden, with mental illness a major source of monetary and productivity losses through direct and indirect costs. The direct costs are not only those of treating depression but also of treating the more severe outcomes of comorbidities, such as cardiovascular disease and diabetes. Depression negatively impacts management of other diseases and yields worse outcomes when co-occurring with them. The indirect costs are mainly the consequence of absenteeism and presenteeism (decreased productivity while at work) (Goetzel et al., 2004). US data puts the additional yearly direct costs to commercial insurers and Medicare of inadequately treated mental illness in the context of physical comorbidity at $132.6 to $351 billion (Melek, Norris, & Paulus, 2014). Additionally, the cost of mental illness has been found to have significant impact at the macroeconomic level, diminishing economic output and inhibiting economic growth, mostly from depressive disorders (Bloom et al., 2011).

Risk Factors for Depression in Persons with Physical Conditions

Identifying the risk factors that contribute to a population becoming more at risk for developing mental-physical comorbidity is essential to adequate and preventative treatment. People at high risk are those who come with the greatest predispositions to depression and physical disorders. Figure 4.2 illustrates potential risk factors that

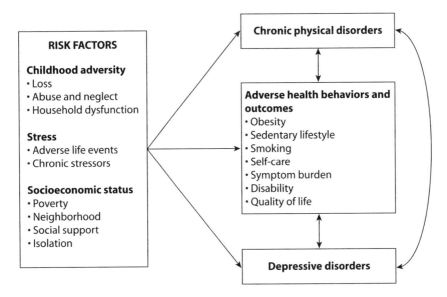

FIGURE 4.2 Risk factors contributing to depression comorbidity with chronic physical disorders

could influence depression comorbidity. Evidence from the WMH Survey initiative has suggested that adversities early in life may trigger a cascade of stressful life experiences and adverse social conditions that evolve into comorbid health outcomes (Scott, 2009). That is, early life environmental stressors can shape behavioral responses and subsequent environmental exposures in a way that increases the risk of disease onset later in life.

A better understanding of the etiology of depression will help us to better identify the risk factors for depression in people with physical conditions. Studies have established that people who already suffer from physical conditions when exposed to a combination of genetic and environmental factors may be more vulnerable to depression (Kang et al., 2015). To reduce the risk factors that may predispose people with physical conditions to depression, early identification of people with specific characteristics would facilitate the early implementation of useful disease management, which may prevent the development of depression.

Treatment of Depression in Persons with Physical Conditions

Depression severely reduces quality of health and social and economic life, and yet it often goes undiagnosed and untreated, mainly due to stigma and other barriers to care (Aguilar-Gaxiola, Kramer, Resendez, & Magaña, 2008; Aguilar-Gaxiola, Loera, Méndez, Sala, & Nakamoto, 2012; Susser & Smith, 2011). A WMH Survey study (Ormel, Petukhova, Von Korff, & Kessler, 2009) revealed that physical disorders were more likely to be treated than mental disorders. For example, in developed countries, 64.4% of all physical disorders were treated compared to 23.7% of all mental disorders. The study found a similar pattern in developing countries, with 51.9% of all physical disorders treated versus only 7.7% of mental disorders. Another study using WMH Survey data found that only 3.4% of people in low / lower-middle-income countries who needed mental health treatment actually sought treatment compared to 12% of people in high-income countries (Wang et al., 2011). While these results highlight the mental-physical treatment gap, they also underscore the need to integrate mental-physical treatment in the same consultation so that there is coordination in our overall approach to treatment of both mental and physical health. Additionally, for an enhanced prevention and early intervention approach, new and creative ways of identifying the relevant environmental and social risk factors are needed to curb depression comorbidity. Prevention and early intervention will be most effective when systemic resources and adequate treatment approaches are targeted at the risk factors and the population groups that are at highest risk and most vulnerable.

Globally, we have a health system in which mental health and physical health are usually not connected. This has created a serious treatment gap for individuals who have both mental and physical conditions. As the literature indicates, individuals have to go to two completely different systems for treatment; if they go to one, in most cases the physical condition will get treated while treatment for the mental disorder rarely occurs. What is needed is a fully integrated approach to incorporate care for the mental aspects of peoples' disorders into the care of physical conditions, and one way is through a collaborative care model (Katon & Unützer, 2006).

Collaborative care is an effective and cost-effective approach to address comorbid conditions, most often consisting of integrated care for persons with depression and commonly co-occurring risk factors and noncommunicable diseases, such as diabetes, cardiovascular disease, and cancer (Druss & Walker, 2011; Katon et al., 2006, 2012; O'Neil et al., 2015). A collaborative model of integrated care consists of key treatment elements critical to closing the mental-physical treatment gap, including combinations of outcome monitoring, stepped treatment options, care coordination, supervision, and self-management. For example, the model focuses on educating and empowering the patient and family through care-provider coordination so that the individual can manage his or her illness. It also emphasizes treatments that combine effective medication management and psychotherapy. Additionally, this model involves mental-physical illness management monitoring and expert consultation for patients who are not making progress. Katon and Unützer (2006) showed that the collaborative care model is an effective approach for treating depression and other mental disorders in primary care settings, and for improving the physical health of patients with a severe mental disorder. Its effectiveness has been established both in the general population and in a variety of subpopulations, such as younger and older adults, women, and low-income patients, with impact on depressive symptoms, quality of life, disability, physical well-being, satisfaction with care, health care costs, and disease-specific outcomes, such as low-density lipoprotein, glycated hemoglobin, and blood pressure (Druss & Walker, 2011; Ell, Aranda, Xie, Lee, & Chou, 2010; Ell et al., 2008; Katon et al., 2006, 2010).

The results of the WMH Survey Initiative support the principle of the integration of mental health care into the primary care system (Caldas de Almeida, Aguilar-Gaxiola, & Loera, 2013) and encourage the adoption of coordinated models of care to address the mental-physical needs of people. In addition, the ongoing work of the WHO and World Bank Group on Service Delivery Platforms for Depression[1] has found that care for depression delivered at the community level, preferably through the primary care network, has shown effectiveness in countries at different stages of development, such as the United States and the United Kingdom, but also Chile, India, Uganda, and many others (Ngo et al., 2013). Integration at the primary care level can be considered a step in the right direction to bridging the gap between physical and mental health services, since it dramatically raises the availability ceiling for mental health

---

1. Increasing attention is being paid to rallying the international community around evidence-based scalable interventions for addressing depression. The WHO and World Bank Group on service delivery platforms for depression will inform a Summit on Mental Health, taking place during the World Bank 2016 Spring meeting, with the goal of promoting an increase in mental health expenditures.

services from a few specialized hospital-based treatment programs to the whole primary care network. Accessibility and quality, however, are also necessary for effective coverage, and a growing body of evidence indicates primary care integration is a sustainable strategy, both from a health outcomes and a cost-effectiveness perspective. In low- and middle-income countries, studies provide evidence of successful delivery of service packages for depression in primary care, relying on locally available human resources who can be trained, mobilized, and supervised to provide psychosocial and pharmacologic interventions. This strategy leverages the potential of community resources (e.g., lay workers, community health promoters, peers) in areas where professional mental health workers are extremely scarce, showing the only viable path for achieving effective coverage scale-up in the short and medium term (Thornicroft & Tansella 2013).

In high- and middle-income countries, adequate mental health services are generally available, but with extreme variations in accessibility and coverage for geographic, ethnic, and socioeconomic groups. Some countries have rolled out coherent strategies aiming at effective coverage of depression and comorbidities (see Chile and the United Kingdom in the following discussion), while others show fragmented approaches, frequently resulting in inconsistencies between the policy and the services delivery level.

In Chile, the government-led Programa Nacional de Diagnóstico y Tratamiento de la Depresión (National Program for the Detection, Diagnosis, and Treatment of Depression), which aims to integrate detection and treatment into primary care in a collaborative approach, has shown impressive results, with a fivefold increase in visits to primary care for mental health and a more than twofold improvement in recovery rates when compared to standard treatment (Araya et al., 2003; Pemjean, 2010). It is also a cost-effective program, obtaining an extra depression-free day at the incremental cost of $1.07 USD (Araya, Flynn, Rojas, Fritsch, & Simon, 2006).

In the United Kingdom, a combination of monetary incentives and scale-up of psychotherapy services provides another path for integration at the primary care level. The quality of outcomes framework provides physical and mental health targets for general practitioners that include a specific quality standard for depression diagnosis and follow-up, while the Improving Access to Psychological Therapies initiative dramatically increased availability of services for depressive and anxiety disorders with 5,000 new therapists trained in the first five years and 900,000 people being treated yearly (Department of Health, 2012). More specific pilot programs are being successfully rolled out, such as the 3 Dimensions of Care for Diabetes (http://mhinnovation .net/innovations/3-dimensions-care-diabetes-3dfd), which integrates medical, psychological, and social care for patients with persistent suboptimal glycemic control and psychological distress. There are also successful examples of integrated NCD and depression programs in the United States, such as the TEAMcare program, which has improved mental health, physical health, and quality of life outcomes through a cost-efficient model of collaborative care (Katon et al., 2010).

Conclusions and Implications

Depression comorbidity is a major cause of disease burden because it leads to (1) increased YLDs, (2) increased years of life lost (YLLs) due to excess all-cause mortality (resulting from suicide and secondary physical comorbidity), and (3) overall loss of health and quality of life. Current GBD methodology significantly underestimates the disease burden of depression, since depression DALYs do not include YLLs (notably, there are zero global deaths attributed yearly to depression). The fact that depression, despite lacking a single YLL attributed to it, is still one of the leading causes of disease burden is a testament to its devastating impact.

The current literature confirms that treatment and services to address depression and physical comorbidity are currently not adequate and are lacking alignment to twenty-first-century public health practices. The vast majority of people with depression and associated physical diseases do not receive care that can greatly improve the quality of their lives. That is, a mental-physical treatment gap still exists, and action is needed to increase intersectoral collaboration or a fully integrated approach to mental-physical care. Bridging this gap is a public health priority, to ensure the reduction in disease burden comprising disability and mortality, and improve the overall health of populations worldwide. The WMH Survey initiative underscores the importance of understanding more about the etiology of the comorbid mental-physical conditions in order to increase the prospect for intervention, prevention, and treatment.

Research Implications

- It is clear that depression is associated with the subsequent development of physical conditions, but more research is required to determine whether that is a causal relationship or whether the relationship comes about through common factors (e.g., early life stressors) giving rise to both depression and physical health problems.
- If depression is causally related to physical ill-health, then we need a better understanding of the temporal sequence and causal pathways. There has been much research into the biological pathways that might link depression with heart disease, but the WMH Surveys findings indicate that depression is associated with a wide variety of chronic physical conditions, so we need to know what generic mechanisms might link depression with subsequent physical ill-health.
- We need a better understanding of what increases the likelihood that those with chronic physical conditions will develop a depressive episode, beyond the known risk factors of past depression history and severity of the physical condition. This research needs to be done with a range of medical patients, as the biological mechanisms and medication effects that can increase the risk of depression vary by physical condition, while psychosocial factors tend to be more generic across

physical conditions. Protective factors that buffer against the development of depression in medical patients should also be studied. This type of research would provide clearer guidance to clinicians and caregivers as to what can be done to make the development of depression less likely.

- Specific research studying delivery platforms of population-level interventions and scale-up of services that have been proven beneficial at the individual level should be prioritized. To effectively address a population-level outcome (e.g., disease burden), it is not enough to just do more of what works at the individual level.

Clinical Implications

- Early detection and treatment of mental disorders would not just reduce depression burden but also contribute to the primary prevention of later chronic physical disease.
- The challenge for primary care is not only to ensure detection and appropriate treatment of mental disorders such as depression but to avoid dichotomous approaches that prioritize either mental or physical health needs. Patients who have been identified as suffering from depression need to have their depression treatment combined with close monitoring of their physical health status and chronic disease risk factors.
- Mental health care clinicians must be aware of the need to routinely assess health behaviors / biomarkers in those with mental disorders. This may be best accomplished with integrative or collaborative care approaches. Although there is awareness of the need to monitor the physical health of people with schizophrenia, for example, there is much less awareness of the need to similarly monitor the physical health of those with depression.
- This dual attention to mental and physical health needs to occur even in young people with mental disorders, as the pathogenesis of most chronic physical conditions starts early in life.
- General health care providers and medical specialists also need to screen for depression and other mental disorders in their medical patients. Holistic approaches based on collaborative care models may be most efficacious for patients with mental-physical comorbidities. When targeting common mental illness, we need to be aware of the dramatic mismatch between the widespread need and the limited clinical resources. With the exception of urban localities in higher-income countries, specialized mental health professionals are inevitably scarce, at least in the short and medium term, and unevenly geographically deployed. Therefore, we need to design, implement, and evaluate clinical interventions that leverage these scarce resources by relying on digital and internet-based interventions that provide support, enhancement, and potentially also alternatives to direct clinical care.

- Given that depression in parents is associated with negative effects on parenting practices and the healthy development of children, when depression is detected in parents in clinical settings, their children should be screened for depression as well (National Research Council and Institute of Medicine, 2009). Primary care providers should be trained to improve their capacity and competence to screen, identify, treat, and prevent depression in parents, and mitigate its effects on children, regardless of their age, by: (1) considering whether the depressed parent has children, (2) considering the impact of the parent's depression on the health and development of his or her children, and (3) screening for depression in children of depressed parents.

Policy Implications

In order to have a roadmap for action, policies should be vision-driven. As we endeavor to move the needle on creating viable solutions to the challenges posed by depression and its associated physical comorbidities toward a population-based public health practice approach, our vision is

> [t]o achieve improved-quality mental health and a high standard of care for all through the provision of integrated, comprehensive, equitable, culturally and linguistically appropriate, and accessible community-based mental health care for all, regardless of class, race/ethnicity, status, and political affiliation. Services will uphold and protect the human rights of people with mental disorders and co-occurring chronic disease conditions. (Aguilar-Gaxiola, 2009, p. 303)

Specific policy considerations include:

- Mental illnesses have traditionally been low priority for decision makers, partly because of an underestimation of their disease and economic burden, a perceived lack of effective and cost-effective interventions, and pervasive stigma. The epidemiologic transition has shifted the bulk of the disease and economic burden from infectious and maternal/child diseases to NCDs, effective and cost-effective interventions are available, and stigma is increasingly acknowledged as a social determinant of mental illness. The first step is to promote academic, advocacy, and policy coalitions capable of systematizing depression's epidemiologic, clinical, and economic data, and presenting a consistent path forward to decision makers.
- The stigma of mental illness affects society at all levels, including decision makers (who would rather allocate resources to other areas), patients (through self-stigma), and health professionals (who frequently provide lower-quality care to patients with mental illness). Specific interventions are necessary to promote acceptance of mental illness and to counter stigma, which is arguably a critical barrier to meaningful social integration, even if services are actually available.

- Investments in multiple societal sectors (e.g., health care, education, workplace, social services, environment/habitat, economic) are critical in disease prevention and health promotion, given the propensity of major depression to strike early in life and its large contribution to the global burden of disease. In order to adequately invest in multiple sectors of society in ways that build community capacity, policy makers must fully understand the social determinants of health outcomes in populations-at-large across the life span (Patel et al., 2016). By investing in the intersectoral linkages, coordination, and integration of society, an expected policy outcome would be increased promotion, prevention, treatment, and rehabilitation services to historically unserved or underserved populations.
- Recognize age patterning, risk factors, and consequences of co-occurrence disorders. From a policy perspective, increase research resources toward addressing the comorbid risk factors throughout the life span because chronic physical / pain conditions increase with age, while mental disorders decrease after midlife. We also must do more to better understand consequences of poor physical health among older adults after age 65.
- Within the health care systems, ensure that responsibility for prevention and management of chronic illness lies within the primary health care service. In the case of organization and health care treatment, primary health care is the setting in which common mental disorders are most likely to be recognized and potentially treated. Therefore, improving the coordination and integration of mental health with physical health care is crucial in treating persons with comorbid mental disorders. Design and implement comprehensive, integrated, effective, and efficient mental health systems that cover promotion, prevention, treatment, rehabilitation, and recovery.
- Address the need for a diverse, culturally and linguistically competent workforce that is effective in addressing comorbid mental and physical conditions. Providers of primary health care services need to be trained in evidence-based practices tailored to target underserved populations and develop capacity and competence to detect and treat people with mental health problems in the community, supported by a network with specialist mental health services and front line workers such as community health promoters.
- New strategies for educating, supporting, and empowering individuals and families are needed, strategies that prevent chronic disease when possible and maximize the ability of individuals with chronic illness to live full and productive lives when chronic disease cannot be prevented.
- Finally, the health care systems of both developed and developing countries need to be reorganized to optimize the abilities to improve population health, focusing on the challenges of managing chronic conditions. In addition, the working practices of primary health care providers and mental health care workers

need to be modernized with new staff roles and responsibilities, requiring changes in values and attitudes, knowledge, and skills, in order to offer effective and efficient care.

References

Aguilar-Gaxiola, S. (2009). Policy implications. In M. Von Korff, K. Scott, & O. Gureje (Eds.), *Global perspectives on mental disorders and physical illness in the WHO World Mental Health surveys* (pp. 302–312). New York, NY: Cambridge University Press.

Aguilar-Gaxiola, S., Kramer, E. J., Resendez, C., & Magaña, C. G. (2008). The context of depression in Latinos in the United States. In S. Aguilar-Gaxiola & T. P. Gullota (Eds.), *Depression in Latinos: Assessment, treatment, and prevention* (pp. 3–28). New York, NY: Springer.

Aguilar-Gaxiola, S., Loera, G., Geraghty, E., Ton, H., Lim, C. W., de Jonge, P., . . . Scott, K. M. (2015). Associations between *DSM-IV* mental disorders and subsequent onset of arthritis. Manuscript submitted for publication.

Aguilar-Gaxiola, S., Loera, G., Méndez, L., Sala, M., & Nakamoto, J. (2012). *Community-defined solutions for Latino mental health care disparities: California Reducing Disparities Project, Latino Strategic Planning Workgroup Population Report.* Davis, CA: University of California.

Alonso, J. (2012). Burden of mental disorders based on the World Mental Health surveys. *Revista Brasileira de Psiquiatria, 34*(1), 7–8.

Alonso, J., Chatterji, S., & He, Y. (Eds.) (2013). *The burdens of mental disorders: Global perspectives from the WHO World Mental Health surveys.* New York, NY: Cambridge University Press.

American Psychiatric Association. (1994). *Diagnostic and statistical manual of mental disorders, 4th edition.* Washington, DC: American Psychiatric Press.

Araya, R., Flynn, T., Rojas, G., Fritsch, R., & Simon, G. (2006). Cost-effectiveness of a primary care treatment program for depression in low-income women in Santiago, Chile. *American Journal of Psychiatry, 163*(8), 1379–1387.

Araya, R., Rojas, G., Fritsch, R., Gaete, J., Rojas, M., Simon, G., & Peters, T. J. (2003). Treating depression in primary care in low-income women in Santiago, Chile: A randomised controlled trial. *The Lancet, 361*(9362), 995–1000.

Atun, R. (2015). Transitioning health systems for multimorbidity. *The Lancet, 6736*(14), 8–9.

Bloom, D. E., Cafiero, E. T., Jané-Llopis, E., Abrahams-Gessel, S., Bloom, L. R., Fathima, S., ... Weinstein, C. (2011). *The global economic burden of noncommunicable diseases.* Geneva: World Economic Forum.

Bromet, E., Andrade, L. H., Hwang, I., Sampson, N. A., Alonso, J., De Girolamo, G., . . . Kessler, R. C. (2011). Cross-national epidemiology of *DSM-IV* major depressive episode. *BMC Medicine, 9*(1), 90.

Caldas de Almeida, J., Aguilar-Gaxiola, S., & Loera, G. (2013). The burdens of mental disorders: Implications for policy. In J. Alonso, S. Chatterji, & Y. He (Eds.), *The burdens of mental disorders: Global perspectives from the WHO World Mental Health surveys* (pp. 230–243). New York, NY: Cambridge University Press.

Carter, R. (2008). Addressing the caregiving crisis. *Preventing Chronic Disease, 5*(1), A02.

Cohen, N., & Galea, S. (2011). Twenty-first century public health practice: Preventing mental illness and promoting mental health. In N. Cohen & S. Galea (Eds.), *Population mental health: Evidence, policy, and public health practice* (pp. 38–50). New York, NY: Routledge.

Costello, E. J., He, J. P., Sampson, N. A., Kessler, R. C., & Merikangas, K. R. (2014). Services for adolescents with psychiatric disorders: 12-month data from the National Comorbidity Survey-Adolescent. *Psychiatric Services, 65*(3), 359–366.

Demyttenaere, K., Bruffaerts, R., Lee, S., Posada-Villa, J., Kovess, V., Angermeyer, M. C., . . . Von Korff, M. (2007). Mental disorders among persons with chronic back or neck pain: Results from the World Mental Health surveys. *Pain, 129*(3), 332–342.

Department of Health. (2012). Improving Access to Psychological Therapies (IAPT) three-year report: The first million patients. Retrieved from http://www.iapt.nhs.uk/silo/files/iapt-3 -year-report.pdf

Druss, B., & Walker, E. R. (2011). *Mental disorders and medical comorbidity: Research synthesis report no. 21.* Princeton, NJ: Robert Wood Johnson Foundation.

Ell, K., Aranda, M. P., Xie, B., Lee, P.-J., & Chou, C.-P. (2010). Collaborative depression treatment in older and younger adults with physical illness: Pooled comparative analysis of three randomized clinical trials. *American Journal of Geriatric Psychiatry, 18*(6), 520–530.

Ell, K., Xie, B., Quon, B., Quinn, D. I., Dwight-Johnson, M., & Lee, P. J. (2008). Randomized controlled trial of collaborative care management of depression among low-income patients with cancer. *Journal of Clinical Oncology, 26*(27), 4488–4496.

Evans, D. L., Charney, D. S., Lewis, L., Golden, R. N., Gorman, J. M., Krishnan, K. R., . . . Valvo, W. J. (2005). Mood disorders in the medically ill: Scientific review and recommendations. *Biological Psychiatry, 58*(3), 175–189.

Frasure-Smith, N., & Lespérance, F. (2008). Depression and anxiety as predictors of 2-year cardiac events in patients with stable coronary artery disease. *Archives of General Psychiatry, 65*(1), 62–71.

Goetzel, R. Z., Long, S. R., Ozminkowski, R. J., Hawkins, K., Wang, S., & Lynch, W. (2004). Health, absence, disability, and presenteeism cost estimates of certain physical and mental health conditions affecting US employers. *Journal of Occupational and Environmental Medicine, 46*(4), 398–412.

Goldston, K., & Baillie, A. J. (2008). Depression and coronary heart disease: A review of the epidemiological evidence, explanatory mechanisms and management approaches. *Clinical Psychology Review, 28*(2), 288–306.

Gotlib, I. H., & Joormann, J. (2010). Cognition and depression: Current status and future directions. *Annual Review Clinical Psychology, 6*, 285–312.

Gureje, O., Von Korff, M., Kola, L., Demyttenaere, K., He, Y., Posada-Villa, J., . . . Alonso, J. (2008). The relation between multiple pains and mental disorders: Results from the World Mental Health Surveys. *Pain, 135*(1), 82–91.

He, Y., Zhang, M., Lin, E. H. B., Bruffaerts, R., Posada-Villa, J., Angermeyer, M. C., . . . Kessler, R. C. (2008). Mental disorders among persons with arthritis: Results from the World Mental Health Surveys. *Psychological Medicine, 38*(11), 1639–1650.

Huffman, J. C., Celano, C. M., Beach, S. R., Motiwala, S. R., & Januzzi, J. L. (2013). Depression and cardiac disease: Epidemiology, mechanisms, and diagnosis. *Cardiovascular Psychiatry and Neurology.* doi: 10.1155/2013/695925. Epub 2013 Apr 7.

Institute for Health Metrics and Evaluation. (2013). *GBD Compare*. Retrieved from http://viz
.healthmetricsandevaluation.org/gbd-compare/

Kang, H. J., Kim, S. Y., Bae, K. Y., Kim, S. W., Shin, I. S., Yoon, J. S., & Kim, J. M. (2015).
Comorbidity of depression with physical disorders: Research and clinical implications.
Chonnam Medical Journal, 51(1), 8–18.

Katon, W. J. (2011). Epidemiology and treatment of depression in patients with chronic
medical illness. *Dialogues in Clinical Neuroscience, 13*(1), 7.

Katon, W. J., Lin, E. H. B., Von Korff, M., Ciechanowski, P., Ludman, E. J., Young, B., . . .
McCulloch, D. (2010). Collaborative care for patients with depression and chronic
illnesses. *New England Journal of Medicine, 363*(27), 2611–2620.

Katon, W. J., Russo, J., Lin, E. H., Schmittdiel, J., Ciechanowski, P., Ludman, E., . . . Von Korff, M.
(2012). Cost-effectiveness of a multi-condition collaborative care intervention. *Archives of
General Psychiatry, 69*(5), 506–514.

Katon, W. J., & Unützer, J. (2006). Collaborative care models for depression: Time to move
from evidence to practice. *Archives of Internal Medicine, 166*(21), 2304–2306.

Katon, W. J., Unützer, J., Fan, M. Y., Williams, J. W., Schoenbaum, M., Lin, E. H. B., &
Hunkeler, E. M. (2006). Cost-effectiveness and net benefit of enhanced treatment of
depression for older adults with diabetes and depression. *Diabetes Care, 29*(2), 265–270.

Keitner, G. I., Ryan, C. E., Miller, I. W., Kohn, R., Bishop, D. S., & Epstein, N. B. (1995). Role of
the family in recovery and major depression. *American Journal of Psychiatry, 152*(7),
1002–1008.

Kendler, K. S. (2005). Toward a philosophical structure for psychiatry. *American Journal of
Psychiatry, 162*(3), 433–440.

Kessler, R. C., Berglund, P., Demler, O., Jin, R., Koretz, D., Merikangas, K. R., . . . Wang, P. S.
(2003). The epidemiology of major depressive disorder: Results from the National
Comorbidity Survey Replication (NCS-R). *Journal of American Medical Association, 289*(23),
3095–3105.

Kessler, R. C., Birnbaum, H., Shahly, V., Bromet, E., Hwang, I., McLaughlin, K. A., . . . Stein, D. J.
(2010). Age differences in the prevalence and comorbidity of *DSM-IV* major depressive
episodes: Results from the WHO World Mental Health Survey Initiative. *Depression and
Anxiety, 27*(4), 351–364.

Kessler, R. C., & Bromet, E. J. (2013). The epidemiology of depression across cultures. *Annual
Review of Public Health, 34,* 119.

Kessler, R. C., Merikangas, K. R., & Wang, P. S. (2008). The prevalence and correlates of
workplace depression in the National Comorbidity Survey Replication. *Journal of Occupational Medicine, 50*(4), 381–390.

Kessler, R. C., & Ustün, T. B. (2004). The World Mental Health (WMH) Survey Initiative
version of the World Health Organization (WHO) Composite International Diagnostic
Interview (CIDI). *International Journal of Methods of Psychiatric Research, 13*(2), 93–121.

Kessler, R. C., Walters, E. E., & Forthofer, M. S. (1998). The social consequences of psychiatric
disorders, III: Probability of marital stability. *American Journal of Psychiatry, 155*(8),
1092–1096.

Kessler, R. C., & Wang P. S. (2009). Epidemiology of depression. In I. H. Gotlib, & C. L.
Hammen (Eds.), *Handbook of depression* (2nd ed., pp. 5–22). New York, NY: Guilford Press.

Kohn, R., Saxena, S., Levav, I., & Saraceno, B. (2004). The treatment gap in mental health care. *Bulletin of the World Health Organization, 82*(11), 858–866.

Kovess-Masfety, V., Alonso, J., Angermeyer, M., Bromet, E., de Girolomo, G., de Jonge, P., . . . Kessler, R. C. (2013). Irritable mood in adult major depressive disorder: Results from the World Mental Health surveys. *Depression and Anxiety, 30*(4), 395–406.

Lépine, J. P., & Briley, M. (2011). The increasing burden of depression. *Neuropsychiatric Disease and Treatment, 7*(1), 3–7.

Mathers, C. D., & Loncar, D. (2006). Projections of global mortality and burden of disease from 2002 to 2030. *PLoS Medicine, 3*(11), e442.

McEwen, B. S. (2003). Mood disorders and allostatic load. *Biological Psychiatry, 54*(3), 200–207.

Melek, S. P., Norris, D. T., & Paulus, J. (2014). Economic impact of integrated medical-behavioral healthcare implications for psychiatry. *Milliman American Psychiatric Association Report.* Denver, CO: Milliman, Inc. Retrieved from http://www.aha.org/content/14 /milliman_economicimpact_behavhealthcare2014.pdf

Merikangas, K. R., Nakamura, E. F., & Kessler, R. C. (2009). Epidemiology of mental disorders in children and adolescents. *Dialogues in clinical neuroscience, 11*(1), 7.

Meyer, C. (2000). Depressive disorders were the fourth leading cause of global disease burden in the year 2000. *Evidence Based Mental Health, 7*(4), 123.

Murray, C. J., Barber, R. M., Foreman, K. J., Ozgoren, A. A., Abd-Allah, F., Abera, S. F., . . . Vos, T. (2015, April 7). Global, regional, and national disability-adjusted life years (DALYs) for 306 diseases and injuries and healthy life expectancy (HALE) for 188 countries, 1990–2013: Quantifying the epidemiological transition. *Lancet.* doi:10.1155/2013/695925.

Murray, C. J., & Lopez, A. D. (Eds.). (1996). *The global burden of disease: A comprehensive assessment of mortality and disability from disease, injuries and risk factors in 1990 and projected to 2020.* Boston, MA: Harvard School of Public Health, World Health Organization, and World Bank.

National Research Council and Institute of Medicine. (2009). *Depression in parents, parenting, and children: Opportunities to improve identification, treatment, and prevention.* Committee on Depression, Parenting Practices, and the Healthy Development of Children. Board on Children, Youth, and Families. Division of Behavioral and Social Sciences and Education. Washington, DC: The National Academies Press.

Naylor, C., Parsonage, M., McDaid, D., Knapp, M., Fossey, M., & Galea, A. (2012). *Long-term conditions and mental health: The cost of co-morbidities.* London: The King's Fund and Center for Mental Health. Retrieved from http://www.kingsfund.org.uk/publications/long-term -conditions-and-mental-health

Ngo, V. K., Rubinstein, A., Ganju, V., Kanellis, P., Loza N., Rabadan-Diehl, C., & Daar, A. S. (2013). Grand challenges: Integrating mental health care into the non-communicable disease agenda. *PLoS Med, 10*(5): doi: 10.1371/journal.pmed.1001443. Epub 2013 May 14.

Nock, M. K., Hwang, I., Sampson, N. A., & Kessler, R. C. (2010). Mental disorders, comorbidity and suicidal behavior: Results from the National Comorbidity Survey Replication. *Molecular Psychiatry, 15*(8), 868–76.

Olfson, M., Fireman, B., Weissman, M. M., Leon, A. C., Sheehan, D. V., Kathol, R. G., . . . Farber, L. (1997). Mental disorders and disability among patients in a primary care group practice. *American Journal of Psychiatry, 154*(12), 1734–1740.

O'Neil, A., Jacka, F. N., Quirk, S. E., Cocker, F., Taylor, C. B., Oldenburg, B., & Berk, M. (2015). A shared framework for the common mental disorders and non-communicable disease: Key considerations for disease prevention and control. *BMC Psychiatry, 15*(1), 1.

Ormel, J., Petukhova, M. V., Von Korff, M. R., & Kessler, R. C. (2009). Disability and treatment of specific mental and physical disorders. In M. R. Von Korff, K. M. Scott, & O. Gureje (Eds.), *Global perspectives on mental-physical comorbidity in the WHO World Mental Health Surveys* (pp. 210–229). New York, NY: Cambridge University Press.

Patel, V., Chisholm, D., Parikh, R., Charlson, F. J., Degenhardt, L., Dua, T., . . . Whiteford, H. (2016). Addressing the burden of mental, neurological, and substance use disorders: Key messages from Disease Control Priorities. *The Lancet, 387*(10028), 1672–1685.

Pemjean, A. (2010). Mental health in primary healthcare in Chile. *International Psychiatry, 7*(1), 7–8.

Perez-Prada, J. (2011). Depression and cardiovascular disease: The need for improved case definition. *Bulletin of Clinical Psychopharamcology, 21*(1), 7–10.

Reddy, M. S. (2010). Depression: The disorder and the burden. *Indian Journal of Psychological Medicine, 32*(1), 1.

Schwartz, S., & Susser, E. (2010). Genome-wide association studies: Does only size matter? *American Journal of Psychiatry, 167*(7), 741–744.

Scott, K. M., Bruffaerts, R., Simon, G. E., Alonso, J., Angermeyer, M., de Girolamo, G., . . . Von Korff, M. (2008a). Obesity and mental disorders in the general population: Results from the World Mental Health Surveys. *International Journal of Obesity, 32*(1), 192–200.

Scott, K. M., Bruffaerts, R., Tsang, A., Ormel, J., Alonso, J., Angermeyer, M. C., . . . Von Korff, M. (2007a). Depression-anxiety relationships with chronic physical conditions: Results from the World Mental Health Surveys. *Journal of Affective Disorders, 103*, 113–120.

Scott, K. M., de Jonge, P., Alonso, J., Viana, M. C., Liu, Z., O'Neill, S., . . . Kessler, R. C. (2013a). Associations between *DSM-IV* mental disorders and subsequent heart disease onset: Beyond depression. *International Journal of Cardiology, 168*(6), 5293–5299.

Scott, K. M., Von Korff, M., Alonso, J., Angermeyer, M., Bromet, E. J., Bruffaerts, R., . . . Williams, D. (2008b). Age patterns in the prevalence of *DSM-IV* depressive/anxiety disorders with and without physical co-morbidity. *Psychological Medicine, 38*(11), 1659–1669.

Scott, K. M., Von Korff, M., Alonso, J., Angermeyer, M. C., Bromet, E., Fayyad, J., . . . Williams, D. (2009). Mental–physical co-morbidity and its relationship with disability: Results from the World Mental Health Surveys. *Psychological Medicine, 39*(1), 33–43.

Scott, K. M., Von Korff, M., Ormel, J., Zhang, M. Y., Bruffaerts, R., Alonso, J., . . . Haro, J. M. (2007b). Mental disorders among adults with asthma: Results from the World Mental Health Survey. *General Hospital Psychiatry, 29*(2), 123–133.

Scott, K. M., Wu, B., Saunders, K., Benjet, C., He, Y., Lépine, J., . . . Von Korff, M. (2013b). Early onset mental disorders and their links to chronic physical conditions in adulthood. In J. Alonso, S. Chatterji, & Y. He (Eds.), *The burdens of mental disorders: Global perspectives from the WHO World Mental Health Surveys* (pp. 87–96). New York, NY: Cambridge University Press.

Spijker, J., Graaf, R., Bijl, R. V., Beekman, A. T., Ormel, J., & Nolen, W. A. (2004). Functional disability and depression in the general population: Results from the Netherlands Mental Health Survey and Incidence Study (NEMESIS). *Acta Psychiatrica Scandinavica, 110*(3), 208–214.

Stein, D. J., Aguilar-Gaxiola, S., Alonso, J., Bruffaerts, R., de Jonge, P., Liu, Z., . . . Scott, K. M. (2014). Associations between mental disorders and subsequent onset of hypertension. *General Hospital Psychiatry, 36*(2), 142–149.

Stein, D. J., Ruscio, A. M., Lee, S., Petukhova, M., Alonso, J., Andrade, L. H., . . . Kessler, R. C. (2010a). Subtyping social anxiety disorder in developed and developing countries. *Depression and Anxiety, 27*(4), 390–403.

Stein, D. J., Scott, K., Haro Abad, J. M., Aguilar-Gaxiola, S., Alonso, J., Angermeyer, M., . . . Von Korff, M. (2010b). Early childhood adversity and later hypertension: Data from the World Mental Health Survey. *Annals of Clinical Psychiatry, 22*(1), 19–28.

Susser, E., & Smith, R. P. (2011). Epidemiology in public mental health. In N. Cohen & S. Galea (Eds.), *Population mental health: Evidence, policy, and public health practice* (pp. 38–50). New York, NY: Routledge.

Thomas, A. J., Kalaria, R. N., & O'Brien, T. J. (2004). Depression and vascular disease: What is the relationship? *Journal of Affective Disorders, 79*(1), 81–95.

Thornicroft, G., & Tansella, M. (2013). The balanced care model for global mental health. *Psychological Medicine, 43*(4), 849–863.

Üstün, T. B., Ayuso-Mateos, J. L., Chatterji, S., Mathers, C., & Murray, C. J. (2004). Global burden of depressive disorders in the year 2000. *British Journal of Psychiatry, 184*(5), 386–392.

Valderas, J. M., Starfield, B., Sibbald, B., Salisbury, C., & Roland, M. (2009). Defining comorbidity: Implications for understanding health and health services. *The Annals of Family Medicine, 7*(4), 357–363.

Viana, M. C., Gruber, M. J., Shahly, V., Alhamzawi, A., Alonso, J., Andrade, L. H., . . . Kessler, R. C. (2013). Family burden related to mental and physical disorders in the world: Results from the WHO World Mental Health (WMH) Survey. *Revista Brasileira de Psiquiatria, 35*(2), 115–125.

Von Korff, M. R., Scott, K. M., & Gureje, O. (Eds.). (2009). *Global perspectives on mental—physical comorbidity: In the WHO World Mental Health Surveys.* New York, NY: Cambridge University Press.

Vos, T., Barber, R. M., Bell, B., Bertozzi-Villa, A., Biryukov, S., Bolliger, I., . . . Murray, C. J. (2015). Global, regional, and national incidence, prevalence, and years lived with disability for 301 acute and chronic diseases and injuries in 188 countries, 1990–2013: A systematic analysis for the Global Burden of Disease Study 2013. *The Lancet, 386*(9995), 743–800. doi:10.1016/S0140-6736(15)00128-2.

Wang, O. S., Aguilar-Gaxiola, S., Al-Hamzawi, A. O., Alonso, J., Andrade, L. H., Angermeyer, M. C., . . . Kessler, R. C. (2011). Treated and untreated prevalence of mental disorders: Results from the World Health Organization World Mental Health (WMH) surveys. In G. Thornicroft, G. Szmukler, K. Mueser, & R. Drake, R. (Eds.), *Oxford textbook of community mental health* (pp. 50–66). London: Oxford University Press.

Wardenaar, K. J., van Loo, H. M., Cai, T., Fava, M., Gruber, M. J., Li, J., . . . Kessler, R. C. (2014). The effects of comorbidity in defining major depression subtypes associated with long-term course and severity. *Psychological Medicine, 44*(15), 3289–3302.

World Health Organization. (2003). *Investing in mental health.* Geneva, Switzerland: WHO Press.

World Health Organization. (2008). *The global burden of disease: 2004 update.* Geneva, Switzerland: WHO Press.

World Health Organization. (2012). *Depression: A global crisis.* Geneva, Switzerland: WHO Press.

CHAPTER 5

Substance Use and Depressive Disorders

Jacquelyn L. Meyers, PhD
Deborah Hasin, PhD

Depressed mood, dysthymia, and major depression have been commonly observed in individuals with substance use disorders (Compton, Thomas, Stinson, & Grant, 2007; Deykin, Levy, & Wells, 1987; Grant & Harford, 1995; Hasin, Stinson, Ogburn, & Grant, 2007; Kessler et al., 1997; Regier et al., 1990). Conversely, rates of substance use disorders have been shown to be extraordinarily high among individuals with depression (Hasin, Endicott, & Lewis, 1985; Hasin, Goodwin, Stinson, & Grant, 2005; Kessler et al., 1996a). In the United States, rates of both disorders are increasing (Grant et al., 2015), indicating that the co-occurrence, or *comorbidity*, of these two conditions is likely to remain a significant public health problem.

As the field of psychiatry entered the modern era of classification systems based on observable symptoms, clinicians were divided on the meaning of co-occurring psychiatric syndromes among substance-dependent individuals (Saunders, Schuckit, Sirovatka, & Regier, 2007). Clinicians primarily involved in treating psychiatric disorders, such as depression, tended to see substance use problems as part of the underlying mood disorder, whereas clinicians mainly involved in the treatment of substance use disorders tended to view depressive symptoms as manifestations of the substance use disorder. Both of these views were reflected in service delivery systems where separate programs existed for treating mental and substance use disorders. These opposing perspectives stimulated decades of research seeking to understand and characterize the relationship between depressive and substance use pathology. However, there are still many unanswered questions.

In the following section, we summarize the scientific literature examining the comorbidity of depressive disorders and substance use disorders. First, we provide an overview of epidemiological and clinical studies that have examined rates of co-occurrence of alcohol, nicotine, and other drug use disorders with depressive disorders, as well as important correlates of these forms of comorbidity. Next, theoretical models of the onset and persistence of depression and substance use disorder comorbidity are considered, followed by a review of various types of studies evaluating these theoretical models. The chapter concludes by examining treatment implications of this comorbidity and suggestions for future research examining co-occurring depressive and substance use disorders.

Evidence for the Comorbidity of Substance Use and Depressive Disorders

Worldwide, studies that have examined the relationship between depression and substance use pathology, including alcohol and other drug use disorders, demonstrate that comorbidity of these disorders is pervasive (Swendsen et al., 1998). This indicates a serious need for mental health researchers and clinicians to understand the presentation, etiology, and treatment of co-occurring major depression and substance use disorder symptoms. In the United States, the prevalence of lifetime substance use disorders among adults with major depression ranges from 24% to 40% (Table 5.1; Hasin et al., 2005; Kessler et al., 2003).

Among individuals with depression, 9%–25% also meet criteria for a current (within a 12-month period) substance use disorder (Compton, Conway, Stinson, & Grant, 2006; Grant, Stinson, et al., 2004; Hasin et al., 2005; Kessler et al., 2003). In the United States, the most prevalent substance use disorders are nicotine and alcohol use disorders; the lifetime prevalence of nicotine use disorders is 17.7%, and the lifetime prevalence of alcohol use disorders is 30.3% (Hasin & Grant, 2015). Given the comparatively lower prevalence of other (i.e., illicit) drug use disorders in the general population (lifetime prevalence: 10.3%), much of the community- or population-based epidemiological literature on the co-occurrence of substance use disorders and depression has focused on *DSM-III* and *DSM-IV* alcohol use disorders (alcohol abuse or dependence), nicotine use disorders, and combined illicit drug use disorders. Historically, relatively few studies have focused on the relationship between major depressive disorder (MDD) and specific drug use disorders; however, this has been rapidly

Table 5.1. Prevalence of lifetime substance use disorders among adults with major depressive disorder (MDD)

Substance use disorder	MDD (lifetime)
Any alcohol use disorder	40.3% (SE: 0.09)
Any drug use disorder	17.2% (SE: 0.64)
Nicotine dependence	30.0% (SE: 0.81)

Source. Hasin et al. (2005).
Note. SE = standard error.

changing within recent years, particularly in the areas of cannabis (Pacek, Martins, & Crum, 2013) and opioid use disorders (Martins et al., 2012).

Epidemiological Studies

In the United States, five primary epidemiologic studies have examined rates and co-occurrences of psychiatric and substance use disorders by conducting nationally representative diagnostic interview surveys of the population, including: the National Institute of Mental Health Epidemiologic Catchment Area (ECA) study, conducted in 1981–1985 (Regier et al., 1990); the National Comorbidity Survey (NCS), conducted in 1991 (Kessler et al., 1994); the National Longitudinal Alcohol Epidemiologic Survey (NLAES), conducted in 1991–1992 (Grant, 1997); the National Epidemiologic Survey of Alcohol and Related Conditions (NESARC), conducted first in 2001–2002 and again in 2004–2005 (Grant, Dawson, et al., 2004); and, most recently, a new survey conducted in 2012–2013, the NESARC-III (Grant et al., 2015). Each of these epidemiologic studies has provided evidence that major depression and substance use disorders commonly co-occur in the US population. An early report from the ECA study indicated that the odds of meeting criteria for *DSM-III* MDD were 1.8 times higher for respondents with *DSM-III* alcohol dependence compared with non-alcohol-dependent individuals (Helzer & Pryzbeck, 1988). Kessler and colleagues (1997) reported a similar pattern of association in the NCS; compared with nondepressed respondents in the NCS, the lifetime odds of *DSM-III-R* alcohol dependence were 2.95 higher for men and 4.05 higher for women with major depression. In addition, NCS data indicated a twofold increase in the lifetime odds of depression among those meeting criteria for alcohol dependence (Kessler et al., 1996a). Results from the NLAES indicated that the lifetime odds of *DSM-IV* alcohol dependence were 3.56 times higher for those with major depression (Grant & Harford, 1995). Further results from the NLAES show that prior *DSM-IV* alcohol dependence increased risk for a current MDD more than fourfold. Importantly, this study also found that the majority of those with depression last used substances two or more years prior to the interview, which precludes acute intoxication or withdrawal effects as an explanation for depression (Hasin & Grant, 2002). Findings from the NESARC indicated that those who were alcohol dependent (*DSM-IV*) had a 1.8 odds of also having past-year or lifetime MDD (Hasin et al., 2005), even after controlling for other psychiatric comorbidity. The NESARC-III assessed diagnoses consistent with *DSM-5* criteria (Hasin et al., 2013), in which alcohol use disorder severity levels were classified as mild, moderate, or severe. In agreement with these previous studies, the odds of MDD ranged from 1.1 to 1.4 for those with *DSM-IV* alcohol use disorder in the NESARC-III (Grant et al., 2015).

Nicotine-dependent individuals are also more likely to have depressive disorders. According to NCS data (obtained in 1991–1992), about 47% of US citizens have smoked cigarettes in their lifetime, with ~17% of the population reporting having depression at any point in their lifetime (Kessler et al., 1994). However, among those who had ever smoked cigarettes in their lifetime, 59% had a major depressive episode (*DSM-III-R*) at some point in their lifetime (Breslau, Kilbey, & Andreski, 1991; Breslau, Novak, & Kessler, 2004). While rates of cigarette smoking have decreased since 1991–1992 (Grant et al., 2015), the relationship between MDD and nicotine dependence remains. For example, recent work in the NESARC has shown that in the United States, individuals with any depressive disorder, including *DSM-IV* MDD, are more likely to use cigarettes and to be nicotine dependent (Goodwin, Zvolensky, Keyes, & Hasin, 2012). Conversely, respondents who are nicotine dependent are between 1.8 and 2.6 times more likely to also meet criteria for MDD (Breslau et al., 1991; Hasin et al., 2005).

Similarly, those with illicit drug dependence have increased odds of meeting current or lifetime *DSM-IV* major depression (odds ratios range between 2.6 and 4.7) (Hasin et al., 2005). While studies that have examined the co-occurrence of depression and specific illicit drugs in the general population are less common, several reports have been published. For example, Grant and Pickering (1998) reported that those with *DSM-IV* MDD were at increased risk for cannabis abuse and dependence in the 1992 NLAES. The association between depression and cannabis use was substantiated in other surveys, including the NCS and NESARC (Grant, 1995; Kessler et al., 1996b). Another study reported that those with *DSM-IV* MDD have ~1.9 greater odds of using nonmedical prescription opioids at some point in their lifetime (Martins et al., 2012).

Clinical Studies

Approximately one-third of individuals who present for major depression treatment also have a recent substance use disorder (Compton et al., 2007; Davis et al., 2007; Grant, 1995; Grant, Stinson, et al., 2004; Hasin et al., 1985; Kessler, Mickelson, & Williams, 1999). Given the particularly high rates of depression and substance use disorder symptoms in clinical populations (Lynskey, 1998), treatment-seeking samples provide important insights into the co-occurrence of these pathologies. However, studies based on treated samples may overestimate the association among substance use disorders and major depression due to the selection of more severe cases into treatment (Wu, Kouzis, & Leaf, 1999); therefore, these rates should not be extrapolated to the general population. In parallel to the epidemiologic literature, several large-scale clinical studies have examined the rates and co-occurrence of psychiatric and substance use disorders. For example, the Sequenced Treatment Alternatives to Relieve Depression (STAR*D) is a multisite study of 4,041 treatment-seeking adults with major depression designed to assess the effectiveness of depression treatments in patients in both primary and specialty care settings. Of the participants in the STAR*D (all of whom had a diagnosis of *DSM-IV* MDD), 9%–25% had a concurrent substance use disorder (McDermut, Mattia, & Zimmerman, 2001), while 30%–43% of participants had a substance use disorder at some point in their lifetimes (Davis et al., 2010). In a survey of 6,355 patients receiving treatment for various addictive disorders, Miller and colleagues (1996) observed that the lifetime prevalence of depression was 43.7%. This high rate is consistent with results from a study conducted in the Collaborative Study on the Genetics of Alcoholism, in which the lifetime prevalence of MDD among treatment-seeking alcoholics was 42.2% (Schuckit, Tsuang, Anthenelli, Tipp, & Nurnberger, 1996). In addition, individuals in treatment with comorbid depressive and substance use disorder symptoms often experience more severe illness, disability, and poorer treatment outcomes than individuals with only major depression or substance use disorder (Burns & Teesson, 2002; Davis et al., 2005; Drake, Price, & Drake, 1996; Najt, Fusar-Poli, & Brambilla, 2011). These data underscore the importance of understanding and treating the co-occurrence of substance use and depressive symptoms.

Heterogeneity in Depression and Substance Use Disorder Relationship

The comorbid relationship between substance use disorders and major depression varies as a function of several factors, including demographic characteristics, diagnosis (abuse vs. dependence), specific substance abused, and time frame of assessment (Grant, 1995). The associations between major depression and substance use disorders are consistently stronger with symptoms of substance dependence as compared with symptoms of substance abuse (Grant et al., 2015), which may indicate that those with more severe symptomology are more likely to have comorbid disorders. Further, the associations between major depression and substance use disorders, when including substance abuse and dependence symptoms, tend to be larger for women as compared with men (Compton et al., 2006). However, these gender effects are largely both substance specific and diagnosis (abuse vs. dependence) specific. For example, associations of major depression and prescription opiate, sedative, tranquilizer, and amphetamine dependence are typically greater for women, whereas the associations between major depression and alcohol, marijuana, cocaine, or hallucinogen dependence are typically greater for men (Grant, 1995). Further, women generally demonstrate stronger relations between substance *abuse* and major depression (Compton et al., 2006), while men generally demonstrate stronger relations between substance *dependence* and major depression (Grant, 1995). In addition, the associations between MDD and substance use disorders are consistently larger for younger adults (aged 18–30), those who have never been married (or are divorced), and non-Hispanic Whites (Compton et al., 2006; Davis et al., 2007; McDermut et al., 2001). In a Minnesota sample that was prospectively assessed at four different times between the ages of 17 and 29, lifetime comorbidity between MDD and substance use disorders increased substantially between ages 17 and 29 (Hamdi & Iacono, 2014). This trend was significant for alcohol dependence and nicotine dependence but not cannabis dependence. In contrast, recent research suggests that in the US adult population, the relationship between major depression and substance disorders may be particularly strong with cannabis (Blanco et al., 2014; Pacek et al., 2013) and nonmedical prescription opioid use (Martins et al., 2012) as compared with more commonly used substances, such as alcohol and nicotine. Further, associations between major depression and polysubstance use disorders (i.e., individuals who have multiple substance use disorders) appear to be larger than the associations observed between major depression and any individual substance use disorder (Pacek et al., 2013). Finally, comorbid MDD/substance use disorder patients typically have greater depressive symptomology and functional impairment, and are at greater risk for dying by suicide (Davis et al., 2005; Davis et al., 2010; Fava et al., 1996; Zimmerman, Chelminski, & McDermut, 2002), again echoing the serious need to address this comorbidity in treatment.

The Question of Temporality

While there is clear evidence for the co-occurrence of major depression and substance use disorders, the temporality of these two disorders (i.e., which disorder came first) remains poorly understood. Several theoretical hypotheses have been proposed to describe the temporal relationship of depression and substance use disorders, and to address their causal relationship, including four primary hypotheses:

1. Depressive symptoms precede pathological substance use and the development of substance use disorders.
2. Substance use disorders precede the onset of depressive symptoms and the development of MDD.
3. The co-occurrence of MDD and substance use disorders is due to shared risk (or protective) factors.
4. Diagnostic criteria for MDD and substance use disorders share common features and symptoms. (Caron & Rutter, 1991)

Phenotypic Causation

The first two hypotheses are termed *phenotypic causation*, as one disorder contributes causally to the other. The first phenotypic causation hypothesis, that depressive symptoms precede the development of substance use disorders, is commonly explained in terms of *self-medication* (Khantzian, 1985). The self-medication hypothesis proposes that individuals experiencing symptoms of depression may use drugs and alcohol to alleviate, or cope with, their negative mood. The self-medication explanation implies that individuals will tend to select drugs that alleviate their specific psychiatric symptoms (Davis, Uezato, Newell, & Frazier, 2008; Markou, Kosten, & Koob, 1998; Quello, Brady, & Sonne, 2005). For example, it has been suggested that individuals experiencing depression may take stimulants (e.g., cocaine) for its energizing properties (Khantzian, 1985; Rounsaville, 2004; Weiss et al., 2007); however, few studies explicitly demonstrating this have been published. One study (Weiss et al., 2007) evaluated motivation for drug use and whether drug use alleviated a negative mood in 494 hospitalized drug abusers. This study found that most patients reported that they used drugs to alleviate symptoms of depression and did indeed experience mood elevation, regardless of their drug of choice. Further, the authors reported that drug use to relieve depressive symptoms was more common in men with MDD, but was equally common in women with and without MDD. Despite a number of studies documenting that relief of depressive symptoms motivates use of cannabis for many individuals (reviewed in Degenhardt, Hall, & Lynskey, 2003), little empirical data has demonstrated that cannabis use alleviates symptoms. One study that explicitly examined this reported that individuals with prior depression are more likely to experience specific *increases* of adverse depressive symptoms while under the influence of cannabis and are less likely to experience specific symptom relief (Arendt et al., 2007). These data suggest that the relationship between depressive symptoms and substance use is complex. Substances *have* been reported to initially decrease or moderate a depressed mood (Degenhardt et al., 2003; Weiss et al., 2007). However, chronic substance abuse and related withdrawal symptoms typically exacerbate depressive (and other psychiatric) symptoms (Arendt et al., 2007). For some individuals, this leads to more substance use and, ultimately, substance use problems or the development of substance use disorders (Quello et al., 2005).

This pathway supports the second phenotypic causation hypothesis, which suggests that depressive symptoms develop in response to the toxic effects of substances when used chronically (i.e., ethanol, cannabis, opioids), or that depressive symptoms themselves are effects of substance withdrawal. For example, alcohol itself can produce negative mood states, especially when consumed in high doses (reviewed in Rohsenow & Howland, 2010). In individuals predisposed to depression (either via genetic or social risk factors), these effects may trigger the expression of depressive symptoms (Wu et al., 2008). Drug addiction has been described by Koob and Le Moal (2005) as a chronically relapsing disorder characterized by a compulsion to seek and take the drug, loss of control in limiting intake, and emergence of a negative emotional state when access to the drug is prevented. The development of the negative emotional state that drives the negative reinforcement of addiction has been defined as the "dark side" of addiction (Koob & Le Moal, 2005) and comprises the *withdrawal / negative affect* stage, consisting of key elements such as chronic irritability, emotional pain, malaise, dysphoria, alexithymia, and loss of motivation for natural rewards (i.e., depressive symptomology). This behavior is observed in animals during withdrawal from all major drugs of abuse (Koob, 2015). Relatedly, depressive symptoms may arise in response to negative psychosocial consequences associated with excessive substance use such as partner or family member's disapproval or loss of employment due to excessive substance use. These life stressors associated with substance abuse may lead to elevations in stress hormones and, consequently, activate brain regions related to negative moods (Childs, O'Connor, & de Wit, 2011; King & Chassin, 2008; Schuckit, Smith, & Kalmijn,

2013). One way to address phenotypic causation is to study the temporal pattern of onset. If the self-medication hypothesis holds, the onset of depressive symptoms should precede increases in substance use and the onset of substance use disorder symptoms. If depressive symptoms are a consequence of excessive substance use, the onset of substance use disorder symptoms should precede the onset of depressive symptoms.

Cross-Sectional Studies

The temporal relationship of substance use disorders and major depression has been examined in several studies, with results showing evidence for both temporal patterns (Deykin et al., 1987; Gratzer et al., 2004). In an early cross-sectional study of college students, Deykin and colleagues (1987) found that the onset of major depression almost always preceded alcohol or substance abuse, supporting the self-medication hypothesis. Further support came from a retrospective, case-control assessment of the drug and depression history of depressed outpatients (Abraham & Fava, 1999), which demonstrated that cocaine dependence occurred about seven years after the first major depressive episode and alcohol dependence about five years after the onset of depression. This led to the conclusion that depression preceded cocaine and alcohol use in this sample, and conformed to a pattern of self-medication. In contrast, data from the Collaborative Study on the Genetics of Alcoholism found that about half of the lifetime depressive episodes in this sample appeared to be substance-induced major depressive episodes (Schuckit, Anthenelli, Bucholz, Hesselbrock, & Tipp, 1995); substance use preceded depression and conformed to the alternative pattern of phenotypic causation (i.e., major depression may develop in reaction to the toxic and depressogenic effects of substances). Further supporting this hypothesis, Hasin and Grant (2002) examined former drinkers from the NLAES that were divided into those with and without past alcohol dependence and were compared on the presence of current MDD. Prior alcohol dependence increased the risk of current major depression more than fourfold. In summary, cross-sectional studies have shown that substance use is associated with increased risk for depressed mood (Abraham & Fava, 1999; Holahan, Moos, Holahan, Cronkite, & Randall, 2003) *and* that chronic substance use has been shown to enhance risk for depression (Schuckit et al., 1997). Further, some studies have shown that there is no evidence that a particular temporal order is more common (Hodgins, el-Guebaly, Armstrong, & Dufour, 1999). This mixed literature led researchers to conduct longitudinal studies that could verify the temporal associations between comorbid disorders, rather than relying on retrospective reports of depressive and substance use pathology assessed in cross-sectional studies.

Longitudinal Studies

Longitudinal studies, or studies that assess the same individual over a given period of time, typically calculate the odds of an onset of one disorder, given lifetime history of another. For example, in an ECA study, two waves of data on 14,480 individuals were used to estimate the odds of either major depression or alcohol dependence being followed by the other disorder after a one-year period. Major depression was associated with symptoms of alcohol dependence at baseline (Odds Ratio: 1.2–4.3), with significantly higher odds observed for females. Conversely, odds ratios indicating the one-year follow-up risk of incident alcohol dependence with depressive symptomatology at baseline were 1.5–7.9, with significantly higher odds for females. These results suggest that both alcohol dependence and major depression pose a significant risk for the development of the other disorder at one year (Gilman & Abraham, 2001). Several recent studies conducted in the NESARC examined the associations between symptomology at Wave 1 (data that was collected in 2001–2002) and Wave 2 (data that was collected in 2004–2005). Two studies assessed whether self-medication of mood disorder symptoms with drugs (Lazareck et al., 2012) and alcohol (Crum et al., 2013) at Wave 1 was associated with substance use disorder incidence and persistence at Wave 2. Both studies found an association of self-medication of mood disorder symptoms at Wave 1 with incident and persistent *DSM-IV* alcohol dependence at Wave 2 (Crum et al., 2013; Crum, Mojtabai, & Sareen, 2014; Lazareck et al., 2012). Pacek and colleagues (2013) found that cannabis use disorders measured in the NESARC Wave 1 were associated with major depression at Wave 2; the odds of having major depression at Wave 2 were about 1.7 for individuals who had a concurrent cannabis abuse diagnosis and about 8.4 for individuals with a cannabis dependence diagnosis at Wave 1. Additionally, positive relationships were observed between Wave 1 depression and cannabis abuse and dependence at Wave 2 (Odds: 2.01–2.67; Pacek et al., 2013). Another study found that those with Wave 1 nonmedical prescription opioid use had greater odds (Odds: 1.7) of having major depression at Wave 2 (Martins et al., 2012). A study from the Christchurch Health and Development Study, a 25-year longitudinal study of a birth cohort of children from New Zealand, found evidence that the association among alcohol abuse/dependence and depression is best explained by a causal model in which alcohol dependence leads to MDD (Fergusson, Boden, & Horwood, 2009). In a longitudinal study of 7,477 Virginia twins (Kuo, Gardner, Kendler, & Prescott, 2006), the age-of-onset distributions of alcohol dependence and major depression differed substantially. Most onsets of alcohol dependence were in young adulthood, whereas onsets of major depression occurred more widely across age. Most twins, especially women, had an onset of major depression preceding alcohol dependence; prior major depression significantly affected risk for developing alcohol dependence, and this risk decreased over time. By contrast, preceding alcohol dependence had negligible effects on the risk for future major depression. Further, this study showed that familial risk was transmitted within disorders but that there was little evidence of additional familial liability shared across disorders, which supports prior findings (Coryell, Winokur, Keller, Scheftner, & Endicott, 1992). Data drawn from a general outpatient population, the Midlife Development in the United States Survey

Waves I and II, was used to examine major depression and cigarette smoking relapse between 1994 and 2005 (Zvolensky, Bakhshaie, Sheffer, Perez, & Goodwin, 2015). Among former smokers, major depression in 1994 was associated with increased odds of smoking relapse by 2005. Further, major depression in 2005 was associated with an even greater risk of relapse within the same year, and depression that persisted from 1994 to 2005 was the greatest predictor of relapse by 2005. A meta-analysis by Boden and Fergusson (2011) examined the literature on the associations between alcohol use disorders and major depression to evaluate the evidence for the existence of a causal relationship between the disorders. The analysis revealed that the presence of either disorder doubled the risks of the second disorder. A large number of clinical trials have examined whether a history of depression is associated with poorer outcomes for substance use disorders treated in randomized clinical trials. As with the longitudinal studies described previously, the clinical trials literature also produces mixed results (Foulds, Adamson, Boden, Williman, & Mulder, 2015).

In summary, this literature has provided evidence for both phenotypic causation hypotheses. That is, some studies show that depressive symptoms precede substance use pathology, supporting the self-medication hypothesis, while other studies show that chronic substance use precedes the onset of depression, supporting the view that heavy substance use exacerbates underlying risk for depression. Further, some studies have shown that there is no evidence that a particular temporal order is more common. Taken together, this body of literature suggests that perhaps neither phenotypic causation hypothesis can fully explain this comorbidity. Alternatively, the mechanisms responsible for the substance use disorder–major depression relationship could vary across individuals and families and represent etiologically distinct subgroups.

Correlated Liability

One potential mechanism might be correlated liability (i.e., two disorders have shared or correlated risk factors), and the onset of an earlier disorder is an earlier manifestation of the liability that is expressed later as other disorder (Neale & Kendler, 1995). One way this hypothesis has been addressed is by examining the familial patterns of substance use disorders and major depression. Family studies use the relationships between individuals to extract information on the (latent) genetic and environmental influences on particular outcomes. Using this design, researchers have reported evidence for shared genetic and environmental liability among psychiatric and substance use disorders. If these two disorders share the same set of genetic or family environmental risk factors, the risk of substance use disorders in relatives of individuals with major depression would be increased, as would the risk of major depression in relatives of individuals with substance use disorders.

Both MDD and substance use disorders have strong familial components (Kendler, Davis, & Kessler, 1997; Kendler, Prescott, Myers, & Neale, 2003). Early family studies suggested that some degree of the transmissible risk for these disorders is shared (Coryell et al., 1992; Merikangas, Weissman, Prusoff, Pauls, & Leckman, 1985). More recently, large twin and family studies have explicitly examined the genetic overlap, or genetic correlation, between MDD and substance use disorders. For example, a study of 5,181 individuals from the Virginia Adult Twin Study of Psychiatric and Substance Use Disorders (Young-Wolff, Kendler, Sintov, & Prescott, 2009) found that the genetic correlation between major depression and alcohol dependence was ~0.20 in females and ~0.08 in males. Stated another way, among females in this sample, about 20% of the genetic variation that contributes to major depression also contributes to alcohol dependence, whereas about 8% of the genetic variation that contributes to major depression also contributes to alcohol dependence among males in this sample.

Other studies conducted in this sample have also demonstrated a shared genetic liability between depression and nicotine use outcomes (Edwards & Kendler, 2012; Edwards, Maes, Pedersen, & Kendler, 2011). In a study of 6,720 males from the Vietnam-Era Twin Registry, Fu and colleagues (2002) found evidence for shared genetic risk among major depression and alcohol dependence, and among major depression and cannabis dependence, some of which operated through genetic risk for antisocial personality disorder. In another study of this sample, a large portion of the genetic correlation between major depression and nicotine dependence was explained by genetic risk factors for conduct disorder (Fu et al., 2007). In addition, several studies have examined the association between specific genetic variants and comorbid depression and substance use outcomes. For example, in an analysis of adolescents aged 14–18 from the National Longitudinal Study of Adolescent Health, Bobadilla, Vaske, and Asberg (2013) found an association between a variant in a dopamine receptor gene (DRD4) and comorbid depression and cannabis abuse. Another study indicated that variation in the brain-derived neurotrophic factor moderated the association between depression severity and nicotine dependence in patients with a current diagnosis of depression or anxiety (Jamal, Van der Does, & Penninx, 2015). Recently, a genome-wide association study of individuals with both depression and alcohol dependence implicated several genes (CDH13, CSMD2, GRIN2, and HTR1B) that have been previously associated with depression, alcohol use disorders, or other addiction-related phenotypes (Edwards et al., 2012).

Cerdá and colleagues (2010) reviewed the genetic and environmental influences on psychiatric comorbidity, including depression and substance abuse, and identified several important social risk factors shared between these disorders. One clear risk factor for both major depression and substance use disorders is trauma exposure (Breslau, 2002; Fetzner, McMillan, Sareen, & Asmundson, 2011; Khoury, Tang, Bradley, Cubells, & Ressler, 2010; Scherrer et al., 2007). Exposure to childhood maltreatment (i.e., abuse, neglect) has been shown to increase risk for many psychiatric disorders, including depressive disorders (Bulik, Prescott, & Kendler, 2001; Kendler et al., 2000;

Widom, DuMont, & Czaja, 2007), alcohol use disorders (Clark, Lesnick, & Hegedus, 1997; Fenton et al., 2013; Fergusson, Boden, & Horwood, 2008; Kendler et al., 2000), and drug use disorders (Afifi, Henriksen, Asmundson, & Sareen, 2012; Clark et al., 1997; Kendler et al., 2000). A 2014 study of individuals in substance use treatment found that higher rates of childhood trauma exposure were associated with elevated rates of depressive disorders, alcohol dependence, and cocaine dependence. Importantly, this study also reported that higher rates of all comorbidity patterns (e.g., comorbid alcohol dependence and depression) were observed among individuals who reported experiencing child abuse (Banducci, Hoffman, Lejuez, & Koenen, 2014). There is also evidence that exposure to trauma in other stages of the life-course increases risk for depression and substance use disorders. Research that examines populations exposed to collective traumas (e.g., terrorist attacks, natural disasters, and war or combat exposure) consistently finds elevated rates of depression and substance use disorders, as well as posttraumatic stress disorder (PTSD) (Bremner, Southwick, Darnell, & Charney, 1996; McCall-Hosenfeld, Mukherjee, & Lehman, 2014; Neria, DiGrande, & Adams, 2011; Norman, Tate, Anderson, & Brown, 2007; Perlman et al., 2011; Rohrbach, Grana, Vernberg, Sussman, & Sun, 2009; Scherrer et al., 2007). For example, a study of all Army soldiers and Marines who completed the routine postdeployment health assessment in 2003 and 2004 on return from deployment to Operation Enduring Freedom in Afghanistan (n = 16,318), Operation Iraqi Freedom (n = 222,620), and other locations (n = 64,967) examined the mental health and service utilization after deployment. This study found that the prevalence of reporting a mental health problem was 19.1% among service members returning from Iraq compared with 11.3% after returning from Afghanistan and 8.5% after returning from other locations; among the most prevalent mental health problems reported were PTSD, depression, and an alcohol or substance use problem (Hoge, Auchterlonie, & Milliken, 2006).

Other risk factors that have been shown to contribute both to depression and substance use disorder risk involve the quality of the family and peer environments (Aseltine, Gore, & Colten, 1998; Kim, Capaldi, & Stoolmiller, 2003; Windle & Davies, 1999; Wu et al., 2006), as well as economic circumstances (Cerdá et al., 2010; de Graaf, Bijl, ten Have, Beekman, & Vollerbergh, 2004; McGee, Williams, Poulton, & Moffitt, 2000). For example, in a study that followed 1,208 adolescents, low family support and high peer pressure differentiated adolescents with comorbid depression and substance abuse from those with depression only. In addition, low levels of family and friend support differentiated adolescents with comorbid depression and substance abuse from those with substance use pathology only (Aseltine et al., 1998). In a sample of 4,796 adults followed for three years, unemployment was the only risk factor that differentiated individuals with substance use pathology and mood disorders (including anxiety and depression) from individuals with mood disorders and no substance use pathology (de Graaf et al., 2004).

Overlap of Diagnostic Criteria

In the *DSM-IV*, two main substance use disorders are included—abuse and dependence. The *DSM-IV* dependence diagnosis includes seven criteria, one of which is withdrawal. *DSM-IV* symptoms of withdrawal from *any* substance include: anxiety, insomnia, vivid or unpleasant dreams, hallucinations, restlessness, shaking, depressed mood, hypersomnia, psychomotor retardation, feeling weak or tired, bad headaches, muscle cramps, runny eyes or nose, yawning, nausea, sweating, fever, and seizures. Several of these criteria (depressed mood, changes in sleep, changes in activity, fatigue or loss of energy) directly overlap with symptoms of MDD. While clinicians are trained to explicitly screen for conditions that may mimic the primary diagnosis (i.e., MDD or substance use disorder), these unclear diagnostic boundaries may contribute to the common co-occurrence of MDD and substance use disorders. In response to concern regarding the reliability of psychiatric diagnoses (i.e., depression) for individuals who drink heavily or use drugs, the Psychiatric Research Interview for Substance and Mental Disorders (PRISM) was designed to improve the reliability for individuals who heavily use substances and may have substance use problems. A 1996 study reported good to excellent test-retest reliability for the PRISM depression and substance use disorder diagnoses (Hasin et al., 1996). In 2006, Hasin and colleagues used the PRISM adopted for *DSM-IV* diagnoses (PRISM-IV) to test the reliability of *DSM-IV*-defined disorders, including primary and substance-induced disorders, in 285 substance-abusing subjects from substance abuse or dual-diagnosis treatment settings and mental health treatment settings. Kappas for primary and substance-induced *DSM-IV* MDD ranged from 0.66 to 0.75, indicating that most *DSM-IV* psychiatric disorders can be assessed in substance-abusing subjects with acceptable to excellent reliability by using specifically designed procedures.

The Dimensional Metastructure

The phenomenon of comorbidity poses a serious challenge to traditional psychiatric classification systems such as the DSM, which conceptualize mental disorders as discrete disorders. Factor analytic studies have characterized observed co-occurrence among common mental disorders in terms of two correlated but distinct factors: *internalizing disorders*, subsuming two related subdimensions of "fear" and "anxious-misery," and *externalizing disorders*. This metastructure has been replicated across a variety of populations across numerous studies (Eaton et al., 2013; Kendler et al., 2003; Kotov et al., 2011; Krueger, 1999; Slade & Watson, 2006; Vollebergh et al., 2001).

Recent studies have expanded our understanding of the metastructure by including additional psychiatric disorders (i.e., thought disorders; Keyes et al., 2013; Kotov et al., 2011) and examining whether the association of risk factors with individual psychiatric disorders could be better expressed in terms of the latent internalizing or externalizing dimensions (Keyes et al., 2012; Meyers et al., 2015). For example, an analysis of the NESARC indicated that the association of childhood maltreatment and individual psychiatric disorders is fully mediated by these latent liability dimensions, with an impact on underlying liability levels to internalizing and externalizing psychopathology rather than specific psychiatric disorders (Keyes et al., 2012). This body of research has both etiologic and clinical implications that challenge the current conceptualization of psychopathology as consisting of specific, individual psychiatric or substance use disorders. These disorders, including MDD and substance use disorders, show considerable comorbidity due to shared variance at an underlying (i.e., latent) level. It has been suggested that clinicians may better serve patients with comorbid mood and substance use disorders if their comorbidity is seen as an indication of high internal (INT) and external (EXT) dimension levels, rather than as multiple specific disorders (Eaton et al., 2015; Livesley, 2008). Additionally, clinical interventions could focus on a cluster of symptoms and behavioral problems instead of using treatments tailored for one particular disorder. Further, research on the etiology of MDD and substance use disorders could focus on understanding genetic and environmental predispositions toward INT and EXT as well as the additional specific factors that may determine how this liability is expressed for each individual (Kendler et al., 2008; Torgersen et al., 2008).

One limitation of this factor analytic approach is that the basis of the moderately large correlation between factors of internalizing and externalizing (i.e., the sources of overlap between disorders in one domain and the other) remains unclear. A complementary approach that has been utilized by researchers in examining comorbidity is *latent-class analysis*. This approach models disorders (that are modeled as dimensions in the metastructure approach) based on "classes" or groups of individuals, rather than as latent dimensions. Modeling data in this manner would help reveal if there are particular patterns among individuals who had comorbid internalizing (e.g., MDD) and externalizing (e.g., substance use disorders) disorders. A 2011 study by Vaidyanathan, Patrick, and Iacono utilized latent-class analysis to characterize patterns of comorbidity exhibited by individuals in two large-scale epidemiological cohorts, the NCS and the NCS-R. The two samples indicated five latent classes exhibiting distinctive profiles of diagnostic comorbidity: (1) a fear class (all phobias and panic disorder), (2) a distress class (including depression, generalized anxiety disorder, and dysthymia), (3) an externalizing class (including alcohol, drug dependence, and conduct disorder), (4) a multimorbid class (highly elevated rates of all disorders), and (5) a few disorders class (very low probability of all disorders). The authors concluded that comorbidity among mental disorders in the general population appears to occur in a finite number of distinct patterns, which can aid in research directed at elucidating the comorbidity of mental disorders. Converging evidence from these alternative approaches increases confidence in the validity of two related internalizing and externalizing dimensions of psychopathology.

Clinical Implications

There are important clinical implications of the epidemiologic research presented in this chapter. Depressive disorders are common in individuals who use alcohol and drugs, especially in those seeking substance abuse treatment. Further, the previous assumptions that depressive symptoms in those with substance use disorders are only an artifact of misdiagnosed intoxication or withdrawal seem unlikely (Hasin & Grant, 2002). Therefore, in the context of traditional psychiatric classification systems such as the DSM, which conceptualizes mental disorders as discrete disorders, the comorbidity of major depression and substance use disorders presents a diagnostic dilemma: is the substance use disorder or the depressive disorder the primary disorder to treat?

The traditional solution is to this dilemma to withhold treatment for depression for a period of time after abstinence is established (usually one month minimum) in order to determine if depressive symptoms are attributable to substance use. However, patients experiencing depression may be unable to establish or sustain abstinence for a month or longer (Aharonovich, Liu, Nunes, & Hasin, 2002; Greenfield et al., 1998; Hasin et al., 2002; Kiefer et al., 2003). For example, a 2003 study found that following inpatient alcohol detoxification, 65% of untreated subjects had consumed alcohol and 50% had returned to heavy drinking within two weeks of discharge (Kiefer et al., 2003). Another study followed patients hospitalized for alcohol dependence for one year after discharge and found that those with major depression at hospitalization entry had a shorter time to first drink and a shorter time to full relapse following discharge (Greenfield et al., 1998). Further, Hasin and colleagues (2002) followed 250 patients hospitalized for cocaine, heroin, or alcohol dependence at 6, 12, and 18 months after discharge, approximately 60% of whom were diagnosed with co-occurring depression. Depressed patients were retrospectively classified into three subgroups: (1) those with major depression prior to the diagnosis of substance use disorder, (2) those meeting criteria for major depression during sustained abstinence during follow-up, or (3) those considered to have exclusively substance-induced depression. Those with premorbid major depression or substance-induced depression (groups 1 and 3) were significantly more likely to meet criteria for substance dependence during the follow-up period. Of the patients who did not use any substances for at least 26 consecutive weeks, those who experienced a major depressive episode during this time were subsequently three times as likely to relapse into dependence during the follow-up period (Hasin et al., 2002). This research demonstrates the difficulty that depressed patients may have abstaining from substance use and suggests that delaying treatment for major depression symptoms until abstinence is achieved may not be the most appropriate course of treatment. Therefore, clinicians in addiction treatment settings must address co-occurring depressive disorders, and clinicians in primary care and mental health settings should assess problematic substance use behavior. However, research guiding clinical decision-making in co-occurring depressive and substance use disorders has been limited. Tolliver and Anton (2015) recently reviewed the existing research and identified several outstanding questions regarding the treatment of individuals with comorbid major depression or substance use disorder diagnoses. They concluded that because individuals with substance use disorders are traditionally excluded from clinical trials for major depression, and likewise most clinical trials of treating substance use disorders exclude other psychiatric conditions, there is limited empirical data to answer questions such as, Can depression be treated successfully in patients who continue to drink or use drugs heavily? Conversely, can patients with severe substance use disorders establish and maintain sobriety without adequate treatment of depression? Can any individual medications effectively treat both conditions, or are combinations of medicines necessary?

In the United States, psychosocial counseling, usually in a combination of group and individual settings, has traditionally been the most common form of substance use disorder treatment. Over the past decade, development of integrated group therapy has shown efficacy in treating individuals with comorbid substance use disorders and mood disorders (Weiss et al., 2007). In addition, established behavioral approaches such as contingency management have been applied to individuals with co-occurring substance use disorders and mood disorders. For example, a randomized controlled design was used to compare outcomes of outpatients with a psychiatric disorder *and* a stimulant use disorder. Although participants in the contingency management condition (three months of contingency management for stimulant abstinence in addition to treatment as usual) were significantly less likely to complete the treatment period than those assigned to the control condition (treatment as usual), they had large reductions in stimulant, injection drug, and alcohol use, with additional benefits for reductions in psychiatric symptoms and hospitalizations (McDonell et al., 2013).

In the case of patients with major depression and comorbid substance use disorders, the majority of previous treatment research has focused on the use of antidepressants. A 2004 meta-analysis by Nunes and Levin (2004) found that of clinical research focusing on comorbid substance use disorders and mood disorders conducted at the time, only one-third (14 of 44) of studies met criteria as adequately placebo-controlled, double-blind, randomized prospective clinical trials. This meta-analysis found evidence for modest treatment effects of antidepressants on mood symptoms in depressed individuals with substance use disorders. Pettinati (2004) reported similar findings in a review of antidepressant trials in depressed individuals with alcohol use disorder, with 75% of the trials finding benefit for reduction of depressive symptoms but only a few studies reporting treatment effects on drinking outcomes. Pettinati and colleagues (2010) reported a significant effect of the combination of sertraline (FDA-approved antidepressant) with the opioid antagonist naltrexone (FDA-approved medication for the treatment of alcohol dependence) in reducing drinking in depressed alcohol-dependent subjects. In this trial, subjects were randomized to sertraline, naltrexone, the combination of sertraline plus naltrexone, or double placebo for 14 weeks while receiving weekly cognitive behavioral therapy. The group receiving the combination of sertraline and naltrexone had a significantly higher rate of abstinence and longer delay to relapse to heavy drinking, and nominally (although not statistically significant) fewer depression symptoms (Pettinati et al., 2010). In another comorbid alcohol dependence and major depression study, Moak and colleagues (2003) found that sertraline in combination with cognitive behavioral therapy reduced drinking and depression in women. These dual-diagnosis treatment research studies are especially important in informing clinical practice for treating individuals with both major depression and substance use disorders.

Conclusion

Co-occurring mood disorders and substance use disorders are common, and tend to have an adverse impact on both mood and substance use outcomes. Diagnostic challenges remain, though longitudinal, clinical, and epidemiological studies conducted over the past two decades have begun to elucidate the prevalence and course of independent versus substance-induced mood disorders in patients with substance use disorders, and have begun to pose questions about the appropriate course of treatment in these patients. Therefore, further research on prognosis and treatment of comorbid depression and substance use disorders is needed.

References

Abraham, H. D., & Fava, M. (1999). Order of onset of substance abuse and depression in a sample of depressed outpatients. *Comprehensive Psychiatry, 40*(1), 44–50.

Afifi, T. O., Henriksen, C. A., Asmundson, G. J. G., & Sareen, J. (2012). Childhood maltreatment and substance use disorders among men and women in a nationally representative sample. *Canadian Journal of Psychiatry: Revue Canadienne de Psychiatrie, 57*(11), 677–686.

Aharonovich, E., Liu, X., Nunes, E., & Hasin, D. S. (2002). Suicide attempts in substance abusers: Effects of major depression in relation to substance use disorders. *American Journal of Psychiatry, 159*(9), 1600–1602.

Arendt, M., Rosenberg, R., Fjordback, L., Brandholdt, J., Foldager, L., Sher, L., & Munk-Jørgensen, P. (2007). Testing the self-medication hypothesis of depression and aggression in cannabis-dependent subjects. *Psychological Medicine, 37*(7), 935–945.

Aseltine, R. H., Gore, S., & Colten, M. E. (1998). The co-occurrence of depression and substance abuse in late adolescence. *Development and Psychopathology, 10*(3), 549–570.

Banducci, A. N., Hoffman, E., Lejuez, C. W., & Koenen, K. C. (2014). The relationship between child abuse and negative outcomes among substance users: Psychopathology, health, and comorbidities. *Addictive Behaviors, 39*(10), 1522–1527.

Blanco, C., Rafful, C., Wall, M. M., Ridenour, T. A., Wang, S., & Kendler, K. S. (2014). Towards a comprehensive developmental model of cannabis use disorders. *Addiction, 109*(2), 284–294.

Bobadilla, L., Vaske, J., & Asberg, K. (2013). Dopamine receptor (D4) polymorphism is related to comorbidity between marijuana abuse and depression. *Addictive Behaviors, 38*(10), 2555–2562.

Boden, J. M., & Fergusson, D. M. (2011). Alcohol and depression. *Addiction, 106*(5), 906–914.

Bremner, J. D., Southwick, S. M., Darnell, A., & Charney, D. S. (1996). Chronic PTSD in Vietnam combat veterans: Course of illness and substance abuse. *American Journal of Psychiatry, 153*(3), 369–375.

Breslau, N. (2002). Epidemiologic studies of trauma, posttraumatic stress disorder, and other psychiatric disorders. *Canadian Journal of Psychiatry: Revue Canadienne de Psychiatrie, 47*(10), 923–929.

Breslau, N., Kilbey, M., & Andreski, P. (1991). Nicotine dependence, major depression, and anxiety in young adults. *Archives of General Psychiatry, 48*(12), 1069–1074.

Breslau, N., Novak, S. P., & Kessler, R. C. (2004). Psychiatric disorders and stages of smoking. *Biological Psychiatry, 55*(1), 69–76.

Bulik, C. M., Prescott, C. A., & Kendler, K. S. (2001). Features of childhood sexual abuse and the development of psychiatric and substance use disorders. *British Journal of Psychiatry, 179*, 444–449.

Burns, L., & Teesson, M. (2002). Alcohol use disorders comorbid with anxiety, depression and drug use disorders: Findings from the Australian National Survey of Mental Health and Well Being. *Drug and Alcohol Dependence, 68*(3), 299–307.

Caron, C., & Rutter, M. (1991). Comorbidity in child psychopathology: Concepts, issues and research strategies. *Journal of Child Psychology and Psychiatry, 32*(7), 1063–1080.

Cerdá, M., Sagdeo, A., Johnson, J., & Galea, S. (2010). Genetic and environmental influences on psychiatric comorbidity: A systematic review. *Journal of Affective Disorders, 126*(1–2), 14–38.

Childs, E., O'Connor, S., & de Wit, H. (2011). Bidirectional interactions between acute psychosocial stress and acute intravenous alcohol in healthy men. *Alcoholism, Clinical and Experimental Research, 35*(10), 1794–1803.

Clark, D. B., Lesnick, L., & Hegedus, A. M. (1997). Traumas and other adverse life events in adolescents with alcohol abuse and dependence. *Journal of the American Academy of Child and Adolescent Psychiatry, 36*(12), 1744–1751.

Compton, W. M., Conway, K. P., Stinson, F. S., & Grant, B. F. (2006). Changes in the prevalence of major depression and comorbid substance use disorders in the United States between 1991–1992 and 2001–2002. *American Journal of Psychiatry, 163*(12), 2141–2147.

Compton, W. M., Thomas, Y. F., Stinson, F. S., & Grant, B. F. (2007). Prevalence, correlates, disability, and comorbidity of DSM-IV drug abuse and dependence in the United States: Results from the National Epidemiologic Survey on Alcohol and Related Conditions. *Archives of General Psychiatry, 64*(5), 566–576.

Coryell, W., Winokur, G., Keller, M., Scheftner, W., & Endicott, J. (1992). Alcoholism and primary major depression: A family study approach to co-existing disorders. *Journal of Affective Disorders, 24*(2), 93–99.

Crum, R. M., Mojtabai, R., Lazareck, S., Bolton, J. M., Robinson, J., Sareen, J., . . . Storr, C. L. (2013). A prospective assessment of reports of drinking to self-medicate mood symptoms with the incidence and persistence of alcohol dependence. *JAMA Psychiatry, 70*(7), 718–726.

Crum, R. M., Mojtabai, R., & Sareen, J. (2014). Does self-medication predict the persistence or rather the recurrence of alcohol dependence?—Reply. *JAMA Psychiatry, 71*(2), 205–206.

Davis, L., Uezato, A., Newell, J. M., & Frazier, E. (2008). Major depression and comorbid substance use disorders. *Current Opinion in Psychiatry, 21*(1), 14–18.

Davis, L. L., Frazier, E. C., Gaynes, B. N., Trivedi, M. H., Wisniewski, S. R., Fava, M., . . . Rush, A. J. (2007). Are depressed outpatients with and without a family history of substance use disorder different? A baseline analysis of the STAR*D cohort. *Journal of Clinical Psychiatry, 68*(12), 1931–1938.

Davis, L. L., Frazier, E., Husain, M. M., Warden, D., Trivedi, M., Fava, M., . . . Rush, A. J. (2010). Substance use disorder comorbidity in major depressive disorder: A confirmatory analysis of the STAR*D cohort. *American Journal on Addictions, 15*(4), 278–285.

Davis, L. L., Rush, J. A., Wisniewski, S. R., Rice, K., Cassano, P., Jewell, M. E., . . . McGrath, P. J. (2005). Substance use disorder comorbidity in major depressive disorder: An exploratory analysis of the Sequenced Treatment Alternatives to Relieve Depression cohort. *Comprehensive Psychiatry, 46*(2), 81–89.

Degenhardt, L., Hall, W., & Lynskey, M. (2003). Exploring the association between cannabis use and depression. *Addiction, 98*(11), 1493–1504.

De Graaf, R., Bijl, R. V., ten Have, M., Beekman, A. T. F., & Vollebergh, W. A. M. (2004). Rapid onset of comorbidity of common mental disorders: Findings from the Netherlands Mental Health Survey and Incidence Study (NEMESIS). *Acta Psychiatrica Scandinavica, 109*(1), 55–63.

Deykin, E. Y., Levy, J. C., & Wells, V. (1987). Adolescent depression, alcohol and drug abuse. *American Journal of Public Health, 77*(2), 178–182.

Drake, R. E., Price, J. L., & Drake, R. E. (1996). Helping depressed clients discover personal power. *Perspectives in Psychiatric Care, 32*(4), 30–35.

Eaton, N. R., Keyes, K. M., Krueger, R. F., Noordhof, A., Skodol, A. E., Markon, K. E., . . . Hasin, D. S. (2013). Ethnicity and psychiatric comorbidity in a national sample: Evidence for latent comorbidity factor invariance and connections with disorder prevalence. *Social Psychiatry and Psychiatric Epidemiology, 48*(5), 701–710.

Eaton, N. R., Rodriguez-Seijas, C., Carragher, N., & Krueger, R. F. (2015). Transdiagnostic factors of psychopathology and substance use disorders: A review. *Social Psychiatry and Psychiatric Epidemiology, 50*(2), 171–182.

Edwards, A. C., Aliev, F., Bierut, L. J., Bucholz, K. K., Edenberg, H., Hesselbrock, V., . . . Dick, D. M. (2012). Genome-wide association study of comorbid depressive syndrome and alcohol dependence. *Psychiatric Genetics, 22*(1), 31–41.

Edwards, A. C., & Kendler, K. S. (2012). A twin study of depression and nicotine dependence: shared liability or causal relationship? *Journal of Affective Disorders, 142*(1–3), 90–97.

Edwards, A. C., Maes, H. H., Pedersen, N. L., & Kendler, K. S. (2011). A population-based twin study of the genetic and environmental relationship of major depression, regular tobacco use and nicotine dependence. *Psychological Medicine, 41*(2), 395–405.

Fava, M., Abraham, M., Alpert, J., Nierenberg, A. A., Pava, J. A., & Rosenbaum, J. F. (1996). Gender differences in Axis I comorbidity among depressed outpatients. *Journal of Affective Disorders, 38*(2–3), 129–133.

Fenton, M. C., Geier, T., Keyes, K., Skodol, A. E., Grant, B. F., & Hasin, D. S. (2013). Combined role of childhood maltreatment, family history, and gender in the risk for alcohol dependence. *Psychological Medicine, 43*(5), 1045–1057.

Fergusson, D. M., Boden, J. M., & Horwood, L. J. (2008). Exposure to childhood sexual and physical abuse and adjustment in early adulthood. *Child Abuse and Neglect, 32*(6), 607–619.

Fergusson, D. M., Boden, J. M., & Horwood, L. J. (2009). Tests of causal links between alcohol abuse or dependence and major depression. *Archives of General Psychiatry, 66*(3), 260–266.

Fetzner, M. G., McMillan, K. A., Sareen, J., & Asmundson, G. J. G. (2011). What is the association between traumatic life events and alcohol abuse/dependence in people with and without PTSD? Findings from a nationally representative sample. *Depression and Anxiety, 28*(8), 632–638.

Foulds, J. A., Adamson, S. J., Boden, J. M., Williman, J. A., & Mulder, R. T. (2015, October). Depression in patients with alcohol use disorders: Systematic review and meta-analysis of outcomes for independent and substance-induced disorders. *Journal of Affective Disorders, 185*, 47–59.

Fu, Q., Heath, A. C., Bucholz, K. K., Lyons, M. J., Tsuang, M. T., True, W. R., & Eisen, S. A. (2007). Common genetic risk of major depression and nicotine dependence: The contribution of antisocial traits in a United States veteran male twin cohort. *Twin Research and Human Genetics, 10*(3), 470–478.

Fu, Q., Heath, A. C., Bucholz, K. K., Nelson, E., Goldberg, J., Lyons, M. J., . . . Eisen, S. A. (2002). Shared genetic risk of major depression, alcohol dependence, and marijuana dependence: Contribution of antisocial personality disorder in men. *Archives of General Psychiatry, 59*(12), 1125–1132.

Gilman, S. E., & Abraham, H. D. (2001). A longitudinal study of the order of onset of alcohol dependence and major depression. *Drug and Alcohol Dependence, 63*(3), 277–286.

Goodwin, R. D., Zvolensky, M. J., Keyes, K. M., & Hasin, D. S. (2012). Mental disorders and cigarette use among adults in the United States. *American Journal on Addictions / American Academy of Psychiatrists in Alcoholism and Addictions, 21*(5), 416–423.

Grant, B. F. (1995). Comorbidity between *DSM-IV* drug use disorders and major depression: Results of a national survey of adults. *Journal of Substance Abuse, 7*(4), 481–497.

Grant, B. F. (1997). Prevalence and correlates of alcohol use and *DSM-IV* alcohol dependence in the United States: Results of the National Longitudinal Alcohol Epidemiologic Survey. *Journal of Studies on Alcohol, 58*(5), 464–473.

Grant, B. F., Dawson, D. A., Stinson, F. S., Chou, S. P., Dufour, M. C., & Pickering, R. P. (2004). The 12-month prevalence and trends in *DSM-IV* alcohol abuse and dependence: United States, 1991–1992 and 2001–2002. *Drug and Alcohol Dependence, 74*(3), 223–234.

Grant, B. F., Goldstein, R. B., Saha, T. D., Chou, S. P., Jung, J., Zhang, H., . . . Hasin, D. S. (2015). Epidemiology of *DSM-5* alcohol use disorder: Results from the National Epidemiologic Survey on Alcohol and Related Conditions III. *JAMA Psychiatry, 72*(8), 757–766.

Grant, B. F., & Harford, T. C. (1995). Comorbidity between *DSM-IV* alcohol use disorders and major depression: Results of a national survey. *Drug and Alcohol Dependence, 39*(3), 197–206.

Grant, B. F., & Pickering, R. (1998). The relationship between cannabis use and *DSM-IV* cannabis abuse and dependence: Results from the National Longitudinal Alcohol Epidemiologic Survey. *Journal of Substance Abuse, 10*(3), 255–264.

Grant, B. F., Stinson, F. S., Dawson, D. A., Chou, S. P., Dufour, M. C., Compton, W., . . . Kaplan, K. (2004). Prevalence and co-occurrence of substance use disorders and independent mood and anxiety disorders: Results from the National Epidemiologic Survey on Alcohol and Related Conditions. *Archives of General Psychiatry, 61*(8), 807–816.

Gratzer, D., Levitan, R. D., Sheldon, T., Toneatto, T., Rector, N. A., & Goering, P. (2004). Lifetime rates of alcoholism in adults with anxiety, depression, or co-morbid depression/anxiety: A community survey of Ontario. *Journal of Affective Disorders, 79*(1–3), 209–215.

Greenfield, S. F., Weiss, R. D., Muenz, L. R., Vagge, L. M., Kelly, J. F., Bello, L. R., & Michael, J. (1998). The effect of depression on return to drinking: A prospective study. *Archives of General Psychiatry, 55*(3), 259–265.

Hamdi, N. R., & Iacono, W. G. (2014). Lifetime prevalence and co-morbidity of externalizing disorders and depression in prospective assessment. *Psychological Medicine, 44*(2), 315–324.

Hasin, D., Endicott, J., & Lewis, C. (1985). Alcohol and drug abuse in patients with affective syndromes. *Comprehensive Psychiatry, 26*(3), 283–295.

Hasin, D. S., Goodwin, R. D., Stinson, F. S., & Grant, B. F. (2005). Epidemiology of major depressive disorder: Results from the National Epidemiologic Survey on Alcoholism and Related Conditions. *Archives of General Psychiatry, 62*(10), 1097–1106.

Hasin, D. S., & Grant, B. F. (2002). Major depression in 6050 former drinkers: Association with past alcohol dependence. *Archives of General Psychiatry, 59*(9), 794–800.

Hasin, D. S., & Grant, B. F. (2015). The National Epidemiologic Survey on Alcohol and Related Conditions (NESARC) Waves 1 and 2: Review and summary of findings. *Social Psychiatry and Psychiatric Epidemiology, 50*(11), 1609–1640.

Hasin, D., Liu, X., Nunes, E., McCloud, S., Samet, S., & Endicott, J. (2002). Effects of major depression on remission and relapse of substance dependence. *Archives of General Psychiatry, 59*(4), 375–380.

Hasin, D. S., O'Brien, C. P., Auriacombe, M., Borges, G., Bucholz, K., Budney, A., . . . Grant, B. F. (2013). *DSM-5* criteria for substance use disorders: Recommendations and rationale. *American Journal of Psychiatry, 170*(8), 834–851.

Hasin, D., Samet, S., Nunes, E., Meydan, J., Matseoane, K., & Waxman, R. (2006). Diagnosis of comorbid psychiatric disorders in substance users assessed with the Psychiatric Research Interview for Substance and Mental Disorders for *DSM-IV*. *American Journal of Psychiatry, 163*(4), 689–696.

Hasin, D. S., Stinson, F. S., Ogburn, E., & Grant, B. F. (2007). Prevalence, correlates, disability, and comorbidity of *DSM-IV* alcohol abuse and dependence in the United States: Results from the National Epidemiologic Survey on Alcohol and Related Conditions. *Archives of General Psychiatry, 64*(7), 830–842.

Hasin, D. S., Trautman, K. D., Miele, G. M., Samet, S., Smith, M., & Endicott, J. (1996). Psychiatric Research Interview for Substance and Mental Disorders (PRISM): Reliability for substance abusers. *American Journal of Psychiatry, 153*(9), 1195–1201.

Helzer, J. E., & Pryzbeck, T. R. (1988). The co-occurrence of alcoholism with other psychiatric disorders in the general population and its impact on treatment. *Journal of Studies on Alcohol, 49*(3), 219–224.

Hodgins, D. C., el-Guebaly, N., Armstrong, S., & Dufour, M. (1999). Implications of depression on outcome from alcohol dependence: A 3-year prospective follow-up. *Alcoholism, Clinical and Experimental Research, 23*(1), 151–157.

Hoge, C. W., Auchterlonie, J. L., & Milliken, C. S. (2006). Mental health problems, use of mental health services, and attrition from military service after returning from deployment to Iraq or Afghanistan. *JAMA, 295*(9), 1023–1032.

Holahan, C. J., Moos, R. H., Holahan, C. K., Cronkite, R. C., & Randall, P. K. (2003). Drinking to cope and alcohol use and abuse in unipolar depression: A 10-year model. *Journal of Abnormal Psychology, 112*(1), 159–165.

Jamal, M., Van der Does, W., & Penninx, B. W. J. H. (2015). Effect of variation in BDNF Val[66]Met polymorphism, smoking, and nicotine dependence on symptom severity of depressive and anxiety disorders. *Drug and Alcohol Dependence, 148*(1), 150–157.

Kendler, K. S., Aggen, S. H., Czajkowski, N., Røysamb, E., Tambs, K., Torgersen, S., . . . Reichborn-Kjennerud, T. (2008). The structure of genetic and environmental risk factors for *DSM-IV* personality disorders: A multivariate twin study. *Archives of General Psychiatry, 65*(12), 1438–1446.

Kendler, K. S., Bulik, C. M., Silberg, J., Hettema, J. M., Myers, J., & Prescott, C. A. (2000). Childhood sexual abuse and adult psychiatric and substance use disorders in women: An epidemiological and cotwin control analysis. *Archives of General Psychiatry, 57*(10), 953–959.

Kendler, K. S., Davis, C. G., & Kessler, R. C. (1997). The familial aggregation of common psychiatric and substance use disorders in the National Comorbidity Survey: A family history study. *British Journal of Psychiatry, 170*, 541–548.

Kendler, K. S., Prescott, C. A., Myers, J., & Neale, M. C. (2003). The structure of genetic and environmental risk factors for common psychiatric and substance use disorders in men and women. *Archives of General Psychiatry, 60*(9), 929–937.

Kessler, R. C., Berglund, P., Demler, O., Jin, R., Koretz, D., Merikangas, K. R., . . . Wang, P. S. (2003). The epidemiology of major depressive disorder: Results from the National Comorbidity Survey Replication (NCS-R). *JAMA, 289*(23), 3095–3105.

Kessler, R. C., Crum, R. M., Warner, L. A., Nelson, C. B., Schulenberg, J., & Anthony, J. C. (1997). Lifetime co-occurrence of *DSM-III-R* alcohol abuse and dependence with other psychiatric disorders in the National Comorbidity Survey. *Archives of General Psychiatry, 54*(4), 313–321.

Kessler, R. C., McGonagle, K. A., Zhao, S., Nelson, C. B., Hughes, M., Eshleman, S., . . . Kendler, K. S. (1994). Lifetime and 12-month prevalence of *DSM-III-R* psychiatric disorders in the United States: Results from the National Comorbidity Survey. *Archives of General Psychiatry, 51*(1), 8–19.

Kessler, R. C., Mickelson, K. D., & Williams, D. R. (1999). The prevalence, distribution, and mental health correlates of perceived discrimination in the United States. *Journal of Health and Social Behavior, 40*(3), 208–230.

Kessler, R. C., Nelson, C. B., McGonagle, K. A., Edlund, M. J., Frank, R. G., & Leaf, P. J. (1996a). The epidemiology of co-occurring addictive and mental disorders: Implications for prevention and service utilization. *American Journal of Orthopsychiatry, 66*(1), 17–31.

Kessler, R. C., Nelson, C. B., McGonagle, K. A., Liu, J., Swartz, M., & Blazer, D. G. (1996b). Comorbidity of *DSM-III-R* major depressive disorder in the general population: Results from the US National Comorbidity Survey. *British Journal of Psychiatry, 30*(suppl.), 17–30.

Keyes, K. M., Eaton, N. R., Krueger, R. F., McLaughlin, K. A., Wall, M. M., Grant, B. F., & Hasin, D. S. (2012). Childhood maltreatment and the structure of common psychiatric disorders. *British Journal of Psychiatry, 200*(2), 107–115.

Keyes, K. M., Eaton, N. R., Krueger, R. F., Skodol, A. E., Wall, M. M., Grant, B., . . . Hasin, D. S. (2013). Thought disorder in the meta-structure of psychopathology. *Psychological Medicine, 43*(8), 1673–1683.

Khantzian, E. J. (1985). The self-medication hypothesis of addictive disorders: Focus on heroin and cocaine dependence. *American Journal of Psychiatry, 142*(11), 1259–1264.

Khoury, L., Tang, Y. L., Bradley, B., Cubells, J. F., & Ressler, K. J. (2010). Substance use, childhood traumatic experience, and posttraumatic stress disorder in an urban civilian population. *Depression and Anxiety, 27*(12), 1077–1786.

Kiefer, F., Jahn, H., Tarnaske, T., Helwig, H., Briken, P., Holzbach, R., . . . Wiedemann, K. (2003). Comparing and combining naltrexone and acamprosate in relapse prevention of alcoholism: A double-blind, placebo-controlled study. *Archives of General Psychiatry, 60*(1), 92–99.

Kim, H. K., Capaldi, D. M., & Stoolmiller, M. (2003). Depressive symptoms across adolescence and young adulthood in men: Predictions from parental and contextual risk factors. *Development and Psychopathology, 15*(2), 469–495.

King, K. M., & Chassin, L. (2008). Adolescent stressors, psychopathology, and young adult substance dependence: A prospective study. *Journal of Studies on Alcohol and Drugs, 69*(5), 629–638.

Koob, G. F. (2015). The dark side of emotion: The addiction perspective. *European Journal of Pharmacology, 753*, 73–87.

Koob, G. F., & Le Moal, M. (2005). Plasticity of reward neurocircuitry and the "dark side" of drug addiction. *Nature Neuroscience, 8*(11), 1442–1444.

Kotov, R., Ruggero, C. J., Krueger, R. F., Watson, D., Yuan, Q., & Zimmerman, M. (2011). New dimensions in the quantitative classification of mental illness. *Archives of General Psychiatry, 68*(10), 1003–1011.

Krueger, R. F. (1999). The structure of common mental disorders. *Archives of General Psychiatry, 56*(10), 921–926.

Kuo, P.-H., Gardner, C. O., Kendler, K. S., & Prescott, C. A. (2006). The temporal relationship of the onsets of alcohol dependence and major depression: Using a genetically informative study design. *Psychological Medicine, 36*(8), 1153–1162.

Lazareck, S., Robinson, J. A., Crum, R. M., Mojtabai, R., Sareen, J., & Bolton, J. M. (2012). A longitudinal investigation of the role of self-medication in the development of comorbid mood and drug use disorders: Findings from the National Epidemiologic Survey on Alcohol and Related Conditions (NESARC). *Journal of Clinical Psychiatry, 73*(5), e588–e593.

Livesley, W. J. (2008). Research trends and directions in the study of personality disorder. *Psychiatric Clinics of North America, 31*(3), 545–559.

Lynskey, M. T. (1998). The comorbidity of alcohol dependence and affective disorders: Treatment implications. *Drug and Alcohol Dependence, 52*(3), 201–209.

Markou, A., Kosten, T. R., & Koob, G. F. (1998). Neurobiological similarities in depression and drug dependence: A self-medication hypothesis. *Neuropsychopharmacology, 18*(3), 135–174.

Martins, S. S., Fenton, M. C., Keyes, K. M., Blanco, C., Zhu, H., & Storr, C. L. (2012). Mood and anxiety disorders and their association with non-medical prescription opioid use and prescription opioid-use disorder: Longitudinal evidence from the National Epidemiologic Study on Alcohol and Related Conditions. *Psychological Medicine, 42*(6), 1261–1272.

McCall-Hosenfeld, J. S., Mukherjee, S., & Lehman, E. B. (2014). The prevalence and correlates of lifetime psychiatric disorders and trauma exposures in urban and rural settings: Results from the National Comorbidity Survey Replication (NCS-R). *PloS One, 9*(11), e112416.

McDermut, W., Mattia, J., & Zimmerman, M. (2001). Comorbidity burden and its impact on psychosocial morbidity in depressed outpatients. *Journal of Affective Disorders, 65*(3), 289–295.

McDonell, M. G., Srebnik, D., Angelo, F., McPherson, S., Lowe, J. M., Sugar, A., . . . Ries, R. K. (2013). Randomized controlled trial of contingency management for stimulant use in community mental health patients with serious mental illness. *American Journal of Psychiatry, 170*(1), 94–101.

McGee, R., Williams, S., Poulton, R., & Moffitt, T. (2000). A longitudinal study of cannabis use and mental health from adolescence to early adulthood. *Addiction, 95*(4), 491–503.

Merikangas, K. R., Weissman, M. M., Prusoff, B. A., Pauls, D. L., & Leckman, J. F. (1985). Depressives with secondary alcoholism: Psychiatric disorders in offspring. *Journal of Studies on Alcohol, 46*(3), 199–204.

Meyers, J. L., Lowe, S. R., Eaton, N. R., Krueger, R., Grant, B. F., & Hasin, D. (2015). Childhood maltreatment, 9/11 exposure, and latent dimensions of psychopathology: A test of stress sensitization. *Journal of Psychiatric Research, 68*, 337–345.

Miller, N. S., Klamen, D., Hoffmann, N. G., & Flaherty, J. A. (1996). Prevalence of depression and alcohol and other drug dependence in addictions treatment populations. *Journal of Psychoactive Drugs, 28*(2), 111–124.

Moak, D. H., Anton, R. F., Latham, P. K., Voronin, K. E., Waid, R. L., & Durazo-Arvizu, R. (2003). Sertraline and cognitive behavioral therapy for depressed alcoholics: Results of a placebo-controlled trial. *Journal of Clinical Psychopharmacology, 23*(6), 553–562.

Najt, P., Fusar-Poli, P., & Brambilla, P. (2011). Co-occurring mental and substance abuse disorders: A review on the potential predictors and clinical outcomes. *Psychiatry Research, 186*(2–3), 159–164.

Neale, M. C., & Kendler, K. S. (1995). Models of comorbidity for multifactorial disorders. *American Journal of Human Genetics, 57*(4), 935–953.

Neria, Y., DiGrande, L., & Adams, B. G. (2011). Posttraumatic stress disorder following the September 11, 2001, terrorist attacks: A review of the literature among highly exposed populations. *American Psychologist, 66*(6), 429–446.

Norman, S. B., Tate, S. R., Anderson, K. G., & Brown, S. A. (2007). Do trauma history and PTSD symptoms influence addiction relapse context? *Drug and Alcohol Dependence, 90*(1), 89–96.

Nunes, E. V., & Levin, F. R. (2004). Treatment of depression in patients with alcohol or other drug dependence: A meta-analysis. *JAMA, 291*(15), 1887–1896.

Pacek, L. R., Martins, S. S., & Crum, R. M. (2013). The bidirectional relationships between alcohol, cannabis, co-occurring alcohol and cannabis use disorders with major depressive disorder: Results from a national sample. *Journal of Affective Disorders, 148*(2–3), 188–195.

Perlman, S. E., Friedman, S., Galea, S., Nair, H. P., Eros-Sarnyai, M., Stellman, S. D., . . . Greene, C. M. (2011). Short-term and medium-term health effects of 9/11. *Lancet, 378*(9794), 925–934.

Pettinati, H. M. (2004). Antidepressant treatment of co-occurring depression and alcohol dependence. *Biological Psychiatry, 56*(10), 785–792.

Pettinati, H. M., Oslin, D. W., Kampman, K. M., Dundon, W. D., Xie, H., Gallis, T. L., . . . O'Brien, C. P. (2010). A double-blind, placebo-controlled trial combining sertraline and naltrexone for treating co-occurring depression and alcohol dependence. *American Journal of Psychiatry, 167*(6), 668–675.

Quello, S. B., Brady, K. T., & Sonne, S. C. (2005). Mood disorders and substance use disorder: A complex comorbidity. *Science and Practice Perspectives, 3*(1), 13–21.

Regier, D. A., Farmer, M. E., Rae, D. S., Locke, B. Z., Keith, S. J., Judd, L. L., & Goodwin, F. K. (1990). Comorbidity of mental disorders with alcohol and other drug abuse. Results from the Epidemiologic Catchment Area (ECA) study. *JAMA, 264*(19), 2511–2518.

Rohrbach, L. A., Grana, R., Vernberg, E., Sussman, S., & Sun, P. (2009). Impact of hurricane Rita on adolescent substance use. *Psychiatry, 72*(3), 222–237.

Rohsenow, D. J., & Howland, J. (2010). The role of beverage congeners in hangover and other residual effects of alcohol intoxication: A review. *Current Drug Abuse Reviews, 3*(2), 76–79.

Rounsaville, B. J. (2004). Treatment of cocaine dependence and depression. *Biological Psychiatry, 56*(10), 803–809.

Saunders, J. B., Schuckit, M. A., Sirovatka, P., & Regier, D. A. (Eds.). (2007). *Diagnostic issues in substance use disorders: Refining the research agenda for* DSM-V. Arlington, VA: American Psychiatric Publishing.

Scherrer, J. F., Xian, H., Lyons, M. J., Goldberg, J., Eisen, S. A., True, W. R., . . . Koenen, K. C. (2007). Posttraumatic stress disorder; combat exposure; and nicotine dependence, alcohol dependence, and major depression in male twins. *Comprehensive Psychiatry, 49*(3), 297–304.

Schuckit, M. A., Anthenelli, R. M., Bucholz, K. K., Hesselbrock, V. M., & Tipp, J. (1995). The time course of development of alcohol-related problems in men and women. *Journal of Studies on Alcohol, 56*(2), 218–225.

Schuckit, M. A., Smith, T. L., & Kalmijn, J. (2013). Relationships among independent major depressions, alcohol use, and other substance use and related problems over 30 years in 397 families. *Journal of Studies on Alcohol and Drugs, 74*(2), 271–279.

Schuckit, M. A., Tipp, J. E., Bergman, M., Reich, W., Hesselbrock, V. M., & Smith, T. L. (1997). Comparison of induced and independent major depressive disorders in 2,945 alcoholics. *American Journal of Psychiatry, 154*(7), 948–957.

Schuckit, M. A., Tsuang, J. W., Anthenelli, R. M., Tipp, J. E., & Nurnberger, J. I. (1996). Alcohol challenges in young men from alcoholic pedigrees and control families: A report from the COGA project. *Journal of Studies on Alcohol, 57*(4), 368–377.

Slade, T., & Watson, D. (2006). The structure of common *DSM-IV* and *ICD-10* mental disorders in the Australian general population. *Psychological Medicine, 36*(11), 1593–1600.

Swendsen, J. D., Merikangas, K. R., Canino, G. J., Kessler, R. C., Rubio-Stipec, M., & Angst, J. (1998). The comorbidity of alcoholism with anxiety and depressive disorders in four geographic communities. *Comprehensive Psychiatry, 39*(4), 176–184.

Tolliver, B. K., & Anton, R. F. (2015). Assessment and treatment of mood disorders in the context of substance abuse. *Dialogues in Clinical Neuroscience, 17*(2), 181–190.

Torgersen, S., Czajkowski, N., Jacobson, K., Reichborn-Kjennerud, T., Røysamb, E., Neale, M. C., & Kendler, K. S. (2008). Dimensional representations of *DSM-IV* cluster B personality disorders in a population-based sample of Norwegian twins: A multivariate study. *Psychological Medicine, 38*(11), 1617–1625.

Vaidyanathan, U., Patrick, C. J., & Iacono, W. G. (2011). Patterns of comorbidity among mental disorders: A person-centered approach. *Comprehensive Psychiatry, 52*(5), 527–535.

Vollebergh, W. A., Iedema, J., Bijl, R. V., de Graaf, R., Smit, F., & Ormel, J. (2001). The structure and stability of common mental disorders: The NEMESIS study. *Archives of General Psychiatry, 58*(6), 597–603.

Weiss, R. D., Griffin, M. L., Kolodziej, M. E., Greenfield, S. F., Najavits, L. M., Daley, D. C., . . . Hennen, J. A. (2007). A randomized trial of integrated group therapy versus group drug counseling for patients with bipolar disorder and substance dependence. *American Journal of Psychiatry, 164*(1), 100–107.

Widom, C. S., DuMont, K., & Czaja, S. J. (2007). A prospective investigation of major depressive disorder and comorbidity in abused and neglected children grown up. *Archives of General Psychiatry, 64*(1), 49–56.

Windle, M., & Davies, P. T. (1999). Depression and heavy alcohol use among adolescents: Concurrent and prospective relations. *Development and Psychopathology, 11*(4), 823–844.

Wu, L. T., Kouzis, A. C., & Leaf, P. J. (1999). Influence of comorbid alcohol and psychiatric disorders on utilization of mental health services in the National Comorbidity Survey. *American Journal of Psychiatry, 156*(8), 1230–1236.

Wu, P., Bird, H. R., Liu, X., Fan, B., Fuller, C., Shen, S., . . . Canino, G. J. (2006). Childhood depressive symptoms and early onset of alcohol use. *Pediatrics, 118*(5), 1907–1915.

Wu, P., Hoven, C. W., Liu, X., Fuller, C. J., Fan, B., Musa, G., . . . Cook, J. A. (2008). The relationship between depressive symptom levels and subsequent increases in substance use among youth with severe emotional disturbance. *Journal of Studies on Alcohol and Drugs, 69*(4), 520–527.

Young-Wolff, K. C., Kendler, K. S., Sintov, N. D., & Prescott, C. A. (2009). Mood-related drinking motives mediate the familial association between major depression and alcohol dependence. *Alcoholism, Clinical and Experimental Research, 33*(8), 1476–1486.

Zimmerman, M., Chelminski, I., & McDermut, W. (2002). Major depressive disorder and Axis I diagnostic comorbidity. *Journal of Clinical Psychiatry, 63*(3), 187–193.

Zvolensky, M. J., Bakhshaie, J., Sheffer, C., Perez, A., & Goodwin, R. D. (2015). Major depressive disorder and smoking relapse among adults in the United States: A 10-year, prospective investigation. *Psychiatry Research, 226*(1), 73–77.

PART II **INFLUENCES**

CHAPTER 6

The Social Epidemiology of Socioeconomic Inequalities in Depression

Helen Cerigo, MSc
Amélie Quesnel-Vallée, PhD

Social determinants of health have been brought to the forefront in recent years with the World Health Organization calling for broad action to achieve health equity (CSDH, 2008). Social inequalities in health have been defined as disparities in health status across different socioeconomic groups. These inequalities are considered unjust because they are created and maintained by societal processes, structures, and institutions (Krieger, 2001). Social inequalities in mental health have been a long-standing interest among sociologists, psychiatrists, and epidemiologists. As with physical health, an inverse relationship between socioeconomic status (SES) and mental health has been consistently and systematically documented (Lorant et al., 2003). In particular, understanding and acting on social inequalities in depression is becoming increasingly important, given how common and disabling the disease can be (Wells et al., 1989). A recent review reported that country-specific lifetime prevalence rates of major depression ranged from 2.0% to 17.1%, with the highest rates in Europe, the Americas, and Australasia (Hasin, Fenton, & Weissman, 2011). Further, it is estimated that by 2030, the leading cause of disability-adjusted life years in high-income countries will be unipolar depressive disorders (Mathers & Loncar, 2005). Yet, although evidence-based clinical solutions exist, access to and quality of mental health services are found to be lagging in most developed countries, notably because of cost barriers (London School of Economics and Political Science, 2006).

In this chapter, we provide an overview of the epidemiology of social inequalities in depression and an exploration of the pathways by which these inequalities are manifested. Indeed, as a relatively recent and authoritative meta-analysis exists on this topic, this chapter does not aim to be a systematic review but rather presents a narrative review aiming at a critical assessment of the literature with the goal to identify knowledge gaps. As such, we notably explore the debate of health selection versus social causation and identify and discuss areas for future research and action. In terms of scope, our focus is primarily on major depression (i.e., major depressive disorder [MDD] or major depressive episode) and dysthymia, though some studies cited focused on depressive symptoms only or mood disorders in general. Social inequalities are conceptualized in terms of both stratification of socioeconomic position and social class, as has been previously suggested (Krieger, Williams, & Moss, 1997; Muntaner, Eaton, & Diala, 2000; Wohlfarth, 1997). Finally, while we focus on high-income countries in this chapter, it is noteworthy that these inequalities have been found to be present globally, both within and between countries (Patel & Kleinman, 2003; World Health Organization and Calouste Gulbenkian Foundation, 2014).

Social Gradient in Depression

The connection between social status and mental health has been explored and documented at least since the nineteenth century, with Edward Jarvis's 1854 survey of the prevalence of mental disorders in Massachusetts (Jarvis, 1855). However, according to Dohrenwend and Dohrenwend (1982), early studies suffered from a variety of methodological limitations, such as using key informants and archival information to ascertain cases. Acknowledging these limitations, epidemiological assessments of population mental health over the past 30 years have increasingly incorporated a number of the following methodological improvements: direct interviews and standardized, validated instruments to identify cases; community-based surveys to identify cases among both the treated and untreated populations; assessment of specific mental disorders and longitudinal study designs (Dohrenwend & Dohrenwend, 1982; Muntaner, Ng, Vanroelen, Christ, & Eaton, 2013). In particular, starting in the 1980s, these limitations motivated the development of the Epidemiologic Catchment Area (ECA) study and the National Comorbidity Survey (NCS), two landmark epidemiological studies conducted in the United States. These were replicated, over the course of the 1990s, by a plethora of other national population-based mental health epidemiological investigations.

The ECA interviewed more than 18,000 participants aged 18 years and older from five different urban communities between 1980 and 1984 (Robins & Regier, 1991). In the analysis of six-month prevalence across all sites, major depression was inversely related with an overall index of SES (Holzer et al., 1986). However, in a separate analysis of risk factors for one-year prevalence, Weissman, Bruce, Leaf, Florio, and Holzer (1991) found an association with dependency on public financial aid and unemployment, but no association with education, income, or occupation, leading to the twin suggestions that the relationship may be specific to certain indicators of socioeconomic position, as well as vary by prevalence period under observation.

Following the ECA, the NCS was the first nationally representative survey to use structured lay interviews to standardize diagnoses of specific mental disorders. In the NCS, which was conducted in 1990–1992 and interviewed more than 8,000 respondents aged 15–54 years, 30-day, 12-month, and lifetime prevalence of affective disorders were reported, with the majority of those classified as major depression. Supporting initial insights from the ECA on differences in the time period under observation, an inverse association was identified with number of years of education and 30-day and 12-month prevalence but not lifetime prevalence of depression (Blazer, Kessler, McGonagle, & Swartz, 1994; Kessler et al., 1994). The association also appeared to depend on the SES indicator, as across all three prevalence rates a significant inverse association with income was found only when comparing the lowest and the highest income groups (Kessler et al., 1994). Finally, in the NCS replication study, which interviewed more than 9,000 respondents in 2001–2002, an association with employment status, education, and income was also reported, although not consistently across lifetime, 12-month MDD, and 12-month severe MDD prevalence (Kessler et al., 2003). Finally, an additional insight gleaned from these large epidemiological surveys is that the association between different measures of SES and depression does not appear to be linear (Holzer et al., 1986; Kessler et al., 2003), which may explain why no social gradients in education and income were found when they were assessed with dichotomous indicators (Weissman et al., 1991).

Following these landmark US studies, other countries, such as in Israel (Dohrenwend et al., 1992), the Netherlands (Bijl, Ravelli, & Van Zessen, 1998; de Graaf, ten Have, van Gool, & van Dorsselaer, 2012), Denmark (Andersen, Thielen, Nygaard, & Diderichsen, 2009), Canada (Bland, Stebelsky, Orn, & Newman, 1988; Wang, Schmitz, & Dewa, 2010), Australia (Wilhelm, Mitchell, Slade, Brownhill, & Andrews, 2003), Sweden (Kosidou et al., 2011), Taiwan (Hwu, Yeh, & Chang, 2007), and the United Kingdom (Meltzer, Gill, Petticrew, & Hinds, 1995), followed suit and also identified social inequalities in depression.

Despite these repeated observations, a more in-depth assessment of the literature, both between studies and within specific studies, reveals the complexity of the relationship between SES and depression. Indeed, conflicting results on the strength and direction of the relationship between SES and depression across a variety of SES indicators has been acknowledged and described in several recent reviews (Fryers, Melzer, & Jenkins, 2003; Kohn, Dohrenwend, & Mirotznik, 1998; Lorant et al., 2003). Specific indicators of SES have shown inconsistent relationships with depression between populations. An inverse association with education, for instance, was identified in a French general population sample (Murcia, Chastang, & Niedhammer, 2015) but not in a Puerto Rican sample (Canino et al., 1987). Similarly, among the studies that have looked at multiple indicators of SES, some found gradients across all indicators investigated (Andersen et al., 2009; Galobardes, Shaw, Lawlor, Lynch, & Smith, 2006a, 2006b), while others reported gradients only among certain indicators (Kessler et al., 1994). The association may also be impacted by depression severity, as it has been suggested that a weaker social gradient exists for dysthymia compared to major depression (Regier et al., 1993).

In light of these debates, a landmark meta-analysis of the association between prevalence, incidence, and persistence of major depression and SES among population-based studies was conducted about a decade ago (Lorant et al., 2003). The SES gradient was assessed by comparing the highest to the lowest socioeconomic group across indicators of education, income, social class, and occupation. Of the 51 prevalence studies identified, 46 identified a social gradient that favored higher depression rates in lower SES groups, with 33 reporting a statistically significant association. Conflictingly, five studies reported a nonsignificant association favoring higher depression among higher SES groups. Overall, those with lower SES had 1.81 higher odds of depression prevalence and 1.24 higher odds of depression incidence compared to those with higher SES. Finally, an important new finding in this study was that SES was not only associated with the occurrence of depression but also with its persistence (odds ratio of 2.06).

Importantly, this meta-analysis demonstrated that the gradient was sensitive to a variety of factors, such as the measurement methods of both depression and SES as well as regional and historical contexts. For example, a lower gradient was found in European studies compared to North American studies, and there was some evidence to suggest that the gradient was decreasing over time (Lorant et al., 2003). However, more recent evidence has allowed us to qualify that finding, as it appears that the effect of time is dependent on context, with some countries reporting a stable (i.e., nondecreasing) gradient over time (Talala, Huurre, Aro, Martelin, & Prättälä, 2009). These observations helped reconcile the mixed results identified within previous reviews. Additionally, a lack of standardized usage of SES indicators and depression diagnosis criteria has been noted, which may impact the consistency of findings (Fryers et al., 2003). Indeed, it is now commonly accepted that different indicators of SES are not interchangeable, as each captures a different set of social circumstances that impact health (Galobardes et al., 2006a, 2006b). Finally, indicators have been found to have effects on each other (Almeida-Filho et al., 2004; Murcia et al., 2015), but these pathways and potential interactions have yet to be fully understood or investigated in the literature, as we discuss later in our concluding section.

Overall, there is enough evidence to conclude that there is a social gradient in depression, with an overrepresentation of depression among those in lower SES strata. Additionally, a strong association with chronicity of depression has been identified, which points to an important target for public health interventions. Thus, although the social gradient in depression prevalence may not be as strong as with other mental disorders or mental health in general (Holzer et al., 1986), it is discernable, particularly when comparing the highest SES strata to the lowest SES strata (Lorant et al., 2003). Furthermore, it appears that the strength and direction of the association between SES and depression varies by the type of socioeconomic indicator, gender, ethnicity, geography, and diagnostic criteria. In the next section, we address the thorny issue of the social causation / mental health selection debate in explaining the roots of these associations.

The Causation-Selection Issue

While an overrepresentation of depression among individuals with lower SES has been repeatedly identified among various populations, the direction of causation has been less clearly defined. This debate features two major competing hypotheses: (1) mental health selection/drift and (2) social causation (Dohrenwend et al., 1992; Eaton, Muntaner, Bovasso, & Smith, 2001). The mental health selection/drift hypothesis posits that predisposition to depression influences SES by either preventing the attainment of higher SES ("selection") or precipitating a downward shift in an individual's SES ("drift"). According to this hypothesis, poor mental health temporally precedes disadvantage. For instance, depression disorders may prevent individuals from attaining higher socioeconomic positions by impeding educational attainment and obtaining and maintaining gainful employment, with attendant consequences for income. The central mechanism through which this is hypothesized to occur is the discrimination of those with poor mental health leading to blocked access to society's opportunity structures and institutions, such as the labor market, education, and health care (West, 1991).

Alternatively, the social gradient in depression may also be explained by the social causation hypothesis, in which the adversity and stresses that are associated with societal disadvantage causally increase an individual's risk of developing depression. This hypothesis underscores the role of the social determinants of health as a cause of depression. As we discuss later in this chapter, a variety of pathways have been identified to explain the social causation of depression, such as greater exposure to stressful life events and heightened reactivity to these stressors, notably due to less access to and recourse to effective coping mechanisms.

Understanding these processes is fundamental for the development of public health interventions. Should interventions target social experiences of disadvantage to prevent incident depression or should people with depression be protected from selection and drift into lower SES (Muntaner, Eaton, Miech, & O'Campo, 2004)? Furthermore, while these may appear to be competing hypotheses, mental health selection and social causation are not necessarily mutually exclusive and can work simultaneously to produce the social gradient identified in cross-sectional studies.

The causation/selection debate was especially contentious when various disorders were conflated, as there is now mounting evidence that these processes may be disorder-specific (Dohrenwend & Dohrenwend, 1982; Johnson, Cohen, Dohrenwend, Link, & Brook, 1999; Kessler, Foster, Saunders, & Stang, 1995; Miech, Caspi, Moffitt, Wright, & Silva, 1999). Hence, disorders with high heritability and severely disabling symptomatology, such as schizophrenia, have been shown to be very consistent with the selection/drift hypothesis (Saraceno, Levav, & Kohn, 2005). However, it has proven more difficult to disentangle the selection and causation processes for depression, which is only moderately influenced by genetic factors (Bierut et al., 1999; Levinson, 2006; Muntaner et al., 2013). An impediment to the determination of the direction of causation is that both SES and depression are strongly influenced by family background *and* both evolve dynamically over the life course, sometimes in parallel with each other but oftentimes in retroactive feedback loops.

Cross-sectional studies have aimed to provide clues to the mechanisms at play through the use of respondent recall of age at disorder onset (Kessler et al., 1995) and time invariant SES predictors (Dohrenwend et al., 1992). For instance, in an analysis of NCS data, the odds of failing to complete school among eighth grade graduates and failing to complete college among those who entered college were 1.5 and 2.9 times higher, respectively, among those with mood disorders (Kessler et al., 1995), providing support for the selection/drift hypothesis. In contrast, Dohrenwend and colleagues' (1992) landmark test of the causation/selection issue assessed mental disorder prevalence in two ethnic groups in Israel, with the assumption that, if the social causation hypothesis was correct, at every level of social stratification the ethnic minority group should have higher levels of mental disorders due to overall discrimination. Evidence was found among women only, but this study design was not able to fully eliminate selection effects due to its cross-sectional nature.

Longitudinal and intergenerational studies provide more robust evidence to the debate, as they have the ability to identify the temporal ordering of SES and depression onset. The Stirling County study found that incident depression was more common among those with low SES at baseline, supporting the causation hypothesis (Murphy et al., 1991). Johnson et al. (1999) tested the selection and causation hypotheses using a community-based sample in New York, followed from 1975 to 1993 with repeated assessments of SES and psychopathology. After controlling for factors such as parental depression, age, gender, and IQ, low family SES (parental education and parental occupation) was associated with increased risk of depression among offspring (9–20 years) (Johnson et al., 1999). No evidence of selection was identified; in fact, offspring with depression were less likely to drop out of high school. Similarly, using an intergenerational design to control for parental depression, Ritsher, Warner, Johnson, and Dohrenwend (2001) found a strong relationship between low parental SES (education and occupation) and later depression in their children but no evidence of selection effects. More recently, a longitudinal study assessed how short-term changes in SES affect depression in a seven-year annual survey of a general population sample from Belgium (Lorant et al., 2007). They found evidence for social causation, as a reduction in material standard of living, measured by financial strain, deprivation, and poverty, between study waves was associated with both an increase in depressive symptoms and major depression.

Interestingly, there has also been some support among longitudinal studies for mental health selection. The follow-up of the ECA Baltimore site more than a decade after the original study found that having depression at baseline had a small negative effect on income at follow-up (Eaton et al., 2001). Similarly, evidence for simultaneous selection and causation processes has been identified in longitudinal samples of Australian and American adults. Dooley, Prause, and Ham-Rowbottom (2000) found that prior depression predicted unemployment, and that joblessness and transition to inadequate employment increased the risk of depression in an assessment of the US National Longitudinal Survey of Youth in 1992 and 1994. Finally, higher levels of psychological distress, as measured by anxiety and depression symptoms in the previous four weeks, were found to be both a cause and effect of poverty among individuals aged 21–59 in Australia (Callander & Schofield, 2015).

As with longitudinal and intergenerational studies, exploiting naturally occurring events to understand the temporal ordering of depression and SES has proven beneficial to disentangle selection and causation effects. Capitalizing on an automobile plant closure, Hamilton, Broman, Hoffman, and Renner (1990) assessed the impact of involuntary unemployment on mental disorders, including depression. Autoworkers who were laid off experienced more depression symptoms than those who remained employed, providing evidence for social causation of depression. Further, they also found a stronger effect among females, black workers with lower education, individuals with lower savings, and individuals with more previous negative life experiences or financial hardships. Another study explored the causation-selection issue by assessing the effects of an income supplement intervention to American Indian families on childhood mental health after the opening of an on-reserve casino (Costello, Compton, Keeler, & Angold, 2003). Initially, a social gradient between many psychiatric symptoms, including depression, was identified; however, moving out of poverty was associated with a reduction in behavioral symptoms but not in depression symptoms. The authors speculated that these findings could be interpreted in support of the selection hypothesis but also cautioned that it may take longer for the effect of moving out of poverty to impact depression levels. Furthermore, Lorant and colleagues (2007) found that negative events had an effect on depression that outweighed that of positive events, suggesting that deprivation and abundance cannot be operationalized merely as inverse statuses. Although natural experiments provide a unique opportunity to isolate the effect of movement between positions of disadvantage and advantage, these types of studies are not commonly found in the literature due to the difficulties in conducting them (Hamilton et al., 1990; Muntaner et al., 2013).

In sum, the current evidence base seems to weigh in the favor of social causation of depression over mental health selection (Lorant et al., 2007; Muntaner et al., 2004). However, it does appear that both causation and selection processes may be operating in the creation and maintenance of the social gradient in depression, but it is likely that these processes will depend on the historical and national context under observation. Similarly, the extent to which the life course stratification process is constrained by family origins and education will also vary along these dimensions (Miech et al., 1999). Thus, future research should aim to replicate current findings in different contexts and with improved and frequent repeated measurements of SES and depression. In the next section, we turn to a more in-depth review of select findings regarding the association of indicators of SES most frequently used in the literature and their hypothesized causal impact on depression.

Specific Indicators of SES

SES can be can be measured through a variety of interconnected concepts, with each indicator measuring a different dimension of social stratification. No indicator alone captures the entire effect of SES, although composite measures incorporating multiple aspects of SES have been used in attempts to measure overall SES. Specific indicators are favored today, as they can provide important hints about the mechanisms of action (Galobardes et al., 2006a) and potential areas for intervention. To provide a fuller understanding of effect of the social gradient, a variety of indicators are often measured instead, although the direction and magnitude of their direction may not always be consistent. We briefly discuss some of the most commonly used measures in the social inequalities of depression literature in the following sections.

Education

Education is one of the most widely used SES indicators, as it is an easily recalled, nonsensitive, and fairly valid indicator (in terms of low measurement error) of an individual's human capital. To wit, in Lorant and colleagues' (2003) meta-analysis, 37 of the 56 studies identified measured the effect of education. The majority of these studies found an inverse association with education and depression, with each additional year of education decreasing the log odds of depression by 3% overall.

Peyrot and colleagues (2015) found that there was almost no genetic correlation between education attainment and MDD, suggesting that other nongenetic factors may play a role in the mechanism that generates this association. Drawing from investigations of mechanisms explaining the association between education and health in general, we find strong plausible evidence for the effects of (1) employment and work conditions, (2) social-psychological resources, and (3) lifestyle factors (Ross & Mirowsky, 1999; Ross & Wu, 1995). Regarding the association between education and employment, education has been shown to be strongly related to an individual's future income and employment, acting as an important contributor to social stratification "sorting" processes (Ross & Mirowsky, 2006; Ross & Wu, 1996). Thus, in a sample of more than 14,000 members of the general population in France, education inequalities in MDD were higher among the general population than among the working population (Murcia et al., 2015), suggesting that employment accounts for some of the effect of education. In addition to the influence on participation in the workforce, education appears to affect the type of job, with those with higher education being more likely to work full time and work in more fulfilling jobs that have a higher degree of control and work creativity. Furthermore, education also has an impact on an individual's nonmaterial, psychosocial resources that protect against depression, such as the sense of control and social support (Ross & Mirowsky, 1999, 2006; Ross & Wu, 1995). Finally, education may also operate through its association with improved lifestyle behaviors and health literacy (Averina et al., 2005; Lincoln et al., 2006), which can serve, respectively, as coping mechanisms and enabling factors facilitating symptom identification and health-seeking behavior in the face of incident depresssion.

Income

Measures of income capture an individual's or household's available economic and material resources. It has long been observed that those with more financial means have lower rates of depression, although research is continuing to elucidate the causal mechanisms through which this gradient emerges. Overall, the effect of income on depression has been shown to be strong, and it was found to have a greater effect than indicators of education (Lorant et al., 2003), perhaps because it is more proximal to the measurement of depression or because it mediates the relationship between education and depression (Quesnel-Vallée & Taylor, 2012). In terms of proposed mechanisms, higher income protects from poverty and the psychological effects of financial stress, and provides a sense of security. Over 29 years in the Alameda County Study, all measures of psychological well-being (purpose in life, self-acceptance, personal growth, environmental mastery, and autonomy) increased as mean income increased (Kaplan, Shema, & Leite, 2008), suggesting one pathway through which income works to prevent depression. Income may also serve as a proxy for the type and status of jobs, as higher-income jobs also tend to offer better working conditions (Zimmerman, Christakis, & Vander Stoep, 2004). In particular, higher-income jobs are also often characterized by greater control over tasks, which could mitigate the potentially negative effects of high psychological demands also associated with these positions (Mausner-Dorsch & Eaton, 2000).

As income potential is influenced by education, occupation, overall health, and individual traits, authors have attempted to decompose and identify causal pathways. For instance, in the 1979 cohort of the National Longitudinal Survey of Youth in the United States, there was some evidence to suggest that the causal effects of income may operate through precursors to income such as employment status and factors stemming from (low) income such as financial strain (Zimmerman & Katon, 2005). However, Costa-Font and Gil (2008) found conflicting results when attempting to isolate the effect of income, with income alone accounting for between 6% and 50% of the depression inequalities across different models. As such, this matter is not settled, and future research should seek to clarify these relationships, notably in identifying other socioeconomic and socioemotional factors that may mediate this relationship.

Finally, beyond income per se, to gain a fuller understanding of economic resources, wealth and debt should also be considered. Wealth indicators capture accumulated physical and financial assets, which tend to be distributed even more unequally than income. However, these indicators are challenging to collect and so are seldom studied. Household wealth has been found to be strongly associated with depression after adjustment for previous poor health and personal income in the Whitehall II study (Martikainen, Adda, Ferrie, Davey, & Marmot, 2003). In a recent systematic review of wealth and health, measures of increased wealth, such as assets, home or car ownership, as well as net worth, were associated with less depression, which led the authors to conclude that failure to measure wealth may underestimate the overall effect of SES (Pollack et al., 2007). Similarly, debt also appears to be a promising (albeit understudied) indicator, as Richardson, Elliott, and Roberts's (2013) meta-analysis found that the odds of depression were 2.77 higher among those with unsecured debt.

(Un)Employment and Occupation

The impact of working life has been captured through a variety of indicators such as unemployment, occupation, and employment contract type. Occupational class measures capture the hierarchical relationships between employers and employees, as well as information about overall social standing (Galobardes et al., 2006b). Both being employed and occupation type are highly correlated with income and therefore part of their mechanism of action is theorized to be through acquisition of material resources. Furthermore, occupational inequalities are partially explained by psychosocial work factors, such as job demands, influence, freedom, development, social relationships, leadership, working hours, job promotion, and workplace violence (Schütte, Chastang, Parent-Thirion, Vermeylen, & Niedhammer, 2015). Similarly, in the Whitehall II study, an inverse gradient in employment grade and depressive symptoms was identified, and the gradient was largely explained by work characteristics, material disadvantage, social support, and health behaviors (Stansfeld, Head, Fuhrer, Wardle, & Cattell, 2003). In other words, current research on occupations tends to support a material perspective.

Paul and Moser's (2009) meta-analysis assessing the association between unemployment and mental health found a large and significant average effect size ($d = 0.50$) for the comparison between unemployed and employed persons and depression. Conversely, finding employment after a period of unemployment was associated with improved mental health. Additionally, gender and occupational class moderated the relationship between poor mental health and unemployment, as men and blue-collar workers were more distressed by unemployment than women and white-collar workers. Not only is job loss bad for depression, but a longer duration of unemployment has been shown to increase the risk of depression and the severity of depression symptoms (Mossakowski, 2009; Paul & Moser, 2009; Stankunas, Kalediene, Starkuviene, & Kapustinskiene, 2006), while other socioeconomic indicators, such as higher income and education, may protect against the risk of depression in both the short and long term (Stankunas et al., 2006).

With recent changes in labor markets in terms of decreasing employment stability and the rise in nonstandard and contract work, researchers have turned to these alternative measures signaling a more precarious position in the labor force (Artazcoz, Benach, Borrell, & Cortès, 2005; Nishimura, 2011; Quesnel-Vallée, DeHaney, & Ciampi, 2010). In the United States, exposure to temporary work in the previous two-year period was associated with an increase in depressive symptoms, even while controlling for the possibility of mental health selection into these positions (Quesnel-Vallée et al., 2010). Similarly, in Spain, some types of insecure and flexible employment contracts (temporary contract and no contract) were associated with poor mental health, especially among manual workers (Artazcoz et al., 2005).

Social Class

In contrast with indicators of income, education, and employment, which "neutrally" describe the rank of individuals within society, indicators of social class underscore the power dynamics between groups in society. Class relations often involve an element of economic exploitation and an asymmetry of power (Krieger et al., 1997). To date, social class indicators are the least commonly used measures of social inequality in the depression literature (Krieger et al., 1997; Muntaner et al., 2013); yet they have been suggested to be promising because of their potential explanatory power to describe the social mechanisms leading to disparities compared to SES indicators (Muntaner, Borrell, Benach, Pasarín, & Fernandez, 2003). Erik Olin Wright's social class measurement scheme measures ownership of productive assets, control/authority, and skill/experience. This scheme predicts a nonlinear association ("contradictory class location") between social class and mental health, with low-level supervisors anticipated to have worse outcomes due to their exposure to high demands, while exerting little control (Wright, 1989). Evidence for the "contradictory class location" has been found consistently in the few studies that investigated this association, with low-level supervisors having a higher degree of depression than both managers and workers (Muntaner et al., 2003; Muntaner, Eaton, Diala, Kessler, & Sorlie, 1998; Prins, Bates, Keyes, & Muntaner, 2015). This early research suggests that relational measures of class may help provide a more complete picture of social inequalities in depression, and researchers should continue to develop these frameworks.

"Master Statuses": Gender and Race and Ethnicity

In sociology, the term *master status* refers to those statuses that overpower all other statuses (Scott & Marshall, 2009). Thus, we end this brief overview of social factors associated with depression with two primary master statuses, namely, gender and race and ethnicity. They are most pertinent to our assessment of inequalities in depression because while these statuses are both associated with disproportionately higher risks of lower socioeconomic status along many of the indicators we discussed previously, their respective associations with depression cannot be subsumed by these associations with particular social locations. Finally, we present these two dimensions under a common overarching rubric to highlight a promising area of study examining the interweaving of deprived social position and discrimination through the lens of intersectionality between gender and race and ethnicity (Raphael & Bryant, 2015). Roxburgh (2009) and Rosenfield (2012) offered examples of the value of this framework as applied to social inequalities in depression and general mental health, respectively, but this is a budding area that merits further investigation.

Gender

Historically, the bulk of research on gender differences in depression has focused on contrasts between women and men. However, more recently, the issue of lesbian, gay, bisexual, and transgender (LGBT) differences in mental health has also garnered increasing attention (Cochran, Sullivan, & Mays, 2003). While we focus primarily in this section on the gender delineation contrasting women and men in recognition of its preeminence in the literature, we also briefly touch on key findings in the LGBT literature in closing this section.

One of the most consistent findings in the depression epidemiology literature is that the risk of depression is about two times higher in females compared to males (Kessler, 2003). This appears to arise from the fact that, while males and females have similar rates of mental disorder overall, they vary in terms of specific disorder prevalence; males are more likely to present externalizing disorders such as substance abuse disorder, while females are more likely to develop internalizing disorders such as depression or anxiety (Seedat et al., 2009). It is currently widely accepted that these differences are neither an artifact of differential reporting or measurement nor are they due to genetic or biological factors (Piccinelli & Wilkinson, 2000). Thus, researchers have turned to the examination of social conditions to explain the large gender differential in depression. While strong social gradients in depression have been identified among both men and women, the gradients appear to vary systematically between the two groups. For example, a significantly stronger effect of education has been identified in women compared to men (Almeida-Filho et al., 2004; Van de Velde, Bracke, & Levecque, 2010). The concepts of gender held by society, which produce gendered power structures and responsibilities, have been suggested to impact vulnerability to and protection from depression differentially. These power structures occur both at work and at home, where women's role in childbearing promotes division of labor and affects their position in society through interruption or postponement of their education or career.

Thus, women typically have a lower social standing compared to males; they receive lower pay than men for similar jobs and tend to have less access to managerial, supervisory, or policy-making jobs (Chonody & Siebert, 2008). While today the majority of women are employed, they continue to perform a lion's share of childcare and housework, creating a double burden of work and role conflict (Lennon & Rosenfield, 1992). Yet, little research has been conducted to understand the impact of gender inequality in work. In a rare example of this type of research, O'Campo, Eaton, and Muntaner (2004) explored the effect of work and gender inequality on health in the ECA Baltimore follow-up sample. While unmarried women and those experiencing financial hardship were more likely to suffer from depression, no associations were found with either work-related factors (large firm, promotion, professional job, and demotion) or gender inequality measures. However, the authors note that the sample was primarily comprised of middle-aged and older women, and the impacts may be different among women early in their careers or across different geographies. Additionally, although women and men tend to face similar levels of stress, lower SES women have been shown to experience more frequent stressful life events and life events that lead to chronic deprivation (Belle, 1990; Brown, Bhrolchain, & Harris, 1975). Similarly, women are more likely than men to face financial hardship, although it has a universal effect on depression (Elliott, 2001).

In addition to the effect of gendered power structures on women's standing in society, women may have reduced decision-making power within the household in terms of finances and division of labor. Although family structure characteristics may be relatively less significant than socioeconomic conditions in the explanation of gender differences in depression, they have been found to be important (Van de Velde et al., 2010). While marriage or living with a partner has been shown to be a buffer against depression among both women and men (O'Campo et al., 2004; Van de Velde et al., 2010), women in relationships with power differentials in decision-making are more likely to be depressed (Byrne & Carr, 2000). Alternatively, female employment and shifts in domestic labor to partners can have a negative effect on husbands' mental health (Rosenfield, 1992).

Women and men also form different types of relationships, impacting their social support. Women tend to form relationships that are more intimate, which, while they provide social support in times of stress, are also more emotionally demanding and leave them more vulnerable to spillover from life events experienced by close relations and friends (Turner & Marino, 1994). Women have access to more social support and may also benefit more from the support they have than men (Elliott, 2001). Other factors such as more effective coping strategies in women, yet lower personal resources such as mastery and self-esteem, have been shown to contribute to differentials (Ennis, Hobfoll, & Schröder, 2000; Meyer, Schwartz, & Frost, 2008). In sum, overall it appears that both socioeconomic and relational factors mediate the relationship between gender and depression but that further research is needed to disentangle these effects.

In more recent developments, researchers have turned to the study of LGBT mental health. As homosexuality was up until the early 1970s classified as a mental disorder, the assessment of inequalities in mental health by LGBT status is fraught with complexities (Meyer, 2003), to which we are undoubtedly unable to do justice in this brief review. However, it is clear that a growing body of evidence suggests that LGB (not enough evidence has been gathered with regard to transgender people) people, and gay men in particular, appear to disproportionately suffer from depression relative to the general population (Cochran & Mays, 2000; Cochran, Sullivan, & Mays, 2003). Meyer (1995) coined the term *minority stress* to refer to the process whereby sexual minorities are subject to chronic stress and stigmatization in heteronormative societies, which results in excess psychopathologies in these populations.

Finally, another important emerging research in the gender area concerns the effect of SES on postpartum depression. Indeed, recent studies suggest that a social gradient in postpartum depression also exists, with lower SES mothers reporting more depressive symptoms postpartum (Mayberry, Horowitz, & Declercq, 2007; Séguin, Potvin, St-Denis, & Loiselle, 1999). Goyal, Gay, and Lee (2010) found that lower income, having less than a college education, being unemployed, and being unmarried were all associated with depressive symptoms at three months postpartum. Furthermore, each additional SES risk factor was associated with an increasing risk of depression, even after controlling for the level of prenatal depression.

Race and Ethnicity

Race and ethnicity are socially constructed concepts, and their social meanings in turn affect individuals' life chances through discrimination and access to material and nonmaterial resources. Racial and ethnic minority groups tend to have lower SES, live in more dangerous neighborhoods, and experience more traumatic events and acute and chronic stressors compared to majority populations (Turner & Avison, 2003; Williams & Collins, 2001; Williams, Yan, Jackson, & Anderson, 1997). Given the known associations between stress, SES, and depression, it is therefore expected that African Americans and nonwhite Hispanics would have higher rates of depression than white Americans. Paradoxically, data from large epidemiological surveys such as the ECA, the NSC replication study, and the National Health and Nutrition Examination Survey III consistently found that black populations report lower or similar rates of depression compared to white populations, even after adjustment for the effects of SES

(Breslau et al., 2006; Kessler et al., 2005; Riolo, Nguyen, Greden, & King, 2005; Williams, Takeuchi, & Adair, 1992).

Several hypotheses have been proposed and explored to understand this unexpected racial patterning of depression. First, a selection hypothesis: epidemiological studies based on general population samples systematically exclude institutionalized individuals, who in the United States are more likely to both be black and to have higher rates of depression (Barnes, Keyes, & Bates, 2013; Nazroo, 2015). Second, there is mixed evidence to suggest that differential measurement and diagnosis of depression across racial and ethnical categories may also contribute to this underestimation, although these relationships are poorly understood due to a paucity of studies (Barnes et al., 2013; Nazroo, 2015). Conversely, some evidence suggests that these patterns may not be artifacts of the data but, rather, may be arising from reliance on coping mechanisms that are specific to this subpopulation and have been poorly studied because of their lack of relevance to the majority population. For example, reliance on "poor" health behaviors such as smoking, alcohol and substance use, and overeating were found in the ECA Baltimore follow-up to moderate the association between stress and depression among blacks but not whites (Mezuk et al., 2010). Similarly, religious participation has also been evoked as a potential fruitful coping mechanism particularly efficacious in this population (Reese, Thorpe, Bell, Bowie, & LaVeist, 2012).

Public Health Intervention and Policy

In this section, we turn to evidence on the potential for action on social inequalities in depression. A first area consists of health policies that could have a direct impact on recovery from depression, as well as potentially a preventive impact on incident cases of clinical depression. Next, we turn to more distal policies that pertain to the structural characteristics of the societies that tend to produce social inequalities that generate the social gradient in depression.

Socioeconomic Status and Mental Health Care

Social advantage and disadvantage can influence mental health though access to mental health care. Given the higher burden of depression among those with lower SES, equitable access to services implies that disadvantaged groups with higher treatment needs should have higher treatment access. Some evidence exists to substantiate this assumption, but it suggests that social inequalities in mental health care for depression vary by the sector of care, with hospital access being reported more frequently by the most disadvantaged while community and outpatient care tend to favor the most advantaged (Alegría, Bijl, Lin, Walters, & Kessler, 2000). Unfortunately, this does not necessarily point to more efficient or equitable use of services. Indeed, compared to outpatient and community services, mental health services within hospitals tend to be sought as a last resort by the most severe or acute cases, which could have resulted from foregone community or outpatient care due to cost. Accordingly, a Canadian study found that rates of hospitalization for depression were higher among those from lower SES areas compared to those from higher SES areas (Canadian Institute for Health Information, 2009). Interestingly though, this study found that once admitted, there was no socioeconomic differential in the length of stay or rate of readmission.

In contrast, regarding community or outpatient mental health services, the literature has consistently shown the reverse gradient holds, with the most advantaged groups being as or more likely to receive these services compared to those in lower SES groups (Alegría et al., 2002; Rhodes, Jaakkimainen, Bondy, & Fung, 2006; Starkes, Poulin, & Kisely, 2005; Steele, Dewa, & Lee, 2007; Steele, Glazier, & Lin, 2006). In Canada, where physician services are generally free at the point of service, a study found that residents in high-SES neighborhoods in Toronto, Ontario, were more likely to both use psychiatric care and use it more frequently than residents of low SES neighborhoods (Steele et al., 2006).

To understand this social gradient in treatment access, Steele and colleagues (2007) explored perceived accessibility, availability, and acceptability barriers among a nationally representative Canadian sample. Individuals with higher income and higher education were less likely to report acceptability barriers to care, although those who were employed were more likely to report these barriers. This may in part explain why education has been found to be a strong predictor of mental health service use in Canada (Rhodes et al., 2006).

Once in treatment, a variety of factors associated with treatment success have been shown to also maintain a social gradient. Falconnier (2009) assessed outcomes and attrition among more than 200 patients across three different treatments for depression (cognitive behavioral therapy, interpersonal psychotherapy, and pharmacotherapy). While there was no effect of SES (as measured by a composite index) on attrition, all treatments appeared to be less effective among those in the lowest SES group compared to the middle SES group. Such findings point to the need for targeted interventions, and indeed, a recent systematic review promisingly identified a range of health care interventions that have been effective in reducing depression among low SES populations both in the short and long term (Rojas-García et al., 2015). Another area of interest has been social inequalities in treatment quality, although few studies have assessed the association for depression treatment specifically (Roy-Byrne, Joesch, Wang, & Kessler, 2009; Young, Klap, Sherbourne, & Wells, 2001). Within the NCS replication study, SES indicators such as education, income, and wealth were weakly associated with receiving adequate treatment for anxiety and depression, although the effects varied by sector (general or specialty medical sector) (Roy-Byrne et al., 2009).

Taken together, there is strong evidence to suggest that there is a social gradient in access to outpatient mental health services and moderate evidence that this gradient persists in factors associated with treatment success and quality.

Social Policies

The clear support in the literature for social causation of depression through factors such as income, education, and employment suggests that improving social and economic circumstances has the potential to alleviate human suffering due to depression. As reported in the World Health Organization's *Closing the Gap in a Generation*, the Priority Public Health Conditions Knowledge Network of the Commission on Social Determinants of Health has outlined intervention targets for mental health (CSDH, 2008). Thus, they recommend interventions that target mental health and its care directly, as well as larger-scale societal change interventions. They call for improved access to care through integration of mental health services into general health care, provision of financially accessible services, and implementation of mental health promotion programs. In turn, larger-scale interventions reach beyond mental health to impact social inequality in general through action on the social determinants of health, such as improved welfare policies, protective labor policies, improved access to credit and saving for the poor, mandating financial support for education, employment programs, and economic policies.

Empirical support for economic and financial policy interventions exists in the literature, as the impact of unemployment on poor mental health has been found to be stronger among countries with weak economic development, unequal income distribution, and weak unemployment protection (Paul & Moser, 2009). Additionally, national economic crises have been shown to impact depression rates, with the prevalence of major depressive episode in Greece doubling in the year after the 2008 financial crisis (Madianos, Economou, Alexiou, & Stefanis, 2011). More generally, Lynch, Smith, Kaplan, and House (2000) expressed support for policies aimed at reducing health inequalities by tackling structural inequalities. Using a neomaterial approach, they called for investments in education, health services, housing, transportation, welfare, and working conditions through a more equitable distribution of public and private resources. Inclusion of personal financial issues as a pertinent component of a patient's medical history has even been suggested as a potential intervention based on a recession case study in the United Kingdom (Jenkins, Fitch, Hurlston, & Walker, 2009). More specifically, the authors argued that, as part of routine assessments, physicians should ask about financial difficulties, screen for depression, and offer referrals for debt counseling. Thus, the current body of literature suggests a variety of avenues for interventions, but implementation and assessment of these types of interventions to date have been lacking.

Finally, an interaction between area-level income inequality and household income has been identified. In the United States, the risk of depression increased among women in low-income households who lived in states with higher income inequality compared to states with a more equal income distribution (Kahn, Wise, Kennedy, & Kawachi, 2000). Conversely, regional income inequality has been shown to confer a higher level of risk among people with higher incomes in Britain (Weich, Lewis, &

Jenkins, 2001). More research is evidently needed to uncover the mechanisms underlying these conflicting findings.

Promising Avenues for Future Research

To conclude this chapter, we highlight two promising areas for future research. This list is obviously not exhaustive but follows from some observations we made in this chapter on important knowledge gaps.

Life Course Processes

Over the past two decades, the life course epidemiology of chronic diseases has gained increasing preeminence as a framework to fruitfully study health inequalities, following, notably, the seminal work of Kuh and Ben-Shlomo (1997). As these concepts resonate with subfields in other related disciplines, such as developmental psychopathology, the study of depression has quickly followed suit (Gilman, 2007). In particular, this area of research has been concerned with identifying whether childhood experiences of social deprivation are associated with adult depression, and by and large, the answer to this question has heretofore been positive. However, a number of questions remain on the agenda.

First, the prevalent modeling strategy in early studies tended to be the estimation of change (expected decreases) in the magnitude of the association between adult SES and adult depression after the inclusion of parents' SES in the model as an implicit assessment of the indirect mediation pathway effects existing between this triad of concepts (Power, Stansfeld, Matthews, Manor, & Hope, 2002). However, this modeling strategy is liable to produce biased estimates in the presence of unmeasured confounding or measurement error when these indirect pathways and the associated covariance structures are not explicitly modeled (Quesnel-Vallée & Taylor, 2012). Given the complex web of mental health selection and social causation that we outlined earlier in this chapter, the study of life course processes of depression is not surprisingly fraught with these risks of measurement error and unmeasured confounding (Gilman, 2007). Furthermore, as has been argued for the study of health inequalities more generally, for the field to progress, a more "vigorous" (though no less rigorous) assessment of the complexity of processes involved in the embodying of social inequalities into health inequalities must occur, notably through the modeling of the dynamic relationship between SES and health (Adler, Bush, & Pantell, 2012).

Pathways

Thus, a first area that is ripe for further development in this field is the study of pathways of SES accumulation, leading (or not) to depression in later life. For example, among the National Longitudinal Survey of Youth 1979 cohort, we found that the greater the parents' education, the fewer the symptoms of depression in their adult children, a relationship that held even after controlling for a family history of depression (Quesnel-Vallée & Taylor, 2012). Through structural equation modeling, we then found that much of that relationship was, in fact, explained by these adult children's own education and income. Using a pathway model, our analysis showed that parents who are more educated also tend to have more educated children, who in turn secure better jobs with higher incomes. This pathway accounted for the entire effect of parents' education on their offspring's depressive symptoms. However, these results may well reflect the specific context from which these relationships emerged: the education and income distribution and labor market opportunities of these youths and their parents, as well as the rigidity of the stratification system. We would not necessarily expect to see the same relationships emerge in other contexts (historical or national) where the relationship between parents' education and children's socioeconomic achievement is weaker (i.e., the more "open" the education system, the weaker the relationship between origins and adult SES). Further research needs to be done to comprehend more fully how these mechanisms work in different stratification systems.

The Stress Process

The second area we found that offered many avenues for further research is in the further examination of the *stress process*. Coined by Pearlin, Menaghan, Morton, and Mullan (1981), this term refers to the interplay between sources of stress and its mediators and manifestations, of which depression was taken as a prime example. With regard to social inequalities, much research has been devoted to determine whether low SES was associated with depression through greater exposure to stressors (e.g., financial strain, job loss) or greater reactivity to stress (e.g., more severe or chronic manifestations). Much research has confirmed both the greater exposure to stressors and greater reactivity hypotheses (McLaughlin, Conron, Koenen, & Gilman, 2010; Thoits, 2010). A rich strand of this research has proposed that this greater reactivity resulted notably from lower availability or lower efficacy of coping resources that could have otherwise buffered the deleterious effects of various sources of stress (Turner & Lloyd, 1999). However, much of this research has operationalized greater reactivity indirectly, through evidence of more severe or chronic manifestations of depression.

More recently, another strand of research has emerged, examining the physiological reactions to stress in an attempt to directly quantify this reactivity. Thus, a growing number of biomarkers plausibly involved in stress and inflammation are increasingly being collected and brought in to explain the relationship between SES and depression, most notably stress hormones and the concept of allostatic load (McEwen, 2000), and other markers of inflammation such as C-reactive protein (Wium-Andersen, Ørsted, Nielsen, & Nordestgaard, 2013). Far from having favored nature over nurture, these investigations, particularly in the more recent field of epigenetics, instead highlight the intertwined reality of individuals as biological, psychological, and social beings, and reaffirm the importance of social processes in the generation of diseases (McEwen & McEwen, 2015). This burgeoning area is therefore prime for interdisciplinary developments.

Conclusion

In summary, we have sought to highlight in this review that although a substantial body of evidence exists to support the association between SES and depression, several knowledge gaps remain. In particular, studying selection *and* causation and their interplay (rather than forcing them to be mutually exclusive), focusing on pathways between various socioeconomic indicators, and delving deeper into the biological-psychological-social nexus that produces the gradient in depression all appeared to us to be particularly fruitful avenues for further research. Finally, an overarching concept that we should all keep in mind when studying the social gradient in depression is that as these relationships are produced by the social context in which they are embedded, they are also likely to be specific to that social context to a large extent. Thus, perhaps the most challenging agenda we set out here is to encourage the comparative study of the impact of the broader social context, consisting notably of policies and the social stratification structure, on the emergence, strength, and persistence of the social gradient in depression.

References

Adler, N., Bush, N. R., & Pantell, M. S. (2012). Rigor, vigor, and the study of health disparities. *Proceedings of the National Academy of Sciences of the United States of America, 109*(Suppl. 2), 17154–17159. doi:10.1073/pnas.1121399109

Alegría, M., Bijl, R. V., Lin, E., Walters, E. E., & Kessler, R. C. (2000). Income differences in persons seeking outpatient treatment for mental disorders: A comparison of the United States with Ontario and The Netherlands. *Archives of General Psychiatry, 57*(4), 383–391. doi:10.1001/archpsyc.57.4.383

Alegría, M., Canino, G., Ríos, R., Vera, M., Calderón, J., Rusch, D., & Ortega, A. N. (2002). Mental health care for Latinos: Inequalities in use of specialty mental health services among Latinos, African Americans, and non-Latino whites. *Psychiatric Services, 53*(12), 1547–1555. doi:10.1176/appi.ps.53.12.1547

Almeida-Filho, N., Lessa, I., Magalhães, L., Araújo, M. J., Aquino, E., James, S. A., & Kawachi, I. (2004). Social inequality and depressive disorders in Bahia, Brazil: Interactions of gender, ethnicity, and social class. *Social Science & Medicine, 59*(7), 1339–1353. doi:10.1016/j.socscimed.2003.11.037

Andersen, I., Thielen, K., Nygaard, E., & Diderichsen, F. (2009). Social inequality in the prevalence of depressive disorders. *Journal of Epidemiology and Community Health, 63*(7), 575–581. doi:10.1136/jech.2008.082719

Artazcoz, L., Benach, J., Borrell, C., & Cortès, I. (2005). Social inequalities in the impact of flexible employment on different domains of psychosocial health. *Journal of Epidemiology and Community Health, 59*(9), 761–767. doi:10.1136/jech.2004.028704

Averina, M., Nilssen, O., Brenn, T., Brox, J., Arkhipovsky, V., & Kalinin, A. (2005). Social and lifestyle determinants of depression, anxiety, sleeping disorders and self-evaluated quality of life in Russia. *Social Psychiatry and Psychiatric Epidemiology, 40*(7), 511–518. doi:10.1007/s00127-005-0918-x

Barnes, D. M., Keyes, K. M., & Bates, L. M. (2013). Racial differences in depression in the United States: How do subgroup analyses inform a paradox? *Social Psychiatry and Psychiatric Epidemiology, 48*(12), 1941–1949. doi:10.1007/s00127-013-0718-7

Belle, D. (1990). Poverty and women's mental health. *American Psychologist, 45*(3), 385. doi:10.1037/0003-066X.45.3.385

Bierut, L. J., Heath, A. C., Bucholz, K. K., Dinwiddie, S. H., Madden, P. A. F., Statham, D. J., . . . Martin, N. G. (1999). Major depressive disorder in a community-based twin sample: Are there different genetic and environmental contributions for men and women? *Archives of General Psychiatry, 56*(6), 557–563.

Bijl, R. V., Ravelli, A., & Van Zessen, G. (1998). Prevalence of psychiatric disorder in the general population: Results of The Netherlands Mental Health Survey and Incidence Study (NEMESIS). *Social Psychiatry and Psychiatric Epidemiology, 33*(12), 587–595. doi:10.1007/s001270050098

Bland, R. C., Stebelsky, G., Orn, H., & Newman, S. C. (1988). Psychiatric disorders and unemployment in Edmonton. *Acta Psychiatrica Scandinavica, 77*(Suppl. 338), 72–80. doi:10.1111/j.1600-0447.1988.tb08550.x

Blazer, D. G., Kessler, R. C., McGonagle, K. A., & Swartz, M.S. (1994). The prevalence and distribution of major depression in a national community sample: The National Comorbidity Survey. *American Journal of Psychiatry, 115*(7), 979–986.

Breslau, J., Aguilar-Gaxiola, S., Kendler, K. S., Su, M., Williams, D., & Kessler, R. C. (2006). Specifying race-ethnic differences in risk for psychiatric disorder in a USA national sample. *Psychological Medicine, 36*(1), 57–68. doi:10.1017/S0033291705006161

Brown, G. W., Bhrolchain, M. N., & Harris, T. (1975). Social class and psychiatric disturbance among women in an urban population. *Sociology, 9*(2), 225–254. doi:10.1177/003803857500900203

Byrne, M., & Carr, A. (2000). Depression and power in marriage. *Journal of Family Therapy, 22*(4), 408–427. doi:10.1111/1467-6427.00161

Callander, E., & Schofield, D. (2015). Psychological distress and the increased risk of falling into poverty: A longitudinal study of Australian adults. *Social Psychiatry and Psychiatric Epidemiology.* Advance online publication. doi:10.3102/0002831209349215

Canadian Institute for Health Information. (2009). *The association between socio-economic status and inpatient hospital service use for depression* (analysis in brief). Retrieved from https://secure.cihi.ca/estore/productSeries.htm?pc=PCC474

Canino, G. J., Bird, H. R., Shrout, P. E., Rubio-Stipec, M., Bravo, M., Martinez, R., . . . Guevara, L. M. (1987). The prevalence of specific psychiatric disorders in Puerto Rico. *Archives of General Psychiatry, 44*(8), 727–735. doi:10.1001/archpsyc.1987.01800200053008

Chonody, J. M., & Siebert, D. C. (2008). Gender differences in depression: A theoretical examination of power. *Affilia, 23*(4), 338–348. doi:10.1177/0886109908323971

Cochran, S. D., & Mays, V. M. (2000). Relation between psychiatric syndromes and behaviorally defined sexual orientation in a sample of the US population. *American Journal of Epidemiology, 151*(5), 516–523.

Cochran, S. D., Sullivan, J. G., & Mays, V. M. (2003). Prevalence of mental disorders, psychological distress, and mental health services use among lesbian, gay, and bisexual adults in the United States. *Journal of Consulting and Clinical Psychology, 71*(1), 53–61. doi:10.1037/0022-006X.71.1.53

Costa-Font, J., & Gil, J. (2008). Would socio-economic inequalities in depression fade away with income transfers? *Journal of Happiness Studies, 9*(4), 539–558. doi:10.1007/s10902-008-9088-3

Costello, E., Compton, S. N., Keeler, G., & Angold, A. (2003). Relationships between poverty and psychopathology: A natural experiment. *JAMA, 290*(15), 2023–2029. doi:10.1001/jama.290.15.2023

CSDH. (2008). *Closing the gap in a generation: Health equity through action on the social determinants of health. Final report of the Commission on Social Determinants of Health.* Geneva, Switzerland: World Health Organization. Retrieved from http://apps.who.int/iris/bitstream/10665/43943/1/9789241563703_eng.pdf

de Graaf, R., ten Have, M., van Gool, C., & van Dorsselaer, S. (2012). Prevalence of mental disorders and trends from 1996 to 2009. Results from the Netherlands Mental Health Survey and Incidence Study-2. *Social Psychiatry and Psychiatric Epidemiology, 47*(2), 203–213. doi:10.1007/s00127-010-0334-8

Dohrenwend, B. P., & Dohrenwend, B. S. (1982). Perspectives on the past and future of psychiatric epidemiology. The 1981 Rema Lapouse lecture. *American Journal of Public Health, 72*(11), 1271–1279.

Dohrenwend, B. P., Levav, I., Shrout, P. E., Schwartz, S., Naveh, G., Link, B. G., . . . Stueve, A. (1992). Socioeconomic status and psychiatric disorders: The causation-selection issue. *Science, 255*(5047), 946–952. doi:10.1126/science.1546291

Dooley, D., Prause, J., & Ham-Rowbottom, K. A. (2000). Underemployment and depression: Longitudinal relationships. *Journal of Health and Social Behavior, 41*(4), 421–436. doi:10.2307/2676295

Eaton, W. W., Muntaner, C., Bovasso, G., & Smith, C. (2001). Socioeconomic status and depressive syndrome: The role of inter- and intra-generational mobility, government assistance, and work environment. *Journal of Health and Social Behavior, 42*(3), 277–294. doi:10.2307/3090215

Elliott, M. (2001). Gender differences in causes of depression. *Women and Health, 33*(3–4), 183–198. doi:10.1300/J013v33n03_11

Ennis, N., Hobfoll, S., & Schröder, K. E. (2000). Money doesn't talk, it swears: How economic stress and resistance resources impact inner-city women's depressed mood. *American Journal of Community Psychology, 28*(2), 149–173. doi:10.1023/A:1005183100610

Falconnier, L. (2009). Socioeconomic status in the treatment of depression. *American Journal of Orthopsychiatry, 79*(2), 148–158. doi:10.1037/a0015469

Fryers, T., Melzer, D., & Jenkins, R. (2003). Social inequalities and the common mental disorders. *Social psychiatry and psychiatric epidemiology, 38*(5), 229–237. doi:10.1007/s00127-003-0627-2

Galobardes, B., Shaw, M., Lawlor, D. A., Lynch, J. W., & Smith, G. D. (2006a). Indicators of socioeconomic position (part 1). *Journal of Epidemiology and Community Health, 60*(1), 7–12. doi:10.1136/jech.2004.023531

Galobardes, B., Shaw, M., Lawlor, D. A., Lynch, J. W., & Smith, G. D. (2006b). Indicators of socioeconomic position (part 2). *Journal of Epidemiology and Community Health, 60*(2), 95–101. doi:10.1136/jech.2004.028092

Gilman, S. E. (2007). Invited commentary: The life course epidemiology of depression. *American Journal of Epidemiology, 166*(10), 1134–1137. doi:10.1093/aje/kwm251

Goyal, D., Gay, C., & Lee, K. A. (2010). How much does low socioeconomic status increase the risk of prenatal and postpartum depressive symptoms in first-time mothers? *Women's Health Issues, 20*(2), 96–104. doi:10.1016/j.whi.2009.11.003

Hamilton, V. L., Broman, C. L., Hoffman, W. S., & Renner, D. S. (1990). Hard times and vulnerable people: Initial effects of plant closing on autoworkers' mental health. *Journal of Health and Social Behavior, 31*(2), 123–140. doi:10.2307/2137167

Hasin, D. S., Fenton, M. C., & Weissman, M. M. (2011). Epidemiology of depressive disorders. In M. T. Tsuang, M. Tohen, & P. Jones (Eds.), *Textbook of psychiatric epidemiology* (3rd ed., pp. 289–309). Hoboken, NJ: John Wiley & Sons.

Holzer, C. E., Shea, B. M., Swanson, J. W., Leaf, P. J., Myers, J. K., George, L., . . . Bednarski, P. (1986). The increased risk for specific psychiatric disorders among persons of low socioeconomic status. *American Journal of Social Psychiatry, 6*(4), 259–271.

Hwu, H. G., Yeh, E. K., & Chang, L. Y. (2007). Prevalence of psychiatric disorders in Taiwan defined by the Chinese Diagnostic Interview Schedule. *Acta Psychiatrica Scandinavica, 79*(2), 136–147. doi:10.1111/j.1600-0447.1989.tb08581.x

Jarvis, E. (1855). *Report on insanity and idiocy in Massachusetts, by the Commission on Lunacy, under resolve of the legislature of 1854.* Boston, MA: White.

Jenkins, R., Fitch, C., Hurlston, M., & Walker, F. (2009). Recession, debt and mental health: Challenges and solutions. *Mental Health in Family Medicine, 6*(2), 85–90.

Johnson, J. G., Cohen, P., Dohrenwend, B. P., Link, B. G., & Brook, J. S. (1999). A longitudinal investigation of social causation and social selection processes involved in the association between socioeconomic status and psychiatric disorders. *Journal of Abnormal Psychology, 108*(3), 490–499. doi:10.1037/0021-843X.108.3.490

Kahn, R. S., Wise, P. H., Kennedy, B. P., & Kawachi, I. (2000). State income inequality, household income, and maternal mental and physical health: Cross sectional national survey. *BMJ: British Medical Journal, 321*(7272), 1311–1315. doi:10.1136/bmj.321.7272.1311

Kaplan, G. A., Shema, S. J., & Leite, M. C. A. (2008). Socioeconomic determinants of psychological well-being: The role of income, income change, and income sources over 29 years. *Annals of Epidemiology, 18*(7), 531–537. doi:10.1016/j.annepidem.2008.03.006

Kessler, R. C. (2003). Epidemiology of women and depression. *Journal of Affective Disorders, 74*(1), 5–13. doi:10.1016/S0165-0327(02)00426-3

Kessler, R. C., Berglund, P., Demler, O., Jin, R., Koretz, D., Merikangas, K. R., . . . Wang, P. S. (2003). The epidemiology of major depressive disorder: Results from the National Comorbidity Survey Replication (NCS-R). *JAMA, 289*(23), 3095–3105. doi:10.1001/jama.289.23.3095

Kessler, R. C., Berglund, P., Demler, O., Jin, R., Merikangas, K. R., & Walters, E. E. (2005). Lifetime prevalence and age-of-onset distributions of *DSM-IV* disorders in the national comorbidity survey replication. *Archives of General Psychiatry, 62*(6), 593–602. doi:10.1001/archpsyc.62.6.593

Kessler, R. C., Foster, C. L., Saunders, W. B., & Stang, P. E. (1995). Social consequences of psychiatric disorders, I: Educational attainment. *American Journal of Psychiatry, 152*(7), 1026–1032.

Kessler, R. C., McGonagle, K. A., Zhao, S., Nelson, C. B., Hughes, M., Eshleman, S., . . . Kendler, K. S. (1994). Lifetime and 12-month prevalence of *DSM-III-R* psychiatric disorders in the United States: Results from the National Comorbidity Survey. *Archives of General Psychiatry, 51*(1), 8–19. doi:10.1001/archpsyc.1994.03950010008002

Kohn, R., Dohrenwend, B. P., & Mirotznik, J. (1998). Epidemiological findings on selected psychiatric disorders. In B. P. Dohrenwend (Ed.), *Adversity, stress, and psychopathology* (pp. 235–284). New York, NY: Oxford University Press.

Kosidou, K., Dalman, C., Lundberg, M., Hallqvist, J., Isacsson, G., & Magnusson, C. (2011). Socioeconomic status and risk of psychological distress and depression in the Stockholm Public Health Cohort: A population-based study. *Journal of Affective Disorders, 134*(1–3), 160–167. doi:10.1016/j.jad.2011.05.024

Krieger, N. (2001). A glossary for social epidemiology. *Journal of Epidemiology and Community Health, 55*(10), 693–700. doi:10.1136/jech.55.10.693

Krieger, N., Williams, D. R., & Moss, N. E. (1997). Measuring social class in US public health research: Concepts, methodologies, and guidelines. *Annual Review of Public Health, 18*, 341–378. doi:10.1146/annurev.publhealth.18.1.341

Kuh, D., & Ben-Shlomo, Y. (1997). *A life course approach to chronic disease epidemiology.* New York, NY: Oxford University Press.

Lennon, M. C., & Rosenfield, S. (1992). Women and mental health: The interaction of job and family conditions. *Journal of Health and Social Behavior, 33*(4), 316–327. doi:10.2307/2137311

Levinson, D. F. (2006). The genetics of depression: A review. *Biological Psychiatry, 60*(2), 84–92. doi:10.1016/j.biopsych.2005.08.024

Lincoln, A., Paasche-Orlow, M. K., Cheng, D. M., Lloyd-Travaglini, C., Caruso, C., Saitz, R., & Samet, J. H. (2006). Impact of health literacy on depressive symptoms and mental health–related quality of life among adults with addiction. *Journal of General Internal Medicine, 21*(8), 818–822. doi:10.1111/j.1525-1497.2006.00533.x

London School of Economics and Political Science. Centre for Economic Performance, Mental Health Policy Group. (2006). *The depression report: A new deal for depression and anxiety disorders.* Retrieved from http://eprints.lse.ac.uk/archive/00000818

Lorant, V., Croux, C., Weich, S., Deliege, D., Mackenbach, J., & Ansseau, M. (2007). Depression and socio-economic risk factors: 7-year longitudinal population study. *The British Journal of Psychiatry, 190*(4), 293–298. doi:10.1192/bjp.bp.105.020040

Lorant, V., Deliège, D., Eaton, W., Robert, A., Philippot, P., & Ansseau, M. (2003). Socioeconomic inequalities in depression: A meta-analysis. *American Journal of Epidemiology, 157*(2), 98–112. doi:10.1093/aje/kwf182

Lynch, J. W., Smith, G. D., Kaplan, G. A., & House, J. S. (2000). Income inequality and mortality: Importance to health of individual income, psychosocial environment, or material conditions. *BMJ: British Medical Journal, 320*(7243), 1200–1204. doi:10.1136/bmj.320.7243.1200

Madianos, M., Economou, M., Alexiou, T., & Stefanis, C. (2011). Depression and economic hardship across Greece in 2008 and 2009: Two cross-sectional surveys nationwide. *Social Psychiatry and Psychiatric Epidemiology, 46*(10), 943–952. doi:10.1007/s00127-010-0265-4

Martikainen, P., Adda, J., Ferrie, J., Davey, S., & Marmot, M. (2003). Effects of income and wealth on GHQ depression and poor self rated health in white collar women and men in the Whitehall II study. *Journal of Epidemiology and Community Health, 57*(9), 718–723. doi:10.1136/jech.57.9.718

Mathers, C. D., & Loncar, D. (2005). *Updated projections of global mortality and burden of disease, 2002–2030: Data sources, methods and results.* Geneva, Switzerland: World Health Organization. Retrieved from http://www.who.int/healthinfo/statistics/bod _projections2030_paper.pdf

Mausner-Dorsch, H., & Eaton, W. W. (2000). Psychosocial work environment and depression: Epidemiologic assessment of the demand-control model. *American Journal of Public Health, 90*(11), 1765–1770. doi:10.2105/AJPH.90.11.1765

Mayberry, L. J., Horowitz, J. A., & Declercq, E. (2007). Depression symptom prevalence and demographic risk factors among US women during the first 2 years postpartum. *Journal of Obstetric, Gynecologic and Neonatal Nursing, 36*(6), 542–549. doi:10.1111/j.1552-6909.2007.00191.x

McEwen, B. S. (2000). Allostasis and allostatic load: Implications for neuropsychopharmacology. *Neuropsychopharmacology, 22*(2), 108–124. doi:10.1016/S0893-133X(99)00129-3

McEwen, B. S., & McEwen, C. A. (2015). Social, psychological, and physiological reactions to stress. In R. A. Scott, S. M. Kosslyn, & N. Pinkerton (Eds.), *Emerging trends in the social and behavioral sciences.* Hoboken, NJ: John Wiley & Sons, Inc. doi:10.1002/9781118900772

McLaughlin, K. A., Conron, K. J., Koenen, K. C., & Gilman, S. E. (2010). Childhood adversity, adult stressful life events, and risk of past-year psychiatric disorder: A test of the stress sensitization hypothesis in a population-based sample of adults. *Psychological Medicine, 40*(10), 1647–1658. doi:10.1017/s0033291709992121

Meltzer, H., Gill, B., Petticrew, M., & Hinds, K. (1995). *OPCS surveys of psychiatric morbidity in Great Britain, Report 1: The prevalence of psychiatric morbidity among adults living in private households.* London, England: HMSO.

Meyer, I. H. (1995). Minority stress and mental health in gay men. *Journal of Health and Social Behavior, 36*(1), 38–56. doi:10.2307/2137286

Meyer, I. H. (2003). Prejudice, social stress, and mental health in lesbian, gay, and bisexual populations: Conceptual issues and research evidence. *Psychological Bulletin, 129*(5), 674–697. doi:10.1037/0033-2909.129.5.674

Meyer, I. H., Schwartz, S., & Frost, D. M. (2008). Social patterning of stress and coping: Does disadvantaged social status confer more stress and fewer coping resources? *Social Science & Medicine, 67*(3), 368–379. doi:10.1016/j.socscimed.2008.03.012

Mezuk, B., Rafferty, J. A., Kershaw, K. N., Hudson, D., Abdou, C. M., Lee, H., . . . Jackson, J. S. (2010). Reconsidering the role of social disadvantage in physical and mental health: Stressful life events, health behaviors, race, and depression. *American Journal of Epidemiology, 172*(11), 1238–1249. doi:10.1093/aje/kwq283

Miech, R. A., Caspi, A., Moffitt, T. E., Wright, B. R. E., & Silva, P. A. (1999). Low socioeconomic status and mental disorders: A longitudinal study of selection and causation during young adulthood. *American Journal of Sociology, 104*(4), 1096–1131. doi:10.1086/210137

Mossakowski, K. N. (2009). The influence of past unemployment duration on symptoms of depression among young women and men in the United States. *American Journal of Public Health, 99*(10), 1826–1832. doi:10.2105/AJPH.2008.152561

Muntaner, C., Borrell, C., Benach, J., Pasarín, M. I., & Fernandez, E. (2003). The associations of social class and social stratification with patterns of general and mental health in a Spanish population. *International Journal of Epidemiology, 32*(6), 950–958. doi:10.1093/ije/dyg170

Muntaner, C., Eaton, W. W., & Diala, C. C. (2000). Social inequalities in mental health: A review of concepts and underlying assumptions. *Health, 4*(1), 89–113. doi:10.1177/136345930000400105

Muntaner, C., Eaton, W. W., Diala, C., Kessler, R. C., & Sorlie, P. D. (1998). Social class, assets, organizational control and the prevalence of common groups of psychiatric disorders. *Social Science and Medicine, 47*(12), 2043–2053. doi:10.1016/S0277-9536(98)00309-8

Muntaner, C., Eaton, W. W., Miech, R., & O'Campo, P. (2004). Socioeconomic position and major mental disorders. *Epidemiologic Reviews, 26*(1), 53–62. doi:10.1093/epirev/mxh001

Muntaner, C., Ng, E., Vanroelen, C., Christ, S., & Eaton, W. W. (2013). Social stratification, social closure, and social class as determinants of mental health disparities. In C. S. Aneshensel, J. C. Phelan, & A. Bierman (Eds.), *Handbook of the sociology of mental health* (2nd ed., pp. 205–227). Dordrecht: Springer.

Murcia, M., Chastang, J.-F., & Niedhammer, I. (2015). Educational inequalities in major depressive and generalized anxiety disorders: Results from the French national SIP study. *Social Psychiatry and Psychiatric Epidemiology, 50*(6), 919–928. doi:10.1007/s00127-015-1010-9

Murphy, J. M., Olivier, D. C., Monson, R. R., Sobol, A. M., Federman, E. B., & Leighton, A. H. (1991). Depression and anxiety in relation to social status: A prospective epidemiologic study. *Archives of General Psychiatry, 48*(3), 223–229. doi:10.1001/archpsyc.1991.01810270035004

Nazroo, J. Y. (2015). Ethnic inequalities in severe mental disorders: Where is the harm? *Social Psychiatry and Psychiatric Epidemiology, 50*(7), 1065–1067. doi:10.1007/s00127-015-1079-1

Nishimura, J. (2011). Socioeconomic status and depression across Japan, Korea, and China: Exploring the impact of labor market structures. *Social Science and Medicine, 73*(4), 604–614. doi:10.1016/j.socscimed.2011.06.020

O'Campo, P., Eaton, W. W., & Muntaner, C. (2004). Labor market experience, work organization, gender inequalities and health status: Results from a prospective analysis of US employed women. *Social Science & Medicine, 58*(3), 585–594.

Patel, V., & Kleinman, A. (2003). Poverty and common mental disorders in developing countries. *Bulletin of the World Health Organization, 81*(8), 609–615.

Paul, K. I., & Moser, K. (2009). Unemployment impairs mental health: Meta-analyses. *Journal of Vocational Behavior, 74*(3), 264–282. doi:10.1016/j.jvb.2009.01.001

Pearlin, L. I., Menaghan, E. G., Morton, A. L., & Mullan, J. T. (1981). The stress process. *Journal of Health and Social Behavior, 22*(4), 337–356. doi:10.2307/2136676

Peyrot, W. J., Lee, S. H., Milaneschi, Y., Abdellaoui, A., Byrne, E. M., Esko, T., . . . Penninx, B. W. (2015). The association between lower educational attainment and depression owing to shared genetic effects? Results in ~25 000 subjects. *Molecular Psychiatry, 20*(6), 735–743. doi:10.1038/mp.2015.50

Piccinelli, M., & Wilkinson, G. (2000). Gender differences in depression: Critical review. *The British Journal of Psychiatry, 177*(6), 486–492. doi:10.1192/bjp.177.6.486

Pollack, C. E., Chideya, S., Cubbin, C., Williams, B., Dekker, M., & Braveman, P. (2007). Should health studies measure wealth? A systematic review. *American Journal of Preventive Medicine, 33*(3), 250–264. doi:10.1016/j.amepre.2007.04.033

Power, C., Stansfeld, S. A., Matthews, S., Manor, O., & Hope, S. (2002). Childhood and adulthood risk factors for socio-economic differentials in psychological distress: Evidence from the 1958 British birth cohort. *Social Science & Medicine, 55*(11), 1989–2004. doi:10.1016/S0277-9536(01)00325-2

Prins, S. J., Bates, L. M., Keyes, K. M., & Muntaner, C. (2015). Anxious? Depressed? You might be suffering from capitalism: Contradictory class locations and the prevalence of depression and anxiety in the USA. *Sociology of Health and Illness*. Advance online publication. doi:10.1111/1467-9566.12315

Quesnel-Vallée, A., DeHaney, S., & Ciampi, A. (2010). Temporary work and depressive symptoms: A propensity score analysis. *Social Science & Medicine, 70*(12), 1982–1987. doi:10.1016/j.socscimed.2010.02.008

Quesnel-Vallée, A., & Taylor, M. (2012). Socioeconomic pathways to depressive symptoms in adulthood: Evidence from the National Longitudinal Survey of Youth 1979. *Social Science & Medicine, 74*(5), 734–743.

Raphael, D., & Bryant, T. (2015). Power, intersectionality and the life-course: Identifying the political and economic structures of welfare states that support or threaten health. *Social Theory Health, 13*(3–4), 245–266. doi:10.1057/sth.2015.18

Reese, A. M., Thorpe, R. J., Jr., Bell, C. N., Bowie, J. V., & LaVeist, T. A. (2012). The effect of religious service attendance on race differences in depression: Findings from the EHDIC-SWB study. *Journal of Urban Health, 89*(3), 510–518. doi:10.1007/s11524-011-9659-1

Regier, D. A., Farmer, M. E., Rae, D. S., Myers, J. K., Kramer, M., Robins, L. N., . . . Locke, B. Z. (1993). One-month prevalence of mental disorders in the United States and sociodemographic characteristics: The Epidemiologic Catchment Area study. *Acta Psychiatrica Scandinavica, 88*(1), 35–47. doi:10.1111/j.1600-0447.1993.tb03411.x

Rhodes, A., Jaakkimainen, R. L., Bondy, S., & Fung, K. (2006). Depression and mental health visits to physicians: A prospective records-based study. *Social Science & Medicine, 62*(4), 828–834. doi:10.1016/j.socscimed.2005.06.039

Richardson, T., Elliott, P., & Roberts, R. (2013). The relationship between personal unsecured debt and mental and physical health: A systematic review and meta-analysis. *Clinical Psychology Review, 33*(8), 1148–1162. doi:10.1016/j.cpr.2013.08.009

Riolo, S. A., Nguyen, T. A., Greden, J. F., & King, C. A. (2005). Prevalence of depression by race/ethnicity: Findings from the National Health and Nutrition Examination Survey III. *American Journal of Public Health, 95*(6), 998–1000. doi:10.2105/AJPH.2004.047225

Ritsher, J. E. B., Warner, V., Johnson, J. G., & Dohrenwend, B. P. (2001). Inter-generational longitudinal study of social class and depression: A test of social causation and social selection models. *The British Journal of Psychiatry, 178*(40), s84–s90. doi:10.1192/bjp.178.40.s84

Robins, L. N., & Regier, D. A. (1991). *Psychiatric disorders in America: The Epidemiologic Catchment Area study.* New York, NY: The Free Press.

Rojas-García, A., Ruiz-Perez, I., Rodríguez-Barranco, M., Bradley, D. C. G., Pastor-Moreno, G., & Ricci-Cabello, I. (2015, June). Healthcare interventions for depression in low socioeconomic status populations: A systematic review and meta-analysis. *Clinical Psychology Review, 38*, 65–78. doi:10.1016/j.cpr.2015.03.001

Rosenfield, S. (1992). The costs of sharing: Wives' employment and husbands' mental health. *Journal of Health and Social Behavior, 33*(3), 213–225.

Rosenfield, S. (2012). Triple jeopardy? Mental health at the intersection of gender, race, and class. *Social Science & Medicine, 74*(11), 1791–1801. doi:10.1016/j.socscimed.2011.11.010

Ross, C. E., & Mirowsky, J. (1999). Refining the association between education and health: The effects of quantity, credential, and selectivity. *Demography, 36*(4), 445–460. doi:10.2307/2648083

Ross, C. E., & Mirowsky, J. (2006). Sex differences in the effect of education on depression: Resource multiplication or resource substitution? *Social Science & Medicine, 63*(5), 1400–1413. doi:10.1016/j.socscimed.2006.03.013

Ross, C. E., & Wu, C.-L. (1995). The links between education and health. *American Sociological Review, 60*(5), 719–745. doi:10.2307/2096319

Ross, C. E., & Wu, C.-L. (1996). Education, age, and the cumulative advantage in health. *Journal of Health and Social Behavior, 37*(1), 104–120. doi:10.2307/2137234

Roxburgh, S. (2009). Untangling inequalities: Gender, race, and socioeconomic differences in depression. *Sociological Forum, 24*(2), 357–381. doi:10.1111/j.1573-7861.2009.01103.x

Roy-Byrne, P. P., Joesch, J. M., Wang, P. S., & Kessler, R. C. (2009). Low socioeconomic status and mental health care use among respondents with anxiety and depression in the NCS-R. *Psychiatric Services, 60*(9), 1190–1197. doi:10.1176/ps.2009.60.9.1190

Saraceno, B., Levav, I., & Kohn, R. (2005). The public mental health significance of research on socio-economic factors in schizophrenia and major depression. *World Psychiatry, 4*(3), 181–185.

Schütte, S., Chastang, J.-F., Parent-Thirion, A., Vermeylen, G., & Niedhammer, I. (2015). Psychosocial work exposures among European employees: Explanations for occupational inequalities in mental health. *Journal of Public Health, 37*(3), 373–388. doi:10.1093/pubmed/fdv044

Scott, J., & Marshall, G. (2009). *A dictionary of sociology* (3rd ed.). New York, NY: Oxford University Press.

Seedat, S., Scott, K. M., Angermeyer, M. C., Berglund, P., Bromet, E. J., Brugha, T. S., . . . Kessler, R. C. (2009). Cross-national associations between gender and mental disorders in the World Health Organization World Mental Health Surveys. *Archieves of General Psychiatry, 66*(7), 785–795. doi:10.1001/archgenpsychiatry.2009.36

Séguin, L., Potvin, L., St-Denis, M., & Loiselle, J. (1999). Socio-environmental factors and postnatal depressive symptomatology: A longitudinal study. *Women and Health, 29*(1), 57–72. doi:10.1300/J013v29n01_05

Stankunas, M., Kalediene, R., Starkuviene, S., & Kapustinskiene, V. (2006). Duration of unemployment and depression: A cross-sectional survey in Lithuania. *BMC Public Health, 6*(174). doi:10.1186/1471-2458-6-174

Stansfeld, S. A., Head, J., Fuhrer, R., Wardle, J., & Cattell, V. (2003). Social inequalities in depressive symptoms and physical functioning in the Whitehall II study: Exploring a common cause explanation. *Journal of Epidemiology and Community Health, 57*(5), 361–367. doi:10.1136/jech.57.5.361

Starkes, J. M., Poulin, C. C., & Kisely, S. R. (2005). Unmet need for the treatment of depression in Atlantic Canada. *Canadian Journal of Psychiatry, 50*(10), 580–590.

Steele, L., Dewa, C., & Lee, K. (2007). Socioeconomic status and self-reported barriers to mental health service use. *Canadian Journal of Psychiatry, 52*(3), 201–206.

Steele, L., Glazier, R. H., & Lin, E. (2006). Inequity in mental health care under Canadian universal health coverage. *Psychiatric Services, 57*(3), 317–324. doi:10.1176/appi.ps.57.3.317

Talala, K., Huurre, T., Aro, H., Martelin, T., & Prättälä, R. (2009). Trends in socio-economic differences in self-reported depression during the years 1979–2002 in Finland. *Social Psychiatry and Psychiatric Epidemiology, 44*(10), 871–879. doi:10.1007/s00127-009-0009-5

Thoits, P. A. (2010). Stress and health: Major findings and policy implications. *Journal of Health and Social Behavior, 51*(Suppl. 1), S41–S53. doi:10.1177/0022146510383499

Turner, R. J., & Avison, W. R. (2003). Status variations in stress exposure: Implications for the interpretation of research on race, socioeconomic status, and gender. *Journal of Health Social Behavior, 44*(4), 488–505. doi:10.2307/1519795

Turner, R. J., & Lloyd, D. A. (1999). The stress process and the social distribution of depression. *Journal of Health and Social Behavior, 40*(4), 374–404. doi:10.2307/2676332

Turner, R. J., & Marino, F. (1994). Social support and social structure: A descriptive epidemiology. *Journal of Health and Social Behavior, 35*(3), 193–212. doi:10.2307/2137276

Van de Velde, S., Bracke, P., & Levecque, K. (2010). Gender differences in depression in 23 European countries. Cross-national variation in the gender gap in depression. *Social Science & Medicine, 71*(2), 305–313. doi:10.1016/j.socscimed.2010.03.035

Wang, J. L., Schmitz, N., & Dewa, C. S. (2010). Socioeconomic status and the risk of major depression: The Canadian National Population Health Survey. *Journal of Epidemiology and Community Health, 64*(5), 447–452. doi:10.1136/jech.2009.090910

Weich, S., Lewis, G., & Jenkins, S. P. (2001). Income inequality and the prevalence of common mental disorders in Britain. *The British Journal of Psychiatry, 178*(3), 222–227. doi:10.1192/bjp.178.3.222

Weissman, M. M., Bruce, L. M., Leaf, P. J., Florio, L. P., & Holzer, C. (1991). Affective disorders. In L. N. Robins & D. A. Regier (Eds.), *Psychiatric disorders in America: The Epidemiologic Catchment Area study* (pp. 53–80). New York, NY: The Free Press.

Wells, K. B., Stewart, A., Hays, R. D., Burnam, M. A., Rogers, W., Daniels, M., . . . Ware, J. (1989). The functioning and well-being of depressed patients: Results from the Medical Outcomes Study. *JAMA, 262*(7), 914–919. doi:10.1001/jama.1989.03430070062031

West, P. (1991). Rethinking the health selection explanation for health inequalities. *Social Science & Medicine, 32*(4), 373–384. doi:10.1016/0277-9536(91)90338-D

Wilhelm, K., Mitchell, P., Slade, T., Brownhill, S., & Andrews, G. (2003). Prevalence and correlates of *DSM-IV* major depression in an Australian national survey. *Journal of Affective Disorders, 75*(2), 155–162. doi:10.1016/S0165-0327(02)00040-X

Williams, D. R., & Collins, C. (2001). Racial residential segregation: A fundamental cause of racial disparities in health. *Public Health Reports, 116*(5), 404–416.

Williams, D. R., Takeuchi, D. T., & Adair, R. K. (1992). Socioeconomic status and psychiatric disorder among blacks and whites. *Social Forces, 71*(1), 179–194. doi:10.1093/sf/71.1.179

Williams, D. R., Yan, Y., Jackson, J. S., & Anderson, N. B. (1997). Racial differences in physical and mental health: Socio-economic status, stress and discrimination. *Journal of Health Psychology, 2*(3), 335–351. doi:10.1177/135910539700200305

Wium-Andersen, M., Ørsted, D., Nielsen, S., & Nordestgaard, B. (2013). Elevated C-reactive protein levels, psychological distress, and depression in 73,131 individuals. *JAMA Psychiatry, 70*(2), 176–184. doi:10.1001/2013.jamapsychiatry.102

Wohlfarth, T. (1997). Socioeconomic inequality and psychopathology: Are socioeconomic status and social class interchangeable? *Social Science & Medicine, 45*(3), 399–410. doi:10.1016/S0277-9536(96)00355-3

World Health Organization and Calouste Gulbenkian Foundation. (2014). *Social determinants of mental health.* Geneva: World Health Organization.

Wright, E. O. (1989). The comparative project on class structure and class consciousness: An overview. *Acta Sociologica, 32*(1), 3–22. doi:10.1177/000169938903200101

Young, A. S., Klap, R., Sherbourne, C. D., & Wells, K. B. (2001). The quality of care for depressive and anxiety disorders in the United States. *Archives of General Psychiatry, 58*(1), 55–61. doi:10.1001/archpsyc.58.1.55

Zimmerman, F. J., Christakis, D. A., & Vander Stoep, A. (2004). Tinker, tailor, soldier, patient: Work attributes and depression disparities among young adults. *Social Science & Medicine, 58*(10), 1889–1901. doi:10.1016/S0277-9536(03)00410-6

Zimmerman, F. J., & Katon, W. (2005). Socioeconomic status, depression disparities, and financial strain: What lies behind the income-depression relationship? *Health Economics, 14*(12), 1197–1215. doi:10.1002/hec.1011

CHAPTER 7

Maternal Depression and the Intergenerational Transmission of Depression

Constance L. Hammen, PhD

Due both to its high prevalence among the world's populations and the high costs it exacts in health and well-being, depression is the leading cause of disability globally and takes an enormous toll on individuals and communities (Kessler & Bromet, 2013; Murray et al., 2012). Depression is commonly recurrent or chronic and is associated with lives lost to suicide, medical morbidity, loss of work productivity, unstable marriages, and social impairment (e.g., Greenberg et al., 2003; Hammen & Shih, 2014; Ormel et al., 2008). But perhaps no aspect is more enduring or potentially tragic than the legacy of depression and psychological maladjustment that is passed on through generations from parent to child. While most forms of mental disorder have a genetic component, sometimes a very substantial one, depression is considered to be only modestly heritable with a significant environmental component and is "inherited" not as a depressive disease in itself but through causal risk factors that affect temperament, cognitive style, reactivity to stress, relational qualities, and coping capabilities that eventuate, through both environmental and biological mechanisms, in depression (for examples of multiple-factor models of depression, see Disner, Beevers, Haigh, & Beck, 2011; Goodman et al., 2011; Hankin, 2015; Kendler & Gardner, 2011). This chapter reviews the evidence of intergenerational transmission of depression, its risk factors, and its implications for public health issues and treatment, with an emphasis on the most current research and new directions.

Defining and Describing Depression

Major depression is generally a disorder of young adult onset, but many cases emerge in adolescence and recur in adulthood (Hankin, 2015; Kessler et al., 2003; Merikangas et al., 2010). Thus, depression is most common in the childbearing years of late adolescence and early adulthood. For many individuals, perhaps most, it is a lifelong disorder marked by recurrent episodes often with incomplete recovery between acute exacerbations (Burcusa & Iocono, 2007; Richards, 2011). Depression is also highly likely to co-occur with other psychological disorders, commonly anxiety, substance use, and eating and other personality and behavioral disorders (e.g., Hasin, Goodwin, Stinson, & Grant, 2005). Depression is debilitating for the individual. Low mood; low energy; problems with concentration and focus; negative outlook about the self, the world, and the future; and loss of enjoyment of typically pleasurable experiences make it difficult to persevere in the tasks of one's roles. Additionally, it also has a negative impact on others and is widely misperceived. The depressed person's irritability or withdrawal, seemingly "irrational" negative thoughts and beliefs ("I'm worthless, un-lovable," "Things will never get better"), and the misperception that depressed people could alter their thoughts and behaviors with effort, distraction, and positive thinking if only they tried often leads to resentment in loved ones. The sufferer's dis-engagement or "complaining" is often experienced as lack of caring, rejection, and weakness of will. In short, depression is often misunderstood and may result in alien-ation from loved ones, often deepening the sadness of the depressed person. Inevita-bly, depression takes a toll on marital and family life, and impairs performance in the parenting role despite a person's wish to be a good parent. Because women are twice as likely to experience depressive disorders as men (Andrade et al., 2003; Kessler et al., 2003; Nolen-Hoeksema & Girgus, 1994), and more likely to be the primary caregiv-ers, most of the studies of parental depression have focused on depressed mothers.

All research on depression, including intergenerational aspects of depression, must be interpreted in light of methodological factors. Importantly, these include measure-ment of depression, whether it refers to diagnoses or symptomatology, and the notable heterogeneity not only of different presentations of symptom profiles but also differ-ences in severity and course of the disorder.

Effects of Maternal Depression on Children

The nature and consequences of maternal depression likely depend on the age of exposure, including prenatal depression, as well as the age of the child and kinds of outcomes that are relevant to measure in preschool-age children compared to older children. Therefore, outcomes are discussed first for school-age children, and then for perinatal exposure and outcomes of young children.

Disorders and Maladjustment in School-Age Offspring

Most of the earliest body of research was conducted on older children and adoles-cents of currently or recently depressed mothers. By the 1990s, research on outcomes of offspring of depressed mothers was increasingly likely to include longitudinal de-signs and assessments of multiple risk factors co-occurring in families. In terms of the overall research findings, largely of school-age (including adolescent) children of depressed parents, a review by Beardslee, Versage, and Gladstone (1998) based mostly on treatment samples suggested that by age 20, a child of a depressed parent had a 40% chance of experiencing an episode of major depressive disorder as well as increased risks of other disorders, including behavioral, substance use, and anxiety disorders. A later meta-analysis of 193 studies (Goodman et al., 2011) comprised both treatment samples and the increasing number of community samples of depressed women, including both diagnosis-based and symptom-based studies. They reported significant small to moderate effect sizes of associations between maternal and child internalizing problems (r = .23), and externalizing problems (r = .21), and the patterns were generally similar in clinically diagnosable depressive conditions and subclinically elevated symptoms.

To highlight results of a few more recent longitudinal community samples that are most representative of the general population of depression, in the Avon (England) Longitudinal Study of Parents and Children, 7,500 mother-child pairs were studied (children were aged 1.5–7.5). The young children of depressed women compared with nondepressed women were found to have significantly higher rates of disorders (1.2% vs. 0.4% depression, 4.1% vs. 1.8% oppositional defiant disorder, 7.7% vs. 2.6% anxiety disorders; Barker, Copeland, Maughan, Jaffee, & Eher, 2012). A longitudinal Canadian community study of depression and anxiety symptoms in young children (n = 1,759) found that trajectories of high sustained and increasing levels of symptoms in children between 1.5 and 5 years was significantly associated with a maternal history of depression (Côté et al., 2009). A community study of women screened for postpartum depression shortly after the birth of their child, with multiple follow-ups, indicated a rate of 40% for any Axis I diagnosis by age 13, including 23% with depressive disorder. The rate of depression was more than 30% for youth whose mother had both postpartum and subsequent depression (Halligan, Murray, Martins, & Cooper, 2007). Hammen and Brennan (2001) studied 815 pairs of 15-year-old children and their depressed or nondepressed mothers selected from a birth cohort sample of more than 5,000 in Queensland, Australia. They found that youth of depressed mothers were diagnosed with past or current major depressive episode at the rate of 18.4% vs. 9.85% for youth of nondepressed women, 9.6% vs. 4.4% anxiety disorders, 4.2% vs. 1.3% conduct disorder. By age 20, offspring of depressed women had a rate of MDE of 39% compared to 28% of children of nondepressed women.

In addition to psychological disorders, the children of depressed women display a variety of problems including cognitive, social-interpersonal, academic, and health issues such as obesity (e.g., Hammen, Brennan, Keenan-Miller, & Herr, 2008; Lampard, Franckle, & Davison, 2014; Weissman et al., 2006).

The majority of studies of effects of maternal depression have been conducted in relatively high-income Western nations. However, Wachs, Black, and Engle (2009) reviewed studies in low- and middle-income countries, noting relatively high rates of maternal depression and significant associations with children's behavioral problems and depression symptoms, difficult temperament, motor and cognitive delays, as well as medical and developmental issues.

It should be noted that there are a few existing long-term follow-ups of children of depressed mothers reporting three-generation patterns. Myrna Weissman's follow-up study found that grandchildren who had both a depressed parent and a depressed grandparent had a 59% chance of psychopathology and were the most impaired (Warner, Weissman, Mufson, & Wickramaratne, 1999; Weissman et al., 2005). The children of depressed parents who did not have a depressed grandparent did not have diagnosed disorders, although they did display impairment of functioning (Weissman et al., 2005). Hammen, Shih, and Brennan (2004) also found that grandparent depression (assessed by mother report) contributed to the prediction of depressive outcomes in offspring of depressed women. In addition, potentially portending a third generation of depression, at age 20 the female offspring of depressed mothers were more likely to have given birth and to be depressed and functioning poorly in the maternal role if they themselves had been depressed by age 15 (Hammen, Brennan, & Le Brocque, 2011). Depressed offspring of depressed mothers also reported higher rates of intimate partner violence between ages 15 and 20 than offspring of nondepressed mothers (Keenan-Miller, Hammen, & Brennan, 2007). In the same follow-up study, the offspring of depressed women who themselves (offspring) had been depressed by age 15 had poorer-quality romantic relations at age 20, as reported by both the youth and the romantic partner, which predicted higher levels of depressive symptoms (Katz, Hammen, & Brennan, 2013). Thus, teen depression among females, especially in the context of histories of maternal depression, appears to portend continuing risk for the transmission of depression into the next generation.

Effects of Maternal Perinatal Depression

In view of extensive research documenting psychological maladjustment in the school-age children of depressed women, investigators have increasingly focused on maternal depression during pregnancy and postpartum. The assumption is that early exposure (prenatal or infancy) might be the most likely to disrupt important infant developmental and parenting processes, and lead to the greatest impairment compared to later exposure (e.g., Goodman et al., 2011). There is clear evidence that mothers' *prenatal* stress, depression, and anxiety may put infants at risk for later depression, operating through mechanisms such as neuroendocrine abnormalities, reduced blood flow to the fetus, fetal neurobehavioral development, and maternal maladaptive health behaviors, among others (reviewed in Goodman & Lusby, 2014). Stein and colleagues (2014) reviewed global research on fetal and neonatal outcomes, finding that prenatal depression is associated with premature birth and low birth weight, especially in low- and middle-income countries compared with high-income countries (see also Surkan, Kennedy, Hurley, & Black, 2011). Longitudinal studies, conducted mostly in high-income countries, reported higher levels of emotional, behavioral, and social difficulties in children of prenatally depressed women and women with postnatal depression (reviewed in Stein et al., 2014), especially those with chronically elevated symptoms (e.g., Cents et al., 2013). Prenatal and postnatal depression are highly correlated with each other, but one large-scale study of 4,500 parents reported independent effects, such that maternal prenatal depression was an independent risk factor for offspring depression at age 18, whereas postnatal depression was a risk factor only in mothers with low levels of education (Pearson et al., 2013).

In addition to assessment of children's symptomatology, investigators have also focused on young children's cognitive, behavioral, and social outcomes that presumably predict future maladjustment. For example, studies of security of infant attachment to the mother have found that prenatal depression is associated with disorganized attachment, independent of postnatal depression (Hayes, Goodman, & Carlson, 2013). A meta-analysis by Martins and Gaffan (2000) on six studies of infants of postnatally depressed women indicated lower levels of secure attachment and higher rates of insecure, especially disorganized, attachment compared to infants of nondepressed women. An additional meta-analysis of 13 studies that included maternal depression also showed significant links with attachment insecurity in young children, especially in more severe clinical samples compared with community samples (Atkinson, Paglia, & Coolbear, 2000).

Cognitive development is another potentially important outcome in young children that is thought to be adversely affected by exposure to perinatal depression. Stein and colleagues (2014) reviewed the literature on IQ, ability to learn, language, and general cognitive development, concluding that both prenatal and postnatal maternal depression predict a range of adverse outcomes, especially among offspring of women with chronic depression (reviewed in Kingston, Tough, & Whitfield, 2012). A large study (n = 1,215 mothers and their infants) from the National Institute of Child Health and Human Development (NICHD) Early Child Care Research Network (1999) found that the children of women with chronic symptoms of depression performed more poorly on cognitive-linguistic measures, and the effects were largely moderated by maternal sensitivity in mother-child interactions.

Moderators and Mediators of Effects of Maternal Depression

Maternal depression clearly is a major risk factor for depression in offspring. However, its effects apply only to some of the children and not others. In the following section, we review recent research that attempts to characterize the conditions under which parent depression is more likely to have adverse consequences for children. Further, in order to fully realize the potential for preventive interventions, it is critical to understand the risk factors and potential mechanisms by which depression in the mother has a negative influence on the children.

Moderators

With respect to moderators, several clinical and demographic factors are associated with worse child outcomes. Overall, chronic depression in the mother has a more negative effect than single episodes. Additionally, the presence of comorbid conditions such as anxiety disorders, substance abuse, and antisocial behavior (Sellars et al., 2013, 2014) generally increases the child's risk for future psychopathology. Further, both younger age of the child's exposure to maternal depression and economic disadvantage (and attendant stress and low educational attainment) are important moderators of the impact of maternal depression on offspring (Goodman et al., 2011; Jaffee et al., 2002; National Research Council and Institute of Medicine, 2009; Stein et al., 2014). These issues are elaborated in the following sections.

Psychosocial Risk Factors and Mechanisms of Depression Transmission

Several overarching themes warrant introduction before presenting research on the risk factors and mediators, and how they contribute to offspring dysfunction. First, parenting styles and practices are typically impaired during depressive episodes and conditions, and dysfunctional parenting is likely the most important—and potentially modifiable—risk factor for youth depression (e.g., reviewed in Goodman, 2007). Indeed, depression commonly takes a toll on functioning in close relationships in general (Hammen & Shih, 2014).

Second, depression typically is a response to stressors in the form of both acute life events such as loss, injury, and failure as well as chronic, ongoing stressful conditions such as marital strife, economic hardship, health problems, and heavy caretaking responsibilities (e.g., Hammen, 2005). To a great extent, depression in adults is a *dysfunctional* response to stress, affecting cognition, emotion, behavior, and neurobiological and genetically influenced responses to the environment that eventuate in depression. For infants and young children especially, environmental stress is funneled through "mom," and the quality of her care has an enormous impact on the child's development (e.g., Tang, Reeb-Sutherland, Romeo, & McEwen, 2014).

A child raised by a depressed and stressed mother "inherits" a stressful family and life environment that may overwhelm both the mother's and the child's coping resources. Unfortunately, depression and the maladaptive cognitions and behaviors that serve as vulnerability factors for depression can also contribute to the further occurrence of stressors, particularly interpersonal stressors (Hammen, 1991). This "stress-generation" pattern portends vicious cycles of interpersonal stress and recurrent or chronic depression (Hammen, 2005; Hammen, Hazel, Brennan, & Najman, 2012; Liu, 2013).

Third, while depression occurs in all segments of the socioeconomic spectrum, those individuals living in poverty typically have not only low income but also low levels of educational attainment and reduced access to other sources of support such as stable spouses and families, and less access to basic health and life-enhancing resources and opportunities. Furthermore, low income is typically highly stressful itself and results in living conditions that are associated with high stress exposure, such as neighborhood danger and increased exposure to unhealthy conditions, unemployment, and disrupted relationships and families. Thus, in the face of stress such parents may experience depression with fewer personal and environmental resources, greatly increasing the challenges of effective child-rearing. It is important to note that economic disadvantage is fairly universally likely to be associated with psychopathology in children, in great part because its attendant stress disrupts effective parenting behaviors (reviewed in Grant, Compas, Stuhlmacher, Thurm, & McMahon, 2003). These elements are discussed in the context of recent research in the following sections.

Parenting Difficulties, Environmental Context, and Offspring Depression

Depression-related symptoms such as low positive and high negative affect; irritability; poor emotion regulation; negative perceptions of the self, others, and the future; low motivation / loss of interest; rumination; and reduced executive functioning (concentration, memory, attention) have been associated with impairments in effective parenting (Psychogiou & Parry, 2014; Stein et al., 2014). Such symptoms, as well as parents' underlying emotional, cognitive, and social vulnerabilities, impede parental warmth, responsiveness, monitoring, and discipline, which undermine children's well-being and effectiveness (Goodman, 2007). Observational studies have noted that depressed, compared to nondepressed, mothers display more negative behaviors toward children, such as criticism and hostility or more withdrawn, disengaged behaviors (reviewed in Lovejoy, Graczyk, O'Hare, & Neuman, 2000). Such patterns are most pronounced in current depression but may remain evident even in women with past depression. Specific patterns commonly observed among depressed women interacting with their infants include intrusive (i.e., harsh, irritated) or withdrawn (i.e., disengaged) styles, or both (Field, Diego, & Hernandez-Reif, 2006).

A large longitudinal study based on the NICHD Study of Early Child Care data found that parenting patterns among chronically depressed mothers could be classified into three groups stable over the first three years: high intrusive, high intrusive / withdrawn, and low intrusive / low withdrawn (Wang & Dix, 2013). These groups did not differ in levels of depression, but the better-functioning mothers (low intrusive / low withdrawn) had more demographic and personal resources (e.g., higher education levels) and less stressful, more supportive environments (e.g., spouses and family support). By age 3, the withdrawn or intrusive patterns were associated with children's poorer language and cognitive development and poorer quality of relationship with the mother. The better-functioning low intrusive, low withdrawn style was associated with cognitive, attachment, and language developmental patterns not significantly different from those of children of nondepressed mothers. However, these children of depressed but better-functioning mothers nonetheless showed more behavioral and social problems than children of nondepressed mothers. Wang and Dix (2013) emphasized the role of demographic and family stress as well as personal and environmental coping resources in moderating the effects of maternal depression on parenting competence.

Numerous studies have tested multiple risk factor models of youth disorders including depression, commonly highlighting the contributions of parental psychopathology, family dysfunction, and stressors (e.g., Côté et al., 2009; Fergusson, Horwood, & Lynskey, 1995; Jaffee et al., 2002: Luby, Belden, & Spitznagel, 2006; Schudlich & Cummings, 2007). Notably, several studies have tested models hypothesizing versions of the idea that the effects of parental depression on children's symptomatology are related to various correlated risk factors including parenting difficulties and family and environmental stress (including marital conflict, absence of supportive relationships, and economic disadvantage). Hammen, Shih, and Brennan (2004) used structural equation modeling and found that maternal depression predicted family and environmental stressors (including marital conflict), with both stress and depression predicting poorer parenting quality, all in turn predicting less youth social competence. These risk factors largely mediated the effect of maternal depression on youth depression. Reising and colleagues (2013) examined families of depressed parents and found support for correlated risk factors (e.g., economic disadvantage, neighborhood stress, and disrupted parenting) predicting both externalizing and internalizing symptoms. When the stress and economic factors were controlled in regression analyses, parenting problems had a significant independent effect. As a further example of multiple risk factor models, Barker and colleagues (2012) examined more than 7,000 pairs of mothers and children, and found evidence that maternal depression was significantly correlated with environmental (socioeconomic), family (relationship conflict, low social support), and lifestyle (early parenthood, low education) risks. A cumulative risk index of the 11 risk factors and maternal depression score at child age 21 months both independently predicted various internalizing and externalizing diagnoses at child age 7.5. Although this study did not specifically measure quality of parenting in infancy, the preponderance of evidence suggests that the measured risk factors are, in fact, highly disruptive of effective parenting (e.g., Grant et al., 2003).

In addition to the direct experiences of nonoptimal parenting that undermine children's healthy development and functioning, the family lives of depressed parents commonly expose children to high levels of stress in which children observe and likely *model* their depressed parent's maladaptive emotional regulation, negative cognitions, and poor problem-solving. Thus, such children may learn and imitate dysfunctional cognitions about self-worth and low expectations of others' reliability, poorer social and problem-solving skills, and often diminished emotional and instrumental support when facing stressors of their own. Children of depressed mothers thus acquire cognitive and social strategies that may put them at risk for depression and impairment in psychosocial functioning. Depressed offspring of depressed mothers show patterns of stress generation, such as contributing to the occurrence of acute stressful life events and selection into chronically stressful situations including early child-rearing and intimate partner violence, as well as impairment in social roles (Adrian & Hammen, 1993; Hammen & Brennan, 2001; Hammen et al., 2011).

Biological Risk Factors and Mechanisms of Depression Transmission

This section presents a selective and general discussion of genetic and neurobiological (neuroendocrine and neural) factors that contribute to depression and maladaptive outcomes in children of depressed mothers. The research largely applies adult models of depression to children and is relatively recent and rapidly evolving. With important exceptions, much of the biological research on depression or risk for depression in children has yet to fully explore and describe developmental processes in biological systems. Moreover, it is also crucially important to consider that prenatal and early life experiences exert critical changes on the developing brain and neuroendocrine system, affecting mechanisms thought to be relevant to depression and other forms of disorder. As noted previously, the role of stressful experiences, including maternal depression, is central to understanding risk for depression. Further, as noted earlier, an infant or young child's experience of environmental stress is buffered (or not) by the quality of maternal care (e.g., Tang et al., 2014). A great deal of basic biological information on early development remains to be probed and enlarged.

Genetic Contributors

Because depression runs in families, a good deal of interest has focused on *genetic* aspects of depression. Depression is known to be modestly heritable (Sullivan, Neale, & Kendler, 2000) albeit far less than rarer severe disorders such as schizophrenia or bipolar disorder. Molecular genetic studies of theoretically predicted candidate genes and hypothesis-free, gene-finding, genome-wide association methods have so far failed to find replicated evidence of single genes as causes of depression, and it is presumed that genetic influences are due to small effects of multiple genes (Flint & Kendler, 2014). As eminent genetic epidemiologist Kenneth Kendler (2005) noted, the "impact of individual genes on risk for psychiatric illness is small, often nonspecific, and embedded in complex causal pathways" (p. 1243). Thus, a search for a "gene for" depression in children of a depressed parent would not provide a useful approach to early prevention or intervention.

Additionally, genetic factors operate in complex ways (bidirectional and dynamic) in concert with multiple levels of neurobiological and environmental/experiential processes (Cohen-Woods, Craig, & McGuffin, 2013; Flint & Kendler, 2014; Hankin, 2015). Presuming that the transmission of depression across generations includes both genetic and environmental factors, it is important to note that there are various kinds of relationships between genes and environments. The effects of genes may be modified by the environment, such that some genetic characteristics confer greater reactivity to the environment (candidate gene-environment interactions). An example relevant to depression is an interaction of the short alleles of the promoter region of the serotonin transporter gene (5HTTLPR) with stress, maltreatment, or high conflict in the family predictive of depression among those with the short allele, but not those who have other expressions of the 5HTTLPR gene (Caspi et al., 2003; Hammen, Brennan, Keenan-Miller, Hazel, & Najman, 2010; Karg, Burmeister, Shedden, & Sen, 2011). Other candidate genes that affect the functioning of the hypothalamic-pituitary-adrenal (HPA) axis also appear to contribute to potential vulnerabilities to developing depression in response to stress (Starr, Hammen, Conway, Raposa, & Brennan, 2014). Additionally, a wide range of genes affect traits in which a child might be more likely to show temperament, cognitive, and neurobiological characteristics that are maladaptive in the face of stress, and serve as precursors to depression or other forms of psychopathology (reviews in Gibb, Beevers, & McGeary, 2013; Hankin, 2015).

Another way in which environments affect the outcomes of genetic characteristics occurs when some genetic attributes are known to promote positive effects under optimal environmental conditions, while the same genetic characteristics confer negative effects under negative environmental conditions, known as plasticity, or differential susceptibility (Belsky & Pluess, 2009). Further, because genes and environments co-occur, it may be difficult to determine the contributions of each one. An example is a child who has heritable traits, such as neuroticism, that predispose toward depressive reactions to stress but also "inherits" parents whose own traits promote punitive or rejecting parenting environments. Another type of gene-environment correlation is exemplified by a child whose heritable traits promote difficult behaviors that elicit punitive and rejecting parenting styles. Jaffee and Price (2007) reviewed research efforts to disentangle common patterns and effects of gene-environment correlations, underscoring the difficulties in ascribing effects to genetic factors.

An additional challenge is that genetic factors in depression likely have different effects at different stages of child development (genes are activated at different stages), as exemplified by findings that adolescent-onset depression is generally considered more heritable compared to childhood-onset depression, which is more environmental (e.g., Rice, 2010). Furthermore, the environment may also alter the effects of genes (*epigenetics*), as when family stress and parenting quality affect gene expression, even from one generation to the next (Hing, Gardner, & Potash, 2014; Romens, McDonald, Svaren, & Pollack, 2015; Weder et al., 2014).

Genetic factors are further complicated because putative "environmental" factors, such as parenting style or experiencing stressful life events, themselves have heritable aspects (Kendler & Baker, 2007). In light of all the obstacles to understanding the separable effects of genes and environments on the transmission of depression, new research designs are being developed that help to separate out genetic versus environmental contributions to offspring depression. For example, there are studies of children who are adopted into homes of nonrelative parents with depression, and among these investigations are studies of adoptees at birth and adoptees studied from conception due to in vitro fertilization. The latter samples provide natural experiments in which it is possible to study the rearing parents, who may or may not be genetically related to the child, and which permit examination of the effects of prenatal as well as postnatal environments. Studies also employ the "children of twins" methods, comparing the monozygotic or dizygotic offspring of twins who are differentially exposed to depression in the twin parents. Overall, in a recent review of such studies of gene-versus-environment effects, Natsuaki and colleagues (2014) concluded that the evidence supported greater effects of environmental risk factors, especially among mothers with chronic depression, affecting a wide range of maladaptive behaviors in babies, and dysfunctions in school-age children, including vulnerability to stress. While the review did not specify precisely what environmental factors are in play, the authors surmised that the negative effects are a product of the contextual challenges associated with parental depression, such as disruption and disengagement in the parenting relationship, adverse life conditions, and negative marital/interparental relationships.

Ultimately, in the current state of knowledge of genetic mechanisms of intergenerational transmission of depression, no genetic test can identify who will be at risk for depression, per se, and no gene-based mechanisms have led to effective treatments for depression. Nonetheless, complex relationships between genetically influenced processes and environmental conditions will doubtless continue to be modeled and inform the understanding of how parental depression, both biologically and environmentally, affects children.

Neurobiological Factors in Intergenerational Transmission

The major focus of neurobiological research relevant to adult depression concerns the potentially maladaptive ways in which the individual responds to stressful experiences (Hammen, 2015). Two major focuses of this work are increasingly being applied to attempt to understand the behaviors of depressed children and children who are at risk due to parental depression. One is the stress response system of the HPA axis, and the second is neural circuits in the brain that characterize the interpretation of stressful events and the mobilization of cognitive processes and physiological reactions to cope with them. Both of these systems are interconnected, affected by thousands of genetic characteristics, and are also interactive with neural hormones and neurotransmitter systems, as well as other neurobiological structures and processes.

It has long been observed that depressed adults have abnormalities in the functioning of the HPA axis, marked by altered basal levels of the steroid hormone, cortisol, which regulates a variety of metabolic and immune processes involved in optimizing the body's responses to stressful challenges. Abnormalities also include disrupted homeostatic mechanisms of the HPA axis and abnormal patterns of reactivity to stressors (Frodl & O'Keane, 2013; Pariante & Lightman, 2008). Increasing evidence linking such glucocorticoid abnormalities to brain circuitry correlated with depressive deficits is accumulating, operating in complex and developmentally programmed ways that affect and are affected by brain structures and functioning. Considerable evidence suggesting that children at risk due to parental depression may display abnormalities in cortisol patterns is also emerging, processes that may be both genetically and environmentally mediated (Gotlib, Joorman, & Foland-Ross, 2014; Lupien et al., 2011; Mackrell et al., 2014; Rao, Hammen, & Poland, 2009; Waters et al., 2013). This research overlaps with findings from studies of genetic factors and early life stress exposure, and their effects on young children's abnormal cortisol levels and variation in limbic system brain volumes (Pagliaccio et al., 2014), and numerous studies of the effects of early life adversities on the developing brain (National Scientific Council on the Developing Child, 2007).

Recent research in adult depression supports a model of a dysfunctional system of emotion regulation involving a neural circuit linking the limbic structures of the brain associated with the processing of emotional stimuli with cortical areas of the brain responsible for executive functioning, planning, and processing. Neuroimaging studies indicate two types of brain abnormalities in depressed compared to nondepressed adults: heightened reactivity to emotional stimuli (e.g., amygdala reactivity; Disner et al., 2011; Drevets, 2001) and hypoactivity in higher-level cortical structures (e.g., dorsolateral prefrontal cortex and related areas; Beevers, Clasen, Stice, & Schnyer, 2010). Depressed individuals, in essence, display highly reactive negative emotional responses and heightened negative perceptions of stressful and threatening information, coupled with difficulties disengaging from the negative material (interpretations, memories, expectations), and deficits in cognitive control over negative thoughts, leading to failure to inhibit irrelevant negative content. Thus, depressed individuals selectively attend to, overinterpret, and ruminate about stressful experiences, and have greater difficulty in "recovering" from negative thoughts (Foland-Ross & Gotlib, 2012; Gotlib & Joorman, 2010). Other circuits of the brain are also implicated in depression, such as reward processing (Gotlib et al., 2014; Pizzagalli, 2014).

A body of research on children at risk due to parental depression has amply demonstrated that the offspring tend to show cognitive bias, such as selective attention to and memory for negative stimuli, even when not yet displaying depression. Neuroimaging studies of such offspring are only recently emerging but display similar patterns in emotion and reward circuitry as shown by depressed adults and children (Gotlib et al., 2014), but whether these are truly markers of mechanisms of eventual depression in the offspring awaits further longitudinal analysis.

Research on Treatments and Preventive Interventions for Families with Parental Depression

Given the high rates of depression among women of childbearing age, a key practical question to consider is whether there may be ways to mitigate the impact of maternal depression on children and to interrupt or prevent the intergenerational transmission of depression. There are numerous implications to consider, ranging from prevention of maternal depression through amelioration of modifiable risk factors (e.g., contributions of poverty to stressful events and circumstances, and supporting parenting skills in samples at risk) to enhancing access to treatments that are effective in reducing maternal depression and that specifically target depression-related dysfunctions that contribute to children's impairments in development and functioning. At the public policy level, the report by the National Research Council and Institute of Medicine of the National Academies titled *Depression in Parents, Parenting, and Children* (2009) identified numerous systemic issues, including barriers to family-oriented screening and treatment due to separate systems of adult and child health and mental health services, lack of comprehensive and integrated service models, and inadequate services and dissemination platforms for vulnerable populations such as low income and culturally and ethnically diverse families, among many others. Approaches to addressing such issues are beyond the scope of this chapter but are vital components of improving mental health.

At the level of treatment and preventive interventions, the following is a brief discussion of several strategies, focused where possible on those subjected to randomized controlled trials. These studies are extremely different in their primary goals, methods of assessing depression and outcome, and in targeted populations, and there are many obstacles to definitive conclusions due mainly to methodological limitations. However, there are several overlapping clusters of studies with common themes, representing key targets and emerging consensus on treatment and prevention potential: prevention-oriented screening for perinatal depression, treatment of parental depression and determining its effects on children, programs targeted to treat family units with a depressed parent, and programs specifically dedicated to supporting parenting in depressed mothers with babies. The following sections briefly note these approaches.

Prevention/Intervention for Postnatal Depression

While the perinatal period may not necessarily be the most prevalent period of likely depression for women, rates of major or minor depression have been estimated to be as high as 19% for the three months postpartum (Gavin et al., 2005). Moreover, as noted previously, depression may disrupt healthy parenting practices during critical periods of infant development, and therefore, many have concluded that interventions to reduce or prevent depression in the early life of the infant should have high priority. O'Hara and McCabe (2013) and Beardslee, Solantaus, Morgan, Gladstone, and Kowalenko (2012) reported on efforts in many Western nations, and in some jurisdictions in the United States, to mandate perinatal screening for depression and provision of treatment and supportive services. A wide variety of studies have examined treatments for women identified (generally in primary care settings) as depressed or at risk due to elevated symptoms. Two meta-analyses (Cuijpers, Brännmark, & van Straten, 2008; Sockol, Epperson, & Barber, 2011) found significant differences in treated versus control women, but the effects either were not maintained during follow-up or no follow-up was conducted. A review of prevention efforts in postpartum women identified as high risk due to low income, prior depression, or minority or low-income status yielded modest evidence for prevention of depression in some samples (O'Hara & McCabe, 2013). Yawn and colleagues (2012) reported on a trial of screening and medication management in 28 family medicine practices in the United States and found favorable outcomes at the 12-month follow-up compared to usual care. Overall, promising results emerge from the limited studies of early identification and treatment in perinatal women, but the results vary greatly by measurement, population, intervention, and setting, warranting considerable further study.

Treatment of Parental Depression: Effects on Children

There are numerous effective treatments for adult depression, including various forms of individual psychotherapy and antidepressant medications. A standard of care in the treatment of depression in adults should be the assessment of possible risks to and distress in children if the parent is depressed (American Psychiatric Association Practice Guidelines), but it is unlikely that this step is followed, much less thoroughly. Moreover, there are relatively few studies that have examined the effects on children associated with treatment of the parent's depression.

Much of the research focus on parental depression has been on the treatment of women with postpartum depression. Several reviews of a limited body of research have shown that treatment does indeed improve the conditions of postpartum depressed women and their children (e.g., Dennis & Hodnett, 2007; O'Hara & McCabe, 2013). A review by Poobalan and colleagues (2007) found improvements in the child's cognitive functioning and mother-child relationships (variously defined in different studies) in treated versus control women but could not determine whether effects were due to improvements in mothers' mood, resulting in more positive reports of relationship quality, or to actual changes in her parenting behaviors.

Gunlicks and Weissman (2008) reviewed 10 studies of the treatment of parental depression that examined symptomatology and social and cognitive functioning in children up to age 18. The majority of studies showed that children of successfully treated mothers showed improvements in symptomatology or diagnoses, better academic or social functioning, and improved parent-child relationships. However, there were no significant associations, especially among the postpartum treatment sample, on attachment, cognitive functioning, and emotionality. Gunlicks and Weissman (2008) provided numerous recommendations for improvements in study design and measurement, as well as the inclusion of moderators and mediators of the links between changes in parents' outcomes and children's outcomes. One well-developed study illustrates several challenges: Coiro, Riley, Broitman, and Miranda (2012) delivered cognitive behavioral therapy to depressed, low-income, predominantly minority mothers of 4- to 11-year-old children. They found that treatment of the mothers was not associated with improved behavioral changes in the children, but that children's improvement was associated with remission of depression in both treated and untreated women. The authors caution that screening low-income, minority women for depression and improving access to treatment may not be sufficient to benefit children.

These studies suggest that it is best for children that their depressed parent have effective treatment, but there are few longitudinal studies that clarify the duration of effects or resolve issues relevant to critical periods of exposure in the child's life and identify moderators and mediators of positive effects. Additional focus on key targets relevant to children is warranted. Coiro and colleagues (2012) also pointed out that there are severe obstacles to access to treatment for low-income, minority women, such as transportation and childcare, that impede consistent and effective participation for standard therapies such as cognitive behavioral therapy, which are likely to limit their effectiveness. Clearly, more work is needed to adapt interventions to such populations to improve their access, success, and sustainability.

A variant of the idea of treating the depressed parent is to treat the high-risk offspring of depressed parents. Garber and colleagues (2009) developed a multisite treatment trial for adolescent offspring of depressed parents who had been identified as at risk because they had previous major depressive episodes or current elevated symptoms. The cognitive behavioral therapy for youth depression intervention was successful in preventing new episodes of depression during a nine-month follow-up compared to the control group, but the positive preventive effect occurred only for youth who did not have a currently depressed parent. Clearly, considerable work is needed to determine how course features of parental depression affect children and how to provide effective services to youth and their parents.

Treatment of Families of a Depressed Parent

Beardslee and colleagues (2003) developed an approach for families with a depressed parent that involved the family meeting together with a clinician for a psychoeducational approach to explaining depression and depression-relevant issues in the individual family. Children and parents were educated on depression, its symptoms and course, children's risk, and the need for promoting resilience processes. For example, children were encouraged to develop positive activities and supportive relationships outside the home. The program was tested in 105 families in a randomized controlled trial comparing clinician-facilitated meetings (a series of 6–11 sessions with parents only, children only, and family together) with an information-only lecture series (two sessions). Beardslee and colleagues (2003) found that parents in the clinician-facilitated intervention reported significantly more changes in their children's behaviors and attitudes at the end of the study and over a 2.5-year follow-up. Children's internalizing (depression/anxiety) symptoms decreased over time, but the treatment groups did not differ significantly. Similar results were reported at the 4.5-year follow-up (Beardslee, Wright, Gladstone, & Forbes, 2007).

Compas and colleagues (2009) combined aspects of cognitive behavioral treatment for at-risk youth with Beardslee's family-based intervention, emphasizing the role of stress in the family due to depression and helping parents and children to cope with the stressful circumstances. The authors tested a family group–based intervention with 111 families with children aged 9–15. Compared to the control group, the family-group intervention was associated with reduced child-reported internalizing symptoms of small to moderate effect sizes but no significant changes in disruptive behavioral symptoms. There were nonsignificant differences in rates of children's depressive diagnoses over the follow-up. Depressed parents reported a significant reduction in symptoms compared to controls, but no differences in diagnoses were observed. Overall, therefore, these two studies suggest modestly positive effects on children of depressed parents from participation in the family interventions, but results fall short of clear evidence of "prevention" of depression in the youth. It remains to be demonstrated what mechanisms may be especially associated with improvements in children's symptoms and functional outcomes, whether improved coping or actual changes in parenting and family interaction behaviors.

Supporting Parenting Skills in Depressed Mothers with Infants

As noted previously, empirical investigations show that parental depression effects on children are mediated significantly by parent-child relational problems, often affecting attachment quality as well as cognitive, social, and emotional functioning. Accordingly, several efforts to specifically target the support of effective parenting have been studied. For example, toddler-parent psychotherapy aims at improving mother-child interaction and maternal responsiveness, and several studies have shown that it has increased attachment security and cognitive development in children of depressed mothers (Cicchetti, Rogosch, & Toth, 2000). Field and colleagues reported success in teaching parenting support and parent massage of their infants in young women with depression, effects that were associated with better emotional and cognitive functioning in the infants compared with the control group (Field, Grizzle, Scafidi, & Schanberg, 1996; Field et al., 2000; see also van Doesum, Riksen-Walraven, Hosman, &

Hoefnagels, 2008). Generally, studies in this area have been based on small samples or lack extensive follow-ups; consequently, considerable research is needed to develop effective ways to disseminate the interventions and make them acceptable to low-income and minority populations.

Conclusions and Future Directions

A great deal of research has shed light on the high rate of depression and other disorders and functional impairment in children of depressed parents, especially depressed mothers. The high incidence of depression in women worldwide, and the likelihood that many cases are chronic or recurring, suggests an enormous need for intervention and effective treatments that promote healthy parenting and healthy children. The empirically established risk factors for depression help to shed light on women especially at risk for depression during their children's lives: those with previous depression, family histories of depression, and exposure to stressful circumstances and life events both in early life and recently. A variety of established vulnerability mechanisms suggest pathways to development of depression in the face of stress: personality traits and temperament, such as negative affectivity and neuroticism, that promote excessively negative emotionality and negative cognitions about the self and environment; inadequate financial, educational, social, relational, and psychological coping resources; and genetic and neurobiological underpinnings of such cognitive, emotional, and behavioral processes that may serve as markers of negative reactivity to the environment. Depression affects all segments of society, but those with high levels of stress combined with diminished personal and situational coping resources are most affected. Similarly, nearly half of all children with depressed mothers experience some diagnosable disorders, suggesting that many children with parental depression exposure are *not* substantially impacted by the depression as such. Research has indicated that those at greatest risk are those with environmental and biological risk factors for depression, and whose families include disruptions in parenting and marital quality. Greater expansion of research on resilience factors is needed as well.

While many of the key factors are known, research has not yet resolved the complex relationships among risk factors and risk mechanisms to the point of certainty in predicting which pregnant women are destined to experience debilitating depression and which children exposed to maternal depression are most likely to benefit from intervention. Greater evidence clarifying the impact of the timing and "dosage" of exposure of depression is needed, along with a fuller understanding of developmental experiences affecting cognitive, affective, and biological processes in children. Such information would permit more specifically targeted and focused treatment timing and content, as well as a more reliable prediction of candidates most likely to benefit.

An even greater gap in knowledge concerns treatment content and treatment delivery. There are considerable obstacles to adapting health care to view both the mother and the child as needing service, and to provide collaborative, integrated, and comprehensive service models (National Research Council, 2009). Dauntingly complex impediments exist in identifying those in need, facilitating access, and providing care that is welcomed and appropriate for low-income and minority populations—and that promotes healthy cognitive and psychosocial development in children in the face of maternal depression and family stress. Optimal integration with educational, community, financial, and related institutional support would promote better coping and resilience, and would ideally reduce the burden of depression itself. Despite the limitations of knowledge to date, solid steps forward and evidence of progress are clear, and what was once a well-hidden "secret" has become a known problem and an important topic of conversation in the public health focus on families.

References

Adrian, C., & Hammen, C. (1993). Stress exposure and stress generation in children of depressed mothers. *Journal of Consulting and Clinical Psychology, 61*(2), 354–359.

Andrade, L., Caraveo-Anduaga, J. J., Berglund, P., Bijl, R. V., De Graaf, R., Vollebergh, W., . . . Wittchen, H.-U. (2003). The epidemiology of major depressive episodes: Results from the International Consortium of Psychiatric Epidemiology (ICPE) Surveys. *International Journal of Methods in Psychiatric Research, 12*(1), 3–21.

Atkinson, L., Paglia, A., & Coolbear, J. (2000). Attachment security: A meta-analysis of maternal mental health correlates. *Clinical Psychology Review, 20*(8), 1019–1040.

Barker, E., Copeland, W., Maughan, B., Jaffee, S., & Uher, R. (2012). Relative impact of maternal depression and associated risk factors on offspring psychopathology. *The British Journal of Psychiatry, 200*(2), 124–129.

Beardslee, W., Gladstone, T., Wright, E., & Cooper, A. (2003). A family-based approach to the prevention of depressive symptoms in children at risk: Evidence of parental and child change. *Pediatrics, 112*(2), 119–131.

Beardslee, W., Solantaus, T., Morgan, B., Gladstone, T., & Kowalenko, N. (2012). Preventive interventions for children of parents with depression: International perspectives. *Medical Journal of Australia, 1*(Suppl. 1), 23–27.

Beardslee, W., Versage, E., & Gladstone, T. (1998). Children of affectively ill parents: A review of the past 10 years. *Journal of the American Academy of Child and Adolescent Psychiatry, 37*(11), 1134–1141.

Beardslee, W., Wright, E., Gladstone, T., & Forbes, P. (2007). Long-term effects from a randomized trial of two public health preventive interventions for parental depression. *Journal of Family Psychology, 21*(4), 703–713.

Beevers, C., Clasen, P., Stice, E., & Schnyer, D. (2010). Depressive symptoms and cognitive control of emotion cues: A functional magnetic resonance imaging study. *Neuroscience, 167*(1), 97–103.

Belsky, J., & Pluess, M. (2009). Beyond diathesis-stress: Differential susceptibility to environmental influences. *Psychological Bulletin, 135*(6), 885–908.

Burcusa, S., & Iacono, W. (2007). Risk for recurrence in depression. *Clinical Psychological Review, 27*(8), 959–989.

Caspi, A., Sugden, K., Moffitt, T. E., Taylor, A., Craig, I. W., Harrington, H., . . . Poulton, R. (2003). Influence of life stress on depression: Moderation by a polymorphism in the 5-HTT gene. *Science, 301*(5631), 386–389.

Cents, R., Diamantopoulou, S., Hudziak, J., Jaddoe, V., Hofman, A., Verhulst, F., . . . Tiemeier, H. (2013). Trajectories of maternal depressive symptoms predict child problem behavior: The Generation R Study. *Psychological Medicine, 43*(1), 13–25.

Cicchetti, D., Rogosch, F., & Toth, S. (2000). The efficacy of toddler-parent psychotherapy for fostering cognitive development in offspring of depressed mothers. *Journal of Abnormal Child Psychology, 28*(2), 135–148.

Cohen-Woods, S., Craig, I., & McGuffin, P. (2013). The current state of play on the molecular genetics of depression. *Psychological Medicine, 43*(4), 673–687.

Coiro, M. J., Riley, A., Broitman, M., & Miranda, J. (2012). Effects on children of treating their mothers' depression: Results of a 12-month follow-up. *Psychiatric Services, 63*(4), 357–363.

Compas, B., Forehand, R., Keller, G., Champion, J., Rakow, A., Reeslund, K., . . . Cole, D. (2009). Randomized controlled trial of a cognitive-behavioral preventive intervention for children of depressed parents. *Journal of Consulting and Clinical Psychology, 77*(6), 1007–1020.

Côté, S., Boivin, M., Liu, X., Nagin, D., Zoccolillo, M., & Tremblay, R. (2009). Depression and anxiety symptoms: Onset, developmental course and risk factors during early childhood. *Journal of Child Psychology and Psychiatry, 50*(10), 1201–1208.

Cuijpers, P., Brännmark, J., & van Straten, A. (2008). Psychological treatment of postpartum depression: A meta-analysis. *Journal of Clinical Psychology, 64*(1), 103–118.

Dennis, C., & Hodnett, E. (2007). Psychosocial and psychological interventions for treating postpartum depression. *Cochrane Database of Systematic Reviews, 4*, CD006116.

Disner, S., Beevers, C., Haigh, E., & Beck, A. (2011). Neural mechanisms of the cognitive model of depression. *Nature Reviews Neuroscience, 12*(8), 467–477.

Drevets, W. (2001). Neuroimaging and neuropathological studies of depression: Implications for the cognitive-emotional features of mood disorders. *Current Opinions in Neurobiology, 11*(2), 240–249.

Du Rocher Schudlich, T., & Cummings, E. M. (2007). Parental dysphoria and children's adjustment: Marital conflict styles, children's emotional security, and parenting as mediators of risk. *Journal of Abnormal Child Psychology, 35*(4), 627–639.

Fergusson, D., Horwood, L. J., & Lynskey, M. (1995). Maternal depressive symptoms and depressive symptoms in adolescents. *Journal of Child Psychology and Psychiatry, 36*(7), 1161–1178.

Field, T., Diego, M., & Hernandez-Reif, M. (2006). Prenatal depression effects on the fetus and newborn: A review. *Infant Behavior and Development, 29*(3), 445–455.

Field, T., Grizzle, N., Scafidi, F., & Schanberg, S. (1996). Massage and relaxation therapies' effects on depressed adolescent mothers. *Adolescence, 31*(124), 903–911.

Field, T., Pickens, J., Prodromidis, M., Malphurs, J., Fox, N., Bendell, D., . . . Kuhn, C. (2000). Targeting adolescent mothers with depressive symptoms for early intervention. *Adolescence, 35*(138), 381–414.

Flint, J., & Kendler, K. (2014). The genetics of major depression. *Neuron, 81*(3), 484–503.

Foland-Ross, L., & Gotlib, I. (2012). Cognitive and neural aspects of information processing in major depressive disorder: An integrative perspective. *Frontiers in Psychology, 3*, 1–17.

Frodl, T., & O'Keane, V. (2013). How does the brain deal with cumulative stress? A review with focus on developmental stress, HPA axis function and hippocampal structure in humans. *Neurobiology of Disease, 52,* 24–37.

Garber, J., Clarke, G., Weersing, V., Beardslee, W., Brent, D., Gladstone, T., . . . Iyengar, S. (2009). Prevention of depression in at-risk adolescents: A randomized controlled trial. *Journal of the American Medical Association, 301*(21), 2215–2224.

Gavin, N., Gaines, B., Lohr, K., Meltzer-Brody, S., Gartlehner, G., & Swinson, T. (2005). Perinatal depression: A systematic review of prevalence and incidence. *Obstetrics and Gynecology, 106*(5), 1071–1083.

Gibb, B., Beevers, C., & McGeary, J. (2013). Toward an integration of cognitive and genetic models of risk for depression. *Cognition and Emotion, 27*(2), 193–216.

Goodman, S. (2007). Depression in mothers. *Annual Review of Clinical Psychology, 3,* 107–135.

Goodman, S., & Lusby, C. (2014). Early adverse experiences and depression. In I. Gotlib and C. Hammen (Eds.), *Handbook of depression* (3rd ed., pp. 220–239). New York, NY: Guilford Press.

Goodman, S. H., Rouse, M. H., Connell, A. M., Broth, M. R., Hall, C. M., & Heyward, D. (2011). Maternal depression and child psychopathology: A meta-analytic review. *Clinical Child and Family Psychology Review, 14*(1), 1–27.

Gotlib, I., & Joorman, J. (2010). Cognition and depression: Current status and future directions. *Annual Review of Clinical Psychology, 6,* 285–312.

Gotlib, I., Joormann, J., & Foland-Ross, L. (2014). Understanding familial risk for depression: A 25-year perspective. *Perspectives on Psychological Science, 9*(1), 94–108.

Grant, K., Compas, B., Stuhlmacher, A., Thurm, A., & McMahon, S. (2003). Stressors and child and adolescent psychopathology: Moving from markers to mechanisms of risk. *Psychological Bulletin, 129*(3), 447–466.

Greenberg, P. E., Kessler, R. C., Birnbaum, H. G., Leong, S. A., Lowe, S. W., Berglund, P. A., & Corey-Lisle, P. K. (2003). The economic burden of depression in the United States: How did it change between 1990 and 2000? *Journal of Clinical Psychiatry, 64*(12), 1465–1475.

Gunlicks, M., & Weissman, M. (2008). Change in child psychopathology with improvement in parental depression: A systematic review. *Journal of the American Academy of Child and Adolescent Psychiatry, 47*(4), 379–389.

Halligan, S., Murray, L., Martins, C., & Cooper, P. (2007). Maternal depression and psychiatric outcomes in adolescent offspring: A 13-year longitudinal study. *Journal of Affective Disorders, 97*(1), 145–154.

Hammen, C. (1991). The generation of stress in the course of unipolar depression. *Journal of Abnormal Psychology, 100*(4), 555–561.

Hammen, C. (2005). Stress and depression. *Annual Review of Clinical Psychology, 1,* 293–319.

Hammen, C. (2015). Stress and depression: Old questions, new approaches. *Current Opinions in Psychology, 4,* 80–85.

Hammen, C., & Brennan, P. (2001). Depressed adolescents of depressed and nondepressed mothers: Tests of an interpersonal impairment hypothesis. *Journal of Consulting and Clinical Psychology, 69*(2), 284–294.

Hammen, C., Brennan, P., & Le Brocque, R. (2011). Youth depression and early childrearing: Stress generation and intergenerational transmission of depression. *Journal of Consulting and Clinical Psychology, 79*(3), 353–363.

Hammen, C., Brennan, P., Keenan-Miller, D., Hazel, N., & Najman, J. (2010). Chronic and acute stress, gender, and serotonin transporter gene-environment interactions predicting depression in youth. *Journal of Child Psychiatry and Psychology, 51*(2), 180–187.

Hammen, C., Brennan, P., Keenan-Miller, D., & Herr, N. (2008). Early onset recurrent subtype of adolescent depression: Clinical and psychosocial correlates. *Journal of Child Psychology and Psychiatry, 49*(4), 433–440.

Hammen, C., Hazel, N., Brennan, P., & Najman, J. (2012). Intergenerational transmission and continuity of stress and depression: Depressed women and their offspring in 20 years of follow-up. *Psychological Medicine, 42*(5), 931–942.

Hammen, C., & Shih, J. (2014). Depression and interpersonal processes. In I. Gotlib and C. Hammen (Eds.), *Handbook of depression*, 3rd edition (pp. 277–295). New York, NY: Guilford Press.

Hammen, C., Shih, J., & Brennan, P. (2004). Intergenerational transmission of depression: Test of an interpersonal stress model in a community sample. *Journal of Consulting and Clinical Psychology, 72*(3), 511–522.

Hankin, B. (2015). Depression from childhood to adolescence: Risk mechanisms across multiple systems and levels of analysis. *Current Opinion in Psychology, 4*, 13–20.

Hasin, D., Goodwin, R., Stinson, F., & Grant, B. (2005). Epidemiology of major depressive disorder: Results from the National Epidemiologic Survey on Alcoholism and Related Disorders. *Archives of General Psychiatry, 62*(10), 10097–11106.

Hayes, L., Goodman, S. H., & Carlson, E. (2013). Maternal antenatal depression and infant disorganized attachment at 12 months. *Attachment and Human Development, 15*(2), 133–153.

Hing, B., Gardner, C., & Potash, J. (2014). Effects of negative stressors on DNA methylation in the brain: Implications for mood and anxiety disorders. *American Journal of Medical Genetics B, 165*(7), 541–554.

Jaffee, S., Moffitt, T., Caspi, A., Fombonne, E., Poulton, R., & Martin, J. (2002). Differences in early childhood risk factors for juvenile-onset and adult-onset depression. *Archives of General Psychiatry, 59*(3), 215–222.

Jaffee, S., & Price, T. (2007). Gene-environment correlations: A review of the evidence and implications for prevention of mental illness. *Molecular Psychiatry, 12*(5), 432–442.

Karg, K., Burmeister, M., Shedden, K., & Sen, S. (2011). The serotonin transporter promoter variant (5-HTTLPR), stress, and depression meta-analysis revisited: Evidence of genetic moderation. *Archives of General Psychiatry, 68*(5), 444–454.

Katz, S., Hammen, C., & Brennan, P. (2013). Maternal depression and the intergenerational transmission of relational impairment. *Journal of Family Psychology, 27*(1), 86–95.

Keenan-Miller, D., Hammen, C., & Brennan, P. (2007). Adolescent psychosocial risk factors for severe intimate partner violence in young adulthood. *Journal of Consulting and Clinical Psychology, 75*(3), 456–463.

Kendler, K. (2005). "A gene for . . .": The nature of gene action in psychiatric disorders. *American Journal of Psychiatry, 162*(7), 1243–1252.

Kendler, K., & Baker, J. (2007). Genetic influences on measures of the environment: A systematic review. *Psychological Medicine, 37*(5), 615–626.

Kendler, K., & Gardner, C. (2011). A longitudinal etiologic model for symptoms of depression and anxiety in women. *Psychological Medicine, 41*(10), 2035–2045.

Kessler, R. C., Berglund, P., Demler, O., Jin, R., Koretz, D., Merikangas, K. R., . . . Wang, P. S. (2003). The epidemiology of major depressive disorder: Results from the National Comorbidity Survey Replication (NCS-R). *Journal of the American Medical Association, 289*(23), 3095–3105.

Kessler, R. C., & Bromet, E. J. (2013). The epidemiology of depression across cultures. *Annual Review of Public Health, 34*, 119–138.

Kingston, D., Tough, S., & Whitfield, H. (2012). Prenatal and postpartum maternal psychological distress and infant development: A systematic review. *Child Psychiatry and Human Development, 43*(5), 683–714.

Lampard, A., Franckle, R,. & Davison, K. (2014). Maternal depression and childhood obesity: A systematic review. *Preventive Medicine, 59*, 60–67.

Liu, R. (2013). Stress generation: Future directions and clinical implications. *Clinical Psychology Review, 33*(3), 406–416.

Lovejoy, M. C., Graczyk, P. A., O'Hare, E., & Neuman, G. (2000). Maternal depression and parenting behavior: A meta-analytic review. *Clinical Psychology Review, 20*(5), 561–592.

Luby, J., Belden, A., & Spitznagel, E. (2006). Risk factors for preschool depression: The mediating role of early stressful life events. *Journal of Child Psychology and Psychiatry, 47*(12), 1292–1298.

Lupien, S., Parent, S., Evans, A., Tremblay, R., Zelazo, P., Corbo, V., . . . Séguin, J. (2011). Larger amygdala but no change in hippocampal volume in 10-year-old children exposed to maternal depressive symptomatology since birth. *Proceedings of the National Academy of Sciences, 108*(34), 14324–14329.

Mackrell, S., Sheikh, H., Kotelnikova, Y., Kryski, K., Jordan, P., Singh, S., & Hayden, E. (2014). Child temperament and parental depression predict cortisol reactivity to stress in middle childhood. *Journal of Abnormal Psychology, 123*(1), 106–116.

Martins, C., & Gaffan, E. (2000). Effects of early maternal depression on patterns of infant-mother attachment: A meta-analytic investigation. *Journal of Child Psychology and Psychiatry, 41*(6), 737–746.

Merikangas, K., He, J.-P., Burstein, M., Swanson, S., Avenevoli, S., Cui, L., . . . Swendsen, J. (2010). Lifetime prevalence of mental disorders in US adolescents: Results from the National Comorbidity Survey Replication-Adolescent Supplement (NCS-A). *Journal of the Academy of Child and Adolescent Psychiatry, 49*, 980–989.

Murray, C. J., Vos, T., Lozano, R., Naghavi, M., Flaxman, A. D., Michaud, C., . . . Memish, Z. (2012). Disability-adjusted life years (DALYs) for 291 diseases and injuries in 21 regions, 1990–2010: A systematic analysis for the Global Burden of Disease Study 2010. *Lancet, 380*(9859), 2197–2223.

National Research Council and Institute of Medicine of the National Academies. (2009). *Depression in parents, parenting, and children: Opportunities to improve identification, treatment, and prevention efforts.* Committee on Depression, Parenting Practices, and Healthy Development of Children. Board on Children, Youth, and Families. Division of Behavioral and Social Sciences and Education. Washington, DC: The National Academies Press.

National Scientific Council on the Developing Child. (2007). *The timing and quality of early experiences combine to shape brain architecture: Working paper no.5.* Retrieved from www .developingchild.harvard.edu

Natsuaki, M., Shaw, D., Neiderhiser, J., Ganiban, J., Harold, G., Reiss, D., & Leve, L. (2014). Raised by depressed parents: Is it an environmental risk? *Clinical Child and Family Psychology Review, 17*(4), 357–367.

NICHD Early Child Care Research Network. (1999). Chronicity of maternal depressive symptoms, maternal sensitivity, and child functioning at 36 months. *Developmental Psychology, 35*(5), 1297–1310.

Nolen-Hoeksema, S. N., & Girgus, J. S. (1994). The emergence of gender differences in depression during adolescence. *Psychological Bulletin, 115*(3), 424–443.

O'Hara, M., & McCabe, J. (2013). Postpartum depression: Current status and future directions. *Annual Review of Clinical Psychology, 9*, 379–407.

Ormel, J., Petukhova, M., Chatterji, S., Aguilar-Gaxiola, S., Alonso, J., Angermeyer, M. C., . . . Kessler, R. C. (2008). Disability and treatment of specific mental and physical disorders across the world. *British Journal of Psychiatry, 192*(5), 368–375.

Pagliaccio, D., Luby, J., Bogdan, R., Agrawal, A., Garrey, M., Belden, A., . . . Barch, D. (2014). Stress-system genes and life stress predict cortisol levels and amygdala and hippocampal volumes in children. *Neuropsychopharmacology, 39*(5), 1245–1253.

Pariante, C., & Lightman, S. (2008). The HPA axis in major depression: Classical theories and new developments. *Trends in Neuroscience, 31*(9), 464–468.

Pearson, R., Evans, J., Kounali, D., Lewis, G., Heron, J., Ramchandani, P., . . . Stein, A. (2013). Maternal depression during pregnancy and the postnatal period: Risks and possible mechanisms for offspring depression at age 18 years. *JAMA Psychiatry, 70*(12), 1312–1319.

Pizzagalli, D. (2014). Depression, stress, and anhedonia: Toward a synthesis and integrated model. *Annual Review of Clinical Psychology, 10*, 393–423.

Poobalan, A., Aucott, L., Ross, L., Smith, W., Helms, P., & Williams, J. (2007). Effects of treating postnatal depression on mother-infant interaction and child development. *British Journal of Psychiatry, 191*(5), 378–386.

Psychogiou, L., & Parry, E. (2014). Why do depressed individuals have difficulty in their parenting role? *Psychological Medicine, 44*(7), 1345–1347.

Rao, U., Hammen, C., & Poland, R. (2009). Risk markers for depression in adolescents: Sleep and HPA measures. *Neuropsychopharmacology, 34*(8), 1936–1945.

Reising, M., Watson, K., Hardcastle, E., Merchant, M., Roberts, L., Forehand, R., & Compas, B. (2013). Parental depression and economic disadvantage: The role of parenting in associations with internalizing and externalizing symptoms in children and adolescents. *Journal of Child and Family Studies, 22*(3), 335–343.

Rice, F. (2010). Genetics of childhood and adolescent depression: Insights into etiological heterogeneity and challenges for future genomic research. *Genome Medicine, 2*(9), 68.

Richards, D. (2011). Prevalence and clinical course of depression: A review. *Clinical Psychology Review, 31*(7), 1117–1135.

Romens, S., McDonald, J., Svaren, J., & Pollack, S. (2015). Associations between early life stress and gene methylation in children. *Child Development, 86*(1), 3030–3309.

Sellars, R., Collishaw, S., Rice, F., Thapar, A. K., Potter, R., Mars, B., . . . Thapar, A. (2013). Risk of psychopathology in adolescent offspring of mothers with psychopathology and recurrent depression. *British Journal of Psychiatry, 202*, 108–114.

Sellars, R., Harold, G., Elam, K., Rhoades, K., Potter, R., Mars, B., . . . Collishaw, S. (2014). Maternal warmth and co-occurring antisocial behavior: Testing maternal hostility and warmth as mediators of risk for offspring psychopathology. *Journal of Child Psychology and Psychiatry, 55*(2), 112–120.

Sockol, L., Epperson, C., & Barber, J. (2011). A meta-analysis of treatments for postpartum depression. *Clinical Psychology Review, 31*(5), 839–849.

Starr, L., Hammen, C., Conway, C., Raposa, E., & Brennan, P. (2014). Sensitizing effect of early adversity on depressive reactions to later proximal stress: Moderation by polymorphisms in serotonin transporter and corticotropin releasing hormone receptor genes in a 20-year longitudinal study. *Development and Psychopathology, 26*(4), 1241–1254.

Stein, A., Pearson, R., Goodman, S., Rapa, E., Rahman, A., McCallum, M., . . . Pariante, C. (2014). Effects of perinatal mental disorders on the fetus and child. *The Lancet, 384*(9956), 1800–1819.

Sullivan, P. F., Neale, M. C., & Kendler, K. S. (2000). Genetic epidemiology of major depression: Review and meta-analysis. *American Journal of Psychiatry, 157*(10), 1552–1562.

Surkan, P., Kennedy, C., Hurley, K., & Black, M. (2011). Maternal depression and early childhood growth in developing countries: Systematic review and meta-analysis. *Bulletin of the World Health Organization, 287*, 607–615D.

Tang, A., Reeb-Sutherland, B., Romeo, R., & McEwen, B. (2014). On the causes of early life experience effects: Evaluating the role of mom. *Frontiers of Neuroendocrinology, 35*(2), 245–251.

Van Doesum, K., Riksen-Walraven, M., Hosman, C., & Hoefnagels, C. (2008). A randomized controlled trial of a home-visiting intervention aimed at preventing relationship problems in depressed mothers and their infants. *Child Development, 79*(3), 547–561.

Wachs, T., Black, M., & Engle, P. (2009). Maternal depression: A global threat to children's health, development, and behavior and to human rights. *Child Development Perspectives, 3*(1), 51–59.

Wang, Y., & Dix, T. (2013). Patterns of depressive parenting: Why they occur and their role in early developmental risk. *Journal of Family Psychology, 27*(6), 884–895.

Warner, V., Weissman, M., Mufson, L., & Wickramaratne, P. (1999). Grandparents, children, and grandchildren at risk for depression: A three-generation study. *Journal of the Academy of Child and Adolescent Psychiatry, 38*(3), 289–296.

Waters, C., van Goozen, S., Phillips, R., Swift, N., Hurst, S.-L., Mundy, L., . . . Hay, D. (2013). Infants at familial risk for depression show a distinct pattern of cortisol response to experimental challenge. *Journal of Affective Disorders, 150*(3), 955–960.

Weder, N., Zhang, H., Jensen, K., Yang, B., Simen, A., Jackowski, A., . . . Kaufman, J. (2014). Child abuse, depression, and methylation in genes involved with stress, neural plasticity, and brain circuitry. *Journal of the American Academy of Child and Adolescent Psychiatry, 53*(4), 417–424.

Weissman, M. M., Wickramaratne, P., Nomura, Y., Warner, V., Pilowsky, D., & Verdeli, H. (2006). Offspring of depressed parents: 20 years later. *American Journal of Psychiatry, 163*(6), 1001–1008.

Weissman, M. M., Wickramaratne, P., Nomura, Y., Warner, V., Pilowsky, D., Verdeli, H., . . . Bruder, G. (2005). Families at high and low risk for depression: A 3-generation study. *Archives of General Psychiatry, 62*(1), 29–36.

Yawn, B., Dietrich, A., Wollan, P., Bertram, S., Graham, D., Huff, J., . . . Pace, W. (2012). TRIPPD: A practice-based network effectiveness study of postpartum depression screening and management. *Annals of Family Medicine, 10*(4), 320–329.

CHAPTER 8

The Influence of Stigma for Depression Care

J. Konadu Fokuo
Patrick W. Corrigan, PsyD

Despite advances in the efficacy of evidence-based mental health treatments and services, people with depression continue to abstain from or display limited "buy in" to mental health treatments and services (Butler, Chapman, Forman, & Beck, 2006; Elkin et al., 1989; Wang et al., 2005). Mental health stigma, which is discrimination against or negative attitudes about people with mental disorders, has often been identified as a major contributor to this phenomenon (Cooper, Corrigan, & Watson, 2003; Corrigan, Morris, Michaels, Rafacz, & Rüsch, 2012). Stigma also exacerbates psychological distress and stunts the achievement of educational and career goals (Pescosolido et al., 2010; Rüsch et al., 2009; Wahl, 1999). To combat the effects of stigma, efforts have been made to increase public knowledge about mental health disorders. Yet, a significant number of people with mental illness continue to report direct experiences of stigma and discrimination from the general public (Corrigan et al., 2012; Parcesepe & Cabassa, 2013).

This chapter begins with a brief definition and conceptualization of mental health stigma, followed by a detailed description of specific manifestations of stigma that impede recovery from depression. These manifestations include: public stigma (discrimination and negative attitudes from society toward people with mental illness), self-stigma (internalized negative attitudes about oneself as it relates to their mental illness), and label avoidance (distancing oneself from places and situations that promote group categorization, such as participating in mental health services). We review the implications of stigma on self-efficacy, recovery, and empowerment as well as public health and conclude by presenting effective ways of combating mental health stigma.

Conceptualization and Origins of Stigma

Erving Goffman (1963) conceptualized stigma as an "attribute that is deeply discrediting" and causes the person labeled as such to be reduced "from a whole and usual person to a tainted, discounted one" (p. 3). Awareness of the attribute results in the belief that a "person with a stigma is not quite human" (p. 5). Goffman's work further distinguishes concealed and overt markers of public stigma. Some stigmas are overt, or externally marked, such as obesity (body size) or ethnicity (skin color). Concealed stigmas are based on "hidden" deviations of personal traits, such as mental illness or homosexuality. Stigma undermines social interactions between individuals with these markers and those who Goffman labels "the normals" (p. 13). This is due to the categorization of individuals into social groups based solely on markers and the assignment of culturally agreed-upon attributes (stereotypes) to all members of the social group by "normals" in that society.

The process of stigmatization (see Figure 8.1) begins with attaching labels to a member of the "out-group," which leads to stereotypes and prejudice (Jacoby, Snape, & Baker, 2005). Stereotypes are attitudes about individuals based on their assignment to a particular group or category. Stereotypes intrinsically rely on generalizations that are often inaccurate or misleading when applied to particular cases. Prejudice refers to negative affective attitudes toward particular groups and implies agreement with derogatory or pejorative stereotypes. People observing an emotionally distraught, unkempt individual, for example, might not only assume that the person has a mental illness (a stereotype) but also might feel anger and fear because of the person's presumed dangerousness (prejudice). Prejudice, which is also considered a cognitive response, leads to discrimination, which is a behavioral (re)action. Discrimination can be exhibited by negative reactions to members of the stigmatized group (out-group) or positive actions toward nonmembers of the stigmatized group (in-group) (Allport, 1958). Discrimination is the behavioral component of stigma and occurs when people act on the basis of prejudiced attitudes or beliefs.

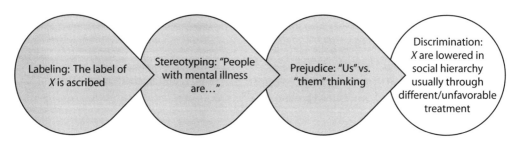

FIGURE 8.1 Sequence of public stigmatization

Public Stigma

Public stigma represents the discrimination and prejudice that the general public exhibit toward people with mental illness. Public stigma is what the public does to people who are labeled with a mental illness (Corrigan & Kleinlein, 2005). The label of mental illness can potentially signal stereotypes and prejudice. Public misconceptions about mental illness and corresponding stigmatizing attitudes often follow certain themes. Media analyses of film and print have identified three: (1) people with mental illness are homicidal maniacs who need to be feared, (2) they have childlike perceptions of the world that should be marveled, or (3) they are responsible for their illness because they have weak character (Evans-Lacko, Henderson, & Thornicroft, 2013; Schomerus et al., 2012; Taylor & Dear, 1981; Wahl, 1999). Results from two independent factor analyses echo these findings (Evans-Lacko et al., 2013; Schomerus et al., 2012):

- *Fear and exclusion*: persons with serious mental illness such as depression should be feared and, therefore, be kept out of most communities;
- *Benevolence*: persons with depression are childlike and need to be cared for;
- *Authoritarianism*: persons with depression are irresponsible, so life decisions should be made by others.

The general public responds most often with acts of discrimination. For example, these attitudes have a deleterious impact on obtaining and keeping employment (Bordieri & Drehmer, 1984; Farina & Felner, 1973; Khalema & Shankar, 2014; Manning & White, 1995; Shankar et al., 2014; Wahl, 1999). Farina and Felner (1973) provided a classic research example of the employment problem. Their study involved male confederates posing as unemployed workers, seeking jobs at 32 businesses. The same work history was reported at each of the job interviews, except 50% of confederates also included information about a past psychiatric hospitalization. Subsequent analyses found that interviewers were less friendly and less supportive of hiring the confederate when they knew about his psychiatric hospitalization.

Discrimination can also appear in public opinion about how to treat people with mental illness. For example, the general public sometimes endorses mandatory treatment for people with mental illness and segregation in health care institutions for people with serious psychiatric disorders (Corrigan & Watson, 2002a). In terms of health care, research indicates that people with mental illness are less likely to benefit from the American health care system than people without these illnesses. Research by Druss and colleagues showed that people with mental illness receive fewer medical services than those not marked with that label (Desai, Rosenheck, Druss, & Perlin, 2002; Druss & Rosenheck, 1997). Moreover, studies suggest that people with mental illness are less likely to receive the same range of insurance benefits as people without mental illness (Druss, Allen, & Bruce, 1998; Druss & Rosenheck, 1998).

Self-Stigma

Self-stigma occurs when individuals perceive themselves to have a stigmatized identity and, being aware of the public's negative attitudes toward this identity, internalize these attitudes; as a result, they experience loss of self-esteem and self-efficacy (Angermeyer & Matschinger, 2003; Corrigan & Watson, 2002b; Rüsch, Angermeyer, & Corrigan, 2005; Watson, Corrigan, Larson, & Sells, 2006). A necessary component of self-stigma is stigma awareness. Most people, including those diagnosed with a mental illness, are cognizant of society's stereotypes about people with mental illness. Identification with the broader "group" of persons who share a stigmatized identity is a key variable that influences how individuals respond to public stigma. For self-stigma to occur, people must then agree with the legitimacy of the stigma. Stereotype agreement occurs when an individual endorses the common public stereotypes (e.g., "People with mental illness are weak"), while a negative outcome (e.g., not being hired) is perceived as legitimate if a stigmatizing expectation (e.g., persons with mental illness are incompetent and will do poorly at work) is perceived as accurate. The process (illustrated in Figure 8.2) specifically becomes self-stigmatizing with the addition of stereotype self-concurrence (application), in which an individual applies the culturally internalized beliefs to him- or herself (e.g., "I am weak because I have a mental illness"). Concurring with the negative belief, in turn, results in diminished self-esteem and self-efficacy. All three *As* of self-stigmatization (awareness, agreement, and application) must occur for this process to be complete. In many cases, people are indifferent to the stigma. In other cases, the process of stigmatization is not complete and the person with mental illness does not endorse self-stigmatizing beliefs.

Self-Esteem and Self-Efficacy

Self-stigma can lead to low self-esteem and self-efficacy, and these are, in turn, linked to negative outcomes. A person who has internalized stereotypes, such as "the depressed have no worth because they have nothing to offer and are only drains on

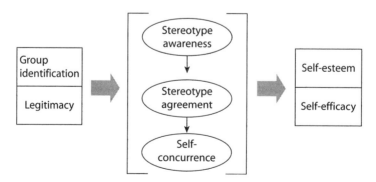

FIGURE 8.2 Theoretical model of self-stigma

society," will struggle to maintain a positive self-concept. Self-esteem here is more than the kind of negative self-statements that are observed in people with depressive symptoms. It is directly linked to applying a derogatory stereotype to one's self. Rosenfield and Neese-Todd (1993) showed that specific domains of quality of life—satisfaction with work, housing, health, and finance—were associated with self-stigma as well as self-esteem. Self-stigma and self-esteem have also been associated with help-seeking behavior (Vogel, Wade, & Haake, 2006).

Self-stigma includes self-efficacy, a cognitive construct that represents a person's confidence in successfully acting on specific situations (Bandura, 1997; Markström et al., 2009). Low self-efficacy has been shown to be associated with failure to pursue work or independent living opportunities at which people with mental illness might otherwise succeed (Gecas, 1989; Link, Cullen, Frank, & Wozniak, 1987; Link, Struening, Neese-Todd, Asmussen, & Phelan, 2014; Livingston & Boyd, 2010; Rosenfield, 1997; Rüsch et al., 2006; Vogel et al., 2006). People with mental illness, such as depression, with low degrees of confidence in managing various circumstances related to their mental illness were found to be unsuccessful in discrete attempts to realize corresponding goals.

The "Why Try" Effect

Self-stigma also yields the "why try" effect (Corrigan, Larson, & Rüsch, 2009): "Why try to seek a job? Someone like me is not worthy"; or, "Why try to live independently? Someone like me is not able." The "why try" effect is based on the relationship between self-stigma (resulting from stereotypes) and life goal achievement, or lack thereof (mediated by self-esteem). People who internalize stereotypes about mental illness experience a loss of self-esteem and self-efficacy (Link et al., 1987; Markowitz, Angell, & Greenberg, 2011; Ritsher & Phelan, 2004).

Label Avoidance

Label avoidance occurs when individuals choose not to seek help for mental health problems in order to avoid negative labels (Corrigan, Roe, & Tsang, 2010). Similar to self-stigma, label avoidance requires an awareness of society's stigmatizing attitudes toward people with mental illness. However, unlike self-stigma, individuals with mental illness also distance themselves from systems related to mental illness, including systems of care and recovery when label avoidance occurs. In order to avoid psychiatric labels, individuals may choose not to associate with mental health clinics or professionals—avoiding diagnosis (Ben-Zeev, Young, & Corrigan, 2010; Corrigan & Kosyluk, 2013; Rüsch et al., 2005; Vogel et al., 2006). Label avoidance has been shown to impact the relationship between help-seeking behaviors and discontinuation of mental health treatment for elderly people with depression (Alexopoulos, 2005). Additionally, because mental illness can be a concealed disorder, some people with mental illness are more likely to "stay in the closet" as opposed to proudly disclosing their mental illness out of fear of discrimination or social harm (Corrigan, Bink, Fokuo, & Schmidt, 2015; Link & Phelan, 2001). Label avoidance, due to its cognitive and behavioral components, may be the most significant barrier to the continuation of treatment for people with mental illness.

How Stigma Interferes with Personal Care-seeking Decisions and Behaviors

Researchers have developed fluid models of care-seeking and treatment participation reflecting the personal psychology of finding and acting on help (Kovandžić et al., 2011; Pescosolido et al., 2010). These models integrate cognitive perspectives (how people make a decision about beginning and staying in care) with social spheres (the interpersonal, familial, and cultural network in which decisions are made and lived out) in an evolving and iterative manner. Care-seeking and participation begin when a person experiences an unsettling physical, emotional, or interpersonal state that is perceived as problematic and in need of care. Labeling the problem as "stress," "psychiatric illness," or "mental health challenge" leads the person to seek care in the broad system of mental health services. Words that comprise labels are important in promoting care-seeking. A college student, early in his or her illness, may be put off by having a "depression" but willing to seek "counsel" for a "mental health challenge." Labeling will likely influence the student to spurn care-seeking in order to avoid stigma (Eisenberg, Downs, Golberstein, & Zivin, 2009). Determination to seek care is influenced by perceived costs and benefits of treatment options. Stigma in its various forms will influence these perceptions (Clement et al., 2013). Costs include stigmatizing labels that arise from treatment and worsened self-stigma and shame. The "why try" consequence of self-stigma may lead the person into believing treatment will not have any real positive impact ("I am not worthy of treatment"; "I am unable to really participate"). People are likely to move forward when benefits seem to outweigh costs, perhaps when the stigma of mental illness is minimized.

Stigma can also undermine treatment participation. People may seek care after a decision to change is made. Unfortunately, many drop out soon after; research suggests that up to 20% of people may discontinue treatment prematurely depending on the type of treatment (e.g., medication versus talk therapy; Corrigan & Fong, 2014; Edlund et al., 2002). As a result of stigma, negative perceptions of mental health and treatment reflecting prejudices of mental illness can reemerge and derail interventions. The sense of poor self-efficacy commensurate with self-stigma harms participation in care. Care-seeking ends when people exit services, that is, when they notify their provider that they have decided to stop treatment or when they discontinue participation without notice. A "cure" requiring no future treatment is not always the goal of ending care. Like all health and wellness considerations, challenges and successes vary depending on the person's age, development, network, and life events.

Changing the Public Stigma of Mental Illness

Three approaches to addressing public stigma have emerged—protest, education, and contact—each with different strengths and limitations (Corrigan & Fong, 2014; Corrigan & Penn, 1999). Protest is defined as an appeal to a moral authority to decrease disrespectful images of mental illness. Typically, an audience is shown egregious images from the media (headline: "Psycho Killer Released from Jail") and instructed to stop thinking that way. Educational programs compare myths about mental illness (e.g., people choose to be mentally ill) with data that challenge the myths (e.g., research shows most serious mental illnesses, such as depression, are biological in origin). Contact facilitates exchanges between people with lived experience and target groups where the former discuss their experiences with mental illness and recovery. The question here is how approaches like these might diminish stigma in order to promote care-seeking.

Protest

Groups protest inaccurate and hostile representations of mental illness as a way to challenge the stigmas they represent. These efforts send two messages: (1) to the media: *stop* reporting inaccurate representations of mental illness; and (2) to the public: *stop* believing negative views about mental illness. Anecdotal evidence suggests that protest campaigns have been effective in getting stigmatizing images of mental illness withdrawn (Corrigan & Watson, 2002b). There is, however, little empirical research on the psychological impact of protest campaigns on stigma and discrimination, suggesting an important direction for future research. Protest is a reactive strategy; it attempts to diminish negative attitudes about mental illness but fails to promote more positive attitudes that are supported by facts.

Education

Educational programs attempt to contrast the myths of mental illness with the facts. They often include the message that mental illnesses are treatable disorders, followed by information regarding service availability in the geographic area. Government and large nongovernmental organizations have rolled this kind of approach into public service campaigns seeking to motivate viewers to ignore stigma and seek out services when in need. Australia's beyondblue has been in place since 2000 (Hickie, 2001), targeting anxiety and depression with programs aimed specifically at young people, men, women, multicultural people, lesbian, gay, bisexual, transgender, transsexual and intersex people, pregnant women and new mothers, and aboriginal people (Dunt et al., 2011).

The public service campaign seems to have significantly penetrated the Australian population. Two separate surveys found that about 40% of teens were aware of the campaign (Jorm, Wright, & Morgan, 2007; Morgan & Jorm, 2009). An additional survey found that 61.9% of the Australian population recognized the campaign (Highet, Luscombe, Davenport, Burns, & Hickie, 2006). Awareness seemed to be related to better recognition of mental illnesses and beliefs about mental health first aid (Yap, Reavley, & Jorm, 2015). Other studies examined beyondblue's effects in Australian states that implemented the program compared to those that did not. Results showed that awareness of the program was about twice as great in states and territories that rolled out the campaign versus those that did not (Jorm, Christensen, & Griffiths, 2005). Awareness seemed to be associated with better recognition of illnesses (Jorm, Christensen, & Griffiths, 2006) and greater understanding of the benefits of treatments such as counseling and medication (Jorm et al., 2005). The link to care-seeking is less clear.

Other countries have rolled out similar campaigns, though research on their penetration and impact is mostly lacking. The Substance Abuse and Mental Health Services Administration (SAMHSA) produced the What a Difference a Friend Makes campaign, designed to encourage young adults to step up and support friends living with mental health problems. The Ad Council reported findings from an online tracking survey on What a Difference and found that 31% of a sample of adults aged 18–25 recognized public service announcements from the campaign in March 2008 and that 28% did so in May 2009 (Corrigan, 2012). Impact, however, is more difficult to assess. One method of assessment has been tracking visits to websites listed at the end of public service announcements. The rationale is that viewers are seeking further information to better learn about and work against stigma; this, in turn, leads to better care-seeking and service engagement. The Ad Council reported website traffic for What a Difference from the launch of the campaign in December 2006 through September 2008, with a monthly median of 64,098 visits. In the first month of the campaign, website visits increased to a high of 102,416 in September 2007. Average time spent on the website was almost eight minutes. However, findings were a bit less sanguine for a second SAMHSA campaign, the Erase the Barriers initiative (Bell, Colangelo, & Pillen, 2005). Monthly visits to the site almost tripled—from 2,743 to 7,627—during its eight-month campaign beginning November 2004, highly significant indeed. The size of effect, however, is quite small. US Census data at the time reported 124 million residents in the eight pilot states of Erase the Barriers. That means that 0.006% of people in these states visited the website. Of additional concern was the finding that 88% of visitors exited the website in less than one minute, and less than 30% of visitors returned to the site in the subsequent months.

One additional concern has emerged from public service campaigns such as these (Corrigan & Fong, 2014). The focus on mental illness being a treatable disease may accentuate the fundamental characteristic of stigma: *difference*, that is, the perception that "people with depression are different than everyone else" (Corrigan et al., 2015; Link & Phelan, 2001). It is unclear whether this kind of unintended consequence undermines the goal of promoting care-seeking; however, it may exacerbate the discrimination that occurs from public stigma. Because "they" are different, employers may not want to hire them, landlords may not want to rent to them, and primary care doctors may provide substandard care. Other public service campaigns seek to combine both agendas, undermining label avoidance and public discrimination. One example is the United Kingdom's Time to Change initiative, which seeks to promote care and challenge discrimination so that people with mental illness have opportunities that are similar to those of everyone else (Smith, 2013). Awareness of Time to Change ranged between 38% and 64% and was associated with greater mental health literacy and less stigmatizing attitudes (Evans-Lacko et al., 2013).

Contact

Educational approaches to stigma change are often augmented by contact: strategic interactions between people with lived experience of mental illness and targeted members of the public (Couture & Penn, 2003). Contact may occur face-to-face or over some medium such as television, Facebook, or YouTube. Contact usually includes "on-the-way-down" summaries of the illness, "on-the-way-up" replies representing recovery, statements of the personally hurtful impact of stigma, and calls to action depending on target group—for example, to psychiatrists, who are called on to provide the same quality of care no matter how psychotic the person. A recent meta-analysis showed contact yielding significantly better effects than education on attitudes about and behavioral intentions toward people with mental illness (Corrigan et al., 2012). The summary also showed that in vivo contact had significantly greater impact than video or online versions. Despite the promise of adding contact to education, no identified research studies have examined its effects on care-seeking.

Changing the Self-Stigma of Mental Illness

Self-stigma and its impact on self-esteem and self-efficacy impacts the care-seeking decisions and behaviors of people with mental illness such as depression. It begins as the personal reaction to the stereotypes of mental illness—people who in some way internalize these attitudes. The depth of self-stigma depends on whether people are aware of and agree with these attitudes, and then apply the stereotypes to themselves. Such personal applications undermine the person's sense of self-esteem and self-efficacy. These kinds of decrements fail to promote the person's pursuits of behaviors related to life goals. As a result, people with mental illness such as depression decide not to engage in opportunities that would hasten work, housing, and other personal aspirations. Alternatively, reactions to stigma may evoke personal empowerment. Generally, these models of self-stigma are fruitful for understanding change strategies meant to decrease stigma's impact.

Group Identity

People engage in activities that directly implicate their group identity in everyday life, such as participating in treatment, mutual-help groups, or mental health advocacy activities. A recent study found a positive correlation between group identification and self-efficacy in people with mental illness (Watson et al., 2006). The same study failed to show such a correlation with self-esteem. These are complex relationships, however. In another study, group identification did not predict self-esteem or empowerment after controlling for depression, but group identification was negatively related to self-esteem (Rüsch et al., 2006).

Data from other social psychological research support the idea that group identification can be a double-edged sword, in this case, for members of stigmatized ethnic minorities (Crabtree, Haslam, Postmes, & Haslam, 2010). In one study, women who received negative feedback on a speech from a male evaluator were subsequently told that the evaluator was either sexist or nonsexist. Women with low gender identification showed higher self-esteem in the sexist condition, because they could attribute negative feedback to the sexism of their evaluator. However, this did not help highly gender-identified women who showed low self-esteem in both conditions. Therefore, when social identity is a core aspect of one's self-concept, individuals seem to become more vulnerable to stigmatizing threats related to this group identity. In a second study, Latin American students were randomly exposed to a text describing pervasive prejudice against their in-group or to a control article (McCoy & Major, 2003). In the control group, baseline ethnic group identification was positively related to self-esteem. However, in the group experiencing the stigmatizing threat, group identification was associated with depressed affect and low self-esteem.

Different reasons could explain these apparent contradictions. If people identify with their in-group and at the same time hold it in high regard, group identification is likely to be associated with high self-esteem. If, on the contrary, an individual holds a negative view of his or her in-group, strong group identification may lead to lower self-esteem. These positive and negative views may reflect perceived legitimacy (Rüsch et al., 2006). In terms of reducing self-stigma and empowerment among persons with mental illness, it is important to acknowledge the risks of identifying with a negatively evaluated in-group. Instead, the goal should be to build a positive group identity. Only the latter is likely to help individuals overcome self-stigma.

Coming Out Proud

Many people with depression opt to avoid self-stigma, thereby diminishing the "why try" effect by keeping their experience with mental illness and corresponding treatment a secret (Stengler-Wenzke, Angermeyer, & Matschinger, 2000). Choosing to participate in consumer-operated services presumes a personal decision about "coming out" into the public with one's mental illness (Corrigan, Kosyluk, & Rüsch, 2013). This may be a narrow decision, only letting the handful of people in the consumer-operated service know of one's background. Conversely, it may be one small step toward being totally out, where the person with serious mental illness broadcasts his or her experiences. Note that coming out may not only include disclosure about one's personal experiences with mental illness but also encounters with the treatment system. Knowing that someone takes a "pill for depression" can be as stigmatizing as awareness that the person is occasionally depressed.

The costs and benefits of coming out vary based on personal goals and decisions. Hence, only persons faced by these decisions are able to consider the costs, benefits, and implications. Prominent disadvantages to coming out include disapproval from coworkers, neighbors, fellow churchgoers, and others when they become aware of the person's psychiatric background. In turn, this disapproval leads to social avoidance. Benefits include the sense of well-being that occurs when the person no longer feels he or she must stay in the closet. This is not meant to be an exhaustive list; people are likely to identify additional consequences when individually considering the costs and benefits.

At the most extreme level, people may stay in the closet through *social avoidance*. This means keeping away from situations where people may find out about one's mental illness. Instead, they only associate with other persons who have mental illness. A second group may choose not to avoid social situations but instead keep their experiences a secret from key agents. When using *selective disclosure*, people differentiate a group of others with whom private information is disclosed versus a group from whom this information is kept secret. People with mental illness may tell peers at work of their disabilities but choose to not make disclosures to their neighbors (Corrigan et al., 2013; Corrigan & Matthews, 2003).

While there may be benefits of selective disclosure, such as an increase in supportive peers, it is still a secret that could represent a source of shame (Brohan, Elgie, Sartorius, & Thornicroft, 2010). People who choose *indiscriminant disclosure* abandon the secrecy altogether. They choose to disregard any of the negative consequences of people finding out about their mental illness. Hence, they make no active efforts to try to conceal their mental health history and experiences. *Broadcasting* one's experience means purposefully and strategically educating people about mental illness. The goal here is to seek out people to share past history and current experiences with mental illness. Broadcasting has additional benefits compared to indiscriminant disclosure. Namely, it fosters a sense of power over the experience of mental illness and stigma.

Conclusion

All of the research discussed in this chapter examines stigma at the individual psychological level. For the most part, these studies have ignored the fact that stigma is inherent in the social structures that make up society. Stigma is evident in the way laws, social services, and the justice system are structured as well as ways in which resources are allocated. Research that focuses on the social structures that maintain stigma and strategies for changing them is sorely needed.

References

Alexopoulos, G. S. (2005). Depression in the elderly. *The Lancet, 365*(9475), 1961–1970.

Allport, G. W. (1958). Personality: Normal and abnormal. *The Sociological Review, 6*(2), 167–180.

Angermeyer, M. C., & Matschinger, H. (2003). The stigma of mental illness: Effects of labelling on public attitudes towards people with mental disorder. *Acta Psychiatrica Scandinavica, 108*(4), 304–309.

Bandura, A. (1997). The anatomy of stages of change. *American Journal of Health Promotion, 12*(1), 8–10.

Bell, J., Colangelo, A., & Pillen, M. (2005). *Final report of the evaluation of the elimination of barriers initiative.* Arlington, VA: James Bell.

Ben-Zeev, D., Young, M. A., & Corrigan, P. W. (2010). DSM-V and the stigma of mental illness. *Journal of Mental Health, 19*(4), 318–327.

Bordieri, J. E., & Drehmer, D. E. (1984). Vietnam veterans: Fighting the employment war. *Journal of Applied Social Psychology, 14*(4), 341–347.

Brohan, E., Elgie, R., Sartorius, N., & Thornicroft, G. (2010). Self-stigma, empowerment and perceived discrimination among people with schizophrenia in 14 European countries: The GAMIAN-Europe study. *Schizophrenia Research, 122*(1–3), 232–238.

Butler, A., Chapman, J., Forman, E., & Beck, A. (2006). The empirical status of cognitive-behavioral therapy: A review of meta-analyses. *Clinical Psychology Review, 26*(1), 17–31.

Clement, S., Lassman, F., Barley, E., Evans-Lacko, S., Williams, P., Yamaguchi, S., . . . Thornicroft, G. (2013). Mass media interventions for reducing mental health-related stigma. *The Cochrane Database of Systematic Reviews, 7*(6), CD009453. Retrieved from http://doi.org/10.1002/14651858.CD009453.pub2

Cooper, A. E., Corrigan, P. W., & Watson, A. C. (2003). Mental illness stigma and care seeking. *The Journal of Nervous and Mental Disease, 191*(5), 339–341.

Corrigan, P. W. (2012). Where is the evidence supporting public service announcements to eliminate mental illness stigma? *Psychiatric Services, 63*(1), 79–82.

Corrigan, P. W., Bink, A. B., Fokuo, J. K., & Schmidt, A. (2015). The public stigma of mental illness means a difference between you and me. *Psychiatry Research, 226*(1), 186–191.

Corrigan, P. W., & Fong, M. W. M. (2014, February). Competing perspectives on erasing the stigma of illness: What says the dodo bird? *Social Science & Medicine, 103*, 110–117.

Corrigan, P. W., & Kleinlein, P. (2005). The impact of mental illness stigma. In P. W. Corrigan (Ed.), *On the stigma of mental illness: Practical strategies for research and social change* (pp. 11–44). Washington, DC: American Psychological Association.

Corrigan, P. W., & Kosyluk, K. A. (2013). Erasing the stigma: Where science meets advocacy. *Basic and Applied Social Psychology, 35*(1), 131–140.

Corrigan, P. W., Kosyluk, K. A., & Rüsch, N. (2013). Reducing self-stigma by coming out proud. *American Journal of Public Health, 103*(5), 794–800.

Corrigan, P. W., Larson, J. E., & Rüsch, N. (2009). Self-stigma and the "why try" effect: Impact on life goals and evidence-based practices. *World Psychiatry, 8*(2), 75–81.

Corrigan, P. W., & Matthews, A. (2003). Stigma and disclosure: Implications for coming out of the closet. *Journal of Mental Health, 12*(3), 235–248.

Corrigan, P. W., Morris, S. B., Michaels, P. J., Rafacz, J. D., & Rüsch, N. (2012). Challenging the public stigma of mental illness: A meta-analysis of outcome studies. *Psychiatric Services, 63*(10), 963–973.

Corrigan, P. W., & Penn, D. L. (1999). Lessons from social psychology on discrediting psychiatric stigma. *American Psychologist, 54*(9), 765–776.

Corrigan, P. W., Roe, D., & Tsang, H. W. H. (2010). *Challenging the stigma of mental illness: Lessons for therapists and advocates.* New York, NY: John Wiley & Sons.

Corrigan, P. W., & Watson, A. C. (2002a). The paradox of self-stigma and mental illness. *Clinical Psychology: Science and Practice, 9*(1), 35–53.

Corrigan, P. W., & Watson, A. C. (2002b). Understanding the impact of stigma on people with mental illness. *World Psychiatry, 1*(1), 16–20.

Couture, S., & Penn, D. (2003). Interpersonal contact and the stigma of mental illness: A review of the literature. *Journal of Mental Health, 12*(3), 291–305.

Crabtree, J. W., Haslam, S. A., Postmes, T., & Haslam, C. (2010). Mental health support groups, stigma, and self-esteem: Positive and negative implications of group identification. *Journal of Social Issues, 66*(3), 553–569.

Desai, M. M., Rosenheck, R. A., Druss, B. G., & Perlin, J. B. (2002). Mental disorders and quality of diabetes care in the Veterans Health Administration. *American Journal of Psychiatry, 159*(9), 1584–1590.

Druss, B. G., Allen, H. M., & Bruce, M. L. (1998). Physical health, depressive symptoms, and managed care enrollment. *American Journal of Psychiatry, 155*(7), 878–882.

Druss, B. G., & Rosenheck, R. A. (1997). Use of medical services by veterans with mental disorders. *Psychosomatics, 38*(5), 451–458.

Druss, B. G., & Rosenheck, R. A. (1998). Mental disorders and access to medical care in the United States. *American Journal of Psychiatry, 155*(12), 1775–1777.

Dunt, D., Robinson, J., Selvarajah, S., Young, L., Highet, N., Shann, C., & Pirkis, J. (2011). beyondblue, Australia's National Depression Initiative: An evaluation for the period 2005–2010. *International Journal of Mental Health Promotion, 13*(3), 22–36.

Edlund, M. J., Wang, P. S., Berglund, P. A., Katz, S. J., Lin, E., & Kessler, R. C. (2002). Dropping out of mental health treatment: Patterns and predictors among epidemiological survey respondents in the United States and Ontario. *American Journal of Psychiatry, 159*(5), 845–851.

Eisenberg, D., Downs, M. F., Golberstein, E., & Zivin, K. (2009). Stigma and help seeking for mental health among college students. *Medical Care Research and Review, 66*(5), 522–541.

Elkin, I., Shea, M. T., Watkins, J. T., Imber, S. D., Sotsky, S. M., Collins, J. F., . . . Docherty, J. P. (1989). National Institute of Mental Health Treatment of Depression Collaborative Research Program: General effectiveness of treatments. *Archives of General Psychiatry, 46*(11), 971–982; discussion 983.

Evans-Lacko, S., Henderson, C., & Thornicroft, G. (2013). Public knowledge, attitudes and behaviour regarding people with mental illness in England 2009–2012. *The British Journal of Psychiatry, 202*(s55), s51–s57.

Farina, A., & Felner, R. D. (1973). Employment interviewer reactions to former mental patients. *Journal of Abnormal Psychology, 82*(2), 268–272.

Gecas, V. (1989). The social psychology of self-efficacy. *Annual Review of Sociology, 15*, 291–316.

Goffman, E. (1963). *Stigma: Notes on the management of spoiled identity*. London: Penguin.

Hickie, I. (2001). beyondblue: The National Depression Initiative. *Australasian Psychiatry, 9*(2), 147–150.

Highet, N. J., Luscombe, G. M., Davenport, T. A., Burns, J. M., & Hickie, I. B. (2006). Positive relationships between public awareness activity and recognition of the impacts of depression in Australia. *The Australian and New Zealand Journal of Psychiatry, 40*(1), 55–58.

Jacoby, A., Snape, D., & Baker, G. A. (2005). Epilepsy and social identity: The stigma of a chronic neurological disorder. *The Lancet Neurology, 4*(3), 171–178.

Jorm, A. F., Christensen, H., & Griffiths, K. M. (2005). The impact of beyondblue: The National Depression Initiative on the Australian public's recognition of depression and beliefs about treatments. *The Australian and New Zealand Journal of Psychiatry, 39*(4), 248–254.

Jorm, A. F., Christensen, H., & Griffiths, K. M. (2006). The public's ability to recognize mental disorders and their beliefs about treatment: Changes in Australia over 8 years. *Australian and New Zealand Journal of Psychiatry, 40*(1), 36–41.

Jorm, A. F., Wright, A., & Morgan, A. J. (2007). Where to seek help for a mental disorder? National survey of the beliefs of Australian youth and their parents. *The Medical Journal of Australia, 187*(10), 556–560.

Khalema, N. E., & Shankar, J. (2014). Perspectives on employment integration, mental illness and disability, and workplace health. *Advances in Public Health, 2014*, e258614.

Kovandžić, M., Chew-Graham, C., Reeve, J., Edwards, S., Peters, S., Edge, D., . . . Dowrick, C. (2011). Access to primary mental health care for hard-to-reach groups: From "silent suffering" to "making it work." *Social Science & Medicine, 72*(5), 763–772.

Link, B. G., Cullen, F. T., Frank, J., & Wozniak, J. (1987). The social rejection of former mental patients: Understanding why labels matter. *American Journal of Sociology, 92*(6), 1461–1500.

Link, B., & Phelan, J. (2001). Conceptualizing stigma. *Annual Review of Sociology, 27*, 363–385. Retrieved from http://www.jstor.org/stable/2678626

Link, B. G., Struening, E. L., Neese-Todd, S., Asmussen, S., & Phelan, J. C. (2014). Stigma as a barrier to recovery: The consequences of stigma for the self-esteem of people with mental illnesses. *Psychiatric Services, 52*(12), 1621–1626.

Livingston, J. D., & Boyd, J. E. (2010). Correlates and consequences of internalized stigma for people living with mental illness: A systematic review and meta-analysis. *Social Science & Medicine, 71*(12), 2150–2161.

Manning, C., & White, P. D. (1995). Attitudes of employers to the mentally ill. *The Psychiatrist, 19*(9), 541–543.

Markowitz, F. E., Angell, B., & Greenberg, J. S. (2011). Stigma, reflected appraisals, and recovery outcomes in mental illness. *Social Psychology Quarterly, 74*(2), 144–165.

Markström, U., Gyllensten, A. L., Bejerholm, U., Björkman, T., Brunt, D., Hansson, L., . . . Eklund, M. (2009). Attitudes towards mental illness among health care students at

Swedish universities—A follow-up study after completed clinical placement. *Nurse Education Today, 29*(6), 660–665.

McCoy, S. K., & Major, B. (2003). Group identification moderates emotional responses to perceived prejudice. *Personality and Social Psychology Bulletin, 29*(8), 1005–1017.

Morgan, A. J., & Jorm, A. F. (2009). Recall of news stories about mental illness by Australian youth: Associations with help-seeking attitudes and stigma. *The Australian and New Zealand Journal of Psychiatry, 43*(9), 866–872.

Parcesepe, A. M., & Cabassa, L. J. (2013). Public stigma of mental illness in the United States: A systematic literature review. *Administration and Policy in Mental Health, 40*(5), 384–399.

Pescosolido, B. A., Martin, J. K., Long, J. S., Medina, T. R., Phelan, J. C., & Link, B. G. (2010). "A disease like any other"? A decade of change in public reactions to schizophrenia, depression, and alcohol dependence. *American Journal of Psychiatry, 167*(11), 1321–1330.

Ritsher, J. B., & Phelan, J. C. (2004). Internalized stigma predicts erosion of morale among psychiatric outpatients. *Psychiatry Research, 129*(3), 257–265.

Rosenfield, S. (1997). Labeling mental illness: The effects of received services and perceived stigma on life satisfaction. *American Sociological Review, 62*(4), 660.

Rosenfield, S., & Neese-Todd, S. (1993). Elements of a psychosocial clubhouse program associated with a satisfying quality of life. *Hospital and Community Psychiatry, 44*(1), 76–78.

Rüsch, N., Angermeyer, M. C., & Corrigan, P. W. (2005). Mental illness stigma: Concepts, consequences, and initiatives to reduce stigma. *European Psychiatry, 20*(8), 529–539.

Rüsch, N., Corrigan, P. W., Wassel, A., Michaels, P., Olschewski, M., Wilkniss, S., & Batia, K. (2009). Ingroup perception and responses to stigma among persons with mental illness: Ingroup perception and stigma. *Acta Psychiatrica Scandinavica, 120*(4), 320–328.

Rüsch, N., Hölzer, A., Hermann, C., Schramm, E., Jacob, G. A., Bohus, M., . . . Corrigan, P. W. (2006). Self-stigma in women with borderline personality disorder and women with social phobia. *The Journal of Nervous and Mental Disease, 194*(10), 766–773.

Schomerus, G., Schwahn, C., Holzinger, A., Corrigan, P. W., Grabe, H. J., Carta, M. G., & Angermeyer, M. C. (2012). Evolution of public attitudes about mental illness: A systematic review and meta-analysis. *Acta Psychiatrica Scandinavica, 125*(6), 440–452.

Shankar, J., Liu, L., Nicholas, D., Warren, S., Lai, D., Tan, S., . . . Sears, A. (2014). Employers' perspectives on hiring and accommodating workers with mental illness. *SAGE Open, 4*(3), 1–13. Retrieved from http://doi.org/10.1177/2158244014547880

Smith, M. (2013). Anti-stigma campaigns: Time to change. *The British Journal of Psychiatry, 202*(s55), s49–s50.

Stengler-Wenzke, K., Angermeyer, M. C., & Matschinger, H. (2000). Depression and stigma. *Psychiatrische Praxis, 27*(7), 330–335.

Taylor, S. M., & Dear, M. J. (1981). Scaling community attitudes toward the mentally ill. *Schizophrenia Bulletin, 7*(2), 225.

Vogel, D. L., Wade, N. G., & Haake, S. (2006). Measuring the self-stigma associated with seeking psychological help. *Journal of Counseling Psychology, 53*(3), 325–337.

Wahl, O. F. (1999). Mental health consumers' experience of stigma. *Schizophrenia Bulletin, 25*(3), 467.

Wang, P. S., Lane, M., Olfson, M., Pincus, H. A., Wells, K. B., & Kessler, R. C. (2005). Twelve-month use of mental health services in the United States: Results from the National Comorbidity Survey Replication. *Archives of General Psychiatry, 62*(6), 629–640.

Watson, A. C., Corrigan, P., Larson, J. E., & Sells, M. (2006). Self-stigma in people with mental illness. *Schizophrenia Bulletin, 33*(6), 1312–1318.

Yap, M. B. H., Reavley, N. J., & Jorm, A. F. (2015). Is the use of accurate psychiatric labels associated with intentions and beliefs about responses to mental illness in a friend? Findings from two national surveys of Australian youth. *Epidemiology and Psychiatric Sciences, 24*(1), 54–68.

PART III RISK, STRATEGIES, AND INTERVENTIONS

CHAPTER 9

Youth Depression
Public Health Implications and Strategies to Address the Problem

Jennifer L. Hughes, PhD

Joan Rosenbaum Asarnow, PhD

Depressive disorders in youth are a major public health concern, causing significant morbidity and mortality, and remaining underdiagnosed and undertreated. Estimates of youth depression range from around 2% in childhood to 4%–8% in adolescence (Avenevoli, Swendsen, He, Burstein, & Merikangas, 2015; Birmaher et al., 2007). Depression is associated with significant impairment in family, social, and academic functioning, as well as other adverse outcomes including substance abuse, suicidality, and future depressive episodes in adulthood (Birmaher et al., 2007). Indeed, depression is currently ranked by the World Health Organization (WHO; 2014) as the leading cause of "illness and disability" for patients aged 10–19 years, and is associated with suicide—the second leading cause of death for adolescents and young adults in the United States (Centers for Disease Control and Prevention, 2014).

There are effective evidence-based interventions to address depression in this age group, but unfortunately many youth do not receive these treatments due to problems with access to care, difficulties with dissemination, and other barriers. Recent changes to the health care system through legislation and financing provide a unique opportunity for addressing youth depression in innovative ways (Asarnow & Miranda, 2014; Asarnow et al., 2015a). This chapter provides an overview of strategies to address youth depression with an emphasis on prevention and population health. The chapter proceeds in four sections: (1) a review of the literature on prevention; (2) a discussion of strategies for integrating evidence-based preventive strategies within our health and behavioral health systems, and the importance of moving toward integrated care; (3) highlighting assessment, measurement-based care, and interventions; and (4) focusing on public health and policy implications, as well as future directions.

Between 11% and 18% of youth will experience a depressive disorder by age 18 (Avenevoli et al., 2015). In childhood, depression occurs at similar rates across gender; after puberty, the rates are twice as high in girls (Birmaher et al., 2007). Major depressive disorder (MDD) in youth is remarkably similar to adult MDD; however, children and adolescents may present with more irritability and impulsivity. Depressed youth have been shown to have negative cognitive functioning, including increased cognitive distortions, negative attributions, hopelessness, and low self-esteem (Asarnow & Bates, 1988; Garber & Hilsman, 1992; Garber, Weiss, & Shanley, 1993; Marton & Kutcher, 1995), school difficulties (Puig-Antich et al., 1993), social impairment (Hamilton, Asarnow, & Tompson, 1997; Hops, Lewinsohn, Andrews, & Roberts, 1990; Puig-Antich et al., 1985a, 1985b), poorer family relationships (Hops et al., 1990; Kashani, Burbach, & Rosenberg, 1988; Puig-Antich et al., 1985a, 1985b, 1993), and more health risk behaviors such as smoking, substance abuse, and risky sexual behavior (Asarnow et al., 2014; Rao et al., 1999; Rohde, Lewinsohn, & Seeley, 1996).

Approximately 90% of children and adolescents recover from an initial episode of MDD within one to two years of onset (Emslie et al., 1997; Kovacs et al., 1984; McCauley et al., 1993; Strober, Lampert, Schmidt, & Morrell, 1993); however, any time spent depressed is impairing during this important time of development. Unfortunately, relapse and recurrence rates are high (Kennard, Emslie, Mayes, & Hughes, 2006), and recent intervention research has focused on developing treatments to address relapse prevention (Emslie et al., 2015; Kennard et al., 2014). Preventing relapse and recurrence in pediatric depression is essential to reduce subsequent difficulties across the life span.

Prevention

The public health concept of disease prevention has historically viewed prevention as primary, secondary, or tertiary based on whether the strategy prevents the onset of the disease, the severity of symptoms or dysfunction, or the severity of the disease and disability once it has occurred. Secondary preventive interventions aim to reduce disease prevalence, whereas tertiary preventive interventions focus on rehabilitation, reducing dysfunction, and relapse prevention. In mental health, due to challenges in identifying the threshold between disorder onset versus offset and need to target risk factors over the course of development, a slightly different nomenclature is often used with distinctions made between universal, selective, and indicated prevention strategies (World Health Organization, 2002). In universal prevention, programs and interventions are developed to target the whole population, regardless of risk profile (e.g., interpersonal problem-solving skills training). In selective prevention, the population is targeted based on a specific, identified risk profile. For example, many youth depression prevention programs focus on youth with a parent who has a mood disorder, as it is known that these children are more at risk for the development of depression. In indicated prevention, the targeted population has demonstrated some of the characteristics of depression; in youth depression, this would be prevention programs targeting youth with subyndromal symptoms.

Reviews of youth depression prevention programs have found strong effects for selective and indicated prevention programs when compared to universal programs (e.g., Ahlen, Lenhard, & Ghaderi, 2015; Horowitz & Garber, 2006; Stice, Shaw, Bohon, Marti, & Rohde, 2009). Although this is likely influenced by the greater challenges in demonstrating preventive effects when only a small subgroup of the population is "truly at risk for disorder," data point to the greatest benefits for interventions that target high-risk individuals, samples that are older and more female, and programs with professional interventionalists and shorter duration more likely to produce larger effects (Stice et al., 2009). Youth depression prevention programs have been implemented across numerous settings, including schools (for review, see Corrieri et al., 2014), primary care, and online (Gladstone, Beardslee, & O'Connor, 2011).

Though there is less empirical support for universal prevention in youth depression, many argue for the inclusion of universal prevention strategies in addressing depression as useful from a public health perspective because selective programs might not be reaching all of those at risk and indicated prevention may be too late. One example of a universal prevention program addressing youth depression and anxiety is the Friends Program in Australia (Barrett & Turner, 2001; Barrett, Farrell, Ollendick, & Dadds, 2006; Lock & Barrett, 2003). This school-based, cognitve behavioral therapy intervention was designed to address child anxiety and depression through coping and problem-solving skills. Initially, there were no differences between the cognitive behavioral therapy (CBT) group and the assessment-only control group on depressive symptoms; these effects emerged at the longer-term follow-up (Lock & Barrett, 2003). This delayed prevention effect has also occurred in other universal prevention programs addressing youth depression (Barrett et al., 2006; Dadds, Spence, Holland, Barrett, & Laurens, 1997; Jaycox, Reivich, Gillham, & Seligman, 1994). Effects on depressive symptoms also appeared stronger in those children who participated in the prevention program at a younger age (sixth grade versus ninth grade); it may be that youth depression universal prevention is most effective earlier in life, as younger children can learn and practice the new skills prior to puberty, when risk of depression increases (Barrett & Turner, 2001; Barrett et al., 2006). A recent school-based prevention project in Europe demonstrated reduced rates of severe suicidal thinking and suicide attempt, both often associated with depression, in students receiving the Youth Aware of Mental Health Programme (YAM), an intervention designed to increase mental health awareness about suicide risk and protective factors, teach about depression and anxiety, and teach skills to counter stress (Wasserman et al., 2015).

The most well-studied youth depression prevention program, which has been used as both universal prevention and selective prevention, is the Penn Resiliency Program (Gillham, Reivich, & Jaycox, 2008). This cognitive behavioral intervention program has been shown to reduce depressive symptoms in school-aged children across different settings and in those of different cultural backgrounds (Brunwasser, Gillham, & Kim, 2009; Gladstone et al., 2011).

With regard to selective prevention, there have been effective prevention programs for youth at risk for depression (Clarke et al., 2001; Stice et al., 2009). Many of these interventions have targeted cognition (e.g., changing explanatory style) and problem solving as a way to prevent future depressive episodes (Gillham et al., 2012; Jaycox et al., 1994; Seligman, Schulman, DeRubeis, & Hollon, 1999), though a review of prevention programs noted that intervention content does not appear to be related to program outcome effect sizes (Stice et al., 2009). In one large multisite study, children of a parent or caregiver who had a depression diagnosis (past or current) received an eight-week (weekly sessions) prevention CBT program. At the nine-month follow-up, those children who received the CBT preventive program had reduced rates of depression onset compared to usual care, but only in those children with a parent who was not suffering from a depressive disorder at the child's program intake (Garber et al., 2009). These reduced depression onset rates were sustained at up to a three-year follow-up, with lower rates of depression diagnosis in those who were treated with the prevention program (Beardslee, Solantaus, Morgan, Gladstone, & Kowalenko, 2013). Those with a currently depressed parent at program intake did not have the same benefit, with average onset rates not differing between the cognitive behavior prevention program and usual care at either follow-up time point (Beardslee et al., 2013; Garber et al., 2009).

In indicated prevention, mostly school- and web-based strategies have been used to prevent more serious and disabling depression in adolescents. One example of a school-based program is from the Netherlands, known as Friends for Life. This program demonstrated reduced anxiety and depressive symptoms in children who had screened positive for either, both during the intervention and at one-year follow-up (Kosters, Chinapaw, Zwaanswijk, van der Wal, & Koot, 2015). One online program, Project CATCH-IT, used a combination of cognitive behavioral, behavioral activation, and interpersonal therapy strategies for children screening positive for depressive symptoms, and demonstrated reduction in the likelihood of a depressive episode when delivered in primary care coupled with motivational interviewing (Landback et al., 2009; Saulsberry et al., 2013; Van Voorhees et al., 2009).

In the United States, the Affordable Care Act places a strong emphasis on prevention and wellness, with hopes of shifting the health care system toward health promotion rather than a system with an intense focus on illness. As such, the Afforable Care Act has increased the need for effective prevention, and there has been a move toward including prevention of *behavioral health problems* (a broad term referring to mental health, substance use, and health behaviors) within pediatric preventive services (see American Academy of Pediatrics Bright Futures Recommendations for Preventive Pediatric Health Care). Because most youths in the United States see a primary care provider annually, integrating mental health care within primary care services has strong protential for improving access to mental health care as well as preventive services for mental health problems (Chevarley, 2001).

Integrated Care

As it is estimated that more than 70% of adolescents are seen in primary care each year in the United States (Newacheck, Brindis, Cart, Marchi, & Irwin, 1999; Ziv, Boulet, & Slap, 1999), primary care presents an optimal chance to identify youths with depressive disorder and provides unique opportunities to connect youths to treatment providers and education about treatment options (Asarnow et al., 2015b; Stancin & Perrin, 2014). In the Youth Partners in Care (YPIC) trial, Asarnow and colleagues developed and tested health information tools and strategies for exporting evidence-based depression care for youths in primary care clinics within five diverse health care organizations. This study demonstrated that enhancing evidence-based depression care was related to positive patient outcomes, including improved depression, functioning, and patient satisfaction, at a six-month follow-up among youths in the intervention condition, as compared to usual care (Asarnow et al., 2005, 2009; Wells, Kataoka, & Asarnow, 2001). The more recent Reaching Out to Adolescents in Distress Study found that, when compared to usual primary care, a collaborative care program similar to that used in YPIC resulted in significantly greater improvements in depression symptom scores, depression response rates (68% vs. 39%), and depression remission rates (50% vs. 21%; Richardson et al., 2014).

Additionally, the greater access to primary versus specialty care among youths in the United States underscores the value of evidence-guided primary care strategies for these major health conditions (Zuckerbrot et al., 2007). To that end, a collaboration among family medicine, pediatrics, psychology, and psychiatry developed clinical guidelines to assist in the management of adolescent depression in primary care, the *Guidelines for Adolescent Depression—Primary Care* (*GLAD-PC*), which address screening, diagnosis, and treatment of depression in youths aged 10–21 (Cheung et al., 2007; Zuckerbrot et al., 2007). Moreover, a recent meta-analysis examining integrated primary and behavioral health care interventions relative to usual primary care (allowing for some enhancements) found a small statistically significant advantage for integrated primary medical-behavioral health care, with the strongest effects for interventions focusing on mental health treatment, particularly for those using collaborative care models (Asarnow, Rozenman, Wiblin, & Zeltzer, 2015).

Assessment and Measurement-Based Care

The diagnostic criteria for youth depression are the same as adult depression; however, there are some key differences in the assessment process and presentation in youths. Children and adolescents usually present for treatment with a caregiver, and clinicians use multiple informants (including the youth, parents, caregivers, and teachers) to understand the duration and nature of symptoms. Generally, youths more accurately report on the internalizing symptoms and caregivers on the more behavioral symptoms. Younger children in particular generally tend to have difficulties reporting the frequency and duration of symptoms; thus, caregiver reports are needed to establish onset dates and course of illness (Emslie, Mayes, Kennard, & Hughes, 2006).

In primary care settings, where providers often have limited time to address multiple patient concerns, self-report screening measures are useful in identifying youths in need of further evaluation. Ideally, a blend of clinician-rated and parent- and self-report rating scales are used to diagnose the presence and severity of depression in the pediatric age group. Measures range from semistructured interviews to short, unstructured interviews specific to depressive symptoms (Elmquist, Melton, Croarkin, & McClintock, 2010). Brief self-report screening measures, such as the Patient Health Questionnaire 9-Adolescent (PHQ-9-A; Kroenke, Spitzer, and Williams, 2001) or the Quick Inventory of Depressive Symptomatology-Self-Report-16 (QIDS-SR-16; Rush et al., 2003), can be used to identify youths in need of further evaluation. Indeed, the PHQ-9-A is currently being considered as a Healthcare Effectiveness Data and Information Set (HEDIS) measure for monitoring depression symptoms in adolescents and adults. Because HEDIS measures are used by more than 90% of US health plans to measure performance on key dimensions, inclusion of systematic screening and monitoring of depressive symptoms is likely to lead to increased attention to the need for depression care—and hopefully increased access to evidence-based, high-quality treatment.

Use of a measurement-based approach to treatment is a critical component of effective management and treatment of depression in youth, as this is a way to systematically evaluate the effects of treatment on symptom response to aid in clinical decision-making (Elmquist et al., 2010). In adult depression treatment, these assessments are now recommended as part of routine clinical care (Harding, Rush, Arbuckle, Trivedi, & Pincus, 2011; Trivedi & Daly, 2007). With a greater emphasis on demonstrating cost-effectiveness and health care outcomes, measurement-based care will become the standard in treatment (Asarnow et al., 2015a). Utilizing ongoing measurement of treatment response in addition to clinical assessment helps achieve that goal in a timely manner (Elmquist et al., 2010). Remission, or essentially few or no remaining symptoms of depression, is the outcome of choice, and clinicians are encouraged to treat symptoms to the point of remission in order to achieve symptom relief and improved functioning, and to prevent relapse (Emslie et al., 2015; Kennard et al., 2006a; Kennard et al., 2014).

Intervention

Effective treatments (psychotherapies and pharmacotherapy) for youth depression are available (for reviews, see Maalouf & Brent, 2012; Sakolsky & Birmaher, 2012; Tompson, Boger, & Asarnow, 2012). Youth presenting with mild depression that does not significantly impact functioning can often be treated through a combination of case management, psychoeducation about depressive symptom monitoring, and supportive therapy. For those youth with moderate to severe depression, more intensive treatment is recommended. To date, the combination of pharmacotherapy and psychotherapy, specifically treatment with selective serotonin reuptake inhibitors (SSRIs) and CBT, appears to be the most efficacious treatment for moderate to severe depression in adolescents (March et al., 2004). Combination treatment serves to enhance the magnitude of response to treatment, and there is some evidence that CBT may play a protective role against suicidality.

Treatment for depression is typically separated into three phases: acute, continuation, and maintenance (Kennard et al., 2006a). Each phase has specified treatment targets, including the reduction or remission of symptoms (acute), further treatment consolidation or response and relapse prevention (continuation), and reducing the likelihood of recurrence (maintenance). Research studies have generally focused on acute treatment, but more recently there has been a shift toward better understanding how to manage depression in a longer-term treatment model, with a focus on preventing relapse (Emslie et al., 2015; Kennard et al., 2014).

With regard to acute treatment, current pharmacological treatment guidelines recommend using SSRIs as first-line antidepressant treatment for youth with depression (Birmaher et al., 2007; Cheung, Emslie, & Mayes, 2005; Hughes et al., 2007). Fluoxetine, the only drug to show benefit over placebo (Bridge et al., 2007), has shown a larger difference between medication and placebo than other antidepressants in adolescents and children younger than 12, and is the only antidepressant with a Food and Drug Administration (FDA) indication for treatment of both children and adolescents (aged 8 years and older) with MDD. At this time, escitalopram also has an FDA indication for adolescents (aged 12 years and older) with MDD. No other antidepressants have an FDA indication for treatment of depression, although some have indications for the treatment of other psychiatric conditions in youth. Approximately 55%–65% of youth will respond to treatment with an SSRI, but remission rates are much lower (around 30%–45%). In a review of three large studies examining psychopharmacological and psychosocial treatment, several clinical characteristics were related to nonresponse to an antidepressant, including more severe depression, poorer functioning, higher rates of suicidal ideation and hopelessness, and more comorbid psychiatric conditions (Emslie, Kennard, & Mayes, 2011). For those youth who do not respond to the first SSRI, guidelines recommend treatment with a second SSRI. No non-SSRI antidepressants have demonstrated efficacy for acute depression, so non-SSRIs are considered third-line treatment options. The only study of treatment-resistant depression in adolescents demonstrated similar improvement rates for a second SSRI or a non-SSRI (venlafaxine), although there was a slightly better adverse event profile with the SSRIs (Brent et al., 2008).

Acute phase psychotherapy treatment studies for the treatment of pediatric depression have demonstrated mixed results. Even with some studies having robust effects, a meta-analysis of 35 randomized controlled trials found the overall effects of psychotherapy for the treatment of youth depression were modest. There was no difference in efficacy between age groups, delivery modality, or type of therapy, and there was no correlation between treatment duration and response (Weisz, McCarty, & Valeri, 2006). Of the various therapeutic modalities, only CBT and interpersonal psychotherapy (IPT) are considered well established at this time (Compton et al., 2004; David-Ferdon & Kaslow, 2008). CBT is the most widely studied psychotherapy for the treatment of pediatric depression, and several studies have shown CBT to be effective even when dealing with comorbid conditions and suicidality.

As family factors are key in youth depression (Sheeber, Hops, & Davis, 2001; Tompson et al., 2012), and family interventions have been useful in preventing depression in youth (Beardslee, Wright, Gladstone, & Forbes, 2007) and in the treatment of youths struggling with suicidality (Asarnow, Berk, Hughes, & Anderson, 2014), treating the family may be an additional approach to treating child depression. Family therapies for depression in children and adolescents show promise. Diamond and colleagues (Diamond, Reis, Diamond, Siqueland, & Issacs, 2002; Diamond & Siqueland, 1995) introduced a model of treatment that included reducing maladaptive interactions between family members through reframing the focus from adolescent symptoms to enhancing adolescent-parent relationships and promoting attachments, as well as enhancing the adolescent's competencies. Thirty-two adolescents with MDD were randomized to this 12-week attachment-based family therapy (ABFT) or a six-week wait-list control group. In this pilot study, 81% of adolescents treated with ABFT no longer met criteria for MDD versus 47% in the wait-list control. In addition, those in the ABFT treatment group demonstrated significant decreases in family conflict, depressive symptoms, and anxiety symptoms (Diamond et al., 2002).

The family has also been more heavily emphasized in the treatment of 23 young children suffering from depression. Although there have only been three studies of children presenting with depressive disorders, all three included strong family components. Tompson and colleagues (2007, 2012, 2016) developed a Family-Focused Treatment for Child Depression (FFT-CD). This approach used an interpersonal model of depression and emphasized developing family strategies for altering interpersonal processes, supporting recovery, and enhancing resilience. While results of a randomized controlled trial (RCT) are currently pending, initial open trial results indicated strong depression recovery rates (66% at posttreatment; 77% by nine months posttreatment; Tompson et al., 2007).

Kovacs and colleagues (Kovacs & Lopez-Duran, 2012; Kovacs et al., 2006) developed a developmentally informed intervention known as contextual emotion regulation therapy (CERT), which specifically targets emotion regulation and mood repair, based on the proposition that recovery from depression requires alleviation of sad/dysphoric/distressed mood. Recognizing the central importance of parents as interpersonal regulatory agents in helping children to develop effective regulatory strategies, parents are included in CERT sessions and play a critical role in treatment. To use a sports analogy, for example, the therapist is the "coach," the parent is the "assistant coach," and the child is the special team "player." While an RCT has not yet been completed of CERT, results of an open trial provide preliminary support for benefits, with 66% of children completing the treatment showing full or partial remission of dysthymia at posttreatment; remission rates of 79% and 92% at 6- and 12-month follow-ups, respectively; and significant declines in child-reported depressive and anxiety symptoms at the end of treatment that persisted throughout follow-up (Kovacs et al., 2006).

Finally, Dietz and colleagues (2015) evaluated the efficacy of family-based interpersonal psychotherapy compared to child-centered therapy in a RCT. This adaptation of interpersonal psychotherapy for adolescents includes a strong parent component, with parents involved in weekly sessions and an emphasis on directly addressing parent-child conflict and interpersonal impairment. Results indicated significant advantages for the family treatment, with higher depression remission rates (66.0% versus 31%), fewer depressive symptoms, and a greater decline in depressive symptoms.

As previously mentioned, few studies have focused on continuation phase treatment in youth depression. It is known that youth who do not continue treatment, particularly those with residual symptoms, experience higher rates of relapse (Emslie et al., 2008). As such, it is recommended that all youth remain in treatment for at least 6–12 months following acute response. If prescribed antidepressants, youth should be followed at regular intervals with emphasis on optimizing medication dose, addressing adherence and side effects, and monitoring treatment response with the goal of treating to remission (Birmaher et al., 2007). Additionally, a relapse prevention treatment for youth depression has been developed and tested with promising results (Kennard et al., 2008a; Kennard, Stewart, Hughes, Jarrett, & Emslie, 2008b). In particular, the RP-CBT program emphasized strategies that promoted health and wellness. The intervention resulted in lower risk of relapse at 30-week follow-up compared to medication management alone, and these results persist at longer-term follow-up (Emslie et al., 2015; Kennard et al., 2014).

Future Directions in Public Health and Policy Implications

Studies of youth depression have resulted in the identification of several efficacious prevention and treatment strategies. Recent changes in the health and behavioral health care systems highlight the need to hold treatment providers and systems accountable for the care they provide, through the use of measurement-based care and the implementation of evidenced-based intervention strategies (Asarnow et al., 2015a). There are an increasing number of dissemination and effectiveness trials in youth depression; however, there are still some identified difficulties in using these evidence-based treatments in real-world practice settings (Atkins, Rusch, Mehta, & Lakind, 2016; Weisz, Ng, & Bearman, 2014).

While several effective treatments have been identified, there has been great difficulty in getting these treatments into clinical practice so that they are widely available to consumers. The emerging field of dissemination and implementation science is attempting to address this problem by better understanding how to distribute information and intervention materials associated with evidence-based interventions to the public health or clinical practice audience while promoting strategies to enhance the adoption and integration of these interventions to change practice patterns in these settings. Several challenges have been identified, including findings that intervention benefits decrease when tested practices are scaled up to these settings, the low relevance of much clinical research to actual clinical practice, and the vast array of evidence-based interventions making it difficult for practice settings to identify or adopt treatments to address their diverse patient needs and preferences (Weisz, Ng, & Bearman, 2014). One way to address this problem has been for treatment developers to partner with community providers during the treatment development stage; this deployment-focused approach often helps to eliminate potential implementation barriers at the outset of treatment development. Additionally, effectiveness trials, in which an intervention that was tested previously in a highly controlled RCT is then tested under usual conditions in a clinical practice setting with community providers, are key to understanding how to effectively move these treatments into other nonlaboratory settings. Additional approaches to addressing these problems have been proposed, including exploring alternative training delivery models using the internet and continuing education systems, and changing the current training models to address the incoming workforce.

Addressing Health

Youth depression is associated with numerous other health risk behaviors, including reduced physical activity, obesity, insomnia, smoking, substance abuse, and unsafe sex (Asarnow et al., 2014). From a public health perspective, it may be useful to integrate health behavior interventions into existing depression treatments to address these commonly associated health risk behaviors. Addressing these health risk behaviors may also result in a decrease in depressive symptoms.

Sleep difficulties are commonly reported in depression, and approximately 75% of those with depression report symptoms of sleep disturbance (Ivanenko, Crabtree, & Gozal, 2004). Insomnia is linked to poorer treatment outcomes and is one of the most common residual symptoms in those youth treated for depression (Emslie et al., 2012; Kennard et al., 2006b). Adolescents who reported having both insomnia and depression were less likely to respond to antidepressant treatment than those without insomnia (Emslie et al., 2012). Insomnia has also been linked to death by suicide in adolescents, the second leading cause of death in this age group (Goldstein, Bridge, & Brent, 2008).

Adult depression treatments that address insomnia have been found to be effective (Manber et al., 2008). While many youth depression treatments include an assessment of sleep and sleep hygiene education, treatments that specifically target insomnia have been recently adapted for depressed adolescents (Clarke & Harvey, 2012). These treatments address dysfunctional thoughts related to sleep, as well as help the youth reassociate the bed with sleep (stimulus control), and sleep restriction strategies to promote sleep and regulate the sleep-and-wake cycle. This intervention utilizes motivational enhancement strategies. The treatment, known as CBT for insomnia, addressing depression and insomnia, has shown promise in improving sleep in depressed adolescents and young adults, compared to a sleep hygiene control condition combined with CBT for depression, in a pilot randomized trial (Clarke & Harvey, 2012; Clarke et al., 2015).

Treatment studies of adult depression have found that high-dose exercise programs can be effective in reducing depressive symptoms (Dunn, Trivedi, Kampert, Clark, & Chambliss, 2002, 2005). Exercise is associated with lower rates of depressive symptoms in youth as well. In a prospective, longitudinal study of a community sample of youth, participants with greater levels of exercise reported lower levels of depressive symptoms (Rothon et al., 2010). Recently, a cognitive behavioral program, the COPE (Creating Opportunities for Personal Empowerment) Healthy Lifestyles TEEN (Thinking, Emotions, Exercise, Nutrition) program, delivered in high schools to encourage 20 minutes of physical activity integrated with a health course, demonstrated effects on lowering body mass index scores and depressive symptoms in those participants who began the program with elevated depressive symptoms (Melnyk et al., 2014). These types of programs are important from a public health standpoint due to relatively low cost, ease of dissemination, and ability to reach youth in their usual environment of school, versus having to go to a treatment clinic. In clinical samples, exercise has been shown to be a promising alternative treatment strategy for depression (Dopp, Mooney, Armitage, & King, 2012; Hughes et al., 2009, 2013). In a RCT of adolescent depression, those treated with exercise, versus a stretch-only control group, had a 100% remission rate at weeks 26 and 52, compared to a 70% remission rate in the stretch-only control group (Hughes et al., 2009, 2013).

Many youth with depression also struggle with substance use, abuse, or dependence. In particular, youth presenting with alcohol or other drug use disorders are at a three- to fourfold increased risk for suicide attempt (Esposito-Smythers & Spirito, 2004), and substance abuse disorders in an adolescent with other mental health problems, such as depression, puts one at an increased risk of future suicidal behavior (Goldston et al., 2009). There is a need for effective interventions to address both youth depression and co-occuring substance abuse, though these service systems have traditionally operated quite separately (Hawkins, 2009). In the Treatment of Adolescents with Depression Study (TADS), participants received treatment for depression and were followed for five years to better understand substance abuse outcomes; response to the depression treatment was unrelated to later alcohol use disorder but did predict lower substance use disorder, regardless of the initial type of depression treatment (Curry et al., 2012). Esposito-Smythers and colleagues (2011) developed an intervention to address both substance abuse and suicidality in adolescents, finding that the integrated outpatient cognitive behavioral intervention was superior to enhanced treatment-as-usual in reducing heavy drinking days, global impairment, suicide attempts, and hospital services use. There were no differences between the groups in rates of depression, however. Future interventions are needed to target both substance use disorders and depression in youth, particularly given the increased risk of suicidal behavior in this population.

Addressing Wellness and Strength

Historically, the focus on treating depression has been on reducing depressive symptoms and promoting remission (or absence of symptoms); however, there has been a recent shift toward promoting health and well-being in those being treated for depression. In mental health, ideally the focus of treatment is not only to achieve the absence of illness but also to promote the presence of wellness. Some of the early important work in the promotion of wellness came from the positive psychology movement (Seligman & Csikszentmihalyi, 2000). This research emphasizes the need for practitioners to focus more attention on amplifying strengths and building positive traits (e.g., optimism) as a means of preventing future illness (Duckworth, Steen, & Seligman, 2005; Kobau et al., 2011). Recently, psychosocial treatments have included more focus on building strengths as opposed to addressing deficits (i.e., decreasing negative mood and cognitions). A wellness-focused approach includes the enhancement of strengths, positive experiences, mood, and cognitions. Strategies that promote health and well-being include mastery, positive self-regard, goal setting, quality relations / social problem solving, and optimism (Jaycox et al., 1994; Ryff & Singer, 1996; Seligman & Csikzentmihalyi, 2000). Specifically, in depressed adolescents, attributions for positive events can help build positive self-worth and optimistic explanatory style (Curry & Craighead, 1990).

This wellness-focused approach to the treatment of depression was first tested in adults. Ryff and Singer (1996) developed a model for defining dimensions of wellness, which was later adapted into intervention strategies for relapse prevention in adults remitted for depression (Fava, Grandi, Zielezny, Canestrari, & Morphy, 1994; Fava, Grandi, Zielezny, Rafanelli, & Canestrari, 1996; Fava, Rafanelli, Grandi, Canestrari, & Morphy, 1998). Continuation phase cognitive behavioral strategies have been found to prevent relapse of depression in adults (Jarrett, Minhajuddin, Gershenfeld, Friedman, & Thasc, 2013; Nierenberg, 2001). Adult studies have also shown that relapse rates can be significantly reduced by combining medication treatments and CBT in the continuation phase of treatment for MDD (Fava et al., 1994, 1996, 1998, 2004; Guidi, Fava, Fava, & Papakostas, 2011; Nierenberg, 2001; Paykel, 2007; Paykel et al., 1999; Teasdale et al., 2000).

A meta-analysis of treatment studies using positive psychology interventions in both youth and adults showed promising results for the treatment of depression (Sin & Lyubomirsky, 2009). In youth depression, more recent work has been done to promote wellness along with adaptive coping strategies to enhance well-being in youth who were successfully treated for depression (Kennard et al., 2008a, 2008b, 2014). Using a continuation phase intevention that included a wellness, strengths-based approach (Relapse Prevention-CBT [RP-CBT]), those who were treated with RP-CBT and continued antidepressant medication had lower relapse rates over a 30-week treatment period compared to those treated with medication only (9% vs. 26.5%). The study also concluded that those who were treated with CBT reported spending more time well (based on percent time well) and required a lower antidepressant dose (Kennard et al., 2014). The results of this study hold up at a longer-term follow-up as well (Emslie et al., 2015).

Conclusion

Depression in children and adolescents continues to go unrecognized and definitely undertreated. Prevention in schools may be an important first step. Additionally, screening for depression in at-risk youth is imperative to early identification, and this can be implemented in primary care settings. A continuum of effective treatments are available, from general health advice (e.g., improved health habits, sleep-wake schedule improvements, and exercise) and relatively inexpensive interventions (e.g., internet-based programs) to more intensive treatment with medication or specific psychotherapies. Measurement-based care is needed to guide clinical decision-making. The need to individualize the treatment based on severity, psychosocial stressors, and family circumstances will inform treatment decisions. Continued work is necessary on identifying barriers from identification to adequate treatment, including accessible, culturally sensitive care, and developing new initiatives to increase the limited numbers of adequately trained professionals.

References

Ahlen, J., Lenhard, F., & Ghaderi, A. (2015). Universal prevention for anxiety and depressive symptoms in children: A meta-analysis of randomized and cluster-randomized trials. *Journal of Primary Prevention, 36*(6), 387–403.

Asarnow, J. R., & Bates, S. (1988). Depression in child psychiatric inpatients: Cognitive and attributional patterns. *Journal of Abnormal Child Psychology, 16*(6), 601–615.

Asarnow, J. R., Berk, M. S., Hughes, J. L., & Anderson, N. L. (2014). The SAFETY Program: A treatment development trial of a cognitive-behavioral family treatment for adolescent suicide attempters. *Journal of Clinical Child and Adolescent Psychology, 44*(1), 194–203.

Asarnow, J. R., Hoagwood, K. E., Stancin, T., Lochman, J. E., Hughes, J. L., Miranda, J. M., . . . Kazak, A. E. (2015a). Psychological science and innovative strategies for informing health care redesign: A policy brief. *Journal of Clinical Child and Adolescent Psychology, 44*(6), 923–932.

Asarnow, J. R., Jaycox, L. H., Duan, N., LaBorde, A. P., Rea, M. M., Murray, P., . . . Wells, K. B. (2005). Effectiveness of a quality improvement intervention for adolescent depression in primary care clinics: A randomized controlled trial. *JAMA, 293*(3), 311–319.

Asarnow, J. R., Jaycox, L. H., Tang, L., Duan, N., LaBorde, A. P., Zeledon, L. R., . . . Wells, K. B. (2009). Long-term benefits of short-term quality improvement interventions for depressed youths in primary care. *American Journal of Psychiatry, 166*(9), 1002–1010.

Asarnow, J. R., & Miranda, J. (2014, March). Improving care for depression and suicide risk in adolescents: Innovative strategies for bringing treatments to community settings. *Annual Review of Clinical Psychology, 10*, 275–303.

Asarnow, J. R., Rozenman, M., Wiblin, J., & Zeltzer, L. (2015b). Integrated medical-behavioral care compared with usual primary care for child and adolescent behavioral health: A meta-analysis. *JAMA Pediatrics, 169*(10), 929–937.

Asarnow, J. R., Zeledon, L. R., D'Amico, E., LaBorde, A., Anderson, M., Avina, C., . . . Shoptaw, S. (2014). Depression and health risk behaviors: Towards optimizing primary care service strategies for addressing risk. *Primary Health Care, 4*(1), 152.

Atkins, M. S., Rusch, D., Mehta, T. G., & Lakind, D. (2016). Future directions for dissemination and implementation science: Aligning ecological theory and public health to close the research to practice gap. *Journal of Clinical Child and Adolescent Psychology, 45*(2), 215–226.

Avenevoli, S., Swendsen, J., He, J. P., Burstein, M., & Merikangas, K. R. (2015). Major depression in the national comorbidity survey-adolescent supplement: Prevalence, correlates, and treatment. *Journal of the American Academy of Child and Adolescent Psychiatry, 54*(1), 37–44.

Barrett, P., Farrell, L., Ollendick, T., & Dadds, M. (2006). Long-term outcomes of an Australian universal prevention trial of anxiety and depression symptoms in children and youth: An evaluation of the friends program. *Journal of Clinical Child and Adolescent Psychology, 35*(3), 403–411.

Barrett, P., & Turner, C. (2001). Prevention of anxiety symptoms in primary school children: Preliminary results from a universal school-based trial. *British Journal of Clinical Psychology, 40*, 399–410.

Beardslee, W. R., Solantaus, T. S., Morgan, B. S., Gladstone, T. R., & Kowalenko, N. M. (2013). Preventive interventions for children of parents with depression: International perspectives. *Medical Journal of Australia, 199*(3 Suppl), S23–25.

Beardslee, W. R., Wright, E. J., Gladstone, T. R. G., & Forbes, P. (2007). Long-term effects from a randomized trial of two public health preventive interventions for parental depression. *Journal of Family Psychology, 21*(4), 703–713.

Birmaher, B., Brent, D., Bernet, B., Bukstein, O., Walter H., Benson, R.S., . . . Medicus, J. (2007). Practice parameter for the assessment and treatment of children and adolescents with depressive disorders. *Journal of the American Academy of Child and Adolescent Psychiatry, 46*(11), 1503–1526.

Brent, D., Emslie, G., Clarke, G., Wagner, K. D., Asarnow, J. R., Keller, M., . . . Zelazny, J. (2008). Switching to another SSRI or to venlafaxine with or without cognitive behavioral therapy for adolescents with SSRI-resistant depression: The TORDIA randomized controlled trial. *JAMA, 299*(8), 901–913.

Bridge, J. A., Iyengar, S., Salary, C. B., Barbe, R. P., Birmaher, B., Pincus, H. A., . . . Brent, D. A. (2007). Clinical response and risk for reported suicidal ideation and suicide attempts in pediatric antidepressant treatment: A meta-analysis of randomized controlled trials. *JAMA, 297*(15), 1683–1696.

Brunwasser, S. M., Gillham, J. E., & Kim, E. S. (2009). A meta-analytic review of the Penn Resiliency Program's effect on depressive symptoms. *Journal of Consulting and Clinical Psychology, 77*(6), 1042–1054.

Centers for Disease Control and Prevention. (2014). Deaths: Final data for 2013. *National Vital Statistics Reports, 64*(2). Retrieved from http://www.cdc.gov/nchs/data/nvsr/nvsr64/nvsr64_02.pdf

Cheung, A., Emslie, G. J., & Mayes, T. L. (2005). Review of the efficacy and safety of antidepressants in youth depression. *Journal of Child Psychology and Psychiatry, 46*(7), 735–754.

Cheung, A. H., Zuckerbrot, R. A., Jensen, P. S., Ghalib, K., Laraque, D., Stein, R. E., & GLAD-PC Steering Group. (2007). Guidelines for Adolescent Depression Primary Care (GLAD-PC): II. Treatment and ongoing management. *Pediatrics, 120*(5), 1313–1326.

Chevarley, F. (2001). *Statistical brief #12: Children's access to necessary health care.* Rockville, MD: Agency for Health Care Quality and Research.

Clarke, G., & Harvey, A. G. (2012). The complex role of sleep in adolescent depression. *Child and Adolescent Psychiatric Clinics of North America, 21*(2), 385–400.

Clarke, G. N., Hornbrook, M., Lynch, F., Polen, M., Beardslee, W. R., O'Connor, E., & Seeley, J. R. (2001). A randomized trial of a group cognitive intervention for preventing depression in adolescent offspring of depressed parents. *Archives of General Psychiatry, 58*(12), 1127–1134.

Clarke, G., McGlinchey, E. L., Hein, K., Gullion, C. M., Dickerson, J. F., Leo, M. C., & Harvey, A. G. (2015). Cognitive-behavioral treatment of insomnia and depression in adolescents: A pilot randomized trial. *Behaviour Research and Therapy, 69*, 111–118.

Compton, S. N., March, J. S., Brent, D., Albano, A. M., Weersing, R., & Curry, J. (2004). Cognitive-behavioral psychotherapy for anxiety and depressive disorders in children and adolescents: An evidence-based medicine review. *Journal of the American Academy of Child and Adolescent Psychiatry, 43*(8), 930–959.

Corrieri, S., Heider, D., Conrad, I., Blume, A., Konig, H., & Riedel-Heller, S. G. (2014). School-based prevention programs for depression and anxiety in adolescence: A systematic review. *Health Promotion International, 29*(3), 427–441.

Curry, J. F., & Craighead, W. E. (1990). Attributional style in clinically depressed and conduct disordered adolescents. *Journal of Consulting and Clinical Psychology, 58*(1), 109–115.

Curry, J., Silva, S., Rohde, P., Ginsburg, G., Kennard, B., Kratochvil, C., . . . March, J. (2012). Onset of alcohol or substance use disorders following treatment for adolescent depression. *Journal of Consulting and Clinical Psychology, 80*(2), 299–312.

Dadds, M. R., Spence, S. H., Holland, D. E., Barrett, P. M., & Laurens, K. R. (1997). Prevention and early intervention for anxiety disorders: A controlled trial. *Journal of Consulting and Clinical Psychology, 55*(4), 627–635.

David-Ferdon, C., & Kaslow, N. J. (2008). Evidence-based psychosocial treatments for child and adolescent depression. *Journal of Clinical Child and Adolescent Psychology, 37*(1), 62–104.

Diamond, G., & Siqueland, L. (1995). Family therapy for the treatment of depressed adolescents. *Psychotherapy: Theory, Research, Practice, Training, 32*, 77–90.

Diamond, G. S., Reis, B. F., Diamond, G. M., Siqueland, L., & Isaacs, L. (2002). Attachment-based family therapy for depressed adolescents: A treatment development study. *Journal of the American Academy of Child and Adolescent Psychiatry, 41*(10), 1190–1196.

Dietz, L. J., Weinberg, R. J., Brent, D. A., & Mufson, L. (2015). Family-based interpersonal psychotherapy for depressed preadolescents: Examining efficacy and potential treatment mechanisms. *Journal of the American Academy of Child and Adolescent Psychiatry, 54*(3), 191–199.

Dopp, R. R., Mooney, A. J., Armitage, R., & King, C. (2012). Exercise for adolescents with depressive disorders: A feasibility study. *Depression Research Treatment, 2012*, 257472.

Duckworth, A. L., Steen, T. A., & Seligman, M. E. (2005). Positive psychology in clinical practice. *Annual Review of Clinical Psychology, 1*, 629–651.

Dunn, A. L., Trivedi, M. H., Kampert, J. B., Clark, C. G., & Chambliss, H. O. (2002). The DOSE study: A clinical trial to examine efficacy and dose-response of exercise as treatment for depression. *Controlled Clinical Trials, 23*, 584–603.

Dunn, A. L., Trivedi, M. H., Kampert, J. B., Clark, C. G., & Chambliss, H. O. (2005). Exercise treatment for depression. *American Journal of Preventive Medicine, 28*(1), 1–8.

Elmquist, J. M., Melton, T. K., Croarkin, P., & McClintock, S. M. (2010). A systematic overview of measurement-based care in the treatment of childhood and adolescent depression. *Journal of Psychiatric Practice, 16*(4), 217–234.

Emslie, G. J., Kennard, B. D., & Mayes, T. L. (2011). Predictors of treatment response in adolescent depression. *Pediatric Annals, 40*(6), 300–306.

Emslie, G. J., Kennard, B. D., Mayes, T. L., Nakonezny, P. A., Moore, J., Jones, J. M., . . . King, J. (2015). Continued effectiveness of relapse prevention cognitive-behavioral therapy following fluoxetine treatment in youth with major depressive disorder. *Journal of the American Academy of Child and Adolescent Psychiatry, 54*(12), 991–998.

Emslie, G. J., Kennard, B. D., Mayes, T. L., Nakonezny, P. A., Zhu, L., Tao, R., . . . Croarkin, P. (2012). Insomnia moderates outcome of serotonin-selective reuptake inhibitor treatment in depressed youth. *Journal of Child and Adolescent Psychopharmacology, 22*(1), 21–28.

Emslie, G. J., Kennard, B. D., Mayes, T. L., Nightingale-Teresi, J., Carmody, T., Hughes, C. W., . . . Rintelmann, J. W. (2008). Fluoxetine versus placebo in preventing relapse of major depression in children and adolescents. *American Journal of Psychiatry, 165*(4), 459–467.

Emslie, G. J., Mayes, T., Kennard, B. D., & Hughes, J. L. (2006). Pediatric mood disorders. In D. J. Stein, D. J. Kupfer, & A. F. Schatzberg (Eds.), *The American psychiatric publishing textbook of mood disorders* (pp. 573–602). Washington, DC: American Psychiatric Publishing, Inc.

Emslie, G. J., Rush, A. J., Weinberg, W. A., Gullion, C. M., Rintelmann, J., & Hughes, C. W. (1997). Recurrence of major depressive disorder in hospitalized children and adolescents. *Journal of the American Academy of Child and Adolescent Psychiatry, 36*, 785–792.

Esposito-Smythers, C., & Spirito, A. (2004). Adolescent substance use and suicidal behavior: A review with implications for treatment research. *Alcoholism: Clinical and Experimental Research, 28*, 77S-88S.

Esposito-Smythers, C., Spirito, A., Kahler, C. W., Hunt, J., & Monti, P. (2011). Treamtent of co-occurring substance abuse and suicidality among adolescents: A randomized trial. *Journal of Consulting and Clinical Psychology, 79*(6), 728–739.

Fava, G., Grandi, S., Zielezny, M., Canestrari, R., & Morphy, M. A. (1994). Cognitive behavioral treatment of residual symptoms in primary major depressive disorder. *American Journal of Psychiatry, 151*(9), 1295–1299.

Fava, G., Grandi, S., Zielezny, M., Rafanelli, C., & Canestrari, R. (1996). Four-year outcome for cognitive behavioral treatment of residual symptoms in major depression. *American Journal of Psychiatry, 153*(7), 945–947.

Fava, G., Rafanelli, C., Grandi, S., Canestrari, R., & Morphy, M. A. (1998). Six-year outcome for cognitive behavioral treatment of residual symptoms in major depression. *American Journal of Psychiatry, 155*(10), 1443–1445.

Fava, G. A., Ruini, C., Rafanelli, C., Finos, L., Conti, S., & Grandi, S. (2004). Six-year outcome of cognitive behavior therapy for prevention of recurrent depression. *American Journal of Psychiatry, 161*(10), 1872–1876.

Garber, J., Clarke, G. N., Weersing, V. R., Beardslee, W. R., Brent, D. A., Gladstone, T. R. G., . . . Iyengar, S. (2009). Prevention of depression in at-risk adolescents: A randomized controlled trial. *JAMA, 301*(21), 2215–2224.

Garber, J., & Hilsman, R. (1992). Cognitions, stress, and depression in children and adolescents. *Child and Adolescent Psychiatric Clinics of North America, 1*(8), 129–167.

Garber, J., Weiss, B., & Shanley, N. (1993). Cognitions, depressive symptoms, and development in adolescents. *Journal of Abnormal Psychology, 102*(1), 47–57.

Gillham, J. E., Reivich, K. J., Brunwasser, S. M., Freres, D. R., Chajon, N. D., Kash-Macdonald, V. M., . . . Seligman, M. E. (2012). Evaluation of a group cognitive-behavioral depression prevention program for young adolescents: A randomized effectiveness trial. *Journal of Clinical Child and Adolescent Psychology, 41*(5), 621–639.

Gillham, J. E., Reivich, K. J., & Jaycox, L. H. (2008). *The Penn Resiliency Program.* Unpublished manuscript. University of Pennsylvania.

Gladstone, T. R. G., Beardslee, W. R., & O'Connor, E. E. (2011). The prevention of adolescent depression. *Psychiatric Clinics of North America, 34*(1), 35–52.

Goldstein, T. R., Bridge, J. A., & Brent, D. A. (2008). Sleep disturbance preceding completed suicide in adolescents. *Journal of Consulting and Clinical Psychology, 76*(1), 84–91.

Goldston, D. B., Daniel, S. S., Erkanli, A., Reboussin, B. A., Mayfield, A., Frazier, P. H., & Treadway, L. (2009). Psychiatric diagnoses as contemporaneous risk factors for suicide attempts among adolescents and youth adults: Developmental changes. *Journal of Consulting and Clinical Psychology, 77*, 281–290.

Guidi, J., Fava, G. A., Fava, M., & Papakostas, G. I. (2011). Efficacy of the sequential integration of psychotherapy and pharmacotherapy in major depressive disorder: A preliminary meta-analysis. *Psychological Medicine, 41*(2), 321–331.

Hamilton, E. B., Asarnow, J. R., & Tompson, M. C. (1997). Social, academic, and behavioral competence of depressed children: Relationship to diagnostic status and family interaction style. *Journal of Youth and Adolescence, 26*, 77–87.

Harding, K. J. K., Rush, A. J., Arbuckle, M., Trivedi, M. H., & Pincus, H. A. (2011). Measurement-based care in psychiatric practice: A policy framework for implementation. *Journal of Clinical Psychiatry, 72*(8), 1136–1143.

Hawkins, E. H. (2009). A tale of two systems: Co-occuring mental health and substance abuse disorders treatments for adolescents. *Annual Review of Psychology, 60*, 197–227.

Hops, H., Lewinsohn, P. M., Andrews, J. A., & Roberts, R. E. (1990). Psychosocial correlates of depressive symptomatology among high school students. *Journal of Clinical Child Psychology, 19*, 211–220.

Horowitz, J. L., & Garber, J. (2006). The prevention of depressive symptoms in children and adolescents: A meta-analytic review. *Journal of Consulting and Clinical Psychology, 74*, 401–415.

Hughes, C. W., Barnes, S., Barnes, C., Defina, L. F., Nakonezny, P., & Emslie, G. J. (2013). Depressed adolescents treated with exercise (DATE): A pilot randomized controlled trial to test feasibility and establish preliminary effect sizes. *Mental Health and Physical Activity, 6*(2). Retrieved from http://doi.10.1016/j.mhpa.2013.06.006

Hughes, C. W., Emslie, G. J., Crismon, M. L., Posner, K., Birmaher, B., Ryan, N., . . . Trivedi, M. H. (2007). Texas Children's Medication Algorithm Project: Update from Texas Consensus Conference Panel on Medication Treatment of Childhood Major Depressive Disorder. *Journal of the American Academy of Child and Adolescent Psychiatry, 46*(6), 667–686.

Hughes, C. W., Trivedi, M. H., Cleaver, J., Greer, T. L., Emslie, G. J., Kennard, B., . . . Barnes, C. (2009). DATE: Depressed adolescents treated with exercise: Study rationale and design for a pilot study. *Mental Health and Physical Activity, 2*(2), 76–85.

Ivanenko, A., Crabtree, V. M., & Gozal, D. (2004). Sleep in children with psychiatric disorders. *Pediatric Clinics of North America, 51*(1), 51–68.

Jarrett, R. B., Minhajuddin, A., Gershenfeld, H., Friedman, E. S., & Thase, M. E. (2013). Preventing depressive relapse and recurrence in higher-risk cognitive therapy responders: A randomized trial of continuation phase cognitive therapy, fluoxetine, or matched pill placebo. *JAMA Psychiatry, 70*(11), 1152–1160.

Jaycox, L. H., Reivich, K. J., Gillham, J., & Seligman, M. E. (1994). Prevention of depressive symptoms in school children. *Behaviour Research and Therapy, 32*(8), 801–816.

Kashani, J. H., Burbach, D. J., & Rosenberg, D. R. (1988). Perception of family conflict resolution and depressive symptomatology in adolescents. *Journal of the American Academy of Child and Adolescent Psychiatry, 27*, 42–48.

Kennard, B. D., Emslie, G. J., Mayes, T. L., & Hughes, J. L. (2006a). Relapse and recurrence in pediatric depression. *Child and Adolescent Psychiatric Clinics of North America, 15*(4), 1057–1079.

Kennard, B. D., Emslie, G. J., Mayes, T. L., Nakonezny, P. A., Jones, J. M., Foxwell, A. A., & King, J. (2014). Sequential treatment with fluoxetine and relapse-prevention CBT to improve outcomes in pediatric depression. *American Journal of Psychiatry, 171*(10), 1083–1090.

Kennard, B. D., Emslie, G. J., Mayes, T. L., Nightingale-Teresi, J., Nakonezny, P. A., Hughes, J. L., . . . Jarrett, R. B. (2008a). Cognitive-behavioral therapy to prevent relapse in pediatric responders to pharmacotherapy for major depressive disorder. *Journal of the American Academy of Child and Adolescent Psychiatry, 47*(12), 1395–1404.

Kennard, B., Silva, S., Vitiello, B., Curry, J., Kratochvil, C., Simons, A., . . . March, J. (2006b). Remission and residual symptoms after short-term treatment in the Treatment of Adolescents with Depression Study (TADS). *Journal of the American Academy of Child and Adolescent Psychiatry, 45*(12), 1404–1411.

Kennard, B. D., Stewart, S. M., Hughes, J. L., Jarrett, R. B., & Emslie, G. J. (2008b). Developing cognitive behavioral therapy to prevent depressive relapse in youth. *Cognitive Behavioral Practice, 15*(4), 387–399.

Kobau, R., Seligman, M. E., Peterson, C., Diener, E., Zack, M. M., Chapman, D., & Thompson, W. (2011). Mental health promotion in public health: Perspectives and strategies from positive psychology. *American Journal of Public Health, 101*(8), 1–9.

Kosters, M. P., Chinapaw, M. J. M., Zwaanswijk, M., van der Wal, M. F., & Koot, H. M. (2015). Indicated prevention of childhood anxiety and depression: Results from a practice-based study up to 12 months after intervention. *American Journal of Public Health, 105*, 2005–2013.

Kovacs, M., Feinberg, T. L., Crouse-Novak, M. A., Paulauskas, S. L., Pollock, M., & Finkelstein, R. (1984). Depressive disorders in childhood: II. A longitudinal study of the risk for a subsequent major depression. *Archives of General Psychiatry, 41*, 643–649.

Kovacs, M., & Lopez-Duran, N. L. (2012). Contextual emotion regulation therapy: A developmentally based intervention for pediatric depression. *Child and Adolescent Psychiatric Clinics of North America, 21*(2), 327–343.

Kovacs, M., Sherrill, J., George, C. J., Pollock, M., Tumuluru, R. V., & Ho, V. (2006). Contextual emotion-regulation therapy for childhood depression: Description and pilot testing of a new intervention. *Journal of the American Academy of Child and Adolescent Psychiatry, 45*(8), 892–903.

Kroenke, K., Spitzer, R. L., & Williams, J. B. W. (2001). The PHQ-9: Validity of a brief depression severity measure. *Journal of General Internal Medicine, 16*, 606–613.

Landback, J., Prochaska, M., Ellis, J., Dmochowska, K., Kuwabara, S. A., Gladstone, T., . . . Van Voorhees, B. W. (2009). From prototype to product: Development of a primary care / internet based depression prevention intervention for adolescents (CATCH-IT). *Community Mental Health Journal, 45*(5), 349–354.

Lock, S., & Barrett, P. M. (2003). A longitudinal study of developmental differences in universal preventive intervention for child anxiety. *Behaviour Change, 20*, 183–199.

Maalouf, F. T., & Brent, D. A. (2012). Child and adolescent depression intervention overview: What works, for whom and how well? *Child and Adolescent Psychiatric Clinics of North America, 21*(2), 299–312.

Manber, R., Edinger, J. D., Gress, J. L., San Pedro-Salcedo, M. G., Kuo, T. F., & Kalista, T. (2008). Cognitive behavioral therapy for insomnia enhances depression outcome in patients with comorbid major depressive disorder and insomnia. *Sleep, 31*(4), 489–495.

March, J., Silva, S., Petrycki, S., Curry, J., Wells, K., Fairbank, J., . . . Treatment for Adolescents with Depression Study (TADS) Team. (2004). Fluoxetine, cognitive-behavioral therapy, and their combination for adolescents with depression: Treatment for Adolescents with Depression Study (TADS) randomized controlled trial. *JAMA, 292*(7), 807–820.

Marton, P., & Kutcher, S. (1995). The prevalence of cognitive distortion in depressed adolescents. *Journal of Psychiatry and Neuroscience, 20*(1), 33–38.

McCauley, E., Myers, K., Mitchell, J., Calderon, R., Schloredt, K., & Treder, R. (1993). Depression in young people: Initial presentation and clinical course. *Journal of the American Academy of Child and Adolescent Psychiatry, 32*, 714–722.

Melnyk, B. M., Jacobson, D., Kelly, S. A., Belyea, M. J., Shaibi, G. Q., Small, L., . . . Marsiglia, F. F. (2014). Twelve-month effects of the COPE Healthy Lifestyles TEEN Program on overweight and depressive symptoms in high school students. *Journal of School Health, 85*(12), 861–870.

Newacheck, P. W., Brindis, C. D., Cart, C. U., Marchi, K., & Irwin, C. E. (1999). Adolescent health insurance coverage: Recent changes and access to care. *Pediatrics, 104*(2 Pt 1), 195–202.

Nierenberg, A. A. (2001). Long-term management of chronic depression. *Journal of Clinical Psychiatry, 62*(Suppl 6), 17–21.

Paykel, E. S. (2007). Cognitive therapy in relapse prevention in depression. *International Journal of Neuropsychopharmacology, 10*(1), 131–136.

Paykel, E. S., Scott, J., Teasdale, J. D., Johnson, A. L., Garland, A., Moore, R., . . . Pope, M. (1999). Prevention of relapse in residual depression by cognitive therapy: A controlled trial. *Archives of General Psychiatry, 56*, 829–835.

Puig-Antich, J., Kaufman, J., Ryan, N., Williamson, D. E., Dahl, R. E., Lukens, E., . . . Nelson, B., (1993). The psychosocial functioning and family environment of depressed adolescents. *Journal of the American Academy of Child and Adolescent Psychiatry, 32*(2), 244–253.

Puig-Antich, J., Lukens, E., Davies, M., Goetz, D., Brennan-Quattrock, M., & Todak, G. (1985a). Psychosocial functioning in prepubertal major depressive disorders I: Interpersonal relationships during the depressive episode. *Archives of General Psychiatry, 42*, 500–507.

Puig-Antich, J., Lukens, E., Davies, M., Goetz, D., Brennan-Quattrock, M., & Todak, G. (1985b). Psychosocial functioning in prepubertal major depressive disorders II: Interpersonal relationships after sustained recovery from affective episode. *Journal of Affective Disorders, 42*, 511–517.

Rao, U., Ryan, N. D., Dahl, R. E., Birmaher, B., Rao, R., Williamson, D. E., & Perel, J. M. (1999). Factors associated with the development of substance use disorder in depressed adolescents. *Journal of the American Academy of Child and Adolescent Psychiatry, 38*, 1109–1117.

Richardson, L. P., Ludman, E., McCauley, E., Lindenbaum, J., Larison, C., Zhou, C., . . . Katon, W. (2014). Collaborative care for adolescents with depression in primary care: A randomized controlled trial. *JAMA, 312*(8), 809–816.

Rohde, P., Lewinsohn, P. M., & Seeley, J. R. (1996). Psychiatric comorbidity with problematic alcohol use in high school students. *Journal of the American Academy of Child and Adolescent Psychiatry, 35*, 101–109.

Rothon, C., Edwards, P., Bhui, K., Viner, R. M., Taylor, S., & Stansfeld, S. A. (2010). Physical activity and depressive symptoms in adolescents: A prospective study. *BMC Medicine, 8*, 32.

Rush, A. J., Trivedi, M. H., Ibrahim, H. M., Carmody, T. J., Arnow, B., Klein, D. N., . . . Keller, M. B. (2003). The 16-item Quick Inventory of Depressive Symptomatology (QIDS) Clinician Rating (QIDS-C) and Self-Report (QIDS-SR): A psychometric evaluation in patients with chronic major depression. *Biological Psychiatry, 54*, 573–583.

Ryff, C. D., & Singer, B. (1996). Psychological well-being: Meaning, measurement, and implications for psychotherapy research. *Psychotherapy and Psychosomatics, 65*(1), 14–23.

Sakolsky, D., & Birmaher, B. (2012). Developmentally informed pharmacotherapy for child and adolescent depressive disorders. *Child and Adolescent Psychiatric Clinics of North America, 21*(2), 313–325.

Saulsberry, A., Marko-Holguin, M., Blomeke, K., Hinkle, C., Fogel, J., Gladstone, T., . . . Van Voorhees, B. W. (2013). Randomized clinical trial of a primary care internet-based intervention to prevent adolescent depression: One-year outcomes. *Journal of the Canadian Academy of Child and Adolescent Psychiatry, 22*(2), 106–117.

Seligman, M., & Csikszentmihalyi, M. (2000). Positive psychology: An introduction. *American Psychologist, 55*, 5–14.

Seligman, M. E., Schulman, P., DeRubeis, R. J., & Hollon, S. D. (1999). The prevention of depression and anxiety. *Prevention and Treatment, 2*, Article 8. Retrieved from http://journals.apa.org/prevention/volume2/pre0020008a.html

Sheeber, L., Hops, H., & Davis, B. (2001). Family processes in adolescent depression. *Clinical Child and Family Psychology Review, 4*(1), 19–35.

Sin, N. L., & Lyubomirsky, S. (2009). Enhancing well-being and alleviating depressive symptoms with positive psychology interventions: A practice-friendly meta-analysis. *Journal of Clinical Psychology, 65*(5), 467–487.

Stancin, T., & Perrin, E. C. (2014). Psychologists and pediatricians: Opportunities for collaboration in primary care. *The American Psychologist, 69*(4), 332–343.

Stice, E., Shaw, H., Bohon, C., Marti, C. N., & Rohde, P. (2009). A meta-analytic review of depression prevention programs for children and adolescents: Factors that predict magnitude of intervention effects. *Journal of Consulting and Clinical Psychology, 77*(3), 486–503.

Strober, M., Lampert, C., Schmidt, S., & Morrell, W. (1993). The course of major depressive disorder in adolescents: I. Recovery and risk of manic switching in a follow-up of psychotic and nonpsychotic subtypes. *Journal of the American Academy of Child and Adolescent Psychiatry, 32*, 34–42.

Teasdale, J. D., Williams, J. M. G., Soulsby, J. M., Segal, Z. V., Ridgeway, V. A., & Lau, M. A. (2000). Prevention of relapse/recurrence in major depression by mindfulness-based cognitive therapy. *Journal of Consulting and Clinical Psychology, 68*(4), 615–625.

Tompson, M. C., Boger, K. D., & Asarnow, J. R. (2012). Enhancing the developmental appropriateness of treatment for depression in youth: Integrating the family in treatment. *Child and Adolescent Psychiatric Clinics of North America, 21*(2), 345–384.

Tompson, M. C., Langer, D. A., Hughes, J. L., & Asarnow, J. R. (2016, June). Family-focused treatment for childhood depression: Model and case illustrations. *Cognitive and Behavioral Practice.* doi:10.1016/j.cbpra.2016.06.003

Tompson, M. C., Pierre, C. B., Haber, F. M., Fogler, J. M., Groff, A. R., & Asarnow, J. R. (2007). Family-focused treatment for childhood-onset depressive disorders: Results of an open trial. *Clinical Child Psychology and Psychiatry, 12*(3), 403–420.

Trivedi, M. H., & Daly, E. J. (2007). Measurement-based care for refractory depression: A clinical decision support model for clinical research and practice. *Drug and Alcohol Dependence, 88*(Supplement), 11.

Van Voorhees, B. W., Fogel, J., Reinecke, M. A., Gladstone, T., Stuart, S., Gollan, J., . . . Bell, C. (2009). Randomized clinical trial of an internet-based depression prevention program for adolescents (Project CATCH-IT) in primary care: 12-week outcomes. *Journal of Developmental and Behavioral Pediatrics, 30*(1), 23–37.

Wasserman, D., Hoven, C. W., Wasserman, C., Wall, M., Eisenberg, R., Hadlaczky, G., . . . Carli, V. (2015). School-based suicide prevention programmes: The SEYLE cluster-randomized, controlled trial. *The Lancet, 385*(9977), 1536–1544.

Weisz, J. R., McCarty, C. A., & Valeri, S. M. (2006). Effects of psychotherappy for depression in children and adolescents: A meta-analysis. *Psychological Bulletin, 132*(1), 132–149.

Weisz, J. R., Ng, M. Y., & Bearman, S. K. (2014). Odd couple? Reenvisioning the relation between science and practice in the dissemination-implementation era. *Clinical Psychological Science, 2*(1), 58–74.

Wells, K. B., Kataoka, S. H., & Asarnow, J. R. (2001). Affective disorders in children and adolescents: Addressing unmet need in primary care settings. *Biological Psychiatry, 49*(12), 1111–1120.

World Health Organization. (2002). *Prevention and promotion in mental health.* Geneva, Switzerland: World Health Organization. Retrieved from http:/www.who.int/mental_health/media/en/545.pdf

World Health Organization. (2014, May 14). *WHO calls for stronger focus on adolescent health.* WHO News Release. Retrieved from http://www.who.int/mediacentre/news/releases/2014/focus-adolescent-health/en/

Ziv, A., Boulet, J. R., & Slap, G. B. (1999). Utilization of physician offices by adolescents in the United States. *Pediatrics, 104*(1), 35–42.

Zuckerbrot, R. A., Cheung, A. H., Jensen, P. S., Stein, R. E., Laraque, D., & GLAD-PC Steering Group. (2007). Guidelines for Adolescent Depression Primary Care (GLAD-PC): I. Identification, assessment, and initial management. *Pediatrics, 120*(5), 1299–1312.

CHAPTER 10

Understanding Adolescent Suicide

Regina Miranda, PhD
Ana Ortin, PhD
Lillian Polanco-Roman, MA, MPhil
Jorge Valderrama, PhD

Over the past decade, suicide has consistently been among the top three leading causes of death in adolescence (Centers for Disease Control and Prevention [CDC], 2016a). Although in 2014, suicide deaths among adolescents aged 12–19 accounted for only about 5% of all suicides in the United States (CDC, 2016b), adolescent suicidal thoughts and behaviors have their highest prevalence during this developmental period. The most recent Youth Risk Behavior Survey (Kann et al., 2016) of high school students in the United States found that in the 12 months preceding the survey, about 18% of teenagers had seriously considered suicide, about 15% reported having made a suicide plan, and about 9% reported having made a suicide attempt, with close to 3% reporting a suicide attempt that required medical attention. However, the relative rarity of actual suicide deaths in this age group makes the prediction of adolescent suicide difficult. Despite a number of contemporary models proposed to explain suicidal behavior (Barzilay & Apter, 2014; O'Connor & Nock, 2014), these models primarily rely on information gathered and observations made with adults. Given that there are no established and empirically validated treatments for the prevention of adolescent suicidal behavior, one important step in improving the identification, measurement, and treatment of adolescent suicidal behavior is to understand the psychological, biological, and sociocultural context in which adolescent suicide occurs. This chapter seeks to provide an overview of adolescent suicide by addressing age, gender, and race-related trends in adolescent suicide, suicide attempts, and suicide ideation, and by examining biological, psychological, and sociocultural risk factors for adolescent suicide. We also review factors that impact the transition from suicide ideation to suicide attempts, along with considerations in the measurement and treatment of suicidal thoughts and behaviors in adolescence.

Defining Suicide Ideation, Suicide Attempts, and Suicide Deaths

The study of adolescent suicide historically has been complicated by lack of precision in defining suicidal behavior. To increase precision in the classification of suicidal behavior, current definitions focus on suicidal intent as the distinguishing feature of nonsuicidal versus suicidal self-injury. Thus, a suicide attempt generally refers to an intentional nonfatal self-injurious behavior with some intent to die. Suicide arises when that behavior results in a person's death. Suicide ideation involves thinking about suicide and can range from passive thoughts about wanting to die to active thoughts involving a suicide plan (Crosby, Ortega, & Melanson, 2011; Silverman, Berman, Sanddal, O'Carroll, & Joiner, 2007). Despite the importance of intent in distinguishing a suicide attempt from other forms of self-injury, it may be difficult to determine suicidal intent in adolescence, as adolescent suicide attempts may be more impulsive, relative to adult attempts, characterized by less knowledge about whether their methods of attempt will result in death, and may be motivated by reasons other than death (Jacobson, Batejan, Kleinman, & Gould, 2013; Parellada et al., 2008). Further difficulty in understanding the nature of adolescent suicidal behavior arises because researchers use a variety of methods to study adolescent suicide ideation and attempts, ranging from single- or multi-item screens (Kann et al., 2016; Shaffer et al., 2004) to more detailed interviews and rating scales (Miranda et al., 2008; Nock, Holmberg, Photos, & Michel, 2007). Despite these limitations, a number of trends and risk factors have been identified that can guide identification and intervention with this vulnerable age group.

Age-Related Trends in Adolescent Suicide Ideation and Attempts

Rates of suicide deaths are low in adolescence (fewer than 7 per 100,000 among 12- to 19-year-olds in the United States during the year 2014) and highest in middle-to-late adulthood (about 20 per 100,000 among 50- to 59-year-olds and close to 17 per 100,000 over age 60 in the year 2014) (CDC, 2016b). However, there are notable developmental trends in the frequency of suicidal behavior. Suicide ideation and attempts are rare in childhood, and rates increase substantially in early adolescence (Bolger, Downey, Walker, & Steininger, 1989; Borges, Benjet, Medina-Mora, Orozco, & Nock, 2008; Nock et al., 2013), peak in middle/late adolescence, and then decrease in adulthood (Boeninger, Masyn, Feldman, & Conger, 2010; Lewinsohn, Rohde, Seeley, & Baldwin, 2001; Nock et al., 2013; Rueter & Kwon, 2005; Steinhausen, Bosiger, & Metzke, 2006). As a result, suicide ideation and attempts reach their highest prevalence during adolescence (Miranda & Shaffer, 2013).

Longitudinal studies support these developmental trends for suicidal behavior in adolescence. For example, the Zurich Epidemiological Study of Child and Adolescent Psychopathology, which followed 593 students over three time points, found that the six-month prevalence of suicide ideation and attempts was about 8% and 2%, respectively, at close to age 14; increased to about 11% and 4%, respectively, at about age 17; and decreased to close to 8% and 2%, respectively, at about age 20 (Steinhausen et al., 2006). However, these developmental trends differ depending on the severity of the suicidal behavior examined (i.e., suicide ideation, suicide plan, or suicide attempt), with suicide ideation increasing earlier and faster than suicide attempts. Using data from the National Comorbidity Survey Replication–Adolescent Supplement, a cross-sectional study of a representative sample of 6,683, 13- to 18-year-old adolescents in the United States, Nock and colleagues (2013) found a lifetime prevalence of suicide ideation, plans, and attempts of about 12%, 4%, and 4%, respectively. The prevalence of suicide ideation was low before age 10, increased slowly through age 12, and then increased more rapidly between ages 12 and 17. The prevalence of suicide plans and attempts was low through age 12 and increased linearly through age 15 and again slowly until age 17 (Nock et al., 2013).

These trends also vary by gender. Girls display an earlier and higher increase in rates of suicidal behavior than boys (Lewinsohn et al., 2001). In a longitudinal study of 1,248 rural European Americans aged 11–19 years, Boeninger and colleagues (2010) found that among girls, the yearly prevalence of suicide ideation and plans followed an inverted-U-shaped trajectory that peaked around age 16. Among boys, the prevalence showed a linear trend through age 19. The gender difference in rates of suicide ideation and suicide plans disappeared in late adolescence. For suicide attempts, girls' yearly prevalence peaked at age 16, and then declined, while for boys, it peaked between ages 16 and 17 before beginning to decline.

Gender Differences in Suicide Ideation and Attempts

Gender differences in suicide ideation and attempts begin to appear in early adolescence. Many studies report no gender differences in suicide ideation and attempts in childhood (Klimes-Dougan et al., 1999; Lewinsohn et al., 2001; Pfeffer, Zuckerman, Plutchik, & Mizruchi, 1984; Taussig, Harpin, & Maguire, 2014). However, research suggests that the gender profile varies by age. One study of 266 children and adolescents referred to a psychiatric emergency department for suicide ideation or an attempt found that of 39 suicidal children aged 11 or younger, 64% were males and 36% were females, while of 227 adolescents aged 12–18, 26% were males and 74% were females (Ben-Yehuda et al., 2012), suggesting a higher prevalence of suicide ideation or attempts among boys than girls in childhood but a higher prevalence among girls in adolescence.

There is a well-established gender paradox in adolescent suicidal behavior, such that while suicide death rates are higher among boys than among girls (3:1 ratio), girls have higher rates of suicide ideation and attempts than boys (Bridge, Goldstein, & Brent, 2006; Evans, Hawton, Rodham, & Deeks, 2005; Reinherz et al., 1995; Wunderlich, Bronisch, Wittchen, & Carter, 2001). Worldwide, rates of suicide attempts are two to three times higher among female than among male adolescents (Krug, Mercy, Dahlberg, & Zwi, 2002; National Adolescent Health Information Center, 2006; World Health Organization, 2012). The 2015 Youth Risk Behavior Survey estimates the 12-month prevalence of seriously considering a suicide attempt, making a suicide plan, and attempting suicide among girls to be about 23%, 19%, and 12%, respectively; while among boys, the 12-month prevalence is 12%, 10%, and 6%, respectively (Kann et al., 2016).

Several explanations for this gender paradox have been proposed, including gender differences in the lethality and reversibility of suicide attempt methods; higher frequency of depression and anxiety disorders among girls versus substance use, conduct disorder, and risk-taking behaviors among boys; earlier pubertal changes in girls; gender differences in socialization practices regarding culturally acceptable forms of self-destructive behaviors; and more accurate and honest reports of suicidal behavior in girls than boys (Canetto & Sakinofsky, 1998; Langhinrichsen-Rohling, Sanders, Crane, & Monson, 1998; Moscicki, 1994). No single explanation appears to adequately account for these differences. Boys, and men in general, tend to employ more lethal methods (e.g., firearms or hanging versus drug overdose) than women (Beautrais et al., 1996; Brezo et al., 2007; King, Hovey, Brand, Wilson, & Ghaziuddin, 1997). Method lethality may explain the higher rate of suicide deaths among boys. Alternatively, girls may have higher rates of suicide ideation and attempts due to their elevated prevalence of depression compared to boys (Brent, Baugher, Bridge, Chen, & Chiappetta, 1999; Kessler, McGonagle, Swartz, Blazer, & Nelson, 1993; Lewinsohn, Rohde, & Seeley, 1993; Lewinsohn et al., 2001; Steinhausen & Metzke, 2004). Research has consistently shown that depression is the diagnosis most strongly associated with suicide ideation and attempts among both adolescents and adults (Brent, Perper, Moritz, Baugher, & Allman, 1993a; Garrison, Addy, Jackson, McKeown, & Waller, 1991; Marttunen, Aro, Henriksson, & Lönnqvist, 1991; Petronis, Samuels, Moscicki, & Anthony, 1990). A longitudinal study of 941 adolescents, aged 14–18, from the Oregon Adolescent Depression Project found that the annual hazard rates for incidence of major depressive disorder (MDD) and suicide attempts increased earlier and reached significantly higher rates among girls than boys during adolescence (Lewinsohn et al., 2001). Women also have higher rates of sexual abuse than men, and sexual abuse increases risk for suicide ideation and attempts, especially in adolescence (Bruffaerts et al., 2010; Silverman, Reinherz, & Giaconia, 1996; Wunderlich et al., 2001). A follow-up study of 9,679 Norwegian students in grades 7–12 examined the effect of gender on suicide attempts, adjusting for variables that have been proposed to explain gender discrepancies, including: depressed mood; eating disorders; self-concept, physical self-concept, and body satisfaction; gender role identification; early pubertal timing; and involvement in romantic relationships. Girls more often endorsed a history of previous suicide attempts (10%) than did boys (6%) and also had slightly higher rates of suicide attempts during the study's two-year follow-up period (3% vs. 2%). At baseline, when depressed mood and disordered eating were entered into the model, the main effect of gender was no longer significant. The association between gender and suicide attempts at follow-up was nonsignificant after accounting for previous suicide attempt history, depressed mood, physical appearance, pubertal timing, and romantic involvement at baseline (Wichstrøm & Rossow, 2002). These results suggest that biological, sociocultural, and psychological factors may mediate the effect of gender on suicidal behavior. Future research is necessary to examine the mediating effects of such variables. In the following sections, we turn our attention to research on neurobiological, sociocultural, and psychological variables associated with suicide ideation and attempts in adolescence.

Neurobiological Mechanisms

Research has indicated various biological markers associated with risk for suicidal behavior in adolescents. Among these are the hypothalamic-pituitary-adrenal (HPA) axis, the serotonergic system, and related genetic variants. This review is intended to summarize our current understanding of the relationship between biological mechanisms and risk for adolescent suicidal behavior.

The HPA Axis System and Adolescent Suicidal Behavior

The HPA axis, the part of the neuroendocrine system that regulates responses to stress, has recently been examined in relation to adolescent suicidal behavior in the context of a stress-diathesis model. The model proposes an epigenetic phenomenon in which HPA axis dysregulation in adolescence is caused by the combination of a genetic predisposition to altered HPA axis functioning and exposure to early life stress. Whether an individual's HPA axis is hyperresponsive or hyporesponsive to stress may be dependent on a variety of factors, including, but not limited to, gender, history of negative life events, and history of depression (Turecki, 2014). Research has revealed both types of dysregulation may be related to adolescent suicidal behavior.

Giletta and colleagues (2015) found that adolescent girls who have an elevated and prolonged cortisol response after exposure to a stressor are more likely to have reported a history of suicide ideation as well as report ideation in a three-month follow-up when compared to adolescent girls who have a normal or hyporesponsive cortisol response. By contrast, a study of 57 adolescent girls with major depression found having a history of repeated self-harm (vs. no self-harm) was associated with a more blunted cortisol response and with greater suicide ideation (Beauchaine, Crowell, & Hsiao, 2015). These findings suggest that whether the HPA axis is hyperresponsive or hyporesponsive to stress might be dependent on self-harm history. Importantly, hyporesponsivity has been found in adults who suffer from posttraumatic stress disorder symptoms (Miller, Chen, & Zhou, 2007), which, in turn, have been found to be associated with adolescent suicidal behavior (Mazza, 2000). In the only study to date to examine the relationship between HPA axis activity and suicidal behavior among both adolescent boys and girls, Mathew and colleagues (2003) found that adolescent boys and girls with high cortisol activity in the late evening hours before sleep were at increased risk for a suicide attempt in young adulthood. Interestingly, adolescent girls displayed significantly higher cortisol activity than boys. Further research is necessary to determine more clearly whether gender differences in HPA axis activity in response to stress may help to explain the gender paradox in suicidal behavior.

Serotonin and Adolescent Suicidal Behavior

Abnormal serotonergic functioning has been implicated in depressed mood and suicidal behavior (Mann, 1999). Much of the research establishing an association between serotonin dysfunction and adolescent suicidal behavior has focused on the serotonin transporter (5-HTT)—in particular, the short variant of the promoter region of 5-HTT, named the 5-HTT gene-linked polymorphic region (5-HTTLPR), as the short variant, or allele, is associated with abnormal and decreased serotonergic functioning (Karg, Burmeister, Shedden, & Sen, 2011).

Findings of the association between variants of 5-HTTLPR and suicidal behavior differ in studies of adolescents versus adults. For example, Zalsman and colleagues (2001) found no relationship between 5-HTT long- versus short alleles and suicidal behavior in a sample of 48 adolescents. By contrast, Caspi and colleagues (2003) found that the short allele was positively associated with increased rates of depression and suicidal behavior in a sample of 847 young adults. However, this association was only present in conjunction with stressful life events, suggesting a "gene x stress" interaction in conferring vulnerability to depression and suicidal behavior. Indeed, a 5-HTT gene-environment interaction was found within a sample of 377 adolescents (Eley et al., 2004). The study compared four groups of adolescents with varying levels of depression and environmental risk. Environmental risk consisted of family social adversity (e.g., problems related to finances, housing, relationships), parental education level, and adverse life events in the previous six months. Increased risk for depression was found only among females with the short allele when they scored high in environmental risk. Such research is consistent with a recent meta-analysis suggesting that the short allele may be associated with increased sensitivity to stress (Karg et al., 2011). Importantly, this research reveals another possible explanation for the gender difference in adolescent suicide ideation and attempts.

Race, Ethnicity, and Cultural Factors

Beyond age and gender, there are racial and ethnic differences in the prevalence of suicide ideation, suicide attempts, and suicide deaths. With the exception of Native American individuals, who have the highest national rates of suicide in the United

States, suicide deaths are most prevalent among white individuals and least common among Asian, black, and Latino individuals. However, adolescence and young adulthood are particularly high-risk periods for suicide deaths among racial and ethnic minority individuals. Whereas the highest proportion of suicide deaths among white individuals occur after age 45, the highest proportion of suicide deaths among Asian, black, and Latino individuals occur among 20- to 29-year-olds, with suicide rates declining thereafter among these groups (CDC, 2016a). Furthermore, data from the 2015 Youth Risk Behavior Survey indicate that the 12-month prevalence of suicide attempts is higher among Latino and black adolescents than among their white counterparts. In fact, the 12-month prevalence of seriously considering suicide, making a suicide plan, and making a suicide attempt is highest among Latina adolescent girls in grades 9–12, with recently estimated rates of 26%, 21%, and 15%, respectively, relative to corresponding rates of 23%, 18%, and 10% among their white counterparts (Kann et al., 2016). Thus, adolescence is a particularly critical period for assessing risk of suicide among racial and ethnic minority individuals.

Such findings have prompted calls for cultural considerations in the study and treatment of suicidal behavior among adolescents, noting the potential role of various cultural factors, including acculturation, religion, and cultural variations in family dynamics and idioms of distress (Goldston et al., 2008). However, relatively little attention has been dedicated to understanding factors that influence racial and ethnic differences in suicidal behavior. Indeed, the impact of culture on risk for suicide among adolescents remains relatively understudied, as more proximal or individual-level factors (e.g., psychiatric disorders, cognitive vulnerabilities such as hopelessness, maladaptive characteristics such as impulsivity or aggression) have garnered much of the attention in the literature (Bridge et al., 2006). However, some scholars have noted the importance of studying individuals' social and cultural environment to understand risk for suicide among adolescents (Ayyash-Abdo, 2002; Goldston et al., 2008; Henry, Stephenson, Hanson, & Hargett, 1994; Langhinrichsen-Rohling, Friend, & Powell, 2009). Further alluding to the importance of understanding cultural influences is the failure of well-documented risk factors, such as alcohol and substance use, to explain racial and ethnic differences in risk for suicidal behavior (Eaton et al., 2011). Additionally, research suggests that racial and ethnic minority adolescents who attempt suicide are less likely to seek mental health care than white adolescents (Freedenthal, 2007; Wu, Katic, Liu, Fan, & Fuller, 2010), further increasing their risk for engaging in future suicidal behavior. Finally, there is evidence of racial and ethnic differences in HPA axis activity, which is associated with suicidal behavior among adolescents and adults (Pandey, 2011). Specifically, DeSantis and colleagues (2007) found that African American and Latino adolescents exhibited a more blunted HPA axis response compared to white adolescents. Understanding the sociocultural context in which suicidal behavior occurs may help to explain racial and ethnic differences in the prevalence of suicide ideation, attempts, and suicide deaths in the United States.

Ecological perspectives on adolescent suicide suggest that the larger cultural environment is one of many systems that may directly or indirectly impact an adolescent's susceptibility to suicidal thoughts and behavior (Ayyash-Abdo, 2002; Henry et al., 1994). For instance, lower suicide rates among black teenagers may be due in part to greater involvement in religious practices and beliefs, which may increase reasons for living and use of effective coping styles (Molock, Puri, Matlin, & Barksdale, 2006). A recent review suggested that integrating suicide prevention resources in churches, such as relying on church members to be gatekeepers of mental health services, may be one way to help reduce the risk for suicide among African American teenagers (Adedoyin & Salter, 2013). Expanding on the ecological framework, Chu and colleagues' (2010) cultural theory and model of suicide suggests that cultural experiences may impact risk for suicide at various junctures. These include the types of stressors to which individuals are exposed (e.g., acculturative stress, racial and ethnic discrimination), the meanings ascribed to stressors and suicide, and the manifestation and expression of suicidal thoughts and behaviors.

Differences in adolescent suicidal behavior have also been observed across various racial and ethnic minority groups by immigration status (for a review, see Langhinrichsen-Rohling et al., 2009). These differences may be accounted for, in part, by acculturation—an adaptive process resulting from frequent exposure to a novel cultural environment (Berry, 2003). A higher level of acculturation has been found to be associated with greater risk for engaging in suicidal thoughts and behaviors (Joe, Baser, Neighbors, Caldwell, & Jackson, 2009; Peña et al., 2008). For instance, in a nationally representative sample of Latino adolescents in the United States, Peña and colleagues (2008) found that US-born Latino teenagers with parents born in the United States had higher odds of attempting suicide than US-born Latino teenagers with immigrant parents, who had higher odds of attempting suicide than immigrant Latino teenagers. Similarly, in a nationally representative sample of black teenagers in the United States, Joe and colleagues (2009) found that African American adolescents had almost five times higher odds of attempting suicide than Caribbean black adolescents, adjusting for other demographic variables and for the concurrent onset of a psychiatric disorder.

While the mechanisms by which acculturation increases risk for suicidal behavior remain unclear, acculturative stress (i.e., stress resulting from acculturation through various experiences such as pressures to assimilate, actual and perceived barriers to advancement, limited social network, and family discord) may provide some insight (Mena, Padilla, & Maldonado, 1987). In fact, researchers have found higher levels of acculturative stress are associated with increases in suicide ideation among racial and ethnic minority teenagers (Gil & Vega, 1996; Hovey & King, 1996).

Racial and ethnic discrimination, or unfair treatment due to race or ethnicity, is another stressor commonly experienced by racial and ethnic minority individuals, and it is akin to a chronic social stressor (Clark, Anderson, Clark, & Williams, 1999;

Harrell, 2000). Racial and ethnic discrimination has been consistently linked to psychiatric symptoms in adults (Chou, Asnaani & Hofmann, 2012; Pascoe & Richman, 2009). More recently, researchers have found that racial and ethnic minority teenagers who reported racial and ethnic discrimination were more likely to report suicide ideation than those who did not (Tobler et al., 2013). Research suggests that adolescence is a vulnerable period for experiencing racial and ethnic discrimination. Longitudinal research suggests that racial and ethnic minority teenagers increasingly perceive experiences of discrimination over time, and this gradual increase is associated with decreases in self-esteem and increases in depressive symptoms (Greene, Way, & Pahl, 2006). Thus, culturally related stressors such as racial and ethnic discrimination and acculturative stress may place racial and ethnic minority teenagers at risk for engaging in suicidal thoughts and behavior.

The family is another system within which an adolescent exists, and family dynamics have garnered significant attention in the literature on adolescent suicide (Bridge et al., 2006). The process of acculturation may contribute to family conflict arising from discrepancies in acculturation between parents and adolescents (Zayas, Lester, Cabassa, & Fortuna, 2005), as parents tend to acculturate at a slower pace than their children (Phinney, Ong, & Madden, 2000; Smokowski, Rose, & Bacallao, 2008). One study reported that Latina teenagers in families with high cohesion and low conflict were less likely to report suicide attempts compared to Latinas in families with low cohesion and high conflict (Peña et al., 2011).

Family also plays a significant role in the development of a racial and ethnic identity, a salient dimension of the self-concept among racial and ethnic minority youth (Phinney, 1990). Neblett and colleagues (2012) proposed that racial and ethnic socialization, or messages about racial and ethnic group affiliation that caregivers transmit to children, may prepare children with necessary tools to cope with culturally related stressors by engendering more adaptive cognitive appraisals and a healthy self-concept. While the research in this area is scarce, one study found that Latina adolescents who developed supportive relationships in response to cultural conflict were less likely to feel alone and isolated and thus less likely to attempt suicide (Gulbas & Zayas, 2015). Thus, racial and ethnic minority parents may help to reduce the risk of suicidal behavior among their adolescent children by encouraging more adaptive ways to confront culturally related stressors.

Transitions from Suicide Ideation to Suicide Attempts

Population-based studies suggest that the transition from suicide ideation to suicide plans and attempts occurs within the first year of the onset of ideation among both adolescents and adults (Borges et al., 2008; McKeown et al., 1998; Nock et al., 2008; Ten Have, van Dorsselaer, & de Graaf, 2013). For example, analyses of the National Comorbidity Survey Replication–Adolescent Supplement showed that the majority of the transitions from suicide ideation to suicide plan (63%) and to suicide attempt (86%) occurred within the first year of onset of suicide ideation, and most of the transitions from a suicide plan to an attempt (88%) also occurred within the year of developing a plan, with the transition occurring similarly by gender (Nock et al., 2013). A study with adolescent inpatients found that suicide ideation decreased in the months following discharge from hospitalization but increased 9–18 months after discharge. Furthermore, such increases in suicide ideation preceded the onset of future suicide attempts (Prinstein et al., 2008).

Psychiatric Disorders Associated with Suicidal Behavior

Psychiatric disorders are strongly associated with suicide ideation, suicide plans, suicide attempts, and suicide deaths. Psychological autopsy studies among adults suggest that 79%–90% of individuals who die by suicide met criteria for a psychiatric disorder—most commonly a mood disorder or substance use disorder—before their deaths (Arsenault-Lapierre, Kim, & Turecki, 2004; Cavanagh, Carson, Sharpe, & Lawrie, 2003), while psychological autopsy studies of adolescents suggest that the most common psychiatric diagnoses among adolescents who die by suicide are mood and conduct disorders (Brent et al., 1999; Shaffer et al., 1996). Depression is among the most commonly studied psychiatric disorders in relation to suicidal behavior (Brent et al., 1993a; Garrison et al., 1991; Lewinsohn et al., 2001; Marttunen et al., 1991; Petronis et al., 1990). However, recent evidence suggests that the associations between psychiatric disorders and suicide ideation, plans, and attempts vary by diagnostic group (Nock et al., 2008; Nock et al., 2009; Nock, Hwang, Sampson, & Kessler, 2010). A study of a representative sample of 3,005 adolescents in Mexico City, aged 12–17, found that while lifetime mood and substance use disorders had the strongest association with the onset of suicide ideation, impulse-control disorders had the strongest association with the onset of suicide plans and attempts (Borges et al., 2008). A study of a convenience sample of 184 adolescents, aged 11–17, found that MDD, but not impulsivity, was significantly associated with suicide ideation, while impulsivity, but not MDD symptoms, was associated with suicide attempts (Javdani, Sadeh, & Verona, 2011). Nock et al. (2013) found diagnostic differences among adolescent suicide ideators who made the transition to either a suicide plan, an unplanned suicide attempt, or a planned suicide attempt. The presence of lifetime MDD or dysthymic disorder was associated with the development of a plan among suicide ideators. In comparison, meeting criteria for lifetime MDD or dysthymia, eating disorders, attention deficit–hyperactivity disorder, and conduct disorders were associated with the transition from suicide ideation to unplanned suicide attempts, while intermittent explosive disorder was associated with the transition from suicide ideation to a planned suicide attempt. Recent findings in adult samples are in line with these results, indicating that while mood disorders are associated with suicide ideation, other disorders characterized by anxiety or agitation and problems with impulse control increase the likelihood that individuals will act on their suicidal thoughts, either by planning or attempting suicide (Nock et al., 2008; Ten Have et al., 2013).

Psychological Correlates of Suicidal Behavior

Until recently, relatively little attention has been paid to understanding what makes adolescents consider and attempt suicide. However, a number of psychological variables have been found to be associated with risk for suicidal behavior. One of the best-studied cognitive predictors of suicide is hopelessness (Beck, Steer, Kovacs, & Garrison, 1985; Brown, Beck, Steer, & Grisham, 2000; Fawcett et al., 1990). While variables such as hopelessness predict suicide over the long term, it has been noted that there has been little attention to understanding the moments immediately leading up to a suicide attempt (Glenn & Nock, 2014; Miranda & Shaffer, 2013).

One type of precipitant examined in the literature is negative life events. Negative life events have been found to precede youth suicides as little as a week prior to and up to within a year of the suicide deaths (Brent et al., 1993b; Cooper, Appleby, & Amos, 2002). Research suggests that a majority of negative life events that precede adolescent suicide attempts involve relationship difficulties or interpersonal conflicts (Beautrais, Joyce, & Mulder, 1997; Dieserud, Gerhardsen, Van den Weghe, & Corbett, 2010; Negron, Piacentini, Graae, Davies, & Shaffer, 1997).

Research also suggests that maladaptive responses to stress increase vulnerability to suicide ideation and attempts. For instance, the tendency to respond to a negative mood by dwelling on the causes, meanings, and consequences of that mood (i.e., to engage in rumination [Nolen-Hoeksema, Wisco, & Lyubomirsky, 2008]) has been found to be associated with increased risk of suicide ideation over a one-year follow-up period in a community sample of adults (Miranda & Nolen-Hoeksema, 2007) and to predict depressive symptoms over time among adolescents (Burwell & Shirk, 2007) and adults (Nolen-Hoeksema et al., 2008). A prospective study of early adolescents and adults found that rumination explained the relationship between stressful life events and anxiety symptoms over time among adolescents and the relationship between stressful life events and depressive symptoms among adults (Michl, McLaughlin, Shepherd, & Nolen-Hoeksema, 2013). Additional research with young adults suggests that rumination increases suicide ideation over time through increases in hopelessness (Smith, Alloy, & Abramson, 2006). Rumination in response to stress may thus increase vulnerability to suicide ideation through increases in cognitive variables such as hopelessness and also through increases in anxiety and depression.

Psychological models of suicide, such as the interpersonal theory of suicide (Joiner, 2005; Van Orden et al., 2010) or the integrated motivational-volitional model of suicide (O'Connor, 2011), suggest that while variables such as life stress and responses to stress, such as rumination, may lead to suicide ideation through other variables (e.g., hopelessness), the transition from suicide ideation to planning and attempts arises through experiences that lead individuals to acquire the capability to engage in potentially lethal self-harm. Psychological characteristics such as impulsivity may lead to such acquired capability by exposing individuals to potentially painful and provocative life experiences that reduce their fear of death and increase their tolerance for physical pain (Van Orden et al., 2010). Indeed, aspects of trait impulsivity have been found to be associated with both suicide ideation and attempts in cross-sectional studies of adolescents (Klonsky & May, 2010; Ortin, Lake, Kleinman, & Gould, 2012) and to prospectively predict suicide attempts among adults (Yen et al., 2009). While additional prospective research is necessary with adolescents, studies of such psychological factors show promise in helping to explain the onset of suicide ideation and the transition to suicide attempts.

Measuring Suicide Risk among Adolescents with a History of Suicide Ideation and Attempts

A history of a previous suicide attempt is one of the best predictors of future suicide attempts among adolescents (Goldston et al., 1999; Hultén et al., 2001; Lewinsohn, Rohde, & Seeley, 1994; Wichstrøm, 2000) and of suicide deaths among adults (Brown et al., 2000; Harris & Barraclough, 1997). Beyond a history of any previous suicide attempt, there is evidence from research with community and clinical samples of adolescents that having a history of more than one previous suicide attempt confers greater risk of making a future attempt than does having a history of only one previous suicide attempt (Goldston et al., 1999; Miranda et al., 2008). Indeed, research has documented differences between adolescents with a history of multiple versus single suicide attempts on variables such as hopelessness, emotion dysregulation (Esposito, Spirito, Boergers, & Donaldson, 2003), aggression (Stein, Apter, Ratzoni, Har-Even, & Avidan, 1998), psychiatric diagnoses (D'Eramo, Prinstein, Freeman, Grapentine, & Spirito, 2004; Miranda et al., 2008), and severity of suicide ideation (D'Eramo et al., 2004). However, psychological autopsy studies indicate that more than half of adolescent suicides occur among teenagers with no previous suicide attempt history (Brent et al., 1999; Shaffer et al., 1996), suggesting that a focus on understanding suicide attempts is not enough. Research with adolescents should also focus on understanding the suicidal thoughts that precede an attempt. Unfortunately, what teenagers think about when they think about killing themselves, and how they think about it, is poorly understood. Given that first-time suicide attempts generally occur within one year after the onset of suicide ideation (Nock et al., 2013), understanding how to assess suicide ideation in a way that is informative about risk for subsequent suicidal behavior is of paramount importance in preventing suicidal thought from leading to action among adolescents.

The measurement of suicide ideation has been limited by the proliferation of measures that either focus on one-item screening questions or by the use of multiple-item measures that generate total scores that only reveal whether ideation is present and whether it is, based on a higher score, more "severe" (Goldston, 2003). While a higher score on a measure of ideation may tell a clinician that there is "more ideation" present than would a lower score, it is not informative about the nature of that ideation. That is, knowing whether a teenager has a high score on a measure of ideation is not informative about *what* they are thinking and *how* they are thinking about it. Further, there is mixed evidence on whether such suicide ideation scores predict future suicide attempts among adolescents (Horwitz, Czyz, & King, 2015; King, Hovey, Brand, & Ghaziuddin, 1997; King, Jiang, Czyz, & Kerr, 2014; Prinstein et al., 2008). For instance, Prinstein and colleagues (2008) found that change in suicide ideation scores predicted future suicide attempts postdischarge among 143 hospitalized teenagers, whereas King and colleagues (2014) found that it did so among adolescent girls but not among boys. In contrast, Horwitz and colleagues (2015) found that total suicide ideation did not predict a future suicide attempt among hospitalized teenagers, but that one question that inquired about duration of suicide ideation did so. Given the limited time afforded to emergency room clinicians conducting suicide risk assessments, knowing which specific features of suicide ideation merit focus would improve clinical care of teenagers who present with suicide ideation or who endorse screening questions about ideation.

There is very little research on specific characteristics of suicide ideation that predict future suicidal behavior. Examination of commonly used measures of ideation, such as the Beck Scale for Suicide Ideation (Beck & Steer, 1991), reveals that these measures of ideation focus on how strongly people wish to die, whether they engage in planning, and, to some degree, the content of their ideation (e.g., whether they have thought of how they will access a method of attempt) (Goldston, 2003). Indeed, on some commonly used measures of suicide ideation, such as the Beck Scale for Suicide Ideation, suicidal desire must be present in order for other elements of ideation (e.g., planning) to be rated (Beck & Steer, 1991). Whether these characteristics that are a focus of measurement actually predict suicide attempts and suicide deaths remains an understudied question. Past research with adults and adolescents who attempted suicide suggests that components of a suicide attempt indicative of planning and preparation may be better predictors of future suicide attempts (Miranda, De Jaegere, Restifo, & Shaffer, 2014a) and suicide deaths (Joiner et al., 2003) than are other circumstances surrounding an attempt or even better than a total score on a suicide intent scale, which has been inconsistent in its prediction of subsequent suicide attempts (Haw, Hawton, Houston, & Townsend, 2003) and suicide deaths (Harriss & Hawton, 2005; Harriss, Hawton, & Zahl, 2005; Suominen, Isometsä, Ostamo, & Lönnqvist, 2004) among adults. Miranda and colleagues (2014a) found that a previous suicide attempt that involved an hour or more of planning predicted whether a teenager went on to make a future suicide attempt.

Previous studies with adults have suggested that suicide ideation can be distinguished by two dimensions: a suicidal desire dimension and a planning and preparation dimension (Beck, Brown, & Steer, 1997; Joiner, Rudd, & Rajab, 1997; Joiner et al., 2003; Witte et al., 2006). The suicidal desire dimension includes characteristics such as wish to die, while the planning and preparation dimension includes characteristics such as means and opportunity, preparations, and intensity and duration of suicide ideation (Joiner, 2005; Joiner, Walker, Rudd, & Jobes, 1999; Witte et al., 2006). In a study with 440 psychiatric outpatient adults with current suicide ideation, Joiner and colleagues (2003) found that suicidal plans (as operationalized by the sum of clinicians' ratings of a group of items reflecting specificity of planning, availability of opportunity, capability, expectancy, and preparation—at an individual's worst-point suicide ideation) predicted eventual suicide. Taken together, the available evidence points to the importance of assessing the degree of suicide planning when assessing risk for future suicidal behavior. At the same time, adult suicide attempts have been found to involve more lethal methods and greater certainty that the attempt will result in death, compared to adolescent attempts, and these differences suggest greater impulsivity in adolescent suicide attempts relative to adult attempts (Parellada et al., 2008). Future research is thus necessary to determine whether characteristics indicative of suicide planning are similarly informative about suicide risk in adolescence as in adulthood.

Interestingly, no measure of suicide ideation of which we are aware focuses on the form that suicide ideation takes—in terms of its frequency (i.e., the actual number of times it occurs on a given day or in a given week) and duration (i.e., the actual number of minutes or hours it lasts). Those who do inquire about these characteristics do so as part of summary scales not meant to focus on these elements of ideation. For instance, the Columbia–Suicide Severity Rating Scale (Posner et al., 2011) includes questions about frequency, duration, and controllability of ideation under a five-item suicide ideation "intensity" subscale that also includes reasons for ideation and the presence of deterrents to making a suicide attempt. The Scale for Suicide Ideation (Beck, Kovacs, & Weissman, 1979) captures frequency and duration of ideation under its "suicidal desire" subscale that also includes ratings of wish to die. The Suicidal Ideation Questionnaire (Reynolds, 1987) assesses how frequently adolescents have thoughts about being better off dead, wishing they were dead, of killing themselves, or of communicating their suicidal intent in the previous month on a scale ranging from "never" to "almost every day." However, the measure does not inquire about how many times per day an individual thinks about suicide or about how long the thoughts last. This is a limitation of current measures, because there is emerging evidence that the form of suicide ideation might be informative about an individual's risk profile. Among teenagers with a previous suicide attempt history, length of suicide planning of greater than an hour leading up to the teenager's most recent attempt (assessed at baseline) was one of the most robust predictors of a reattempt during a follow-up period of four to six years (Miranda et al., 2014a). Another study found that among teenagers who endorsed suicide ideation in the previous three to six months, length of their most recent ideation predicted whether they went on to make a suicide attempt during a four- to six-year follow-up period, independently of wish to die, even adjusting for depressive symptoms and for history of a previous suicide attempt. Further, even among those who reported suicide ideation without a previous suicide attempt history, length of an ideation episode greater than an hour predicted earlier onset of a future attempt (within one year), relative to ideation length of less than an hour (within three to four years) (Miranda, Ortin, Scott, & Shaffer, 2014b). Finally, a recent study of hospitalized adolescents found three trajectories of suicide ideation over a 12-month follow-up period: subclinical ideation, elevated ideation that rapidly declined, and suicide ideation that was chronically elevated (i.e., in terms of total score on a self-report measure of ideation). A trajectory involving chronically elevated suicide ideation more strongly predicted a future attempt and rehospitalization, compared to subclinical and rapidly declining ideation (Czyz & King, 2015). Taken together, these findings suggest that among teenagers who endorse suicide ideation, knowing the form their ideation takes—in terms of length and pattern—is informative about their vulnerability to future suicidal behavior.

These findings are also consistent with research with adults that suggests different patterns of suicide ideation preceding attempts. Bagge and colleagues (2013) found that suicide attempts that were characterized as more impulsive (i.e., defined by less than three hours of planning before the attempt) tended to be preceded by a negative life event within the 24 hours prior to the attempt, more so than did suicide attempts that were preceded by more than three hours of planning. This finding might suggest that impulsive suicide attempts are triggered by negative life events, whereas suicide attempts that were preceded by a longer period of suicide ideation do not require an external trigger such as an event preceding the attempt. Further research of this type is needed with adolescents.

Contemporary psychological models suggest ways that suicide ideation may, over time, lower the threshold for the onset of future suicidal episodes. Wenzel and Beck (2008) suggested that vulnerable individuals will transition from suicide ideation to suicide attempts during times of distress when they are unable to disengage from their suicide-related thoughts. A key element of the interpersonal theory of suicide is the idea that people acquire the ability to engage in lethal self-injury through practice (Joiner, 2005). This acquired ability affects the transition from suicidal desire to suicidal intent (Van Orden et al., 2010). Rudd's fluid vulnerability theory suggests that previous suicide attempts and suicide ideation lower the threshold for triggering a "suicidal mode," as the connections between suicide-related thoughts, feelings, and behaviors increase in memory (Rudd, 2006). The longer an individual's suicide ideation episode lasts, the more an individual may acquire the ability to engage in suicidal behavior as a result of practice (i.e., mental rehearsal) and habituation to the idea of lethal self-harm, and such practice in thinking about suicide may lower the threshold for triggering a future suicidal episode. Additional prospective studies should thus focus on understanding whether the onset of suicide ideation in adolescence, followed by a pattern of more persistent ideation over time, confers increased vulnerability to suicide through such mechanisms involving habituation or sensitization.

Assessing Suicide Risk via Indirect Methods

The assessment of suicide risk in adolescence is complicated by the fact that individuals at highest risk of engaging in suicidal behavior may also be those less likely to disclose their suicidal thoughts (Horesh, Zalsman, & Apter, 2004). Given the difficulty in assessing risk for suicidal behavior via direct inquiry, some research over the past decade has focused on the development of indirect methods of assessing risk for suicidal behavior via the use of techniques developed in laboratories. One line of research focuses on examining suicide-related cognitions via reaction time–based tasks. Nock and colleagues have developed and tested two such methods for assessing risk for future suicide attempts: the Self-Injury and Death/Suicide Implicit Association Tests (SI-IAT; Nock & Banaji, 2007; and Suicide-IAT; Nock et al., 2010) and the Suicide Stroop test (Cha, Najmi, Park, Finn, & Nock, 2010). The SI-IAT and Suicide-IAT measure the degree to which individuals associate self-injury or suicide-related words (vs. neutral stimuli) with themselves. Research with adolescents has found that degree of self-injury-related bias in implicit associations distinguishes adolescents with a suicide attempt history from those without a suicide attempt history (Nock & Banaji, 2007). Furthermore, a study of adults recruited from a psychiatric emergency department found that degree of suicide-related bias in implicit associations predicts future suicide attempts over a six-month follow-up period, beyond depression, suicide attempt history, and both clinician and patient predictions (Nock et al., 2010). Similarly, the Suicide Stroop test measures semantic interference from suicide-related words, relative to neutral words, in a color-naming test. Adapted from emotion-related Stroop tests (Williams, Mathews, & MacLeod, 1996), the Suicide Stroop requires that individuals name the colors of words that appear, one by one, on a computer screen as quickly as possible. Individuals with a history of suicide attempts have been found to show more semantic interference from suicide-related words (e.g., *death*), relative to neutral words. In addition, such a suicide-related bias on the Suicide Stroop test predicts future suicide attempts among adults over a six-month follow-up period, beyond clinician predictions, patients' own predictions, and known risk factors, such as the presence of a mood disorder and having a history of multiple suicide attempts (Cha et al., 2010). These tasks thus show promise in helping clinicians to identify individuals at risk of making the transition from suicidal thoughts to suicidal behavior.

Treatment of Adolescent Suicidal Behavior

Few psychological interventions are effective in the long-lasting reduction of suicidal behavior among adolescents (Ougrin, Tranah, Stahl, Moran, & Asarnow, 2015;

Tarrier, Taylor, & Gooding, 2008). Most of these interventions focus on addressing distal and proximal risk factors for suicidal behavior, such as depression (Asarnow et al., 2011; Brent et al., 2009; Spirito, Esposito-Smythers, Wolff, & Uhl, 2011; Stanley et al., 2009), substance use (Esposito-Smythers, Spirito, Kahler, Hunt, & Monti, 2011), distress tolerance and emotion dysregulation (Canadian Agency for Drugs and Technologies in Health, 2010; Rossouw & Fonagy, 2012), and familial problems (Diamond et al., 2010; Huey et al., 2004), with reduction in suicidal behavior being a secondary consideration. Other interventions, such as safety planning, aim to identify and implement strategies that adolescents can undertake when they experience any thoughts of suicide or self-harm (Stanley & Brown, 2012). A review by Tarrier and colleagues (2008) suggested that treatments for suicidal behavior might be more effective if they focused specifically on actually reducing some aspect of suicidal behavior, rather than focusing on associated symptoms (e.g., depression). Such treatments might, for instance, focus on training individuals to disengage from or reduce the length of their suicide ideation, given that length of ideation is associated with earlier transition from ideation to an attempt (Miranda et al., 2014b).

Conclusion

Adolescence is a period in which individuals are most at risk for the onset of suicide ideation and attempts, with gender differences emerging in ideation, attempts, and suicides during this period of development. The available evidence indicates that one of the best predictors of future suicidal behavior is past suicidal behavior, and the highest risk of the transition from suicidal thought to action seems to be within a year of the onset of ideation. Early identification of those adolescents who think about suicide is crucial to curb its progression, especially when more than half of adolescents who die by suicide are first-time attempters. Despite some of the limitations in understanding how suicide ideation emerges, current evidence suggests that a number of psychological variables are associated with suicide ideation, including depression, ruminative thinking, and hopelessness-related cognitions. Further research is necessary to understand the transition from suicide ideation to attempts, although recent research findings suggest that psychological variables such as impulsivity, along with impulse control–related disorders, may be associated with the transition to suicide attempts. Further, we have evidence that HPA axis dysregulation and abnormal serotonergic functioning are critical biomarkers for adolescent suicidal behavior. Despite limited research examining these systems in adolescence, our current knowledge suggests that theoretical models of suicidal behavior should include biological systems in conjunction with other known risk factors. Additionally, an emerging literature on the sociocultural context of suicide may help to explain racial and ethnic variability in suicide attempts relative to suicide deaths. Indeed, an integrative approach to understanding adolescent suicidal behavior appears to be the best avenue for developing treatments and interventions in the prevention of suicide. Finally, future research should attempt to better understand what adolescents actually think about when they think about suicide, along with the form that their suicide ideation takes. Such approaches, combined with laboratory-based methods, may substantially improve suicide risk assessment in adolescence and guide the development and improvement of treatments.

References

Adedoyin, A. C., & Salter, S. N. (2013). Mainstreaming black churches into suicide prevention among adolescents: A literature review. *Ethnicity and Inequalities in Health and Social Care, 6*, 43–53.

Arsenault-Lapierre, G., Kim, C., & Turecki, G. (2004). Psychiatric diagnoses in 3275 suicides: A meta-analysis. *BMC Psychiatry, 4*, 37. Retrieved from http://doi:10.1186/1471-244X-4-37

Asarnow, J. R., Porta, G., Spirito, A., Emslie, G., Clarke, G., Wagner, K. D., . . . Brent, D. A. (2011). Suicide attempts and non-suicidal self-injury in the treatment of resistant depression in adolescents: Findings from the TORDIA study. *Journal of the American Academy of Child and Adolescent Psychiatry, 50*, 772–781.

Ayyash-Abdo, H. (2002). Adolescent suicide: An ecological approach. *Psychology in the Schools, 39*, 459–475.

Bagge, C. L., Glenn, C. R., & Lee, H.-J. (2013). Quantifying the impact of recent negative life events on suicide attempts. *Journal of Abnormal Psychology, 122*, 359–368.

Barzilay, S., & Apter, A. (2014). Psychological models of suicide. *Archives of Suicide Research, 18*, 295–312.

Beauchaine, T. P., Crowell, S. E., & Hsiao, R. C. (2015). Post-dexamethasone cortisol, self-inflicted injury, and suicidal ideation among depressed adolescent girls. *Journal of Abnormal Child Psychology, 43*, 619–632.

Beautrais, A. L., Joyce, P. R., & Mulder, R. T. (1997). Precipitating factors and life events in serious suicide attempts among youths aged 13 through 24 years. *Journal of the American Academy of Child and Adolescent Psychiatry, 36*, 1543–1551.

Beautrais, A. L., Joyce, P. R., Mulder, R. T., Fergusson, D. M., Deavoll, B. J., & Nightingale, S. K. (1996). Prevalence and comorbidity of mental disorders in persons making serious suicide attempts: A case-control study. *American Journal of Psychiatry, 153*, 1009–1014.

Beck, A. T., Brown, G. K., & Steer, R. A. (1997). Psychometric characteristics of the Scale for Suicide Ideation with psychiatric outpatients. *Behavior Research and Therapy, 35*, 1039–1046.

Beck, A. T., Kovacs, M., & Weissman, A. (1979). Assessment of suicidal intention: The Scale for Suicide Ideation. *Journal of Consulting and Clinical Psychology, 47*, 343–352.

Beck, A. T., & Steer, R. A. (1991). *Manual for the Beck Scale for Suicide Ideation.* San Antonio, TX: Psychological Corporation.

Beck, A. T., Steer, R. A., Kovacs, M., & Garrison, B. (1985). Hopelessness and eventual suicide: A 10-year prospective study of patients hospitalized with suicidal ideation. *American Journal of Psychiatry, 142*, 559–563.

Ben-Yehuda, A., Aviram, S., Govezensky, J., Nitzan, U., Levkovitz, Y., & Bloch, Y. (2012). Suicidal behavior in minors: Diagnostic differences between children and adolescents. *Journal of Developmental and Behavioral Pediatrics, 33*, 542–547.

Berry, J. W. (2003). Conceptual approaches to acculturation. In K. M. Chun, P. B. Organista, & G. Marin (Eds.), *Acculturation: Advances in theory, measurement, and applied research* (pp. 17–37). Washington, DC: American Psychological Association.

Boeninger, D. K., Masyn, K. E., Feldman, B. J., & Conger, R. D. (2010). Sex differences in developmental trends of suicide ideation, plans, and attempts among European American adolescents. *Suicide and Life-Threatening Behavior, 40*, 451–464.

Bolger, N., Downey, G., Walker, E., & Steininger, P. (1989). The onset of suicidal ideation in childhood and adolescence. *Journal of Youth and Adolescence, 18*, 175–190.

Borges, G., Benjet, C., Medina-Mora, M. E., Orozco, R., & Nock, M. (2008). Suicide ideation, plan, and attempt in the Mexican adolescent mental health survey. *Journal of the American Academy of Child and Adolescent Psychiatry, 47*, 41–52.

Brent, D. A., Baugher, M., Bridge, J., Chen, T., & Chiappetta, L. (1999). Age- and sex-related risk factors for adolescent suicide. *Journal of the American Academy of Child and Adolescent Psychiatry, 38*, 1497–1505.

Brent, D. A., Greenhill, L. L., Compton, S., Emslie, G., Wells, K., Walkup, J. T., . . . Turner, J. B. (2009). The Treatment of Adolescent Suicide Attempters study (TASA): Predictors of suicidal events in an open treatment trial. *Journal of the American Academy of Child and Adolescent Psychiatry, 48*, 987–996.

Brent, D. A., Perper, J., Moritz, G., Baugher, M., & Allman, C. (1993a). Suicide in adolescents with no apparent psychopathology. *Journal of the American Academy of Child and Adolescent Psychiatry, 32*, 494–500.

Brent, D. A., Perper, J. A., Moritz, G., Baugher, M., Roth, C., Balach, L., & Schweers, J. (1993b). Stressful life events, psychopathology, and adolescent suicide: A case control study. *Suicide and Life-Threatening Behavior, 23*, 179–187.

Brezo, J., Paris, J., Barker, E. D., Tremblay, R., Vitaro, F., Zoccolillo, M., . . . Turecki, G. (2007). Natural history of suicidal behaviors in a population-based sample of young adults. *Psychological Medicine, 37*, 1563–1574.

Bridge, J. A., Goldstein, T. R., & Brent, D. A. (2006). Adolescent suicide and suicidal behavior. *Journal of Child Psychology and Psychiatry, 47*, 372–394.

Brown, G. K., Beck, A. T., Steer, R. A., & Grisham, J. R. (2000). Risk factors for suicide in psychiatric outpatients: A 20-year prospective study. *Journal of Consulting and Clinical Psychology, 68*, 371–377.

Bruffaerts, R., Demyttenaere, K., Borges, G., Haro, J. M., Chiu, W. T., Hwang, I., . . . Nock, M. K. (2010). Childhood adversities as risk factors for onset and persistence of suicidal behaviour. *British Journal of Psychiatry, 197*, 20–27.

Burwell, R. A., & Shirk, S. R. (2007). Subtypes of rumination in adolescence: Associations between brooding, reflection, depressive symptoms, and coping. *Journal of Clinical Child and Adolescent Psychology, 36*, 56–65.

Canadian Agency for Drugs and Technologies in Health. (2010). Dialectical behaviour therapy in adolescents for suicide prevention: Systematic review of clinical-effectiveness. *CADTH Technology Overviews, 1*, e0104. Retrieved from https://www.cadth.ca/dialectical-behaviour -therapy-adolescents-suicide-prevention

Canetto, S. S., & Sakinofsky, I. (1998). The gender paradox in suicide. *Suicide and Life- Threatening Behavior, 28*, 1–23.

Caspi, A., Sugden, K., Moffitt, T. E., Taylor, A., Craig, I. W., Harrington, H., . . . & Poulton, R. (2003). Influence of life stress on depression: Moderation by a polymorphism in the 5-HTT gene. *Science, 301*, 386–389.

Cavanagh, J. T. O., Carson, A. J., Sharpe, M., & Lawrie, S. M. (2003). Psychological autopsy studies of suicide: A systematic review. *Psychological Medicine, 33*, 395–405.

Centers for Disease Control and Prevention. (2016a). *Leading causes of death reports, national and regional, 1999–2014. National Centers for Injury Prevention and Control, Web-based Injury Statistics Query and Reporting System (WISQARS)*. Retrieved from http://webappa.cdc.gov /sasweb/ncipc/leadcaus10_us.html

Centers for Disease Control and Prevention. (2016b). *Fatal injury reports, national and regional, 1999–2014. National Centers for Injury Prevention and Control, Web-based Injury Statistics Query and Reporting System (WISQARS)*. Retrieved from http://webappa.cdc.gov/sasweb /ncipc/mortrate10_us.html

Cha, C. B., Najmi, S., Park, J. M., Finn, C. T., & Nock, M. K. (2010). Attentional bias toward suicide-related stimuli predicts suicidal behavior. *Journal of Abnormal Psychology, 119*, 616–622.

Chou, T., Asnaani, A., & Hofmann, S. G. (2012). Perception of racial discrimination and psychopathology across three US ethnic minority groups. *Cultural Diversity and Ethnic Minority Psychology, 18*, 74–81.

Chu, J. P., Goldblum, P., Floyd, R., & Bongar, B. (2010). The cultural theory and model of suicide. *Applied and Preventive Psychology, 14*, 25–40.

Clark, R., Anderson, N. B., Clark, V. R., & Williams, D. R. (1999). Racism as a stressor for African Americans: A biopsychosocial model. *American Psychologist, 54*(10), 805–816.

Cooper, J., Appleby, L., & Amos, T. (2002). Life events preceding suicide by young people. *Social Psychiatry and Psychiatric Epidemiology, 37*, 271–275.

Crosby, A. E., Ortega, L., & Melanson, C. (2011). *Self-directed violence surveillance: Uniform definitions and recommended data elements, Version 1.0*. Atlanta, GA: Centers for Disease Control and Prevention, National Center for Injury Prevention and Control.

Czyz, E. K., & King, C.A. (2015). Longitudinal trajectories of suicidal ideation and subsequent suicide attempts among adolescent inpatients. *Journal of Clinical Child and Adolescent Psychology, 44*, 181–193.

D'Eramo, K. S., Prinstein, M. J., Freeman, J., Grapentine, W. L., & Spirito, A. (2004). Psychiatric diagnoses and comorbidity in relation to suicidal behavior among psychiatrically hospitalized adolescents. *Child Psychiatry and Human Development, 35*, 21–35.

DeSantis, A. S., Adam, E. K., Doane, L. D., Mineka, S., Zinbarg, R. E., & Craske, M. G. (2007). Racial/ethnic differences in cortisol diurnal rhythms in a community sample of adolescents. *Journal of Adolescent Health, 41*, 3–13.

Diamond, G. S., Wintersteen, M. B., Brown, G. K., Diamond, G. M., Gallop, R., Shelef, K., & Levy, S. (2010). Attachment-based family therapy for adolescents with suicidal ideation: A randomized controlled trial. *Journal of the American Academy of Child and Adolescent Psychiatry, 49*, 122–131.

Dieserud, G., Gerhardsen, R. M., Van den Weghe, H., & Corbett, K. (2010). Adolescent suicide attempts in Baerum, Norway, 1984–2006: Trends, triggers, and underlying reasons. *Crisis, 3*, 255–264.

Eaton, D. K., Foti, K., Brener, N. D., Crosby, A. E., Flores, G., & Kann, L. (2011). Associations between risk behaviors and suicidal ideation and suicide attempts: Do racial/ethnic variations in associations account for increased risk of suicidal behaviors among Hispanic/Latina 9th- to 12th-grade female students? *Archives of Suicide Research, 15*, 113–126.

Eley, T. C., Sugden, K., Corsico, A., Gregory, A. M., Sham, P., McGuffin, P., . . . & Craig, I. W. (2004). Gene–environment interaction analysis of serotonin system markers with adolescent depression. *Molecular Psychiatry, 9*, 908–915.

Esposito, C., Spirito, A., Boergers, J., & Donaldson, D. (2003). Affective, behavioral, and cognitive functioning in adolescents with multiple suicide attempts. *Suicide and Life-Threatening Behavior, 33*, 389–399.

Esposito-Smythers, C., Spirito, A., Kahler, C. W., Hunt, J., & Monti, P. (2011). Treatment of co-occurring substance abuse and suicidality among adolescents: A randomized trial. *Journal of Consulting and Clinical Psychology, 79*, 728–739.

Evans, E., Hawton, K., Rodham, K., & Deeks, J. (2005). The prevalence of suicidal phenomena in adolescents: A systematic review of population-based studies. *Suicide and Life-Threatening Behavior, 35*, 239–250.

Fawcett, J., Scheftner, W. A., Fogg, L., Clark, D. C., Young, M. A., Hedeker, D., & Gibbons, R. (1990). Time-related predictors of suicide in major affective disorder. *American Journal of Psychiatry, 147*, 1189–1194.

Freedenthal, S. (2007). Racial disparities in mental health service use by adolescents who thought about or attempted suicide. *Suicide and Life-Threatening Behavior, 37*, 22–34.

Garrison, C. Z., Addy, C. L., Jackson, K. L., McKeown, R. E., & Waller, J. L. (1991). A longitudinal study of suicidal ideation in young adolescents. *Journal of the American Academy of Child and Adolescent Psychiatry, 30*, 597–603.

Gil, A. G., & Vega, W. A. (1996). Two different worlds: Acculturation stress and adaptation among Cuban and Nicaraguan families. *Journal of Social and Personal Relationships, 13*, 435–456.

Giletta, M., Calhoun, C. D., Hastings, P. D., Rudolph, K. D., Nock, M. K., & Prinstein, M. J. (2015). Multi-level risk factors for suicidal ideation among at-risk adolescent females: The role of hypothalamic-pituitary-adrenal axis responses to stress. *Journal of Abnormal Child Psychology, 43*, 807–820.

Glenn, C. R., & Nock, M. K. (2014). Improving the short-term prediction of suicidal behavior. *American Journal of Preventive Medicine, 47*, S176–S180.

Goldston, D. B. (2003). *Measuring suicidal behavior and risk in children and adolescents.* Washington, DC: American Psychological Association.

Goldston, D. B., Daniel, S. S., Reboussin, D. M., Reboussin, B. A., Frazier, P. H., & Kelley, A. E. (1999). Suicide attempts among formerly hospitalized adolescents: A prospective naturalistic study of risk during the first 5 years after discharge. *Journal of the American Academy of Child and Adolescent Psychiatry, 38*, 660–671.

Goldston, D., Molock, S., Whitbeck, L., Murakami, J., Zayas, L., & Hall, G. (2008). Cultural considerations in adolescent suicide prevention and psychosocial treatment. *American Psychologist, 63*, 14–31.

Greene, M. L., Way, N., & Pahl, K. (2006). Trajectories of perceived adult and peer discrimination among Black, Latino, and Asian American adolescents: Patterns and psychological correlates. *Developmental Psychology, 42*, 218–236.

Gulbas, L. E., & Zayas, L. H. (2015). Examining the interplay among family, culture, and Latina teen suicidal behavior. *Qualitative Health Research, 25*, 689–699.

Harrell, S. P. (2000). A multidimensional conceptualization of racism-related stress: Implications for the well-being of people of color. *American Journal of Orthopsychiatry, 70*, 42–57.

Harris, E. C. & Barraclough, B. (1997). Suicide as an outcome for mental disorders: A meta-analysis. *British Journal of Psychiatry, 170*, 205–228.

Harriss, L., & Hawton, K. (2005). Suicidal intent in deliberate self-harm and the risk of suicide: The predictive power of the Suicide Intent Scale. *Journal of Affective Disorders, 86*, 225–233.

Harriss, L., Hawton, K., & Zahl, D. (2005). Value of measuring suicidal intent in the assessment of people attending hospital following self-poisoning or self-injury. *British Journal of Psychiatry, 186*, 60–66.

Haw, C., Hawton, K., Houston, K., & Townsend, E. (2003). Correlates or relative lethality and suicidal intent among deliberate self-harm patients. *Suicide and Life-Threatening Behavior, 33*, 353–364.

Henry, C. S., Stephenson, A. L., Hanson, M. F., & Hargett, W. (1994). Adolescent suicide and families: An ecological approach. *Family Therapy, 21*, 63–80.

Horesh, N., Zalsman, G., & Apter, A. (2004). Suicidal behavior and self-disclosure in adolescent psychiatric inpatients. *The Journal of Nervous and Mental Disease, 192*, 837–842.

Horwitz, A. G., Czyz, E. K., & King, C. A. (2015). Predicting future suicide attempts among adolescent and emerging adult psychiatric emergency patients. *Journal of Clinical Child and Adolescent Psychology, 44*, 751–761.

Hovey, J. D., & King, C. A. (1996). Acculturative stress, depression, and suicidal ideation among immigrant and second-generation Latino adolescents. *Journal of the American Academy of Child and Adolescent Psychiatry, 35*, 1183–1192.

Huey, S. J., Jr., Henggeler, S. W., Rowland, M. D., Halliday-Boykins, C. A., Cunningham, P. B., Pickrel, S. G., & Edwards, J. (2004). Multisystemic therapy effects on attempted suicide by youths presenting psychiatric emergencies. *Journal of the American Academy of Child and Adolescent Psychiatry, 43*, 183–190.

Hultén, A., Jiang, G.-X., Wasserman, D., Hawton, K., Hjelmeland, H., De Leo, D., . . . Schmidtke, A. (2001). Repetition of attempted suicide among teenagers in Europe: Frequency, timing, and risk factors. *European Child and Adolescent Psychiatry, 10*, 161–169.

Jacobson, C., Batejan, K., Kleinman, M., & Gould, M. (2013). Reasons for attempting suicide among a community sample of adolescents. *Suicide and Life-Threatening Behavior, 43*, 646–662.

Javdani, S., Sadeh, N., & Verona, E. (2011). Suicidality as a function of impulsivity, callous-unemotional traits, and depressive symptoms in youth. *Journal of Abnormal Psychology, 120*, 400–413.

Joe, S., Baser, R. S., Neighbors, H. W., Caldwell, C. H., & Jackson, J. S. (2009). 12-month and lifetime prevalence of suicide attempts among black adolescents in the National Survey of American Life. *Journal of the American Academy of Child and Adolescent Psychiatry, 48*, 271–282.

Joiner, T. E. (2005). *Why people die by suicide.* Cambridge, MA: Harvard University Press.

Joiner, T. E., Rudd, M. D., & Rajab, M. H. (1997). The Modified Scale for Suicidal Ideation: Factors of suicidality and their relation to clinical and diagnostic variables. *Journal of Abnormal Psychology, 106*, 260–265.

Joiner, T. E., Steer, R. A., Brown, G., Beck, A. T., Pettit, J. W., & Rudd, M. D. (2003). Worst-point suicidal plans: A dimension of suicidality predictive of past suicide attempts and eventual death by suicide. *Behaviour Research and Therapy, 41*, 1469–1480.

Joiner, T. E., Walker, R. L., Rudd, M. D., & Jobes, D. A. (1999). Scientizing and routinizing the assessment of suicidality in outpatient practice. *Professional Psychology: Research and Practice, 30*, 447–453.

Kann, L., McManus, T., Harris, W., Shanklin, S. L., Flint, K. H., Hawkins, J., . . . Zaza, S. (2016). Youth Risk Behavior Surveillance—United States, 2015. *Morbidity and Mortality Weekly Report, 65*, 1–174.

Karg, K., Burmeister, M., Shedden, K., & Sen, S. (2011). The serotonin transporter promoter variant (5-HTTLPR), stress, and depression meta-analysis revisited: Evidence of genetic moderation. *Archives of General Psychiatry, 68*, 444–454.

Kessler, R. C., McGonagle, K. A., Swartz, M., Blazer, D. G., & Nelson, C. B. (1993). Sex and depression in the National Comorbidity Survey I: Lifetime prevalence, chronicity and recurrence. *Journal of Affective Disorders, 29*, 85–96.

King, C. A., Hovey, J. D., Brand, E., & Ghaziuddin, N. (1997). Prediction of positive outcomes for adolescent psychiatric inpatients. *Journal of the American Academy of Child and Adolescent Psychiatry, 36*, 1434–1442.

King, C. A., Hovey, J. D., Brand, E., Wilson, R., & Ghaziuddin, N. (1997). Suicidal adolescents after hospitalization: Parent and family impacts on treatment follow-through. *Journal of the American Academy of Child and Adolescent Psychiatry, 36*, 85–93.

King, C. A., Jiang, Q., Czyz, E. K., & Kerr, D. C. (2014). Suicidal ideation of psychiatrically hospitalized adolescents has one-year predictive validity for suicide attempts in girls only. *Journal of Abnormal Child Psychology, 42*, 467–477.

Klimes-Dougan, B., Free, K., Ronsaville, D., Stilwell, J., Welsh, C. J., & Radke-Yarrow, M. (1999). Suicidal ideation and attempts: A longitudinal investigation of children of depressed and well mothers. *Journal of the American Academy of Child and Adolescent Psychiatry, 38*, 651–659.

Klonsky, E. D., & May, A. (2010). Rethinking impulsivity in suicide. *Suicide and Life- Threatening Behavior, 40*, 612–619.

Krug, E. G., Mercy, J. A., Dahlberg, L. L., & Zwi, A. B. (2002). The world report on violence and health. *The Lancet, 360*, 1083–1088.

Langhinrichsen-Rohling, J., Friend, J., & Powell, A. (2009). Adolescent suicide, gender, and culture: A rate and risk factor analysis. *Aggression and Violent Behavior, 14*, 402–414.

Langhinrichsen-Rohling, J., Sanders, A., Crane, M., & Monson, C. M. (1998). Gender and history of suicidality: Are these factors related to US college students' current suicidal thoughts, feelings, and actions? *Suicide and Life-Threatening Behavior, 28*, 127–142.

Lewinsohn, P. M., Rohde, P., & Seeley, J. R. (1993). Psychosocial characteristics of adolescents with a history of suicide attempt. *Journal of the American Academy of Child and Adolescent Psychiatry, 32*, 60–68.

Lewinsohn, P. M., Rohde, P., & Seeley, J. R. (1994). Psychosocial risk factors for future adolescent suicide attempts. *Journal of Consulting and Clinical Psychology, 62*, 297–305.

Lewinsohn, P. M., Rohde, P., Seeley, J. R., & Baldwin, C. L. (2001). Gender differences in suicide attempts from adolescence to young adulthood. *Journal of the American Academy of Child and Adolescent Psychiatry, 40*, 427–434.

Mann, J. J. (1999). Role of the serotonergic system in the pathogenesis of major depression and suicidal behavior. *Neuropsychopharmacology, 21,* 99S-105S.

Marttunen, M. J., Aro, H. M., Henriksson, M. M., & Lonnqvist, J. K. (1991). Mental disorders in adolescent suicide. *DSM-III-R* axes I and II diagnoses in suicides among 13- to 19-year-olds in Finland. *Archives of General Psychiatry, 48,* 834–839.

Mathew, S. J., Coplan, J. D., Goetz, R. R., Feder, A., Greenwald, S., Dahl, R. E., . . . Weissman, M. M. (2003). Differentiating depressed adolescent 24 h cortisol secretion in light of their adult clinical outcome. *Neuropsychopharmacology, 28,* 1336–1343.

Mazza, J. J. (2000). The relationship between posttraumatic stress symptomatology and suicidal behavior in school based adolescents. *Suicide and Life-Threatening Behavior, 30,* 91–103.

McKeown, R. E., Garrison, C. Z., Cuffe, S. P., Waller, J. L., Jackson, K. L., & Addy, C. L. (1998). Incidence and predictors of suicidal behaviors in a longitudinal sample of young adolescents. *Journal of the American Academy of Child and Adolescent Psychiatry, 37,* 612–619.

Mena, F. J., Padilla, A. M., & Maldonado, M. (1987). Acculturative stress and specific coping strategies among immigrant and later generation college students. *Hispanic Journal of Behavioral Sciences, 9,* 207–225.

Michl, L. C., McLaughlin, K. A., Shepherd, K., & Nolen-Hoeksema, S. (2013). Rumination as a mechanism linking stressful life events to symptoms of depression and anxiety: Longitudinal evidence in early adolescents and adults. *Journal of Abnormal Psychology, 122,* 339–352.

Miller, G. E., Chen, E., & Zhou, E. S. (2007). If it goes up, must it come down? Chronic stress and the hypothalamic-pituitary-adrenocortical axis in humans. *Psychological Bulletin, 133,* 25–45.

Miranda, R., De Jaegere, E., Restifo, K., & Shaffer, D. (2014a). Longitudinal follow-up study of adolescents who report a suicide attempt: Aspects of suicidal behavior that increase risk of a future attempt. *Depression and Anxiety, 31,* 19–26.

Miranda, R., & Nolen-Hoeksema, S. (2007). Brooding and reflection: Rumination predicts suicidal ideation at 1-year follow-up in a community sample. *Behaviour Research and Therapy, 45,* 3088–3095.

Miranda, R., Ortin, A., Scott, M., & Shaffer, D. (2014b). Characteristics of suicidal ideation that predict the transition to future suicide attempts in adolescents. *Journal of Child Psychology and Psychiatry, 55,* 1288–1296.

Miranda, R., Scott, M., Hicks, R., Wilcox, H. C., Harris Munfakh, J. L., & Shaffer, D. (2008). Suicide attempt characteristics, diagnoses, and future attempts: Comparing multiple attempters to single attempters and ideators. *Journal of the American Academy of Child and Adolescent Psychiatry, 47,* 32–40.

Miranda, R., & Shaffer, D. (2013). Understanding the suicidal moment in adolescence. *Annals of the New York Academy of Sciences, 1304,* 14–21.

Molock, S. D., Puri, R., Matlin, S., & Barksdale, C. (2006). Relationship between religious coping and suicidal behaviors among African American adolescents. *Journal of Black Psychology, 32,* 366–389.

Moscicki, E. K. (1994). Gender differences in completed and attempted suicides. *Annals of Epidemiology, 4,* 152–158.

National Adolescent Health Information Center. (2006). *2006 Fact Sheet on Suicide: Adolescents and Young Adults.* Retrieved from http://nahic.ucsf.edu/downloads/Suicide.pdf

Neblett, E. W., Rivas-Drake, D., & Umaña-Taylor, A. J. (2012). The promise of racial and ethnic protective factors in promoting ethnic minority youth development. *Child Development Perspectives, 6*, 295–303.

Negron, R., Piacentini, J., Graae, F., Davies, M., & Shaffer, D. (1997). Microanalysis of adolescent suicide attempters and ideators during the acute suicidal episode. *Journal of the American Academy of Child and Adolescent Psychiatry, 36*, 1512–1519.

Nock, M. K., & Banaji, M. R. (2007). Prediction of suicide ideation and attempts among adolescents using a brief performance-based test. *Journal of Consulting and Clinical Psychology, 75*, 707–715.

Nock, M. K., Borges, G., Bromet, E. J., Alonso, J., Angermeyer, M., Beautrais, A., . . . Williams, D. (2008). Cross-national prevalence and risk factors for suicidal ideation, plans and attempts. *British Journal of Psychiatry, 192*, 98–105.

Nock, M. K., Green, J. G., Hwang, I., McLaughlin, K. A., Sampson, N. A., Zaslavsky, A. M., & Kessler, R. C. (2013). Prevalence, correlates, and treatment of lifetime suicidal behavior among adolescents: Results from the National Comorbidity Survey Replication Adolescent Supplement. *JAMA Psychiatry, 70*, 300–310.

Nock, M. K., Holmberg, E. B., Photos, V. I., & Michel, B. D. (2007). Self-injurious thoughts and behaviors interview: Development, reliability, and validity in an adolescent sample. *Psychological Assessment, 19*, 309–317.

Nock, M. K., Hwang, I., Sampson, N. A., & Kessler, R. C. (2010). Mental disorders, comorbidity and suicidal behavior: Results from the National Comorbidity Survey Replication. *Molecular Psychiatry, 15*, 868–876.

Nock, M. K., Hwang, I., Sampson, N., Kessler, R. C., Angermeyer, M., Beautrais, A., . . . Williams, D. R. (2009). Cross-national analysis of the associations among mental disorders and suicidal behavior: Findings from the WHO World Mental Health Surveys. *PLoS Medicine, 6*, e1000123.

Nock, M. K., Park, J. M., Finn, C. T., Deliberto, T. L., Dour, H. J., & Banaji, M. R. (2010). Measuring the suicidal mind: Implicit cognition predicts suicidal behavior. *Psychological Science, 21*, 511–517.

Nolen-Hoeksema, S., Wisco, B. E., & Lyubomirsky, S. (2008). Rethinking rumination. *Perspectives on Psychological Science, 3*, 400–424.

O'Connor, R. C. (2011). The integrated motivational-volitional model of suicidal behavior. *Crisis, 32*, 295–298.

O'Connor, R. C., & Nock, M. K. (2014). The psychology of suicidal behavior. *Lancet Psychiatry, 1*, 73–85.

Ortin, A., Lake, A. M., Kleinman, M., & Gould, M. S. (2012). Sensation seeking as risk factor for suicidal ideation and suicide attempts in adolescence. *Journal of Affective Disorders, 143*, 214–222.

Ougrin, D., Tranah, T., Stahl, D., Moran, P., & Asarnow, J. R. (2015). Therapeutic interventions for suicide attempts and self-harm in adolescents: Systematic review and meta-analysis. *Journal of the American Academy of Child and Adolescent Psychiatry, 54*, 97–107.

Pandey, G. N. (2011). Neurobiology of adult and teenage suicide. *Asian Journal of Psychiatry, 4*, 2–13.

Parellada, M., Saiz, P., Moreno, D., Vidal, J., Llorente, C., Alvarez, M., . . . Bobes, J. (2008). Is attempted suicide different in adolescent and adults? *Psychiatry Research, 157*, 131–137.

Pascoe, E. A., & Richman, L. S. (2009). Perceived discrimination and health: A meta-analytic review. *Psychological Bulletin, 135*, 531–554.

Peña, J. B., Kuhlberg, J. A., Zayas, L. H., Baumann, A. A., Gulbas, L., Hausmann-Stabile, C., & Nolle, A. P. (2011). Familism, family environment, and suicide attempts among Latina youth. *Suicide and Life-Threatening Behavior, 41*, 330–341.

Peña, J. B., Wyman, P. A., Brown, C. H., Matthieu, M. M., Olivares, T. E., Hartel, D., & Zayas, L. H. (2008). Immigration generation status and its association with suicide attempts, substance use, and depressive symptoms among Latino adolescents in the USA. *Prevention Science, 9*, 299–310.

Petronis, K. R., Samuels, J. F., Moscicki, E. K., & Anthony, J. C. (1990). An epidemiologic investigation of potential risk factors for suicide attempts. *Social Psychiatry and Psychiatric Epidemiology, 25*, 193–199.

Pfeffer, C. R., Zuckerman, S., Plutchik, R., & Mizruchi, M. S. (1984). Suicidal behavior in normal school children: A comparison with child psychiatric inpatients. *Journal of the American Academy of Child and Adolescent Psychiatry, 23*, 416–423.

Phinney, J. S. (1990). Ethnic identity in adolescents and adults: Review of research. *Psychological Bulletin, 108*, 499–514.

Phinney, J. S., Ong, A., & Madden, T. (2000). Cultural values and intergenerational value discrepancies in immigrant and non-immigrant families. *Child Development, 71*, 528–539.

Posner, K., Brown, G. K., Stanley, B., Brent, D. A., Yershova, K. V., Oquendo, M. A., . . . Mann, J. J. (2011). The Columbia-Suicide Severity Rating Scale: Initial validity and internal consistency findings from three multisite studies with adolescents and adults. *American Journal of Psychiatry, 168*, 1266–1277.

Prinstein, M. J., Nock, M. K., Simon, V., Aikins, J. W., Cheah, C. S., & Spirito, A. (2008). Longitudinal trajectories and predictors of adolescent suicidal ideation and attempts following inpatient hospitalization. *Journal of Consulting and Clinical Psychology, 76*, 92–103.

Reinherz, H. Z., Giaconia, R. M., Silverman, A. B., Friedman, A., Pakiz, B., Frost, A. K., & Cohen, E. (1995). Early psychosocial risks for adolescent suicidal ideation and attempts. *Journal of the American Academy of Child and Adolescent Psychiatry, 34*, 599–611.

Reynolds, W. M. (1987). *Suicidal Ideation Questionnaire (SIQ): Professional Manual*. Odessa, FL: Psychological Assessment Resources.

Rossouw, T. I., & Fonagy, P. (2012). Mentalization-based treatment for self-harm in adolescents: A randomized controlled trial. *Journal of the American Academy of Child and Adolescent Psychiatry, 51*, 1304–1313.

Rudd, D. M. (2006). Fluid vulnerability theory: A cognitive approach to understanding the process of acute and chronic suicide risk. In T. E. Ellis (Ed.), *Cognition and suicide: Theory, research, and therapy* (pp. 355–360). Washington, DC: American Psychological Association.

Rueter, M. A., & Kwon, H. (2005). Developmental trends in adolescent suicidal ideation. *Journal of Research on Adolescence, 15*, 205–222.

Shaffer, D., Gould, M. S., Fisher, P., Trautman, P., Moreau, D., Kleinman, M., & Flory, M. (1996). Psychiatric diagnosis in child and adolescent suicide. *Archives of General Psychiatry, 53*, 339–348.

Shaffer, D., Scott, M., Wilcox, H., Maslow, C., Hicks, R., Lucas, C., . . . Greenwald, S. (2004). The Columbia Suicide Screen: Validity and reliability of a screen for youth suicide and depression. *Journal of the American Academy of Child and Adolescent Psychiatry, 43*, 71–79.

Silverman, A. B., Reinherz, H. Z., & Giaconia, R. M. (1996). The long-term sequelae of child and adolescent abuse: A longitudinal community study. *Child Abuse and Neglect, 20*, 709–723.

Silverman, M. M., Berman, A. L., Sanddal, N. D., O'Carroll, P. W., & Joiner, T. E. (2007). Rebuilding the Tower of Babel: A revised nomenclature for the study of suicide and suicidal behaviors part 2: Suicide-related ideations, communications, and behaviors. *Suicide and Life-Threatening Behavior, 37*, 264–277.

Smith, J. M., Alloy, L. B., & Abramson, L. Y. (2006). Cognitive vulnerability to depression, rumination, hopelessness, and suicidal ideation: Multiple pathways to self-injurious thinking. *Suicide and Life-Threatening Behavior, 36*, 443–454.

Smokowski, P. R., Rose, R., & Bacallao, M. L. (2008). Acculturation and Latino family processes: How cultural involvement, biculturalism, and acculturation gaps influence family dynamics. *Family Relations, 57*, 295–308.

Spirito, A., Esposito-Smythers, C., Wolff, J., & Uhl, K. (2011). Cognitive-behavioral therapy for adolescent depression and suicidality. *Child and Adolescent Psychiatric Clinics of North America, 20*, 191–204.

Stanley, B., & Brown, G. K. (2012). Safety planning intervention: A brief intervention to mitigate suicide risk. *Cognitive and Behavioral Practice, 19*, 256–264.

Stanley, B., Brown, G., Brent, D. A., Wells, K., Poling, K., Curry, J., . . . Hughes, J. (2009). Cognitive-behavioral therapy for suicide prevention (CBT-SP): Treatment model, feasibility, and acceptability. *Journal of the American Academy of Child and Adolescent Psychiatry, 48*, 1005–1013.

Stein, D., Apter, A., Ratzoni, G., Har-Even, D., & Avidan, G. (1998). Association between multiple suicide attempts and negative affects in adolescents. *Journal of the American Academy of Child and Adolescent Psychiatry, 37*, 488–494.

Steinhausen, H. C., Bosiger, R., & Metzke, C. W. (2006). Stability, correlates, and outcome of adolescent suicidal risk. *Journal of Child Psychology and Psychiatry, 47*, 713–722.

Steinhausen, H. C., & Metzke, C. W. (2004). The impact of suicidal ideation in preadolescence, adolescence, and young adulthood on psychosocial functioning and psychopathology in young adulthood. *Acta Psychiatrica Scandinavica, 110*, 438–445.

Suominen, K., Isometsä, E., Ostamo, A., & Lönnqvist, J. (2004). Level of suicidal intent predicts overall mortality and suicide after attempted suicide: A 12-year follow-up study. *BMC Psychiatry, 4*, 11.

Tarrier, N., Taylor, K., & Gooding, P. (2008). Cognitive-behavioral interventions to reduce suicide behavior: A systematic review and meta-analysis. *Behavior Modification, 32*, 77–108.

Taussig, H. N., Harpin, S. B., & Maguire, S. A. (2014). Suicidality among preadolescent maltreated children in foster care. *Child Maltreatment, 19*, 17–26.

Ten Have, M., van Dorsselaer, S., & de Graaf, R. (2013). Prevalence and risk factors for first onset of suicidal behaviors in the Netherlands Mental Health Survey and Incidence Study-2. *Journal of Affective Disorders, 147*, 205–211.

Tobler, A. L., Maldonado-Molina, M. M., Staras, S. A., O'Mara, R. J., Livingston, M. D., & Komro, K. A. (2013). Perceived racial/ethnic discrimination, problem behaviors, and mental health among minority urban youth. *Ethnicity and Health, 18*, 337–349.

Turecki, G. (2014). Epigenetics and suicidal behavior research pathways. *American Journal of Preventive Medicine, 47*, S144–S151.

Van Orden, K. A., Witte, T. K., Cukrowicz, K. C., Braithwaite, S., Selby, E. A., & Joiner, T. E. (2010). The interpersonal theory of suicide. *Psychological Review, 117*, 575–600.

Wenzel, A., & Beck, A. T. (2008). A cognitive model of suicidal behavior: Theory and treatment. *Applied and Preventive Psychology, 12,* 189–201.

Wichstrøm, L. (2000). Predictors of adolescent suicide attempts: A nationally representative longitudinal study of Norwegian adolescents. *Journal of the American Academy of Child and Adolescent Psychiatry, 39,* 603–610.

Wichstrøm, L., & Rossow, I. (2002). Explaining the gender difference in self-reported suicide attempts: A nationally representative study of Norwegian adolescents. *Suicide and Life-Threatening Behavior, 32,* 101–116.

Williams, J. M. G., Mathews, A., & MacLeod, C. (1996). The emotional Stroop task and psychopathology. *Psychological Bulletin, 120,* 3–24.

Witte, T. K., Joiner, T. E., Brown, G. K., Beck, A. T., Beckman, A., Duberstein, P., & Conwell, Y. (2006). Factors of suicidal ideation and their relation to clinical and other indicators in older adults. *Journal of Affective Disorders, 94,* 165–172.

World Health Organization (WHO). (2012). *Mental health. Suicide data.* Retrieved from http://www.who.int/mental_health/prevention/suicide/suicideprevent/en/

Wu, P., Katic, B. J., Liu, X., Fan, B., & Fuller, C. J. (2010). Mental health service use among suicidal adolescents: Findings from a US national community survey. *Psychiatric Services, 61,* 17–24.

Wunderlich, U., Bronisch, T., Wittchen, H. U., & Carter, R. (2001). Gender differences in adolescents and young adults with suicidal behaviour. *Acta Psychiatrica Scandinavica, 104,* 332–339.

Yen, S., Shea, M. T., Sanislow, C. A., Skodol, A. E., Grilo, C. M., Edelen, M. O., . . . Gunderson, J. G. (2009). Personality traits as prospective predictors of suicide attempts. *Acta Psychiatrica Scandinavica, 120,* 222–229.

Zalsman, G., Frisch, A., Bromberg, M., Gelernter, J., Michaelovsky, E., Campino, A., . . . & Weizman, A. (2001). Family based association study of serotonin transporter promoter in suicidal adolescents: No association with suicidality but possible role in violence traits. *American Journal of Medical Genetics, 105,* 239–245.

Zayas, L. H., Lester, R. J., Cabassa, L. J., & Fortuna, L. R. (2005). Why do so many Latina teens attempt suicide? A conceptual model for research. *American Journal of Orthopsychiatry, 75,* 275–287.

CHAPTER 11

Interrelationship of Suicidality with Depressive Disorders and Its Implications for Suicide Prevention Strategies at the Population and Individual Levels

Beth Han, MD, PhD, MPH
Wilson M. Compton, MD, MPE
Richard McKeon, PhD, MPH

Suicide is a major public health problem in the United States. Despite frequent misclassification and underreporting (Rockett, 2010), it was the tenth leading cause of death in the United States (American Foundation for Suicide Prevention, 2016; US Department of Health and Human Services, 2012). In 2013, there were approximately 41,149 reported deaths by suicide in the United States. Suicide costs the United States more than $34.6 billion a year in combined medical and work loss costs (Centers of Disease Control and Prevention [CDC], 2015). Also in 2013, 9.3 million adults aged 18 or older had serious thoughts of suicide (suicidal ideation) in the previous 12 months, 2.7 million made a suicide plan, and 1.3 million attempted suicide (Substance Abuse and Mental Health Services Administration [SAMHSA], 2014). Among persons aged 15–54, approximately 60% of planned first suicide attempts occurred within the first year of having the onset of suicidal ideation (Kessler, Borges, & Walters, 1999). Furthermore, a suicide attempt history is the strongest known clinical predictor of death by suicide (US Department of Health and Human Services, 2012). The overall annual suicide rate in the United States increased from 10.4 per 100,000 persons in 2000 to 13.0 per 100,000 persons in 2013 (CDC, 2015).

To improve the effectiveness of detecting and intervening with people at high risk of suicide, it is critical to better understand and modify specific risk factors associated with suicidality. Importantly, the presence of depressive disorders is one of the strongest risk factors for suicidal ideation (Borges et al., 2006; Conner et al., 2007; Han, Compton, Gfroerer, & McKeon, 2015a; Han, McKeon, & Gfroerer, 2014a; Joe, Baser, Breeden, Neighbors, & Jackson, 2006; Kessler et al., 1999; Nock, Hwang, Sampson, & Kessler, 2010), suicide attempt (Bolton & Robinson, 2010; Borges et al., 2006; Joe et al., 2006; Kessler et al., 1999; Nock et al., 2010; Nock et al., 2013), and death by suicide (Cavanagh, Carson, Sharpe, & Lawrie, 2003; Finkelstein et al., 2015; Harris & Barraclough, 1997).

Depressive disorders are common in the United States. Using data from 9,282 respondents aged 18 or older who participated in the National Comorbidity Survey Replication (NCS-R, nationally representative data on the prevalence of *DSM-IV* disorders among the US adult population), Kessler and colleagues (2005a, 2009) estimated that the prevalence of major depressive disorder (MDD) for lifetime was 16.6% and for 12 months was 6.7%; dysthymia for lifetime was 2.5% and for 12 months was 1.5%; bipolar I or II for lifetime was 3.9% and for 12 months was 2.6%; and any mood disorder for lifetime was 20.8% and for 12 months was 9.5%.

Also based on the NCS-R data, Kessler and colleagues (2005b) estimated that among respondents with 12-month suicidal ideation, 61.0% had a mood disorder in the past year, including 38.9% for 12-month MDD, 8.0% for 12-month dysthymia, and 22.1% for 12-month bipolar I or II disorders. Among respondents with 12-month suicide plan, 83.1% had a mood disorder in the past year, including 51.3% for 12-month MDD, 12.10% for 12-month dysthymia, and 31.8% for 12-month bipolar I or II disorders. Among respondents with 12-month suicide attempt, 69.9% had a mood disorder in the past year, including 38.9% for 12-month MDD, 7.4% for 12-month dysthymia, and 31.0% for 12-month bipolar I or II disorders.

Because depressive disorders are widely distributed in the US population and because suicidality is common among individuals with depressive disorders, it is critical to understand the complex interrelationship of suicidality with depressive disorders. Importantly, knowing the complex interrelation will help us draw its implications for suicide prevention strategies at the population and individual levels. We subsequently review data on the relationship of depressive disorders with different aspects of suicidality: ideation, overall attempts, attempts among those with and without a suicide plan, and death by suicide.

Interrelationship of Suicidal Ideation with Depressive Disorders

Since targeted suicide prevention and treatment strategies focus on populations at risk for suicide, suicide risk assessments usually begin after having evidence of suicidal ideation (Mann et al., 2005; US Department of Health and Human Services, 2012). Many studies have consistently shown strong associations between depressive disorders and suicidal ideation (Borges et al., 2006; Han et al., 2014a; Kessler et al., 1999; Nock et al., 2010).

Based on the data from 5,877 respondents aged 15–54 who participated in the National Comorbidity Survey (NCS, a nationally representative population survey carried out from 1990 to 1992), Kessler and colleagues (1999) estimated that the lifetime prevalence of suicidal ideation was 13.5%. After controlling for person-year, sociodemographic factors, and individual lifetime *DSM-III-R* disorders, those with lifetime dysthymia and those with lifetime major depressive episode (MDE) were 7.7–9.6 (adjusted odds ratios [AORs] = 7.7–9.6) times more likely to have subsequent first onset of suicidal ideation than those without the corresponding disorder. AOR is a statistical tool that quantifies how strongly property A is associated with property B in a given population after controlling for covariates. MDE was defined using diagnostic criteria in the *DSM-III-R*, specifying that at least five symptoms must be present during the same two-week period and must present a change from previous functioning. At least one of the symptoms must be either depressed mood or loss of interest.

Using the data from 5,692 persons aged 18 or older who participated in the NCS-R, Borges and colleagues (2006) examined the associations between individual 12-month mental disorders and 12-month suicidal ideation. After controlling for sociodemographics, respondents' history of prior suicidal behavior, parental psychopathology, and individual 12-month *DSM-IV* disorders, they found that adults with 12-month dysthymic disorder, MDD, and bipolar disorder were 6.2–9.6 (AORs = 6.2–9.6) times more likely to have 12-month suicidal ideation than adults without the corresponding disorder. Using the same dataset, Nock and colleagues (2010) examined the associations between individual lifetime mental disorders and subsequent first occurrence of suicidal ideation. After adjusting for age, age-squared, age cohort, sex, person-year, and individual lifetime *DSM-IV* disorders, they found that adults with lifetime bipolar disorder or lifetime MDD were 2.2–2.3 (AORs = 2.2–2.3) times more likely to have subsequent first onset of suicidal ideation than adults without the corresponding disorder.

Based on data from 183,100 persons aged 18 years or older (including 9,800 sampled adults with past-year suicidal ideation) who participated in the 2008–2011 National Survey on Drug Use and Health (NSDUH), Han and colleagues (2014a) found that the 12-month prevalence of suicidal ideation was 26.3% among adults with a 12-month MDE. By contrast, it was 2.1% among adults without an MDE in the past 12 months. NSDUHs are a series of annual, cross-sectional, nationally representative surveys of the US civilian, noninstitutionalized population aged 12 years or older conducted by the SAMHSA (SAMHSA, 2014). In the NSDUHs, the 12-month prevalence of suicidal ideation showed an age-related gradation: 6.6% among those aged 18–25 years, 4.0% among those aged 26–49 years, and 2.5% among adults aged 50 years or older.

Han and colleagues (2014a) also found that factors associated with 12-month suicidal ideation varied by age and 12-month MDE status. MDE was defined using diagnostic criteria stipulated in the *DSM-IV*, which specified a period of two weeks or longer during which there is either depressed mood or loss of interest or pleasure and at least four other symptoms that reflect a change in functioning, such as problems with sleep, eating, energy, concentration, and self-image. Those aged 50 or older who had 12-month MDE were 4.3 (AOR = 4.3) times more likely to have 12-month suicidal ideation than their age counterparts without MDE. Moreover, those aged 18–49 who had 12-month MDE were 5.4–6.4 (AORs = 5.4–6.4) times more likely to have 12-month suicidal ideation than others in their age group without MDE. Moreover, adults aged 18–49 who had 12-month MDE were more likely to have 12-month suicidal ideation than their counterparts aged 50 or older.

Interrelationship of Suicide Attempt with Depressive Disorders

Several studies have consistently found that depressive disorders were highly prevalent among suicide attempters and were associated with increased risk for suicide attempt (Bolton & Robinson, 2010; Kessler et al., 1999; Korczak & Goldstein, 2009; Nock et al., 2010; Nock et al., 2013). Based on data from the 1991–1992 National Longitudinal Alcohol Epidemiologic Survey (n = 42,862) and the 2001–2002 National Epidemiologic Survey on Alcohol and Related Conditions (NESARC, n = 43,093), Baca-Garcia and colleagues (2010) estimated that the lifetime prevalence of suicide attempt was 2.4% among adults aged 18 or older in the United States. Using data from 6,778 respondents aged 18 or older who had MDD and participated in the 2001–2002 NESARC, Korczak and Goldstein (2009) found that childhood onset (i.e., prior to age 13) of MDD was associated with a greater number of MDD episodes, longer episode duration, and an increased risk for lifetime suicide attempt.

Based on data from the 6,483 adolescents aged 13–18 who participated in the National Comorbidity Survey Replication–Adolescent Supplement, Nock and colleagues (2013) found that the lifetime prevalence of suicide attempt among youths was 4.1%. Among youths with lifetime suicide attempts, the lifetime prevalence of MDD or dysthymia was 75.5%. Moreover, youths with MDD or dysthymia were 6.2 (AOR = 6.2) times more likely to have first onset of suicide attempt than their counterparts without the corresponding disorder (Nock et al., 2013).

Based on the NCS data, Kessler and colleagues (1999) estimated that the lifetime prevalence of suicide attempt among persons aged 15–54 was 4.6%. After controlling for person-year, sociodemographic factors, and individual lifetime *DSM-III* disorders, they found that those with lifetime dysthymia and those with lifetime MDE were 7.8–11.0 (AORs = 7.8–11.0; n = 272) times more likely to have subsequent first onset of suicide attempt than those without the corresponding mood disorder.

Using the NCS-R data, Nock and colleagues (2010) examined the associations between individual lifetime mental disorders and subsequent first occurrence of suicide attempt among adults aged 18 or older. After adjusting for age, age-squared, age cohort, sex, person-year, and individual lifetime *DSM-IV* disorders, they found that adults with MDD and adults with bipolar disorder were 2.0–2.3 (AORs = 2.0–2.3; n = 5692) times more likely to have subsequent first onset of suicide attempt than those without the corresponding mood disorder.

Using the data from 34,653 respondents aged 20 or older who participated in the 2004–2005 NESARC, Bolton and Robinson (2010) examined the population-attributable fraction (PAF, also known as the population-attributable risk) of *DSM-IV*

Axis I and Axis II disorders for suicide attempt. PAF is a statistical tool used to better quantify the effect of risk factors on a given outcome at the population level. After adjusting for sociodemographic factors, physical disability, physical diseases, and individual lifetime *DSM-IV* disorders, the highest proportion of suicide attempts was attributable to MDD, which independently accounted for 26.6% of all suicide attempts in the sample (PAF = 26.6%). Bipolar I and dysthymic disorder each independently accounted for 1.6% and 2.9% (PAFs = 1.6–2.9%, respectively) of all suicide attempts in the sample. Additionally, borderline personality disorder, nicotine dependence, and posttraumatic stress disorder were the other disorders that accounted for substantial proportions of the suicide attempts (PAF = 18.1%, 8.4%, and 6.3%, respectively).

In summary, these studies consistently suggest the interrelationship of suicide attempt with depressive disorders. Depressive disorders are highly prevalent among suicide attempters and are associated with increased risk for suicide attempt. People with MDD or MDE are often more likely to attempt suicide than those without the corresponding mood disorder.

Interrelationship of Suicide Attempt with Depressive Disorders among Ideators with a Suicide Plan

Having a suicide plan is considered a psychiatric emergency because it is related to an imminent lethal attempt and high suicide risk (Coryell & Young, 2005; Han et al., 2015a; Nakagawa et al., 2009). The theoretical continuum of risk for attempting suicide, beginning with passive suicidal ideation (desire for death) or active suicidal ideation, then progressing to suicide plan, and eventually to suicide attempt, is not always supported by empirical data (Baca-Garcia et al., 2011). Many people attempt suicide without a suicide plan. In 2013, although 1.1 million adults reported planning and attempting suicide, about 20% (0.2 million) reported attempting suicide without a suicide plan (SAMHSA, 2014). To reduce suicide risk, it is important to understand how factors triggering the progression from suicide plan to suicide attempt differ from factors triggering the transition from suicidal ideation directly to suicide attempt (Han et al., 2015a; Nock et al., 2010).

After controlling for person-year, sociodemographic factors, and individual lifetime *DSM-III-R* disorders, Kessler and colleagues (1999) found that among persons aged 15–54 who had a suicide plan (n = 127), those with lifetime dysthymia and those with lifetime MDE were 1.8–2.1 (AORs = 1.8–2.1) times more likely to have subsequent first onset of suicide attempt than those without the corresponding mood disorder. However, this result is inconsistent with the recent study result by Nock and colleagues (2010).

Based on the NCS-R data, Nock and colleagues (2010) examined the associations between individual lifetime mental disorders and subsequent first occurrence of suicide attempt among adult suicide ideators with a plan (n = 504). After adjusting for age, age-squared, age cohort, sex, person-year, and individual lifetime *DSM-IV* disorders, they found that adults with lifetime bipolar disorder were 2.2 (AOR = 2.2) times more likely to have subsequent first onset of suicide attempt than those without bipolar disorder. Neither lifetime MDD nor lifetime dysthymia was associated with subsequent first onset of planned suicide attempt among suicidal ideators aged 18 or older. In contrast, lifetime anxiety disorders and impulse-control disorders were associated with subsequent first onset of planned suicide attempt among adult suicidal ideators.

Han and colleagues (2015a) examined data from 229,600 persons aged 18 years or older who participated in the 2008–2012 NSDUHs, including 12,300 sampled adults with past-year suicidal ideation and 2,000 sampled adults with past-year suicide attempt. They found that among past-year suicidal ideators, 13.2% attempted suicide in the past 12 months. The 12-month prevalence of suicide attempt among past-year suicidal ideators with 12-month MDE was higher than among their counterparts without 12-month MDE (14.1% vs. 12.0%). Moreover, the 12-month prevalence of suicide attempt was more common among ideators with a 12-month suicide plan than among ideators without a 12-month suicide plan (37.0% vs. 3.7%). The 12-month prevalence of suicide attempt was higher among ideators with a plan but without MDE than among ideators with a plan and MDE (42.1% vs. 32.9%).

Furthermore, after adjusting for sociodemographic factors, self-rated health, substance use disorders, and the number of times a participant was arrested or booked in the past year, adult suicidal ideators with a plan and MDE were less likely to have 12-month suicide attempt than their counterparts with a plan but without MDE (Han et al., 2015a). The presence of a suicide plan was a more important predictor of a suicide attempt than MDE itself. Additionally, their multivariate results revealed that 12-month hallucinogen use and hallucinogen use disorders were associated with increased risk for 12-month suicide attempt among adult suicidal ideators with a plan. These results confirmed the previous findings by Nock and colleagues (2010) that major depression may not trigger further progression from ideation to plan and attempt and highlighted the important role that suicide planning plays during the dangerous behavioral progression among some adult suicide ideators.

Interrelationship of Suicide Attempt with Depressive Disorders among Ideators without a Suicide Plan

Based on the NCS data, after controlling for person-year, sociodemographic factors, and individual lifetime *DSM-III* disorders, Kessler and colleagues (1999) found that among persons aged 15–54 who did not have a suicide plan (n = 145), those with lifetime MDE were 1.9 (AOR = 1.9) times more likely to have subsequent first onset of suicide attempt than those without MDE. Again, this result was also inconsistent with the recent study results by Nock and colleagues (2010).

Using the NCS-R data, Nock and colleagues (2010) examined the associations between individual lifetime mental disorders and subsequent first occurrence of suicide attempt among adult suicide ideators without a plan (n = 842). After adjusting for age, age-squared, age cohort, sex, person-year, and individual lifetime *DSM-IV* disorders, they found that none of the lifetime mood disorders (MDD, dysthymia, and bipolar disorders) were associated with subsequent first onset of unplanned suicide attempt among suicidal ideators aged 18 or older. In contrast, lifetime impulse-control disorder, posttraumatic stress disorder, and alcohol use disorders were associated with subsequent first onset of unplanned suicide attempt.

Han and colleagues (2015a) investigated the associations between 12-month MDE and 12-month suicide attempt among adult suicidal ideators without a plan (n = 8,600). After adjusting for sociodemographic factors, self-rated health, substance use disorders, and the number of times a participant was arrested or booked in the past year, they found that among adult suicidal ideators without a plan, MDE was not associated with 12-month suicide attempt. Instead, their multivariate results also revealed that 12-month alcohol use and alcohol use disorders were associated with increased risk for 12-month suicide attempt. Conner and colleagues (2007) also found that alcohol-related aggression was uniquely related to unplanned suicide attempt. These results were consistent with the findings by Nock and colleagues (2010) that major depression may not trigger further progression from suicidal ideation directly to suicide attempt.

In summary, many studies have consistently shown strong associations between depressive disorders and suicidal ideation (Borges et al., 2006; Han et al., 2014a; Kessler et al., 1999; Nock et al., 2010) as well as strong associations between depressive disorders and suicide attempt (Bolton & Robinson, 2010; Kessler et al., 1999; Korczak & Goldstein, 2009; Nock et al., 2010, 2013). The recent studies conducted by Nock and colleagues (2010) and Han and colleagues (2015a) further show that depressive disorders are associated with the development of suicidal ideation, while other disorders marked by agitation, aggressiveness, or impulse-control deficits rather than depressive disorders are associated with increased likelihood of "acting" on suicidal ideation (i.e., attempting suicide).

Interrelationship of Death by Suicide with Depressive Disorders

Suicidal ideators (those with ideation only), suicide attempters, and those who die by suicide may be three interrelated but distinct groups (Ginera et al., 2013; Molock et al., 2014; Smith, Cukrowicz, Poindexter, Hobson, & Cohen, 2010). Although factors associated with suicide attempt may differ from factors related to death by suicide (Ginera et al., 2013), MDD and other depressive syndromes were the most commonly identified Axis I diagnoses among individuals who die by suicide (Bostwick & Pankratz, 2000; Conwell et al., 1996; Henriksson et al., 1993; Sher, Oquendo, & Mann, 2001). For individuals with bipolar disorder, most deaths by suicide occurred during depressive episodes (Isometsa, Henriksson, Aro, & Lönnqvist, 1994; Rihmer, 2005;

Tondo, Isacsson, & Baldessarini, 2003). More than two-thirds of individuals who died by suicide had (mostly untreated) current MDE (Henriksson et al., 1993; Rihmer, 1996, 2005, 2007).

Based on 249 papers published between 1966 and 1993, Harris and Barraclough (1997) conducted a meta-analysis and found that individuals with dysthymia, bipolar disorder, and MDD had twelvefold to twentyfold increases in risk for death by suicide (standardized mortality ratios [SMRs] = 12.1–20.4). SMRs here reflect relative mortality from suicide among individuals with a particular mental disorder, compared with the general population. Although the suicide rate is greatest near the age of mental disorder onset, suicide risk persists throughout the illness course among people with bipolar disorder and MDD (Angst, Stassen, Clayton, & Angst, 2002). In older studies, the estimated lifetime suicide rate was 15.5% among those with bipolar disorder and 14.6% among those with MDD (Harris & Barraclough, 1997). However, these estimates have been revised downward in newer studies, primarily related to the severity of the cases included in the samples. For example, Inskip, Harris, and Barraclough (1998) reported that lifetime death by suicide rate among people with affective disorder was 6%. Blair-West, Mellsop, and Eyeson-Annan (1997) reported lifetime death by suicide rate was 3.5% among people with MDD if outpatients were taken into account in the estimation. The lifetime death by suicide rate was 2.2% among mixed inpatient and outpatient populations and was less than 0.5% among the nonaffectively ill population (Bostwick & Pankratz, 2000).

Risk for death by suicide increased among patients who were once hospitalized for mood disorders. Using longitudinal data from the Danish Psychiatric Case Register, Hoyer, Mortensen, and Olesen (2000) found that standardized mortality rates were comparable for patients with MDD and bipolar disorder (SMRs = 19.33 and 18.09, respectively). Based on longitudinal data from the Swedish Inpatient Register, Osby and colleagues (2001) found that SMRs were higher among women and patients with MDD (15.0 for male patients with bipolar disorder, 20.9 for male patients with MDD, 22.4 for female patients with bipolar disorder, and 27.0 for female patients with MDD). Among psychiatric patients, suicide risk was highest immediately after hospital or emergency department discharge (US Department of Health and Human Services, 2012).

Death by suicide is a complex, multicausal human behavior with biological, psychological, sociological, and cultural components. Although depressive disorders are consistently identified as a significant risk factor for suicide, other factors are likely to modify that risk, including psychiatric factors (e.g., specific type, severity, and duration of the mood disorder, treatment history, and other comorbid mental disorders characterized by agitation, aggression, and impulsiveness), biological factors (e.g., disruptions in the functioning of the inhibitory neurotransmitter serotonin, abnormal molecular and hormonal responses to stressful events, and altered expression of micro ribonucleic acids), psychosocial factors (e.g., the occurrence of stressful life events and lack of social support), and demographic factors (e.g., gender, sexual orientation, race, and education) (Denney et al., 2009; Nock et al., 2008; Rihmer, 2007; Sher et al., 2001; Turecki, 2014; Van Orden et al., 2010; Vyssoki et al., 2014). For example, the presence of severe anxiety or agitation is a major factor for death by suicide among individuals with depressive disorders. Among hospital dischargees who died by suicide, 79% had episodes of severe anxiety or agitation in the week prior to their suicide (Busch, Fawcett, & Jacobs, 2003). Ilgen and colleagues (2009) examined 887,859 Veterans Affairs health system patients treated for depression between 1999 and 2004, and identified the following characteristics of depressed patients who were at highest risk for death by suicide: co-occurring substance use disorder diagnosis, non–African American race, and past-year psychiatric hospitalization. Cherpitel, Borges, and Wilcox (2004) conducted a systematic review of the existing literature and found that a median of 37% of suicides and 40% of suicide attempts were preceded by alcohol use. A recent study found that suicide completers were more likely to be male and suffer from alcohol abuse, health problems (e.g., somatic illness), and narcissistic personality disorder compared with suicide attempters (Ginera et al., 2013).

Implications for Suicide Prevention Strategies at the Population and Individual Levels
Enhanced Receipt and Effectiveness of Mental Health Treatment for Depressive Disorders and Suicidality

Major depression is one of the most common mental disorders in the United States. In addition to suicidal ideation, attempt, and death by suicide, MDD is associated with significant disability, morbidity, and early mortality (Eaton et al., 2008), and is projected to become one of the three leading causes of global burden of disease by 2030 (Mathers & Loncar, 2006). MDD is costly to both individuals and society (Kessler, 2012). Although frequently diagnosed and treated in the primary care setting (Kessler et al., 2003), MDD is underdiagnosed and undertreated because many patients do not report depressive symptoms to their primary care physicians and many physicians do not screen for or recognize MDD in their patients (Mojtabai & Olfson, 2008; Unützer & Park, 2012). Based on NCS-R data, Kessler and colleagues (2003) found that among adults with 12-month MDD, 57.3% received some type of treatment in the past 12 months. They also found that treatment met criteria for being at least minimally adequate in 64.3% of cases in the specialty mental health sector and 41.3% of cases in the general medical sector (Kessler et al., 2003).

Also, using the NCS-R data, in addition to estimating 12-month mental health services received by adults with 12-month MDD, Wang and colleagues (2005) estimated that among adults with 12-month dysthymia, 67.5% received mental health services of some type in the past 12 months. Among adults with 12-month bipolar I or II disorders, 55.5% received some type of mental health treatment in the past year. Among adults with any 12-month mood disorder, 56.4% received mental health services of some type in the past 12 months. They found that only about 38.5% of adults with any 12-month mood disorder who received mental health services from the health care treatment sector in the past year met treatment criteria for at least minimally adequate care. Consequently, Wang and colleagues (2005) concluded that a majority of patients with mood disorders remained either untreated or poorly treated.

Recently, evidence-based collaborative programs, in which primary care providers work closely with special mental health providers, have been shown to be significantly more effective in treating MDD than usual primary care (Jacob et al., 2012; Olfson, Pincus, & Pardes, 2013; Thota et al., 2012; Unützer & Park, 2012). Moreover, based on results from a randomized controlled trial, Bruce and colleagues (2004) found that treatment guidelines tailored for the elderly with a care management intervention were effective in reducing suicidal ideation among depressed older primary care patients, regardless of their depression severity. In the intervention group, more than two-thirds of patients with suicidal ideation were no longer suicidal at four months of treatment, an improvement rate similar to the specialty mental health sector (Bruce et al., 2004). Similarly, Unützer and colleagues (2006) found that primary care–based collaborative care programs for depression significantly reduced suicidal ideation among older primary care patients. O'Connor and colleagues (2013) conducted a systematic review on screening for and treatment of suicide risk relevant to primary care and found that psychotherapy may reduce suicide attempts in some high-risk adults. These results highlighted the critical role of primary care intervention as a prevention strategy to reduce suicide risk.

Aspirational Goal 4 of the National Action Alliance for Suicide Prevention's Research Prioritization Task Force (2014) is to ensure that people at risk for suicide receive effective psychosocial interventions and medications. Brown and Jager-Hyman (2014) conducted a brief review of the science of psychotherapeutic interventions for suicide prevention and found the following psychotherapies effective for preventing suicide attempts among adults: cognitive therapy for suicide prevention, cognitive behavioral therapy, dialectical behavior therapy, problem-solving therapy, mentalization-based treatment, and psychodynamic interpersonal therapy. For example, a recent study found a lower risk of repeated deliberate self-harm and general mortality in recipients of psychosocial therapy after short-term and long-term follow-up, and a protective effect for suicide after long-term follow-up, indicating the effect of psychosocial therapy interventions after deliberate self-harm (Erlangsen et al., 2015)

The role of pharmacotherapy is also important in suicide prevention. There is reasonably strong evidence that lithium may reduce the risk of suicide among patients with bipolar disorder (Bowden, 2003; Oquendo et al., 2011), and discontinuation of lithium contributing to increased risk for suicidal behavior in bipolar disorder (Goodwin et al., 2003; Yerevanian, Koek, & Mintz, 2003, 2007). The role of antidepressants in suicide prevention is controversial. Certain antidepressant medications, the selective serotonin reuptake inhibitors, may be related to a reduced risk of suicide among depressed adults aged 26 or older, but it may increase suicide risk among children, adolescents, and young adults (Bridge et al., 2007; Gibbons, Hur, Bhaumik, & Mann, 2006; Olfson, Marcus, & Shaffer, 2006; Simon, Savarino, Operskalski, & Wang, 2006).

Importantly, treating depressive disorders and other underlying conditions may not always remove suicide risk. Achieving the goal of suicide prevention is improved when treatments for the underlying conditions are combined with strategies addressing suicide risk directly (US Department of Health and Human Services, 2012).

Focused Suicide Prevention during High-Risk Time Periods

Among psychiatric patients, suicide risk was highest immediately after hospital discharge (US Department of Health and Human Services, 2012). Based on data from 1979 to 1986 from a population-based study in the United Kingdom, Goldacre, Seagroatt, and Hawton (1993) found that more than one-third (38%) of all suicides in the first year following psychiatric hospital discharge occurred in the first 28 days. Among a national sample from England and Wales (1996–1998), of those who died by suicide within 12 months of contact with mental health services and who were psychiatric inpatients, about 23% of the suicides occurred in the first week after admission, and approximately 40% of the suicides occurred when discharge was being planned (Appleby et al., 1999).

A recent observational study found that after the implementation of mental health service recommendations (including a seven-day follow-up after psychiatric hospital discharge) in England and Wales, the suicide rate declined from 24.8 to 19.5 per 100,000 persons (While et al., 2012). Moreover, a significant reduction in death by suicide was found in Taiwan after that country implemented a nationwide aftercare program for suicide attempters (Pan et al., 2013). In contrast, in the United States, only about half of psychiatric inpatients received outpatient mental health care during the first week following hospital discharge, and only about two-thirds received mental health care during the first month (Olfson, Marcus, & Bridge, 2014). Furthermore, a recent study based on the 2008–2012 NSDUH data revealed that approximately half of past-year suicide attempters who received mental health treatment perceived unmet treatment needs, indicating that they might have received insufficient care (Han, Compton, Gfroerer, & McKeon, 2014b). Brown and Green (2014) conducted a review of evidence-based follow-up care for suicide prevention and found that clinicians who reached out to patients using caring letters to express concern and support may help to reduce the rate of suicide following discharge from a psychiatric hospital.

These results reinforce that more follow-up and continuity of suicide-specific mental health treatment are needed among psychiatric patients and patients with suicidal ideation or behavior. This notion is emphasized in the 2012 National Strategy for Suicide Prevention (US Department of Health and Human Services, 2012) and Aspirational

Goal 9 of the National Action Alliance for Suicide Prevention's Research Prioritization Task Force (2014). In addition, continuity of care is important to strengthen patient connectedness and reduce social isolation through a collaborative engagement approach among patients, outpatient mental health providers, community organizations, and supportive family members (Olfson et al., 2014; US Department of Health and Human Services, 2012).

Improved Clinical Insight and Greater Help-seeking and Mental Health Treatment among Individuals with Depressive Disorders and Suicidal Ideation or Behavior

Based on the 2008–2011 NSDUH data, Han and colleagues (2014a) found that among community-dwelling adults with 12-month suicidal ideation in the United States, less than half (48.5%) received mental health treatment at some point in the past 12 months. While 12.8% of suicidal ideators did not receive treatment but perceived unmet treatment need, 38.1% of adults with suicidal ideation neither received mental health treatment nor perceived unmet treatment need. Based on the 2008–2012 NSDUH data, Han and colleagues (2014b) found that among community-dwelling adults with 12-month suicide attempt in the United States, only 56.3% received mental health treatment at some point during the past year. Over one-third of past 12-month suicide attempters neither receive mental health treatment nor perceived unmet treatment need. Based on the NCS-R data, Kessler and colleagues (2005b) also estimated that among 12-month suicidal ideators, 43.9% received mental health treatment at some point during the past year. And among 12-month suicide attempters in the United States, 61.3% received mental health treatment at some point during the past year.

Thus, efforts are needed to promote effective public awareness programs about mental disorders, suicidal ideation and behavior, and mental health treatment in such diverse settings as schools, universities, workplaces, emergency departments, primary care settings, specialty substance use treatment facilities, the criminal justice system, mental health clinics, and American Indian reservations (Caine, 2013; Han et al., 2014b). Among suicidal individuals, the lack of clinical insight or low awareness of perceived need for mental health treatment might contribute to their low prevalence of receipt of mental health treatment (Han et al., 2014b). Consequently, these suicidal adults do not recognize the warning signs for needing mental health treatment. Lack of insight may stem from a combination of primary symptoms, neurocognitive deficits, and cognitive style, which is associated with treatment nonadherence (Williams, Olfson, & Galanter, 2015). Amador and David (1998) summarized five core components of insight: awareness of having a disorder, awareness of symptoms, attribution of symptoms to the disorder, recognizing the consequences of symptoms, and appreciation of need for treatment. It is essential for suicidal adults to understand these components and understand that effective mental health treatment is available

(Bruce et al., 2004; Unützer et al., 2006; US Department of Health and Human Services, 2012).

Awareness programs and outreach efforts must be culturally and linguistically appropriate to effectively promote seeking help among minority suicidal individuals (Range et al., 1999). Sociocultural norms, which can either facilitate or inhibit suicidal behavior or death by suicide (Orbach, 1997), may be related to receipt of mental health treatment among suicidal individuals. For example, Han and colleagues (2014b) found that among 12-month suicide attempters who did not perceive unmet need, non-Hispanic blacks were less likely to receive mental health treatment in the past year than non-Hispanic whites. Among 12-month suicide attempters who did not receive medical attention resulting from a suicide attempt, Hispanics and non-Hispanic blacks were less likely to receive mental health treatment in the past year than non-Hispanic whites.

Even among suicide attempters who perceived unmet need for mental health treatment but did not receive treatment, almost half reported that they could not afford the treatment costs, and almost 30% did not know where to go for treatment (Han et al., 2014b). These results were consistent with findings from recent studies on barriers to mental health treatment reported by suicidal hotline callers in the United States (Gould, Munfakh, Kleinman, & Lake, 2012) and on low acceptance rates for all health insurance types by psychiatrists compared with other specialty physicians (Bishop, Press, Keyhani, & Pincus, 2014).

Significant policy changes with the potential to increase access to mental health treatment since 2008 may influence future mental health treatment–seeking patterns among individuals with depressive disorders and suicidality. First, the Mental Health Parity and Addiction Equity Act of 2008 required any group health plan that covers more than 50 employees and offers mental health and substance use disorders coverage to provide that coverage with no greater financial requirements (i.e., co-pays, deductibles, annual or lifetime dollar limits) or treatment limitations (i.e., number of visits) than those requirements the plan applies to its medical and surgical benefits (US Department of Health and Human Services, 2013). Second, the Medicare Improvements for Patients and Providers Act of 2008 addressed the inequity of a 50% copayment by beneficiaries for Part B outpatient psychiatric services, compared with a 20% copayment for general medical care (US Government Printing Office, 2008). Third, under the Medicaid expansion and insurance exchange programs of the Affordable Care Act of 2010, some uninsured individuals with depressive disorders and suicidality might be eligible for Medicaid or private insurance enrollment (Han et al., 2015b). Fourth, starting in 2011 (for generic drugs) and 2013 (for brand-name drugs), the Affordable Care Act reduced the amount that Medicare Part D enrollees were required to pay for their prescriptions when they reached the coverage gap between the initial coverage limit and the catastrophic-coverage threshold (Centers for Medicare and Medicaid Services, 2008). Aspirational Goal 8 of the National Action Alliance for

Suicide Prevention's Research Prioritization Task Force (2014) is to ensure that people at risk for suicidal risk can access affordable care that works, no matter where they are. Future studies are needed to continue to monitor mental health treatment patterns among adults with depressive disorders and suicidal ideation or behavior as the aforementioned health care reforms are more fully implemented.

To identify and treat individuals with high suicide risk, it is also critical to improve the knowledge, attitudes, and practice of health care providers. This is consistent with Aspirational Goal 7 of the National Action Alliance for Suicide Prevention's Research Prioritization Task Force (2014), which states that health care providers and others in the community must be well trained in how to find and treat those at risk of suicide. Patients with high suicide risk are not uncommon in clinical practice. However, suicidal individuals frequently present with somatic complaints and may not talk about their suicidal ideation, plan, or attempt unless asked directly. Moreover, Betz and colleagues (2013) found that many providers did not feel that they had the skills to assess the severity of suicide risk, provide counseling, or even refer patients appropriately to specialty services. In Sweden, systematic education and training of primary care providers in the detection and treatment of depression on the island of Gotland resulted in fewer suicides among women compared with other regions of Sweden (Rutz, von Knorring, Pihlgren, Rihmer, & Walinder, 1995; Rutz, von Knorring, & Walinder, 1989). Additionally, a suicide prevention program implemented in the US Air Force focused on increasing gatekeeper training for suicide prevention and improving treatment of depression by primary care physicians reduced suicide rates (Knox, Litts, Talcott, Feig, & Caine, 2003).

Using an objective and improved assessment of suicide risk may increase precision in diagnosis, treatment, and prediction of risk and may help clinicians monitor suicidal behavior (Boudreaux & Horowitz, 2014; Hughes, 2011). For example, the Columbia–Suicide Severity Rating Scale (C-SSRS), designed to quantify the severity of suicidal ideation and behavior, has been found to be a suitable assessment tool. C-SSRS demonstrated good convergent and divergent validity with high sensitivity and specificity for suicidal behavior classifications (Posner et al., 2011). In addition, the *DSM-5* has a suicide assessment procedure for the use of clinicians in section III of the manual, which may increase the clinician's attention to suicide risk assessment (Fawcett, 2013).

Enhanced Focus on Public Health Prevention, Strengthened Resiliency, and Well-Being of the Population

Preventing suicide is everyone's business and can be successful (US Department of Health and Human Services, 2012). A comprehensive approach that addresses individual, family and peer, community, and societal-level factors can lead to a sustained decline in suicide rates and other adverse outcomes. One such program implemented by the US Air Force (Knox et al., 2003) included public awareness campaigns designed to alert the community to the issues of mental illness as well as to available prevention and treatment resources. Moreover, the US Air Force effort trained clinicians to better identify and treat mental disorders, and provided programs to promote individual social connectedness and coping skills. Knox and colleagues (2013) observed a 33% reduction in relative risk for death by suicide after the implementation of this comprehensive approach.

Consistent with Aspirational Goal 11 of the National Action Alliance for Suicide Prevention's Research Prioritization Task Force (2014), it is critical to develop and deliver prevention programs that can build resilience through social connections and reduce risk in broad-based populations. An earlier study found that adolescents with consistent and healthy attachments to family and school were less likely to have suicidal ideation and suicide attempts (Borowsky, Ireland, & Resnick, 2001). Additionally, school-based prevention programs targeting risk factors such as delinquency, depression, and substance use showed reductions in hopelessness, suicidal ideation, and suicide attempts (Wilcox et al., 2008). Moreover, a recent study found that women who were socially well integrated had a more than threefold lower risk for suicide after 18 years of follow-up (Tsai, Lucas, & Kawachi, 2015). More research is needed to better understand how individual social integration affects a person's mindset when he or she is suicidal (Caine, 2015). Furthermore, although adults with full-time employment are at lower risk for suicidal ideation and suicide attempt, the utility of workplace prevention and intervention programs should not be ignored because they represent more than one-fourth of adult suicide attempters (annual average based on the 2008–2012 NSDUH data) in the United States (Colpe & Pringle, 2014).

In addition to helping foster a sense of connection and belonging, community-based programs need to promote effective coping skills and provide critically needed services. For people with a history of suicide attempt, religious belief and practice, companionship, and a social network of family and peers were the main coping strategies (Alexander, Haugland, Ashenden, Knight, & Brown, 2009). Spirituality and religion were associated with access to social supports, resilience to stress, emotional stability, and low suicide risk (Rasic et al., 2009). Higher score on moral or religious objections to suicide was associated with fewer suicidal acts in depressed bipolar patients (Dervic et al., 2011). In addition, prevention programs are needed to deal with fundamental factors, such as family turmoil, employment adversity, and serious medical comorbidities, which may precede suicidal ideation.

Although many settings focus on detecting and managing imminent or short-term suicide risk, it is essential from a public health perspective to detect and manage lifetime risk. It is critical to reduce the prevalence of adversities that drive human vulnerabilities toward distress and disease. For example, results from a recent meta-analysis found that individuals who experienced early emotional or physical childhood abuse were three times more likely to attempt suicide (Norman et al., 2012). In addition, studies showed that interpersonal violence was associated with death by suicide and other adverse outcomes (Conner et al., 2001; Webb et al., 2011). To reduce suicide risk, it is important to mitigate, reduce, and prevent child abuse and neglect as well as interpersonal violence in the United States.

Government agencies at all levels, schools, not-for-profit organizations, and businesses have initiated programs and public awareness campaigns to address suicide risk. For example, SAMHSA's National Suicide Prevention Lifeline program, a toll-free suicide prevention hotline that provides free and confidential crisis counseling to anyone anytime, encourages timely treatment-seeking, particularly among suicidal ideators (Gould et al., 2012; Han et al., 2014a). The Garrett Lee Smith Memorial Act, focusing on persons aged 10–24 in states, tribes, and colleges, has funded numerous suicide prevention programs since 2005 (Goldston et al., 2010). The implementation of the Garrett Lee Smith Memorial Act suicide prevention programs has shown an important reduction in youth suicide rates (Walrath, Garraza, Reid, Goldston, & McKeon, 2015).

Another major public health initiative for suicide prevention is means restriction or control (Barber & Miller, 2014; Yip et al., 2012). At the population level, means restriction proves most effective when the method is common and highly lethal. For example, after the Sri Lankan government placed restrictions on sales of the most highly human-toxic pesticides in the 1990s, the overall national suicide rate dropped by 50% (Gunnell et al., 2007). At the individual level, clinicians could speak with family members about the removal of potential lethal methods from the reach of suicidal kin.

Although suicidality most commonly occurs in people with depressive disorders, it also occurs in individuals with schizophrenia, substance use disorders, personality disorders, and anxiety disorder. In addition, approximately 10% of those who die by suicide or who attempt suicide may not have identifiable mental disorders (Cavanagh et al., 2003; Harris & Barraclough, 1997; Sher et al., 2001). Thus, the absence of major depression should not be mistaken for the absence of suicide risk (Han et al., 2015a; Oquendo, Baca-Garcia, Mann, & Giner, 2008). Suicide prevention efforts need to target nondepressed ideators with a suicide plan as well (Han et al., 2015a). Another recent study also indicated that remission of one specific disorder (e.g., MDE) may be insufficient to reduce suicide risk if an adult has co-occurring psychiatric comorbidity (Hoertel et al., 2015).

It is important for suicidal individuals to receive timely mental health treatment. Aspirational Goal 2 of the National Action Alliance for Suicide Prevention's Research Prioritization Task Force (2014) is to determine the degree of suicide risk among individuals in diverse populations and in diverse settings through feasible and effective screening and assessment approaches. After effective screening and assessment by trained clinicians, referral is necessary, but it is not sufficient for patients to actually connect to the mental health treatment. Specific outreach programs can be more effective in increasing the receipt of mental health treatment with continuity of care among suicidal individuals. Comprehensive suicide prevention approaches are needed to addresses individual, family and peer, community, and societal-level factors. It is also essential to deliver programs that can build resilience through social connections, promote effective coping skills, and reduce suicide risk in broad-based populations.

Disclaimers: The findings and conclusions of this study are those of the authors and do not necessarily reflect the views of the Substance Abuse and Mental Health Services Administration, the National Institute on Drug Abuse of the National Institutes of Health, or the US Department of Health and Human Services.

References

Alexander, M. J., Haugland, G., Ashenden, P., Knight, E., & Brown, I. (2009). Coping with thoughts of suicide: Techniques used by consumers of mental health services. *Psychiatric Services, 60*(9), 1214–1221.

Amador, X. F., & David, A. S. (1998). *Insight and psychosis.* New York, NY: Oxford University Press.

American Foundation for Suicide Prevention. (2016). *Facts and figures.* Retrieved from https://www.afsp.org/understanding-suicide/facts-and-figures

Angst, F., Stassen, H. H., Clayton, P. J., & Angst, J. (2002). Mortality of patients with mood disorders: Follow-up over 34–38 years. *Journal of Affective Disorders, 68*(2–3), 167–181.

Appleby, L., Shaw, J., Amos, T., McDonnell, R., Harris, C., McCann, K., . . . Parsons, R. (1999). Suicide within 12 months of contact with mental health services: National clinical survey. *British Journal of Psychiatry, 318*(7193), 1235–1239.

Baca-Garcia, E., Perez-Rodriguez, M. M., Keyes, K. M., Oquendo, M. A., Hasin, D. S., Grant, B. F., & Blanco, C. (2010). Suicidal ideation and suicide attempts in the United States: 1991–1992 and 2001–2002. *Molecular Psychiatry, 15*(3), 250–259.

Baca-Garcia, E., Perez-Rodriguez, M. M., Oquendo, M. A., Keyes, K. M., Hasin, D. S., Grant, B. F., & Blanco, C. (2011). Estimating risk for suicide attempt: Are we asking the right questions? Passive suicidal ideation as marker for suicidal behavior. *Journal of Affective Disorder, 134*(1–3), 327–332.

Barber, C. W., & Miller, M. J. (2014). Reducing a suicidal person's access to lethal means of suicide. *American Journal of Preventive Medicine, 47*(3 Suppl. 2), S264–S272.

Betz, M. E., Sullivan, A. F., Manton, A. P., Espinola, J. A., Miller, I., Camargo, C. A., & Boudreaux, E. D. (2013). Knowledge, attitudes, and practices of emergency department providers in the care of suicidal patients. *Depression and Anxiety, 30*(10), 1005–1012.

Bishop, T. F., Press, M. J., Keyhani, S., & Pincus, H. A. (2014). Acceptance of insurance by psychiatrists and the implications for access to mental health care. *JAMA Psychiatry, 71*(2), 176–181.

Blair-West, G. W., Mellsop, G. W., & Eyeson-Annan, M. L. (1997). Down-rating lifetime suicide risk in major depression. *Acta Psychiatrica Scandinavica, 95*(3), 259–263.

Bolton, J. M., & Robinson, J. (2010). Population-attributable fractions of Axis I and Axis II mental disorders for suicide attempts: Findings from a representative sample of the adults, noninstitutionalized US population. *American Journal of Public Health, 100*(12), 2473–2480.

Borges, G., Angst, J., Nock, M. K., Ruscio, A. M., Walters, E. E., & Kessler, R. C. (2006). A risk index for 12-month suicide attempts in the National Comorbidity Survey Replication (NCS-R). *Psychological Medicine, 36*(12), 1747–1757.

Borowsky, I. W., Ireland, M., & Resnick, M. D. (2001). Adolescent suicide attempts: Risks and protectors. *Pediatrics, 107*(3), 485–493.

Bostwick, J. M., & Pankratz, V. S. (2000). Affective disorders and suicide risk: A reexamination. *American Journal of Psychiatry, 157*(12), 1925–1932.

Boudreaux, E. D., & Horowitz, L. M. (2014). Suicide risk screening and assessment. *American Journal of Preventive Medicine, 47*(3 Suppl. 2), S163–S169.

Bowden, C. L. (2003). Acute and maintenance treatment with mood stabilizers. *International Journal of Neuropsychopharmacology, 6*(3), 269–275.

Bridge, J. A., Iyengar, S., Salary, C. B., Barbe, R. P., Birmaher, B., Pincus, H. A., . . . Brent, D. A. (2007). Clinical response and risk for reported suicidal ideation and suicide attempts in pediatric antidepressant treatment: A meta-analysis of randomized controlled trials. *Journal of the American Medical Association, 297*(15), 1683–1696.

Brown, G. K., & Green, K. L. (2014). A review of evidence-based follow-up care for suicide prevention. *American Journal of Preventive Medicine, 47*(3 Suppl. 2), S209–S2015.

Brown, G. K., & Jager-Hyman, S. (2014). Evidence-based psychotherapies for suicide prevention. *American Journal of Preventive Medicine, 47*(3 Suppl. 2), S186–S194.

Bruce, M. L., Ten Have, T. R., Reynolds, C. F., Katz, I. I., Schulberg, H. C., Mulsant, B. H., . . . Alexopoulos, G. S. (2004). Reducing suicidal ideation and depressive symptoms in depressed older primary care patients. *Journal of the American Medical Association, 291*(9), 1081–1091.

Busch, K. A., Fawcett, J., & Jacobs, D. (2003). Clinical correlates of inpatient suicide. *Journal of Clinical Psychiatry, 64*(1), 14–19.

Caine, E. D. (2013). Forging an agenda for suicide prevention in the United States. *American Journal of Public Health, 103*(5), 822–829.

Caine, E. D. (2015). Suicide and social processes. *JAMA Psychiatry, 72*(10), 965–967.

Cavanagh, J. T., Carson, A. J., Sharpe, M., & Lawrie, S. M. (2003). Psychological autopsy studies of suicide: A systematic review. *Psychological Medicine, 33*(3), 395–405.

Centers for Disease Control and Prevention. (2015). *Fatal injury reports, 1999–2013, for national, regional, and states* (restricted). Retrieved from http://webappa.cdc.gov/cgi-bin/broker.exe

Centers for Medicare and Medicaid Services. (2008). *Medicare prescription drug benefit manual.* Retrieved from http://www.cms.gov/Medicare/PrescriptionDrugCoverage/Prescription-DrugCovContra/Downloads/MemoPDBManualChapter5_093011.pdf

Cherpitel, C. J., Borges, G. L. G., & Wilcox, H. C. (2004). Acute alcohol use and suicidal behavior: A review of the literature. *Alcoholism: Clinical and Experimental Research, 28*(5 Suppl.), S18–S28.

Colpe, L. J., & Pringle, B. A. (2014). Data for building a national suicide prevention strategy. What we have and what we need. *American Journal of Preventive Medicine, 47*(3 Suppl. 2), S130–S136.

Conner, K. R., Cox, C., Duberstein, P. R., Tian, L., Nisbet, P. A., & Conwell, Y. (2001). Violence, alcohol, and completed suicide: A case-control study. *American Journal of Psychiatry, 158*(10), 1701–1705.

Conner, K. R., Hesselbrock, V. M., Meldrum, S. C., Schuckit, M. A., Bucholz, K. K., Gamble, S. A., . . . Kramer, J. (2007). Transitions to, and correlates of, suicidal ideation, plans, and unplanned and planned suicide attempts among 3,729 men and women with alcohol dependence. *Journal of Studies on Alcohol and Drugs, 68*(5), 654–662.

Conwell, Y., Duberstein, P. R., Cox, C., Herrmann, J. H., Forbes, N. T., & Caine, E. D. (1996). Relationships of age and Axis I diagnoses in victims of completed suicide: A psychological autopsy study. *Am J Psychiatry, 153*(8), 1001–1008.

Coryell, W., & Young, E. A. (2005). Clinical predictors of suicide in primary major depressive disorder. *Journal of Clinical Psychiatry, 66*(4), 412–417.

Denney, J. T., Rogers, R. G., Krueger, P. M., & Wadsworth, T. (2009). Adult suicide mortality in the United States: Marital status, family size, socioeconomic status, and differences by sex. *Social Science Quarterly, 90*(5), 1167–1185.

Dervic, K., Carballo, J. J., Baca-Garcia, E., Galfalvy, H. C., Mann, J. J., Brent, D. A., & Oquendo, M. A. (2011). Moral or religious objections to suicide may protect against suicidal behavior in bipolar disorder. *Journal of Clinical Psychiatry, 72*(10), 1390–1396.

Eaton, W. W., Martins, S. S., Nestadt, G., Bienvenu, O. J., Clarke, D., & Alexandre, P. (2008). The burden of mental disorders. *Epidemiologic Reviews, 30*(1), 1–14.

Erlangsen, A., Lind, B. D., Stuart, E. A., Qin, P., Stenager, E., Larsen, K. J., . . . Nordentoft, M. (2015). Short-term and long-term effects of psychosocial therapy for people after deliberate self-harm: A register-based, nationwide multicentre study using propensity score matching. *Lancet Psychiatry, 2*(1), 49–58.

Fawcett, J. (2013). The cutting edge: Suicide and anxiety in *DSM-5*. *Depression and Anxiety, 30*(10), 898–901.

Finkelstein, Y., Macdonald, E. M., Hollands, S., Sivilotti, M. L. A., Huston, J. R., Mamdani, M. M., . . . Juurlink, D. N. (2015). Risk of suicide following deliberate self-poisoning. *JAMA Psychiatry, 72*(6), 570–575.

Gibbons, R. D., Hur, K., Bhaumik, D. K., & Mann, J. J. (2006). The relationships between antidepressant prescription rates and rate of early adolescent suicide. *American Journal of Psychiatry, 163*(11), 1898–1904.

Ginera, L., Blasco-Fontecillab, H., Perez-Rodriguezc, M., Garcia-Nietod, R., Ginera, J., Guijaa, J. A., . . . Baca-Garcia, E. (2013). Personality disorders and health problems distinguish suicide attempters from completers in a direct comparison. *Journal of Affective Disorders, 151*(2), 474–483.

Goldacre, M., Seagroatt, V., & Hawton, K. (1993). Suicide after discharge from psychiatric inpatient care. *Lancet, 342*(8866), 283–286.

Goldston, D. B., Walrath, C. M., McKeon, R., Puddy, R. W., Lubell, K. M., Potter, L. B., & Rodi, M. S. (2010). The Garrett Lee Smith Memorial Suicide Prevention Program. *Suicide and Life-Threating Behavior, 40*(3), 245–256.

Goodwin, F. K., Fireman, B., Simon, G. E., Hunkeler, E. M., Lee, J., & Revicki, D. (2003). Suicide risk in bipolar disorder during treatment with lithium and divalproex. *Journal of the American Medical Association, 290*(11), 1467–1473.

Gould, M. S., Munfakh, J. L., Kleinman, M., & Lake, A. M. (2012). National suicide prevention lifeline: Enhancing mental health care for suicidal individuals and other people in crisis. *Suicide and Life-Threating Behavior, 42*(1), 22–35.

Gunnell, D., Fernando, R., Hewagama, M., Priyangika, W. D., Konradsen, F., & Eddleston, M. (2007). The impact of pesticide regulations on suicide in Sri Lanka. *International Journal of Epidemiology, 36*(6), 1235–1242.

Han, B., Compton, W. M., Gfroerer, J., & McKeon, R. (2014b). Mental health treatment patterns among adults with recent suicide attempts in the United States. *American Journal of Public Health, 104*(12), 2359–2368.

Han, B., Compton, W. M., Gfroerer, J., & McKeon, R. (2015a). Prevalence and correlates of past 12-month suicide attempt among adults with past-year suicidal ideation in the United States. *Journal of Clinical Psychiatry, 76*(3), 295–302.

Han, B., Gfroerer, J., Kuramoto, S. J., Ali, M., Woodward, A. M., & Teich, J. (2015b). Medicaid expansion under the Affordable Care Act: Potential changes in receipt of mental health treatment among low-income nonelderly adults with serious mental illness. *American Journal of Public Health, 105*(10), 1982–1989.

Han, B., McKeon, R., & Gfroerer, J. (2014a). Suicidal ideation among community-dwelling adults in the United States. *American Journal of Public Health, 104*(3), 488–497.

Harris, E. C., & Barraclough, B. (1997). Suicide as an outcome for mental disorders: A meta-analysis. *British Journal of Psychiatry, 170*(3), 205–228.

Henriksson, M. M., Aro, H. M., Mattunen, M. J., Heikkinen, M. E., Isometsa, E. T., Kuoppasalmi, K. I., & Lönnqvist, J. K. (1993). Mental disorders and comorbidity in suicide. *American Journal of Psychiatry, 150*(6), 935–940.

Hoertel, N., Franco, S., Wall, M. M., Oquendo, M. A., Kerridge, B. T., Limosin, F., & Blanco, C. (2015). Mental disorders and risk of suicide attempt: A national prospective study. *Molecular Psychiatry, 20*(6), 718–726.

Hoyer, E. H., Mortensen, P. B., & Olesen, A. V. (2000). Mortality and causes of death in a total national sample of patients with affective disorders admitted for the first time between 1973 and 1993. *British Journal of Psychiatry, 176*(1), 76–82.

Hughes, C. W. (2011). Objective assessment of suicide risk: Significant improvements in assessment, classification, and prediction. *American Journal of Psychiatry, 168*(12), 1233–1234.

Ilgen, M. A., Downing, K., Zivin, K., Hoggatt, K. J., Kim, H. M., Ganoczy, D., . . . Valenstein, M. (2009). Identifying subgroups of patients with depression who are at high risk for suicide. *Journal of Clinical Psychiatry, 70*(11), 1495–1500.

Inskip, H. M., Harris, E. C., & Barraclough, B. (1998). Lifetime risk of suicide for affective disorder, alcoholism and schizophrenia. *British Journal of Psychiatry, 172*(1), 35–37.

Isometsa, E. T., Henriksson, M. M., Aro, H. M., & Lönnqvist, J. K. (1994). Suicide in bipolar disorder in Finland. *American Journal of Psychiatry, 151*(7), 1020–1024.

Jacob, V., Chattopadhyay, S. K., Sipe, T. A., Thota, A. B., Byard, G. J., Chapman, D. P., & Community Preventive Services Task Force. (2012). Economics of collaborative care for management of depressive disorders: A community guide systematic review. *American Journal of Preventive Medicine, 42*(5), 539–549.

Joe, S., Baser, R. E., Breeden, G., Neighbors, H. W., & Jackson, J. S. (2006). Prevalence of and risk factors for lifetime suicide attempts among blacks in the United States. *Journal of the American Medical Association, 296*(17), 2112–2123.

Kessler, R. C. (2012). The costs of depression. *Psychiatric Clinics of North America, 35*(1), 1–14.

Kessler, R. C., Berglund, P., Borges, G., Nock, M., & Wang, P. S. (2005b). Trends in suicide ideation, plans, gestures, and attempts in the United States, 1990–1992 to 2001–2003. *Journal of the American Medical Association, 293*(20), 2487–2495.

Kessler, R. C., Berglund, P., Demler, O., Jin, R., Koretz, D., Merikangas, K. R., . . . Wang, P. S. (2003). The epidemiology of major depressive disorder: Results from the National

Comorbidity Survey Replication. *Journal of the American Medical Association, 289*(23), 3095–3105.

Kessler, R. C., Berglund, P., Demler, O., Jin, R., Merikangas, K. R., & Walters, E. E. (2009). Lifetime prevalence and age-of-onset distributions of *DSM-IV* disorders in the National Comorbidity Survey Replication. *Archives of General Psychiatry, 62*(6), 593–602.

Kessler, R. C., Borges, G., & Walters, E. E. (1999). Prevalence of and risk factors for lifetime suicide attempts in the National Comorbidity Survey. *Archives of General Psychiatry, 56*(7), 617–626.

Kessler, R. C., Chiu, W. T., Demler, O., & Walters, E. E. (2005a). Prevalence, severity, and comorbidity of twelve-month *DSM-IV* disorders in the National Comorbidity Survey Replication (NCD-R). *Archives of General Psychiatry, 62*(6), 617–627.

Knox, K. L., Litts, D. A., Talcott, G. W., Feig, J. C., & Caine, E. D. (2003). Risk of suicide and related adverse outcomes after exposure to a suicide prevention programme in the US Air Force: Cohort study. *British Journal of Psychiatry, 327*(7428), 1376–1378.

Korczak, D. J., & Goldstein, B. I. (2009). Childhood onset major depressive disorder: Course of illness and psychiatric comorbidity in a community sample. *Journal of Pediatrics, 155*(1), 118–123.

Mann, J. J., Apter, A., Bertolote, J., Beautrais, A., Currier, D., Haas, A., . . . Hendin, H. (2005). Suicide prevention strategies: A systematic review. *Journal of the American Medical Association, 294*(16), 2064–2074.

Mathers, C. D., & Loncar, D. (2006). Projections of global mortality and burden of disease from 2002 to 2030. *PLoS Med, 3*(11), e442.

Mojtabai, R., & Olfson, M. (2008). National patterns in antidepressant treatment by psychiatrists and general medical providers: Results from the National Comorbidity Survey Replication. *Journal of Clinical Psychiatry, 69*(7), 1064–1074.

Molock, S. D., Heekin, J. M., Matlin, S. G., Barksdale, C. L., Gray, E., & Booth, C. L. (2014). The baby or the bath water? Lessons learned from the National Action Alliance for Suicide Prevention Research Prioritization Task Force literature review. *American Journal of Preventive Medicine, 47*(3 Suppl. 2), S115–S121.

Nakagawa, A., Grunebaum, M. F., Oquento, M. A., Burke, A. K., Kashima, H., & Mann, J. J. (2009). Clinical correlates of planned, more lethal suicide attempts in major depressive disorder. *Journal of Affective Disorders, 112*(1–3), 237–242.

National Action Alliance for Suicide Prevention Research Prioritization Task Force. (2014). *A prioritized research agenda for suicide prevention: An action plan to save lives.* Rockville, MD: National Institute of Mental Health and Research Prioritization Task Force.

Nock, M. K., Borges, G., Bromet, E. J., Cha, C. B., Kessler, R. C., & Lee, S. (2008). Suicide and suicidal behavior. *Epidemiologic Reviews, 30*(1), 133–153.

Nock, M. K., Green, J. G., Hwang, I., McLaughlin, K. A., Sampson, N. A., Zaslavsky, A. M., & Kessler, R. C. (2013). Prevalence, correlates, and treatment of lifetime suicidal behavior among adolescents. *JAMA Psychiatry, 70*(3), 300–310.

Nock, M. K., Hwang, I., Sampson, N. A., & Kessler, R. C. (2010). Mental disorders, comorbidity and suicidal behavior: Results from the National Comorbidity Survey Replication. *Molecular Psychiatry, 15*(8), 868–876.

Norman, R. E., Byambaa, M., De, R., Butchart, A., Scott, J., & Vos, T. (2012). The long-term health consequences of child physical abuse, emotional abuse, and neglect: A systematic review and meta-analysis. *PLoS Medicine, 9*(11), e1001349.

O'Connor, E., Gaynes, B. N., Burda, B. U., Soh, C., & Whitlock, E. P. (2013). Screening for and treatment of suicide risk relevant to primary care: A systematic review for the US Preventive Services Task Force. *Annals of Intern Medicine, 158*(10), 741–754.

Olfson, M., Marcus, S. C., & Bridge, J. A. (2014). Focusing suicide prevention on periods of high risk. *Journal of the American Medical Association, 311*(11), 1107–1108.

Olfson, M., Marcus, S. C., & Shaffer, D. (2006). Antidepressant drug therapy and suicide in severely depressed children and adults. *Archives of General Psychiatry, 63*(8), 865–872.

Olfson, M., Pincus, H. A., & Pardes, H. (2013). Investing in evidence-based care for the severely mentally ill. *Journal of the American Medical Association, 310*(13), 1345–1346.

Oquendo, M. A., Baca-Garcia, E., Mann, J. J., & Giner, J. (2008). Issues for *DSM-V*: Suicidal behavior as a separate diagnosis on a separate axis. *American Journal of Psychiatry, 165*(11), 1383–1384.

Oquendo, M. A., Galfalvy, H. C., Currier, D., Grunebaum, M. F., Sher, L., Sullivan, G. M., . . . Mann, J. J. (2011). Treatment of suicide attempters with bipolar disorder: A randomized clinical trial comparing lithium and valproate in the prevention of suicidal behavior. *American Journal of Psychiatry, 168*(10), 1050–1056.

Orbach, I. (1997). A taxonomy of factors related to suicidal behavior. *Clinical Psychology: Science and Practice, 4*(1), 208–224.

Osby, U., Brandt, L., Correia, N., Ekbom, A., & Sparen, P. (2001). Excess mortality in bipolar and unipolar disorder in Sweden. *Archives of General Psychiatry, 58*(9), 844–850.

Pan, Y. J., Chang, W. H., Lee, M. B., Chen, C. H., Liao, S. C., & Caine, E. D. (2013). Effectiveness of a nationwide aftercare program for suicide attempters. *Psychological Medicine, 43*(7), 1447–1454.

Posner, K., Brown, G. K., Stanley, B., Brent, D. A., Yeshova, K. V., Oquendo, M. A., . . . Mann, J. J. (2011). The Columbia-Suicide Severity Rating Scale: Initial validity and internal consistency findings from three multisite studies with adolescents and adults. *American Journal of Psychiatry, 168*(12), 1266–1277.

Range, L. M., Leach, M. M., McIntyre, D., Posey-Deters, P. B., Marion, M. S., Kovac, S. H., . . . Vigil J. (1999). Multicultural perspectives on suicide. *Aggression and Violent Behavior, 4*(4), 413–430.

Rasic, R. T., Belik, S., Elias, B., Katz, L. Y., Enns, M., Sareen, J., & Swampy Cree Suicide Prevention Team. (2009). Spirituality, religion and suicidal behavior in a nationally representative sample. *Journal of Affective Disorders, 114*(1–3), 32–40.

Rihmer, Z. (1996). Strategies for suicide prevention: Focus on healthcare. *Journal of Affective Disorders, 39*(2), 83–91.

Rihmer, Z. (2005). Prediction and prevention of suicide in bipolar disorders. *Clinical Neuropsychiatry, 2*(1), 48–54.

Rihmer, Z. (2007). Suicide risk in mood disorders. *Current Opinion in Psychiatry, 20*(1), 17–22.

Rockett, I. R. H. (2010). Counting suicides and making suicide count as a public health problem. *Crisis, 31*, 227–230.

Rutz, W., von Knorring, L., Pihlgren, H., Rihmer, Z., & Walinder, J. (1995). Prevention of male suicides: Lessons from Gotland study. *Lancet, 345*(8948), 524.

Rutz, W., von Knorring, L., & Walinder, J. (1989). Frequency of suicide on Gotland after systematic postgraduate education of general practitioners. *Acta Psychiatrica Scandinavica, 80*(2), 151–154.

Sher, L., Oquendo, M. A., & Mann, J. J. (2001). Risk of suicide in mood disorders. *Clinical Neuroscience Research, 1*(5), 337–344.

Simon, G. E., Savarino, J., Operskalski, B., & Wang, P. (2006). Suicide risk during antidepressant treatment. *Journal of Psychiatry, 163*(1), 41–47.

Smith, P. N., Cukrowicz, K. C., Poindexter, E. K., Hobson, V., & Cohen, L. M. (2010). The acquired capability for suicide: A comparison of suicide attempters, suicide ideators, and non-suicidal controls. *Depression and Anxiety, 27*(9), 871–877.

Substance Abuse and Mental Health Services Administration. (2014). *Results from the 2013 National Survey on Drug Use and Health: Mental health findings.* HHS Publication No. SMA 14-4887. Rockville, MD: Substance Abuse and Mental Health Services Administration.

Thota, A. B., Sipe, T. A., Byard, G. B., Zometa, C. S., Hahn, R. A., McKnight-Eily, L. R., . . . Community Preventive Services Task Force. (2012). Collaborative care to improve the management of depressive disorders. *American Journal of Preventive Medicine, 42*(5), 525–538.

Tondo, L., Isacsson, G., & Baldessarini, R. J. (2003). Suicide behavior in bipolar disorder: Risk and prevention. *CNS Drugs, 17*(7), 491–511.

Tsai, A. C., Lucas, M., & Kawachi, I. (2015). Association between social integration and suicide among women in the United States. *JAMA Psychiatry, 72*(10), 987–993.

Turecki, G. (2014). Epigenetics and suicidal behavior research pathways. *American Journal of Preventive Medicine, 47*(3 Suppl. 2), S144–151.

Unützer, J., & Park, M. (2012). Older adults with severe, treatment-resistant depression. *Journal of the American Medical Association, 308*(9), 909–918.

Unützer, J., Tang, L., Oishi, S., Katon, W., Williams J. W., Hunkeler, E., . . . Langston, C. (2006). Reducing suicidal ideation in depressed older primary care patients. *Journal of the American Geriatrics Society, 54*(10), 1550–1556.

US Department of Health and Human Services. Office of the Surgeon General and National Action Alliance for Suicide Prevention. (2012). *The 2012 national strategy for suicide prevention: Goals and objectives for action.* Retrieved from https://www.ncbi.nlm.nih.gov/books/NBK109917/

US Department of Health and Human Services. (2013). *Administration issues final mental health and substance use disorder parity rule.* Retrieved from http://www.hhs.gov/news/press/2013pres/11/20131108b.html

US Government Printing Office. (2008). *Medicare improvements for patient and providers act of 2008.* Retrieved from http://www.gpo.gov/fdsys/pkg/PLAW-110publ275/pdf/PLAW-110publ275.pdf

Van Orden, K. A., Witte, T. K., Cukrowicz, K. C., Braithwaite, S., Selby, E. A., & Joiner, T. E. (2010). The interpersonal theory of suicide. *Psychological Review, 117*(2), 575–600.

Vyssoki, B., Kapusta, N. D., Praschak-Rieder, N., Dorffner, G., & Willert, M. (2014). Direct effect of sunshine on suicide. *JAMA Psychiatry, 71*(11), 1231–1237.

Walrath, C., Garraza, L. G., Reid, H., Goldston, D. B., & McKeon, R. (2015). Impact of the Garrett Lee Smith youth suicide prevention program on suicide mortality. *American Journal of Public Health, 105*(5), 986–993.

Wang, P. S., Lane, M., Olfson, M., Pincus, H. A., Wells, K. B., & Kessler, R. C. (2005). Twelve-month use of mental health services in the United States: Results from the National Comorbidity Survey Replication. *Archives of General Psychiatry, 62*(6), 629–640.

Webb, R. T., Qin, P., Stevens, H., Mortensen, P. B., Appleby, L., & Shaw, L. (2011). National study of suicide in all people with a criminal justice history. *Archives of General Psychiatry, 68*(6), 591–599.

While, D., Bickley, H., Roscoe, A., Windfuhr, K., Rahman, S., Shaw, J., . . . Kapur, N. (2012). Implementation of mental health service recommendations in England and Wales and suicide rates, 1997–2006: A cross-sectional and before-and-after observational study. *Lancet, 379*(9820), 1005–1012.

Wilcox, D., Kellam, S. G., Brown, C. H., Poduska, J. M., Ialongo, N. S., Wang, W., & Anthony, J. C. (2008). The impact of two universal randomized first- and second-grade classroom intervention on young adult suicide ideation and attempts. *Drug and Alcohol Dependence, 95*(Suppl. 1), S60–S73.

Williams, A. R., Olfson, M., & Galanter, M. (2015). Assessing and improving clinical insight among patients "in denial." *JAMA Psychiatry, 72*(4), 303–304.

Yerevanian, B. L., Keok, R. J., & Mintz, J. (2003). Lithium, anticonvulsants, and suicidal behavior in bipolar disorder. *Journal of Affective Disorders, 73*(3), 223–228.

Yerevanian, B. L., Keok, R. J., & Mintz, J. (2007). Bipolar pharmacotherapy and suicidal behavior. Part I: Lithium, divalproex, and carbamazepine. *Journal of Affective Disorders, 103*(1–3), 5–11.

Yip, P. S., Caine, E., Yousulf, S., Change, S. S., Su, K. C., & Chen, Y. Y. (2012). Means restriction for suicide prevention. *Lancet, 379*(9834), 2393–2399.

CHAPTER 12

Mindfulness-Based Approaches for Promoting Mental Health in Urban Youth

Tamar Mendelson, PhD
April Joy Damian, MSc

Mindfulness-based interventions are increasingly being implemented with children and adolescents, including those living in urban communities characterized by high rates of crime and poverty. This chapter provides an overview of mindfulness-based approaches for improving social, emotional, and academic functioning in youth, with particular attention to urban youth. In the following sections, we summarize key mental health issues among urban youth, describe the rationale for use of mindfulness-based strategies with this population, review emerging research on mindfulness programs in school and other youth-serving settings, and discuss practice and research considerations relevant for this area of work.

Mental Health in Urban Youth

Lifetime prevalence of major depressive disorder (MDD) among adolescents aged 15–18 was found to be between 11% and 14% in nationally representative studies, with an estimated 20% of adolescents experiencing MDD by age 18 (Avenevoli, Swendson, He, Burstein, & Merikangas, 2015; Kessler & Walters, 1998). In addition, approximately one-quarter of adolescents endorse subthreshold depressive symptoms that cause impairment in daily functioning (Klein, Shankman, Lewinsohn, & Seeley, 2009).

Youth exposed to community or interpersonal violence are at heightened risk for depression and other forms of psychopathology, with risk for depression increasing as the number of exposures increases (Cisler et al., 2012; Slopen, Fitzmaurice, Williams, & Gilman, 2012). Forty-six million children in the United States—more than 60%—were estimated to have experienced violence, abuse, and crime in 2012 alone (Listenbee et al., 2012). Chronic stress and trauma exposure are particularly prevalent in disenfranchised communities. For instance, more than 85% of youth from disadvantaged urban communities were estimated to witness some form of violence in their life-times, and as many as 69% have reported direct victimization (McDonald & Rich-mond, 2008). Inner-city youth are at high risk for a range of traumatic exposures that also includes family conflict and disruption, housing instability, and other adversities linked to poverty and neighborhood disadvantage (Breslau, Wilcox, Storr, Lucia, & Anthony, 2004; Buka, Stichick, Birdthistle, & Earls, 2001; Evans, 2004).

Exposure to chronic stress and trauma results in elevated risk not only for depres-sive symptoms and disorders but also for broad-based negative effects on physiologi-cal and psychological functioning. A growing body of research demonstrates that stress and trauma exposure have harmful effects on the developing brain and stress response systems (Anda et al., 2006; Lupien, McEwen, Gunnar, & Heim, 2009). Chronic stress and trauma negatively impact brain regions associated with self-regulatory capacities such as executive functioning and emotion regulation (Compas, 2006; McEwen, 2005); this in turn impairs an individual's ability to respond effectively to stress (Com-pas, 2006) and increases risks for developing emotional and behavioral problems (Romeo, 2010). Negative effects of stress and trauma exposure may be especially acute during adolescence (Spear, 2009). Neurobiological changes during puberty increase stress reactivity (Gunnar, Wewerka, Frenn, Long, & Griggs, 2009), worsening effects of poor self-regulation skills and increasing risks for emotional issues, including de-pression and trauma symptoms (Romeo, 2010; Spear, 2009).

Unaddressed emotional problems have been associated with academic difficulties (Hinshaw, 1992; Needham, Crosnoe, & Muller, 2004; Reid, Gonzalez, Nordness, Trout, & Epstein, 2004). Students who experience chronic stress and trauma generally come to school tense and "on edge" and often lack skills for identifying and regulat-ing difficult emotions. As a result, they are likely to have trouble paying attention in class, learning and remembering course material, and communicating their needs effectively. Studies on youth residing in low-income housing have found low levels of school engagement, difficulty getting along with teachers, disobedience at school, bul-lying other students, and hyperactivity and restlessness (Popkin & McDaniel, 2013). At a population level, low-income and minority youth face many challenges in achieving their academic potential; achievement disparities by class and race are well documented (Heckman & LaFontaine, 2010; Roderick, Nagaoka, & Coca, 2009). Living in a disad-vantaged neighborhood, for example, was found to decrease probability of high school graduation by 20% for African American youth (Wodtke, Harding, & Elwert, 2011). Problems with cognitive and emotion regulation stemming from stress exposure are likely a critical factor contributing to school problems for disadvantaged adolescents. Other downstream effects of these exposures include substance use, involvement in delinquent and criminal activities, and poor physical health (Ruchkin, Henrich, Jones, Vermeiren, & Schwab-Stone, 2007; Sampson, 2012).

Policy reforms to reduce systemic structural inequities in social and economic re-sources are required to address fundamental causes of these health disparities. There is also potential to benefit youth by implementing strength-based interventions that increase youths' resilience to stress by enhancing their natural capacities for self-regulation, positive coping, and stress management. This chapter addresses the potential of mindfulness-based strategies to increase youth resilience.

Mindfulness: What Is It, and Why Might It Be Helpful for Urban Youth?

Mindfulness practices derive from Eastern contemplative traditions and are aimed at improving attention, awareness, and equanimity (Brown & Ryan, 2003). The concept of mindfulness dates back 2,500 years to Buddhist spiritual practices. Mindfulness is said to have played a key role in Buddhist traditions focused on achieving an end to personal suffering. Although mindfulness is most often associated with Buddhism, it is also at the core of other Eastern contemplative practices, traditionally described by the Sanskrit word *dharma*, which carries the meaning of *lawfulness*, as in "the laws of physics" or simply "the way things are," as in the Chinese notion of *Tao* (Kabat-Zinn, 2003). While specific practices vary considerably across traditions, at its core mindfulness refers to nonjudgmental awareness and openness to the present.

Mindful awareness practices—which include meditation, yoga, and tai chi—encourage awareness and acceptance of the present moment, including challenging emotional and physical states. Acceptance can be a powerful way to reduce the additional suffering that may arise when we ruminate and worry about painful emotions (Linehan, 1993). Accepting thoughts, feelings, and bodily sensations can be a first step in becoming less reactive to these stimuli and better able to tolerate and manage stress.

Dr. Jon Kabat-Zinn was a pioneer in the adaptation of mindfulness approaches for use in contemporary secular Western contexts. The Mindfulness-Based Stress Reduction Program he developed in 1979 is one of the most widely used and extensively studied mindfulness interventions in the West. Mindfulness has also been incorporated into other Western clinical interventions. Dialectical behavior therapy, an empirically supported intervention to reduce emotional dysregulation, integrates mindfulness skills to promote acceptance, distress tolerance, and emotion regulation with cognitive behavioral approaches that address behavioral change (Linehan, 1993). Mindfulness-based cognitive therapy (Segal, Williams, & Teasdale, 2002) and mindfulness-based relapse prevention (Bowen, Chawla, & Marlatt, 2010) combine mindfulness skills and CBT strategies to prevent recurrence of major depression and substance abuse relapse, respectively.

A growing body of research suggests that mindfulness-based interventions reduce symptoms of distress and psychiatric disorders in adults. Recent meta-analyses of meditation programs and mindfulness-based therapies indicate that these interventions are effective for reducing depressive and anxiety symptoms (Goyal et al., 2014; Hofmann,

Sawyer, Witt, & Oh, 2010; Khoury et al., 2013). In addition, meta-analyses of mindfulness-based cognitive therapy found that the intervention reduced major depression recurrence in patients with multiple prior episodes (Chiesa & Serretti, 2011; Piet & Hougaard, 2011).

Research with adults indicates that mindfulness-based practices enhance self-regulatory capacities such as the ability to inhibit cognitive and emotional processes, such as rumination, that can increase or maintain stress (Brefczynski-Lewis, Lutz, Schaefer, Levinson, & Davidson, 2007). Self-regulatory capacities such as enhanced attention and awareness appear to have beneficial effects on the ability to cope with stress without adverse psychological or physical outcomes (i.e., resilience). The preponderance of evidence from studies using neuroimaging, EEG, and performance on cognitive tasks shows that mindfulness-based practices enhance components of self-regulation, such as attention (e.g., Chiesa & Serretti, 2009; Lutz et al., 2008; Manna et al., 2010), which underlie key aspects of cognitive, social-emotional, and behavioral functioning. Further, significant improvements in self-regulation and attentional capacity are evident even after brief periods of mindfulness training and with novices (Tang et al., 2009). For instance, an eight-week mindfulness training was found to improve the ability to maintain a state of focused attention and concentration during cognitive testing among individuals without prior training in mindfulness practices (Jha, Krompinger, & Baime, 2007).

There is growing interest in the use of mindfulness-based practices with children and adolescents, although research on these populations is far less advanced than for adults. Given the evidence that mindfulness enhances capacities for self-regulation in adults, it may hold particular promise for use with chronically stressed urban youth at risk for emotional and behavioral issues. Emerging research provides preliminary support for benefits of mindfulness with youth, although there are still significant methodological limitations in this work. In the following discussion, we highlight key developments in research on mindfulness with youth.

Mindfulness Interventions for Youth

Mindfulness-based programs for youth have become increasingly popular and are offered at a growing number of schools, after-school programs, and other youth-serving settings. Few of these programs have been subjected to study, and as Greenberg and Harris (2011) noted: "Enthusiasm for promoting such practices outweighs the current evidence supporting them" (p. 161). While still in the early stages of development, the evidence base for mindfulness practices with youth is also expanding rapidly. A number of reviews and meta-analyses have now been published on this literature, and—while all highlight significant methodological limitations—findings also consistently suggest that mindfulness-based practices show promise in promoting certain benefits for youth and merit additional rigorous study (Black, 2015; Greenberg & Harris, 2011; Harnett & Dawe, 2012; Meiklejohn et al., 2012; Zenner, Herrnleben-Kurz, & Walach, 2014; Zoogman, Goldberg, Hoyt, & Miller, 2014).

Intervention Benefits for Youth

Psychological Functioning

A number of studies have reported that mindfulness-based interventions improved psychological functioning in youth, including reductions in depressive and anxiety symptoms (Biegel, Brown, Shapiro, & Schubert, 2009; Liehr & Diaz, 2010). A meta-analysis of studies on mindfulness programs delivered in a range of settings reported significant intervention impacts on psychological symptoms; the effect size—a measure of the strength of program impact—was larger on average for psychological symptoms than for other outcomes (Zoogman et al., 2014). Similarly, another review concluded that mindfulness training can be categorized as "probably efficacious" for decreasing depressive and anxiety symptoms in nonclinical youth because at least two randomized controlled trials (RCTs) reported those outcomes, and quasi-experimental findings have tended to support those results (Black, 2015). By contrast, a recent meta-analysis focusing only on school-based mindfulness programs (Zenner et al., 2014) reported that these programs had a small and nonsignificant impact on emotional problems. It is possible that lower average levels of emotional symptoms in the school-based samples in Zenner and colleagues' review attenuated the ability to detect program effects in this domain.

Cognitive Performance

A number of studies have evaluated whether mindfulness training improves children's executive functions, particularly attention. Measures used to assess executive functions have included cognitive tests (e.g., computerized tests of attention) and, more frequently, parent or teaching rating scales. Zenner and colleagues' (2014) meta-analysis of school-based mindfulness interventions reported that the average effect size for improvements in cognitive performance (Hedges's $g = 0.80$) was larger than that of any other outcome domain. At least two RCTs have found positive effects on cognitive outcomes, with quasi-experimental findings generally supporting these results, indicating that mindfulness training is "probably efficacious" for enhancing executive functions related to attention in children (Black, 2015).

Stress-Related Outcomes

Zenner and colleagues' (2014) meta-analysis of school-based mindfulness studies found small to medium effect sizes for improvements in stress (Hedges's $g = 0.39$) and resilience (Hedges's $g = 0.36$) in studies that primarily used self-report scales to measure these constructs. A few studies have also evaluated biological or physiologic stress responses, although the literature would benefit from more attention to these sorts of objective measures. For instance, one school-based study found that levels of the stress hormone cortisol increased for control group participants but remained constant for intervention participants, a pattern consistent with predictions (Sibinga et al., 2013). Evidence from RCTs also suggests that mindfulness training is "probably efficacious" for reducing blood pressure and heart rate in African American youth with normal or elevated blood pressure (Black, 2015).

Settings for Intervention

Most mindfulness programs for youth have been implemented and studied in schools. Schools offer unique potential for reaching many youth and for enhancing their opportunity to engage productively in academic activities. Implementing mindfulness programming in schools, if integrated effectively into the curriculum, holds potential for shifting educational practices and school climate. Indeed, researchers have advocated for the integration of mindfulness into schools as a way not only to impact youth diversity but also to transform educational contexts into safe and supportive environments that nurture learning (Davidson et al., 2012; Greenberg & Harris, 2011). To achieve this goal, we must implement feasible and effective mindfulness interventions, and identify school contexts that are conducive to successfully implementing and maintaining these programs.

Some school-based programs have focused on teaching mindfulness skills directly to youth, using either expert mindfulness instructors from external agencies (e.g., Mendelson et al., 2010) or teachers trained to deliver the program (e.g., Schonert-Reichl & Lawlor, 2010). Some researchers have utilized DVDs, CDs, and other teaching aids to standardize intervention instruction by teachers and enhance the likelihood that mindfulness concepts will be effectively communicated despite the fact that most teachers have no background in this area (e.g., Parker, Kupersmidt, Mathis, Scull, & Sims, 2013). Learning to BREATHE and MindUp are examples of mindfulness-based programs with well-developed curricula that can be delivered in school settings (see Boxes 12.1 and 12.2).

By contrast, other programs have targeted teachers as *participants* in mindfulness-based interventions (Ancona & Mendelson, 2014; Jennings, Frank, Snowberg, Coccia, & Greenberg, 2013; Roeser et al., 2013). These programs provide teachers with skills for self-care and emotion regulation, with the aim of improving teachers' classroom performance. For example, Cultivating Awareness and Resilience in Education is a teacher professional development program that promotes teachers' social-emotional competence using mindful awareness practices as well as activities to strengthen compassion. Findings from a randomized controlled trial indicated that Cultivating Awareness and Resilience in Education improved teacher outcomes, including well-being, efficacy, and stress (Jennings et al., 2013). These outcomes are significant from a public health

---

Box 12.1. Learning to BREATHE

Learning to BREATHE is a mindfulness program for adolescents that can be delivered during school, after school, or in clinical facilities (Broderick, 2013; Broderick & Frank, 2014).

- The program contains six core themes:
  1. Body awareness
  2. Understanding and working with thoughts
  3. Understanding and working with feelings
  4. Integrating awareness of thoughts, feelings, and bodily sensations
  5. Reducing harmful self-judgments
  6. Integrating mindful awareness into daily life
- Each program session includes a brief introduction, group activities, discussion, and meditation practice. Students are given workbooks and CDs to promote a home meditation practice.
- The number and length of sessions is flexible and can be tailored to the school setting (e.g., 6, 12, 18). Teachers can be trained to deliver the program.
- The program was found to improve emotion regulation and other aspects of emotional functioning in studies with high school and middle school students (Bluth et al., 2015; Broderick & Metz, 2009; Fung, Guo, Jin, Bear, & Lau, 2016; Metz et al., 2013).

Box 12.2. MindUp

MindUp (Hawn Foundation, 2008) is a social-emotional learning program for elementary school children.

- The curriculum includes mindfulness practices as well as activities to promote executive functioning, positive mood, and kindness.
- The 12-session program can be administered by teachers in weekly sessions of 45–50 minutes.
- In a randomized controlled study with 99 fourth and fifth graders, the program was found to improve:
  1. cognitive control, measured using computer-based tests of executive function;
  2. stress physiology, measured using salivary cortisol;
  3. peer acceptance, measured using peer ratings; and
  4. various self-reported aspects of well-being (Schonert-Reichl et al., 2015).

---

perspective given high prevalence and negative effects of teacher stress and burnout (Johnson et al., 2005), particularly in low-income schools where teachers are responsible for managing students with higher average rates of student academic and behavioral problems.

If successful, teacher-focused interventions have potential not only to enhance teachers' personal well-being but also to create classroom environments in which teachers model "mindful behavior" and respond in socially and emotionally competent ways to students, facilitating improvement of students' self-regulation skills (Jennings & Greenberg, 2009). Ultimately, a combination of teacher- and student-focused mindfulness training may be most effective, but this integration has not yet been rigorously studied and will require greater resources for implementation.

Mindfulness training has also been implemented in other settings, including after-school programs, summer programs, clinic settings, and correctional facilities. For instance, Sibinga and colleagues (2011) provided a mindfulness intervention to urban youth who were patients in a pediatric primary care clinic. Primary care and other clinical contexts offer a unique opportunity to reach youth at risk for stress and psychological distress who may also have physical health issues.

Incarcerated youth are another population at risk for poor outcomes. While it is often difficult to conduct randomized controlled designs in correctional settings, emerging research suggests that implementing mindfulness programs may be feasible and have benefits for participants (Bowen et al., 2006; Himelstein, Hastings, Shapiro, & Heery, 2012). For example, one recent study randomly assigned dormitories of incarcerated adolescents to participate in either an intervention involving mindfulness training and cognitive behavioral therapy (Power Source) or a program about substance use attitudes and beliefs (Leonard et al., 2013). While adolescents in both study groups experienced reductions in attention capacity—likely due to the stress of incarceration—those in Power Source experienced a lower rate of decline in attention, and more time spent practicing mindfulness was associated with better capacities for attention.

Universal versus Targeted Intervention Approaches

Some mindfulness interventions have been implemented with a universal focus, offered to all youth in a given setting without screening for risk factors or symptoms. Other programs have been delivered in a more targeted fashion to youth with risk factors, elevated symptoms, or clinical disorders. For instance, mindfulness training has been tested with youth diagnosed with ADHD (e.g., van der Oord, Bogels, & Peijnenburg, 2012) and with youth in residential treatment for psychiatric issues (e.g., Biegel et al., 2009). Intervention effect sizes were reported to be larger for programs offered to clinical as compared with nonclinical samples (del = 0.50 versus 0.20, $p < 0.05$) (Zoogman et al., 2014). This pattern may reflect the fact that there is more room for symptom reduction in symptomatic populations, whereas nonclinical populations may show "floor effects" for symptom scales on which they do not endorse many items at baseline.

Interventions delivered in schools serving highly disadvantaged communities can be conceptualized as taking a targeted, or selective, approach in that they are delivered to a population of youth with a high prevalence of risk factors for depression and other emotional and behavioral issues. For instance, our team worked with urban public schools serving Baltimore City communities with high rates of violence and crime (Mendelson et al., 2010). The students were not screened for trauma exposure or psychological distress symptoms. Data gathered in our baseline surveys, however, indicated that most students had experienced traumatic stressors, such as hearing gunshots, seeing drug deals, and witnessing beatings, with reported exposure to some of these events as high as 93% in some schools and age groups. These high prevalence rates highlight the pervasive nature of stress and trauma exposure in some low-resourced urban areas.

Implementing and Studying Mindfulness-Based Interventions for Youth
Implementation Considerations

Implementing mindfulness-based programs successfully with youth requires navigating a number of hurdles. Selection of an appropriate setting for intervention delivery is critical. The setting must be appropriate for engaging youth (e.g., schools) and also conducive to formation of effective working partnerships between the intervention developers and organization administrators, as well as researchers, if applicable.

Effective Partnerships

Effective partnerships involve a mutual understanding of the goals of the intervention, how it will be delivered, and what role the organization and its personnel will play in program delivery. For instance, our team found that lack of support from principals and teachers was a critical barrier to intervention implementation at some of our partner schools (Mendelson et al., 2013). While principals and teachers were generally enthusiastic about the intervention in theory, they were often unable to provide the logistical support needed to promote student attendance and maintain effective communication with program instructors. It was also difficult to secure an appropriate room for intervention sessions on a consistent basis in some public schools. These basic supports are necessary to maximize the likelihood that an intervention can be delivered as intended; thus, it is important to assess whether a school or other organization has the resources and readiness for an effective partnership before moving forward with implementation.

Intervention Delivery

As noted previously, programs can be delivered by expert instructors or by on-site personnel; each of these methods has strengths and limitations. Programs taught by expert instructors are likely to be of high quality given instructors' extensive training in mindfulness practices. Instructors are often not well trained in classroom management, however, which may result in disruptions due to poorly handled student behavioral issues. In addition, this delivery method involves expenses of hiring outside personnel to deliver a program, which can reduce program sustainability and potential for dissemination. It is also often more difficult to positively impact the climate at a school or other youth-serving setting if teachers, administrators, or other relevant organization personnel are not involved in intervention delivery.

Utilizing personnel at the target organization to deliver a program (e.g., gym or health teachers) is generally more cost-effective and has potential to increase organizational engagement and ownership of the intervention, facilitating shifts in organization climate and promoting sustainability. Training, however, must be brief enough to be feasible for busy personnel but thorough enough to ensure high-quality instruction, often a challenge when training individuals without prior experience with mindfulness practices. Ongoing supervision and monitoring is also important to ensure that instructors maintain fidelity of implementation. While frequent supervision is ideal, this is more costly and may not be feasible from a time management or financial perspective.

Dosage and Frequency

Developers of mindfulness-based interventions for youth need to determine how many sessions to offer, as well as session length and spacing. These decisions must reflect both the developers' hypotheses about maximum program benefits for youth and practical constraints of the setting for intervention delivery. For instance, our team wanted to offer an intervention twice per week over 24 weeks to urban middle schools, but after accounting for participant recruitment, assessments, and school standardized testing, only 16 weeks of intervention were feasible.

The intensity of a program (i.e., the amount of mindfulness practice participants engage in through the program) was found to be a key predictor of program benefits in the meta-analysis of school-based mindfulness interventions by Zenner and colleagues (2014). Zoogman and colleagues' (2014) meta-analysis of mindfulness interventions for youth across diverse contexts, however, did not find that youth outcomes varied systematically as a function of program intensity, duration, or outside practice of skills. There is currently limited data on program dosage and frequency, and their association with various outcomes, and research clarifying these associations would greatly benefit the field (Black, 2015; Cook-Cottone, 2013; Greenberg & Harris, 2011).

Developmental Fit

Mindfulness-based interventions are becoming increasingly popular in schools and other settings, with programs offered to children of all ages. Little is currently known, however, about whether the potential to benefit from mindfulness practices varies by age or how such practices should be modified to be maximally effective for different age groups (Greenberg & Harris, 2011). Intervention developers must be well informed about child development so as to offer programming that is developmentally appropriate. If intervention developers specify the ages they are targeting, as well as how the program is tailored cognitively and physically for the target age group, this will facilitate the ability of researchers to investigate program effects and mechanisms of action for different ages.

Research Considerations

Research on mindfulness programs for youth is expanding rapidly, but most empirical investigations in this area have been pilot feasibility studies with serious methodological limitations. We outline areas that merit further development in the empirical literature in the following sections.

Rigorous Study Designs

Emerging research on mindfulness for youth is increasingly using randomized designs, rather than pre-post assessments without control groups. Only a few studies, however, have used active control conditions (e.g., Schonert-Reichl et al., 2015; Sibinga et al., 2013). This is an important next step in research, as studies without active control conditions cannot rule out the possibility that variables such as attention, relationships with instructors, and involvement in a "special" program were fully or partially responsible for intervention effects. Randomized controlled studies with active control conditions are more costly and resource-intensive but are the next critical step for advancing research about programs that have proven promising in pilot feasibility studies.

Fidelity of Implementation

It is critical that we study not only program outcomes but also the extent to which programs are faithfully delivered to avoid incorrectly concluding that an intervention is not effective when, in fact, it simply was not delivered according to plan (Domitrovich & Greenberg, 2000). To that end, it is critical that researchers identify program core components—the hypothesized "active ingredients" of the intervention—and specify how these core components are anticipated to produce changes in youth functioning. Core components, in turn, must be operationalized and assessed using a systematic method for coding fidelity so that their implementation can be evaluated. The process of operationalizing and assessing core components is an iterative one that should begin in the early stages of intervention implementation and testing and continue through large-scale efficacy and effectiveness trials (Feagans Gould et al., 2014). This process can lead to refinements in the intervention logic model. A systematic review of school-based mindfulness studies by our team indicated that only 10% of studies specified core intervention components or logic models, and only 20% reported on any aspect of implementation fidelity other than participant dosage (Feagans Gould, Dariotis, Greenberg, & Mendelson, 2015). Almost no studies, moreover, evaluated the extent to which implementation fidelity of mindfulness interventions was associated with outcomes, despite evidence that outcomes of youth interventions are impacted significantly by fidelity of implementation (Durlak & Dupre, 2008).

Appropriate Outcome Measures

Many studies on mindfulness-based programs for youth have assessed intervention impacts using self-report measures of constructs such as mood, stress, and coping. While self-report measures are useful, they are also subject to recall bias and social desirability bias. Youth may also lack the insight and metacognitive perspective needed to self-report on emotional and mental shifts in their functioning as a result of participation in mindfulness-based programs. Indeed, reporting on these sorts of changes may be challenging for adults as well, given the nuanced nature of the experience. Engagement with mindfulness practices may also not produce a linear improvement in symptoms; for instance, mindfulness practice may initially increase symptoms of distress as an individual becomes more aware of emotions and internal states he or she may have previously avoided.

Some studies using a mixture of qualitative and quantitative methods (e.g., Sibinga et al., 2011) have found that qualitative data (e.g., participant focus groups) indicated program improvements, whereas quantitative data (e.g., self-report surveys) did not show significant changes. Discrepancy between quantitative and qualitative measures may reflect some of the difficulties with self-report scales outlined earlier and may also suggest a need for new quantitative measures to more accurately capture youths' perspectives. Inclusion of qualitative data—particularly at early stages of intervention implementation and testing—provides a more nuanced perspective from participants that is generally not captured by self-report measures and that may guide subsequent intervention or measurement refinements.

Inclusion of multiple reporters (e.g., teachers, parents, observers) can add a valuable perspective to data from youth, indicating whether others in a child's environment observe changes in his or her social and emotional functioning. Use of cognitive tests to assess aspects of executive functioning such as attention, response inhibition, and working memory can provide important data on how mindfulness practices influence performance on tasks relevant to academic success. Finally, biological and physiological measures—including cortisol and heart rate variability—can offer insight into how mindfulness may impact the stress response system and capacity to respond to stressful stimuli. Inclusion of multiple modalities of measurement is the strongest approach, when feasible, as it allows for triangulation of data, facilitating a more comprehensive understanding of intervention effects.

Moderators and Mediators

As studies begin to employ randomized controlled designs with larger sample sizes, it becomes increasingly feasible to evaluate intervention *moderation* (which youth may benefit most or least from a mindfulness-based intervention) and *mediation* (which mechanisms drive intervention effects). The types of self-reports, teacher reports, cognitive tests, and biological or physiological measures described previously have the potential to provide rich data for exploration of these questions. For instance, some findings suggest that youth with low baseline levels of executive functioning may benefit more from mindfulness intervention than those with higher levels of executive functioning (Flook et al., 2010), a potential moderator that may help intervention developers target which youth should receive a particular program. Many researchers have hypothesized that improvements in self-regulation may mediate reductions in emotional and behavioral problems (e.g., Mendelson et al., 2010), but we currently have limited research rigorously evaluating mediating pathways.

Long-Term Follow-ups

Very few mindfulness-based studies with youth have included long-term follow-up assessments to determine whether effects were maintained over time. It is often challenging to follow youth for 12 or more months due to school transfers and changes in address and phone numbers; frequent relocations are particularly common for low-income urban youth, making this a more difficult-to-reach population. Long-term follow-ups, however, are needed to provide data about the extent to which program effects persist, increase, or decline after an intervention ends; these data can inform decisions about whether, for example, to offer an intervention over multiple years in a school setting or to provide booster sessions.

Conclusion

The use of mindfulness-based interventions with youth is an exciting area of practice and research. Mindfulness practices offer experiential means of training one's attention and awareness and show potential for promising effects on stress management and emotional well-being. These practices seem a logical fit for promoting positive development in youth and may offer particular advantages for chronically stressed urban youth at risk for emotional and behavioral problems. At present, intervention development and implementation outpace empirical knowledge about the efficacy of mindfulness-based practices for youth, but research in this area is growing rapidly.

While still in its early stages, the field is poised to launch increasingly rigorous studies that will elucidate key questions about intervention effects, mechanisms, and moderators.

References

Ancona, M. R., & Mendelson, T. (2014). Feasibility and preliminary outcomes of a yoga and mindfulness intervention for school teachers. *Advances in School Mental Health Promotion, 7*, 156–170.

Anda, R. F., Felitti, V. J., Bremner, J. D., Walker, J. D., Whitfield, C., Perry, B. D., . . . Giles, W. H. (2006). The enduring effects of abuse and related adverse experiences in childhood: A convergence of evidence from neurobiology and epidemiology. *European Archives of Psychiatry and Clinical Neuroscience, 256*, 174–186.

Avenevoli, S., Swendson, J., He, J., Burstein, M., & Merikangas, K. R. (2015). Major depression in the National Comorbidity Survey-Adolescent Supplement: Prevalence, correlates, and treatment. *American Academy of Child and Adolescent Psychiatry, 54*, 37–44.

Biegel, G. M., Brown, K. W., Shapiro, S. L., & Schubert, C. M. (2009). Mindfulness-based stress reduction for the treatment of adolescent psychiatric outpatients: A randomized clinical trial. *Journal of Consulting and Clinical Psychology, 77*, 855–866.

Black, D. S. (2015). Mindfulness training for children and adolescents: A state-of-the-science review. In K. Brown, D. Creswell, & R. Ryan (Eds.), *Handbook of mindfulness: Theory and research* (pp. 283–310). New York, NY: Guilford Press.

Bluth, K., Campo, R. A., Pruteanu-Malinici, S., Reams, A., Mullarkey, M., & Broderick, P. C. (2015). A school-based mindfulness pilot study for ethnically diverse at-risk adolescents. *Mindfulness, 7*, 90–104.

Bowen, S., Chawla, N., & Marlatt, G. A. (2010). *Mindfulness-based relapse prevention for addictive behaviors: A clinician's guide.* New York, NY: The Guilford Press.

Bowen, S., Witkiewitz, K., Dilworth, T. M., Chawla, N., Simpson, T. L., Ostafin, B. D., . . . Marlatt, G. A. (2006). Mindfulness meditation and substance use in an incarcerated population. *Psychology of Addictive Behaviors, 20*, 343–347.

Brefczynski-Lewis, J. A., Lutz, A., Schaefer, H. S., Levinson, D. B., & Davidson, R. J. (2007). Neural correlates of attentional expertise in long-term meditation practitioners. *Proceedings of the National Academy of Sciences, 104*, 11483–11488.

Breslau, N., Wilcox, H. C., Storr, C. L., Lucia, V. C., & Anthony, J. C. (2004). Trauma exposure and posttraumatic stress disorder: A study of youths in urban America. *Journal of Urban Health, 81*, 530–544.

Broderick, P. C. (2013). *Learning to BREATHE: A mindfulness curriculum for adolescents to cultivate emotion regulation, attention, and performance.* Oakland, CA: New Harbinger Publications.

Broderick, P. C., & Frank, J. L. (2014). Learning to BREATHE: An intervention to foster mindfulness in adolescence. *New Directions in Youth Development, 142*, 31–44.

Broderick, P. C., & Metz, S. (2009). Learning to BREATHE: A pilot trial of a mindfulness curriculum for adolescents. *Advances in School Mental Health Promotion, 2*, 35–46.

Brown, K. W., & Ryan, R. M. (2003). The benefits of being present: Mindfulness and its role in psychological well-being. *Journal of Personality and Social Psychology, 84*, 822–848.

Buka, S. L., Stichick, T. L., Birdthistle, I., & Earls, F. J. (2001). Youth exposure to violence: Prevalence, risks, and consequences. *American Journal of Orthopsychiatry, 71*, 298–310.

Chiesa, A., & Serretti, A. (2009). A systematic review of neurobiological and clinical features of mindfulness meditations. *Psychological Medicine, 27*, 1–14.

Chiesa, A., & Serretti, A. (2011). Mindfulness based cognitive therapy for psychiatric disorders: A systematic review and meta-analysis. *Psychiatry Research, 187*, 441–453.

Cisler, J. M., Begle, A. M., Amstadter, A. B., Resnick, H. S., Danielson, C. K., Saunders, B. E., & Kilpatrick, D. G. (2012). Exposure to interpersonal violence and risk for PTSD, depression, delinquency, and binge drinking among adolescents: Data from the NSA-R. *Journal of Traumatic Stress, 25*, 33–40.

Compas, B. E. (2006). Psychobiological processes of stress and coping: Implications for resilience in children and adolescents—comments on the papers of Romeo and McEwen and Fisher et al. *Annals of the New York Academy of Sciences, 1094*, 226–234.

Cook-Cottone, C. (2013). Dosage as a critical variable in yoga therapy research. *International Journal of Yoga Therapy, 23*, 11–12.

Davidson, R. J., Dunne, J. D., Eccles, J. S., Engle, A., Greenberg, M., Jennings, P. A., . . . Vago, D. (2012). Contemplative practices and mental training: Prospects for American education. *Child Development Perspectives, 6*, 146–153.

Domitrovich, C. E., & Greenberg, M. T. (2000). The study of implementation: Current findings from effective programs that prevent mental disorders in school-aged children. *Journal of Educational and Psychological Consultation, 11*, 193–221.

Durlak, J. A., & Dupre, E. P. (2008). Implementation matters: A review of research on the influence of implementation on program outcomes and the factors affecting implementation. *American Journal of Community Psychology, 41*, 327–350.

Evans, G. W. (2004). The environment of child poverty. *American Psychologist, 59*, 77–92.

Feagans Gould, L., Dariotis, J. K., Greenberg, M., & Mendelson, T. (2015). Assessing fidelity of implementation (FOI) for school-based mindfulness and yoga interventions: A systematic review. *Mindfulness, 7*(1), 5–33.

Feagans Gould, L., Mendelson, T., Dariotis, J. K., Ancona, M., Smith, A. S. R., Gonzalez, A. A., . . . Greenberg, M. T. (2014). Assessing fidelity of core components in a mindfulness and yoga intervention for urban youth: The CORE process. *New Directions for Youth Development, 142*, 58–81. doi:10.1002/yd.20097

Flook, L., Smalley, S. L., Kitil, M. J., Galla, B. M., Kaiser-Greenland, S., Locke, J., . . . Kasari, C. (2010). Effects of mindful awareness practices on executive functions in elementary school children. *Journal of Applied School Psychology, 26*, 70–95.

Fung, J., Guo, S., Jin, J., Bear, L., & Lau, A. (2016). A pilot randomized trial evaluating a school-based mindfulness intervention of ethnic minority youth. *Mindfulness, 4*, 819–828.

Goyal, M., Singh, S., Sibinga, E. M., Gould, N. F., Rowland-Seymour, A., Sharma, R., . . . Haythornthwaite, J. A. (2014). Meditation programs for psychological stress and well-being: A systematic review and meta-analysis. *JAMA Internal Medicine, 174*, 357–368.

Greenberg, M. T., & Harris, A. R. (2011). Nurturing mindfulness in children and youth: Current state of research. *Child Development Perspectives, 6*, 161–166.

Gunnar, M. R., Wewerka, S., Frenn, K., Long, J. D., & Griggs, C. (2009). Developmental changes in HPA activity over the transition to adolescence: Normative changes and associations with puberty. *Development and Psychopathology, 21*, 69–85.

Harnett, P. H., & Dawe, S. (2012). The contribution of mindfulness-based therapies for children and families and proposed conceptual integration. *Child and Adolescent Mental Health, 17*, 195–208.

Hawn Foundation. (2008). *Mindfulness education*. Miami Beach, FL: Author.

Heckman, J. J., & LaFontaine, P. A. (2010). The American high school graduation rate: Trends and levels. *The Review of Economics and Statistics, 92*, 244–262.

Himelstein, S., Hastings, A., Shapiro, S., & Heery, M. (2012). A qualitative investigation of the experience of a mindfulness-based intervention with incarcerated adolescents. *Child and Adolescent Mental Health, 17*, 231–237.

Hinshaw, S. P. (1992). Academic underachievement, attention deficits, and aggression: Comorbidity and implications for intervention. *Journal of Consulting and Clinical Psychology, 60*, 893–903.

Hofmann, S. G., Sawyer, A. T., Witt, A. A., & Oh, D. (2010). The effect of mindfulness-based therapy on anxiety and depression: A meta-analytic review. *Journal of Consulting and Clinical Psychology, 78*, 169–183.

Jennings, P. A., Frank, J. L., Snowberg, K. E., Coccia, M. A., & Greenberg, M. T. (2013). Improving classroom learning environments by Cultivating Awareness and Resilience in Education (CARE): Results of a randomized controlled trial. *School Psychology Quarterly, 28*, 374–390.

Jennings, P. A., & Greenberg, M. (2009). The prosocial classroom: Teacher social and emotional competence in relation to student and classroom outcomes. *Review of Educational Research, 79*, 491–525.

Jha, A. P., Krompinger, J., & Baime, M. J. (2007). Mindfulness training modifies subsystems of attention. *Cognitive, Affective, and Behavioral Neuroscience, 7*, 109–119.

Johnson, S., Cooper, C., Cartwright, S., Donald, I., Taylor, P., & Millet, C. (2005). The experience of work-related stress across occupations. *Journal of Managerial Psychology, 20*, 178–187.

Kabat-Zinn, J. (2003). Mindfulness-based interventions in context: Past, present, and future. *Clinical Psychology: Science and Practice, 10*, 144–156.

Kessler, R. C., & Walters, E. E. (1998). Epidemiology of *DSM-III-R* major depression and minor depression among adolescents and young adults in the National Comorbidity Survey. *Depression and Anxiety, 7*, 3–15.

Khoury, B., Lecomte, T., Fortin, G., Masse, M., Therien, P., Bouchard, V., . . . Hofmann, S. G. (2013). Mindfulness-based therapy: A comprehensive meta-analysis. *Clinical Psychology Review, 33*, 763–771.

Klein, D. N., Shankman, S. A., Lewinsohn, P. M., & Seeley, J. R. (2009). Subthreshold depessive disorder in adolescents: Predictors of escalation to full-syndrome depressive disorders. *Journal of the American Academy of Child and Adolescent Psychiatry, 48*, 703–710.

Leonard, N. R., Jha, A., Casarjian, B., Goolsarran, M., Garcia, C., Cleland, C. M., . . . Massey, Z. (2013). Mindfulness training improves attentional task performance in incarcerated youth: A group randomized controlled intervention trial. *Frontiers in Psychology, 4*, 1–10.

Liehr, P., & Diaz, N. (2010). A pilot study examining the effect of mindfulness on depression and anxiety for minority children. *Archives of Psychiatric Nursing, 24*, 69–71.

Linehan, M. (1993). *Cognitive-behavioral treatment of borderline personality disorder*. New York, NY: The Guilford Press.

Listenbee, R. L., Torre, J., Boyle, G. S. J., Cooper, S. W., Deer, S., Durfee, D. T., . . . Taguba, A. (2012). *Report of the attorney general's National Task Force on Children Exposed to Violence.* Washington, DC: US Department of Justice.

Lupien, S. J., McEwen, B. S., Gunnar, M. R., & Heim, C. (2009). Effects of stress throughout the lifespan on the brain, behaviour and cognition. *Nature Reviews Neuroscience, 10,* 434–445.

Lutz, A., Slagter, H. A., Dunne, J. D., & Davidson, R. J. (2008). Attention regulation and monitoring in meditation. *Trends in Cognitive Sciences, 12,* 163–169.

Manna, A., Raffone, A., Perrucci, M. G., Nardo, D., Ferretti, A., . . . Tartaro, A. (2010). Neural correlates of focused attention and cognitive monitoring in meditation. *Brain Research Bulletin, 82,* 46–56.

McDonald, C. C., & Richmond, T. R. (2008). The relationship between community violence exposure and mental health symptoms in urban adolescents. *Journal of Psychiatric and Mental Health Nursing, 15,* 833–849.

McEwen, B. S. (2005). Glucocorticoids, depression, and mood disorders: Structural remodeling in the brain. *Metabolism, 54,* 5 (Supplement), 20–23.

Meiklejohn, J., Phillips, C., Freedman, M. L., Griffin, M. L., Biegel, G., Roach, A., . . . Saltzman, A. (2012). Integrating mindfulness training into K-12 education: Fostering the resilience of teachers and students. *Mindfulness, 3,* 291–307.

Mendelson, T., Dariotis, J. K., Feagans Gould, L., Smith, A. S. R., Smith, A. A., Gonzalez, A. A., & Greenberg, M. T. (2013). Implementing mindfulness and yoga in urban schools: A community-academic partnership. *Journal of Children's Services, 8,* 276–291.

Mendelson, T., Greenberg, M. T., Dariotis, J. K., Gould, L. F., Rhoades, B. L., & Leaf, P. J. (2010). Feasibility and preliminary outcomes of a school-based mindfulness intervention for urban youth. *Journal of Abnormal Child Psychology, 38,* 985–994.

Metz, S., Frank, J. L., Reibel, D., Cantrell, T., Sanders, R., & Broderick, P. C. (2013). The effectiveness of the Learning to BREATHE program on adolescent emotion regulation. *Research in Human Development, 10,* 252–272.

Needham, B., Crosnoe, R., & Muller, C. (2004). Academic failure in secondary school: The interrelated role of health problems and educational context. *Social Problems, 51,* 569–586.

Parker, A. E., Kupersmidt, J. B., Mathis, E. T., Scull, T. M., & Sims, C. (2013). The impact of mindfulness education on elementary school students: Evaluation of the Master Mind program. *Advances in School Mental Health Promotion, 7,* 184–204.

Piet, J., & Hougaard, E. (2011). The effect of mindfulness-based cognitive therapy for prevention of relapse in recurrent major depressive disorder: A systematic review and meta-analysis. *Clinical Psychology Review, 31,* 1032–1040.

Popkin, S. J., & McDaniel, M. (2013). *HOST: Can public housing be a platform for change?* Washington, DC: Urban Institute.

Reid, R., Gonzalez, J., Nordness, P. D., Trout, A., & Epstein, M. H. (2004). A meta-analysis of the academic status of students with emotional/behavioral disturbance. *Journal of Special Education, 38,* 130–143.

Roderick, M., Nagaoka, J., & Coca, V. (2009). College readiness for all: The challenge for urban high schools. *The Future of Children, 19,* 185–210.

Roeser, R. W., Schonert-Reichl, K. A., Jha, A., Cullen, M., Wallace, L., Wilensky, R., . . . Harrison, J. L. (2013). Mindfulness training and reductions in teacher stress and burnout:

Results from two ransomized, waitlist-control field trials. *Journal of Educational Psychology, 105*, 787–804.

Romeo, R. D. (2010). Adolescence: A central event in shaping stress reactivity. *Developmental Psychobiology, 52*, 244–253.

Ruchkin, V., Henrich, C. C., Jones, S. M., Vermeiren, R., & Schwab-Stone, M. (2007). Violence exposure and psychopathology in urban youth: The mediating role of posttraumatic stress. *Journal of Abnormal Child Psychology, 35*, 578–593.

Sampson, R. J. (2012). *Great American city: Chicago and the enduring neighborhood effect*. Chicago, IL: University of Chicago Press.

Schonert-Reichl, K. A., & Lawlor, M. S. (2010). The effects of a mindfulness-based education program on pre- and early adolescents' well-being and social and emotional competence. *Mindfulness, 1*, 137–151.

Schonert-Reichl, K. A., Oberle, E., Lawlor, M. S., Abbot, R. D., Thompson, E. A., Oberlander, T. F., & Diamond, A. (2015). Enhancing cognitive and social-emotional development through a simple-to-administer mindfulness-based school program for elementary school children: A randomized controlled trial. *Developmental Psychology, 51*, 52–66.

Segal, Z. V., Williams, M. G., & Teasdale, J. D. (2002). *Mindfulness-based cognitive therapy for depression*. New York, NY: Guilford Press.

Sibinga, E. M. S., Kerrigan, D., Stewart, M., Johnson, K., Magyari, T., & Ellen, J. M. (2011). Mindfulness-based stress reduction for urban youth. *The Journal of Alternative and Complementary Medicine, 17*, 213–218.

Sibinga, E. M. S., Perry-Parrish, C., Chung, S. E., Johnson, S. B., Smith, M., & Ellen, J. M. (2013). School-based mindfulness instruction for urban male youth: A small randomized controlled trial. *Preventive Medicine, 57*, 799–801.

Slopen, N., Fitzmaurice, G. M., Williams, D. R., & Gilman, S. E. (2012). Common patterns of violence experiences and depression and anxiety among adolescents. *Social Psychiatry and Psychiatric Epidemiology, 47*, 1591–1605.

Spear, L. P. (2009). Heightened stress responsivity and emotional reactivity during pubertal maturation: Implications for psychopathology. *Development and Psychopathology, 21*, 87–97.

Tang, Y.-Y., Ma, Y., Fan, Y., Feng, H., Wang, J., Feng, S., . . . Fan, M. (2009). Central and autonomic nervous system interaction is altered by short-term meditation. *Proceedings of the National Academy of Sciences, 106*, 8865–8870.

van der Oord, S., Bogels, S. M., & Peijnenburg, D. (2012). The effectiveness of mindfulness training for children with ADHD and mindful parenting for their parents. *Journal of Child and Family Studies, 21*, 775–787.

Wodtke, G. T., Harding, D. J., & Elwert, F. (2011). Neighborhood effects in temporal perspective: The impact of long-term exposure to concentrated disadvantage on high school graduation. *American Sociological Review, 76*, 713–736.

Zenner, C., Herrnleben-Kurz, S., & Walach, H. (2014). Mindfulness-based interventions in schools: A systematic review and meta-analysis. *Frontiers in Psychology, 5*. doi:10.3389/fpsyg.2014.00603

Zoogman, S., Goldberg, S. B., Hoyt, W. T., & Miller, L. (2014). Mindfulness interventions with youth: A meta-analysis. *Mindfulness, 6*, 290–302.

CHAPTER 13

Maternal Depression in Pregnancy

Amelia R. Gavin, PhD
Rebecca Rebbe, MSW

Major depression, a common and debilitating psychiatric disorder, is a major public health problem. Worldwide it is estimated that major depression will become the second most significant cause of disease burden by the year 2020 (World Health Organization, 2000). In the United States, one of the most consistent findings in this literature is women are nearly twice as likely as men to experience unipolar major depression (Kessler, 2003). The prevalence of major depression is highest among women between the ages of 25 and 44. The median age of onset for major depression therefore occurs during the childbearing years, which suggests many women are likely to experience major depression during pregnancy (Spinelli, 1998).

For some time, pregnancy was considered to be a time period in a woman's life where she was "protected" against the development of depression, in part due to the lower suicide rate during pregnancy and during the two years after childbirth (Oates, 2003). The idea that pregnancy was protective against depression probably contributed to research and clinical efforts to primarily focus on postpartum depression (Boyce, Galbally, Snellen, & Buist, 2014). More recently, we know that depression in pregnancy is a public health concern for a number of reasons. First, there has been recognition that depression during pregnancy is a common condition that often goes undetected and untreated (Ko, Farr, Dietz, & Robbins, 2012) despite the fact that the majority of pregnant women regularly obtain prenatal care services (Payne, 2012). Second, the rates of *DSM-IV*-defined major depression are relatively similar among pregnant, postpartum, and nonpregnant women (Vesga-López et al., 2008). Finally, depression in pregnancy is unique from depression occurring during other phases of a woman's life course because of potential short- and long-term effects on pregnancy outcomes, fetal development, and infant outcomes (Flynn, 2010; Waters, Hay, Simmonds, & van Goozen, 2014).

Consequences of Maternal Depression in Pregnancy

Maternal depression in pregnancy, either assessed as major depression using diagnostic criteria or as elevated depression symptoms, is highly prevalent during the antenatal period (Meltzer-Brody, 2011) and is associated with adverse outcomes for women, their offspring, and their families.

Maternal depression in pregnancy affects a woman's quality of life by adversely influencing her ability to fulfill her roles as a worker, mother, and partner (Yonkers, Vigod, & Ross, 2011a). Among pregnant women, major depression and elevated depression symptoms are associated with functional impairment, which may result in limitations in their ability to fully engage in social activities, occupational activities (Borri et al., 2008), and home management (Orr, Blazer, James, & Reiter, 2007), and may lead to increased health care service utilization (Bixo, Sundström-Poromaa, Björn, & Åström, 2001; Malmenström, Bixo, Björn, Åström, & Poromaa, 2006). It has been posited that the association between elevated depression symptoms and diminished health in pregnancy may in part explain increased risk of poor pregnancy outcomes (Orr et al., 2007).

A shared feature of both major depression and pregnancy is changes in appetite, which may result in substandard prenatal nutrition. Women who experience depression in pregnancy may eat a poor diet as a coping mechanism, or they may have a reduced motivation to maintain a healthy diet during pregnancy. Additionally, poor nutrition in pregnancy may also be linked to the development of mental health problems (Baskin, Hill, Jacka, O'Neil, & Skouteris, 2015). Evidence suggests that women who experience elevated depression symptoms in pregnancy are more likely to report poor maternal nutritional intake, which in the short term may result in suboptimal fetal development (Pina-Camacho, Jensen, Gaysina, & Barker, 2015).

Maternal depression in pregnancy is one of the strongest predictors of postpartum depression (Robertson, Grace, Wallington, & Stewart, 2004). Further, postpartum depression has a negative impact on maternal sensitivity, which may result in insecure maternal-offspring bonding and attachment (Campbell et al., 2004). As a result, depressed mothers are more likely to be intrusive and harsh with their infants (Campbell et al., 2004; NICHD Early Child Care Research Network, 1999) and less likely to engage in infant safety practices (Flynn, Davis, Marcus, Cunningham, & Blow, 2004) and healthy child development practices (Paulson, Dauber, & Leiferman, 2006).

Major depression and elevated depression symptoms in pregnancy have been directly associated with adverse birth outcomes, such as preterm birth, low birth weight, small-for-gestational-age, and cesarean delivery (Bansil et al., 2010; Grigoriadis et al., 2013c; Grote et al., 2010; Mei-Dan, Ray, & Vigod, 2015). Additionally, major depression in pregnancy has been indirectly linked to poor birth outcomes via substance use behaviors (e.g., pre-pregnancy substance use disorder, prenatal smoking), comorbid psychiatric disorders (e.g., anxiety), and pregnancy complications (e.g., gestational/pre-pregnancy diabetes, pre-pregnancy hypertension) (Mei-Dan et al., 2015; Räisänen et al., 2014; Winkel et al., 2015).

Moreover, offspring of women who experience major depression or elevated depression symptoms during pregnancy experience adverse outcomes that extend beyond parturition. Findings from prospective, longitudinal cohort studies, including the Avon (England) Longitudinal Study of Parents and Children, the Maternal Health Study, the Mater University Study of Pregnancy, and the South London Child Development Study, reported that maternal elevated depression symptoms in pregnancy predicted offspring developmental delay at 18 months of age (Deave, Heron, Evans, & Emond, 2008), child dysregulation at age 7 (Pina-Camacho et al., 2015), offspring mental health problems (Barker, Jaffee, Uher, & Maughan, 2011; Betts, Williams, Najman, & Alati, 2014; Pawlby, Hay, Sharp, Waters, & O'Keane, 2009), increased emotional and behavioral problems (Giallo, Woolhouse, Gartland, Hiscock, & Brown, 2015; Leis, Heron, Stuart, & Mendelson, 2014), and offspring depression in adulthood (Betts, Williams, Najman, & Alati, 2015; Pearson et al., 2013; Plant, Pariante, Sharp, & Pawlby, 2015). Furthermore, elevated depression symptoms during pregnancy significantly predicted offspring reporting engagement in violent acts or diagnosis of conduct disorder during adolescence (Hay, Pawlby, Waters, Perra, & Sharp, 2010).

Detection and Prevalence of Major Depression in Pregnancy

Despite the growing public health significance of maternal depression in pregnancy, there is less clarity on its exact prevalence. This may be due in part to the absence of mandatory routine screening protocols for prenatal depression in the United States. In the United States, obstetricians and gynecologists are frequently the primary care providers for women during their childbearing years. Therefore, these health care providers are most likely to care for women when they experience a depressive disorder (Yonkers et al., 2011a). As such, in 2010 (and most recently in 2015), the American College of Obstetrics and Gynecologists (ACOG) Committee on Obstetric Practice recommended, but did not mandate, routine screening for both prenatal and postpartum depression (ACOG, 2010, 2015). This lack of mandatory standards is also reflected in the extant literature; the prevalence estimates for maternal depression in pregnancy vary based on which definition of depression is used (major depression, minor depression, and elevated depressive symptomatology), the timing of depression assessment during pregnancy, characteristics of the sample population, and whether clinical depression or elevated depression symptoms were assessed (Gavin et al., 2005; Gaynes et al., 2005).

In the case of major depression, prior studies have either diagnosed major depression in pregnancy using a rigorous interview protocol such as the Structured Clinical Interview for *DSM* diagnoses (Spitzer, Williams, Gibbon, & First, 1992), confirmed diagnosis via physician-assigned diagnostic codes from patient records, or assumed a depression diagnosis based on the presence of an antidepressant medication prescription in the patient's medical record. This varied approach to identification of depression diagnoses may in part explain the varied estimates of major depression in pregnancy. For example, a systematic review of 28 prevalence studies conducted by Gavin and colleagues (2005) found that 12.7% of women experienced an episode of major depression during pregnancy. Additionally, the point prevalence of major depression was 3.8% in the first trimester, 4.9% in the second trimester, and 3.1% in the third trimester. Data from incidence studies suggest that 7.5% of women experience a new episode of major depression during the prenatal period. A meta-analysis of 30 studies revealed that the point prevalence estimates for major depression during pregnancy ranged from 3.1% to 4.9% (Gaynes et al., 2005). In a nationally representative sample of women from the National Epidemiological Survey on Alcohol and Related Conditions, Vesga-López and colleagues (2008) used the National Institute on Alcohol Abuse and Alcoholism's Alcohol Use Disorder and Associated Disabilities Interview Schedule-*DSM-IV* version to assess the 12-month prevalence of major depression during pregnancy. The authors reported 8.4% of the women in their study experienced major depression during pregnancy. Another study used data from the 2005–2009 National Surveys on Drug Use and found the 12-month prevalence of major depressive episode among pregnant women was 7.7% (Ko et al., 2012). However, in a large population-based study of 32.2 million women, hospital discharge data from the Nationwide Inpatient Sample revealed that only 0.8% of women had ICD-9-CM physician-diagnosed depressive disorders at the time of hospitalization for delivery (Bansil et al., 2010). Among 4,398 women continuously enrolled in a HMO practice, 6.9% had ICD-9-CM physician-diagnosed depressive disorders during pregnancy (Dietz et al., 2007).

Detection and Prevalence of Elevated Depression Symptoms in Pregnancy

In pregnancy, screening is a common method used to assess whether women have an elevated likelihood of being currently depressed. Screening for depressive symptoms does not establish a diagnosis of depression. Rather, screening for elevated depressive symptoms is determined as exceeding a cut point on a brief, self-reported depression symptom measure (O'Hara & Wisner, 2014). Prenatal screening for depressive symptoms is clinically important for a number of reasons. First, prenatal elevated depression symptoms are one of the strongest risk factors for postpartum depression symptoms (Paschetta et al., 2014). Given the well-documented negative effects of postpartum depression symptoms on maternal and offspring outcomes, it is vital to screen for depression in pregnancy. Second, women who report elevated depressive symptoms that fall short of a diagnostic threshold may still experience deleterious effects that adversely affect the course of pregnancy (Sidebottom, Harrison, Godecker, & Kim, 2012). Therefore, screening for depressive symptoms in pregnancy aims to identify women at risk for depression who may benefit from treatment in order to reduce maternal distress with improved pregnancy outcomes. Second, prenatal screening for depression symptoms is less expensive and time-consuming than conducting a diagnostic assessment because screening identifies a subgroup of women with elevated symptoms to better target diagnostic assessments (Milgrom & Gemmill, 2014). Lastly, depressive disorders and pregnancy share some features such as disturbed sleep, appetite changes, and decreased energy and interest levels. Because of the adverse consequences of elevated depression symptoms in pregnancy, screening is imperative to discriminate somatic symptoms of pregnancy from depression symptoms (Pereira et al., 2014).

Depression Screening Instruments in Pregnancy

The majority of epidemiologic data on depression in pregnancy has been documented using brief, self-administered instruments that assess elevated depression symptoms in pregnancy. Nearly all screening instruments used to assess depression symptoms in pregnancy were originally designed to assess elevated depressive symptoms among nonpregnant populations. Consequently, these screening instruments include symptoms of depression such as fatigue, appetite changes, and sleep problems, which are common features of pregnancy. Thus, the inclusion of somatic symptoms in depression screening scales make it difficult to distinguish depression symptoms from typical experiences of pregnancy, which may result in a higher prevalence of depressive symptoms among pregnant women compared to the prevalence of major depression (Castro E Couto et al., 2015; Sidebottom et al., 2012). Therefore, in order for screening to accurately identify a high prevalence group to which diagnostic assessments can then be offered, screening tools must be precise in determining the cutoff points above which pregnant women are at risk for elevated depressive symptoms (Milgrom & Gemmill, 2014).

A variety of tools have been validated for use as screening assessments for depression symptoms among pregnant women: these include the Primary Care Evaluation of Mental Disorders (PRIME-MD) Patient Health Questionnaire (PHQ), the Beck Depression Inventory (BDI), the Centers for Epidemiologic Studies Depression Scale (CES-D), and the Edinburgh Postnatal Depression Scale (EPDS).

The PRIME-MD is a clinician-administered diagnostic instrument that was developed and validated for use among primary care patients to assess mood, anxiety, eating, alcohol, and somatoform disorders (Spitzer et al., 1994; Spitzer, Williams, Kroenke, Hornyak, & McMurray, 2000). Given the resources needed to administer the PRIME-MD, the self-administered PRIME-MD PHQ was developed. Validated among 3,000 obstetric-gynecologic patients, the PRIME-MD PHQ was designed to assess disorders common among women, including postpartum mood disorders (Spitzer et al., 2000). The PHQ-9, a nine-item, self-administered depression module from the PRIME-MD PHQ, has been validated for use among obstetrics-gynecology patients and generates reliable criteria-based diagnoses of depressive disorders as well as depression severity. A score of 5–9 indicates mild depression, a score of 10–14 indicates moderate depression, a score of 15–19 indicates moderate to severe depression, and a score greater than 19 indicates severe depression (Kroenke, Spitzer, & Williams, 2001). In a validation study that assessed the PHQ-9 among a prenatal sample of 745 women, a PHQ-9 score of 10 or more indicated sensitivity (85%) and specificity (84%) rates for depression diagnoses (Sidebottom et al., 2012).

The BDI, a 21-item, self-administered questionnaire, was developed to assess the severity of depression symptomatology in psychiatric populations (Beck, Ward, Mendelson, Mock, & Erbaugh, 1961). Validated for use in 105 pregnant women, a score greater than 16 yielded sensitivity (83%) and specificity (89%) rates to detect current depression (Holcomb, Stone, Lustman, Gavard, & Mostello, 1996).

The CES-D is a widely used instrument to screen for depression symptoms among the general population. The CES-D is a 20-item, self-report scale designed to assess depression symptomatology during the past week (Radloff, 1977). A CES-D score of 16 or greater identifies those at increased risk for depression. However, some argue that a higher cutoff is needed because the CES-D contains features of depression symptoms that are similar to somatic complaints in pregnancy. Therefore, an alternative cutoff of 23 or higher has been used to identify those at risk for major depression (Wilusz, Peters, & Cassidy-Bushrow, 2014). The CES-D has been shown to be a valid measure among pregnant women, especially among different racial groups (Canady, Stommel, & Holzman, 2009).

The EPDS, the most widely used screening questionnaire in the perinatal period, was originally designed to detect postpartum depression symptoms (Bunevicius, Kusminskas, Pop, Pedersen, & Bunevicius, 2009; Cox, Holden, & Sagovsky, 1987). The EPDS is a 10-item instrument that assesses depression symptoms during the past seven days. An EPDS score of 12 or greater suggests being at risk for probable major depression, and a score of 10 or greater suggests being at risk for depression (includes major and minor depression combined). Unlike other depression symptom screeners, the EPDS excludes some somatic symptoms (e.g., changes in appetite and sleeping patterns) that are common features of the perinatal period (Milgrom & Gimmell, 2014). The EPDS has been increasingly used to screen for depression symptoms during pregnancy (Ji et al., 2011), as well as to identify those at risk for developing depression during pregnancy (Ji et al., 2011; Thoppil, Riutcel, & Nalesnik, 2005). Given the scale's extensive use during the prenatal period, it has been renamed the Edinburgh Depression Scale (EDS). A systematic review of 11 EDS validation studies revealed sensitivity and specificity estimates ranging from 64% to 100% and 73% to 100%, respectively. Despite the heterogeneity present among studies included in the review, the EDS is still considered a valid measure to assess depression symptoms in pregnancy (Kozinszky & Dudas, 2015).

Given the variation in depression screening instruments, determining the exact prevalence of elevated depression symptoms in pregnancy remains a challenge. In light of this challenge, Bennett and colleagues (2004) estimated the prevalence of elevated depression symptoms in pregnancy via a meta-analysis using 16 studies that screened for depression using either the EPDS or the BDI. The researchers reported that 14.2% of women reported elevated depression symptoms in the first trimester, 13.9% in the second trimester, and 13.2% in the third trimester (Bennett, Einarson, Taddio, Koren, & Einarson, 2004).

Maternal Risk Factors for Depression in Pregnancy
Risk Factors for Major Depression during Pregnancy

Clinically, it is important to determine the risk factors associated with depression in pregnancy because this may enable health professionals to more easily identify women who are at risk for developing the illness (Lancaster et al., 2010). For example, one of the most significant predictors of postpartum depression is maternal depression in pregnancy (O'Hara & Swain, 1996). Identifying women at risk for developing maternal depression during pregnancy appeared to be an important strategy to treat the illness as well as to prevent postpartum depression (Boyce et al., 2014). However, few studies have examined the risk factors for major depression in pregnancy, and these studies commonly rely on depression diagnoses from administrative data records. For example, a population-based, cross-sectional study of more than 500,000 pregnant women who gave birth between 2002 and 2010 used data from three national health registries to examine risk factors associated with physician-diagnosed major depression as defined by ICD-10 codes. Results from the study revealed that women with physician-diagnosed major depression during pregnancy were more likely to report a history of depression prior to pregnancy, low SES, and single marital status; were fearful of childbirth; and smoked during pregnancy (Räisänen et al., 2014). In another study, major depression during pregnancy was identified from medical records using physician-diagnosed major depression, defined by ICD-9 codes as well as treatment for major depression (antidepressant medication use or at least one mental health visit). Study findings suggest that 54.2% of women with physician-diagnosed depression in pregnancy reported a history of major depression prior to their pregnancy (Dietz et al., 2007). Among 192 low-income women, not having a cohabitating partner was found to heighten the risk for major depression during pregnancy (Hobfoll, Ritter, Lavin, Hulsizer, & Cameron, 1995). Elevated pre-pregnancy body mass index was also associated with major depression in pregnancy in a sample of 242 women (Bodnar, Wisner, Moses-Kolko, Sit, & Hanusa, 2009).

Risk Factors for Depression Symptoms during Pregnancy

Based on the extant obstetric literature, a number of risk factors have been identified for elevated depression symptoms during the prenatal period. Commonly observed risk factors include race and ethnicity, young maternal age, poor overall health, alcohol use, prenatal smoking, perceived racial discrimination, psychosocial stress, lack of social support, low educational attainment, unemployment, receipt of government-funded insurance, intimate partner violence, social conflict, pregnancy intent, and suicidal ideation (Bennett, Culhane, McCollum, Mathew, & Elo, 2007; Dayan et al., 2010; Ertel et al., 2012; Fellenzer & Cibula, 2014; Gavin et al., 2011; Leigh & Milgrom, 2008; Marcus, Flynn, Blow, & Barry, 2003; Melville, Gavin, Guo, Fan, & Katon, 2010; Mora et al., 2009; Westdahl et al., 2007).

Research studies have also shown that women who report certain risk factors prior to the pregnancy period are at significant risk for depression during pregnancy. These risk factors include a history of depression, childhood maltreatment, chronic health conditions (e.g., diabetes, hypertension, asthma, or cardiovascular problems), economic and psychosocial problems, and prior fetal loss (Armstrong, 2004; Gavin et al., 2011; Holzman et al., 2006; Leigh & Milgrom, 2008; Melville et al., 2010).

A recent systematic review of 57 studies reported that life stress (defined as psychologically significant events that occur in women's lives), negative life events, domestic violence, and lack of support from an intimate partner were significant risk factors for depression symptoms in pregnancy. Despite the strength of this review, limitations exist due to the significant heterogeneity present among the included studies, which precluded the authors from using meta-analytic procedures. First, studies used a variety of depression screening instruments, each of which had different cutoff points to indicate clinically significant depression symptoms. Second, the studies examined a wide range of risk factors for elevated depression symptoms in pregnancy, with one-third of the studies failing to control for confounders in their multivariate analyses (Lancaster et al., 2010).

Maternal Depression in Pregnancy: Treatment Strategies and Issues

Given the short- and long-term negative consequences associated with maternal depression during pregnancy for women, their offspring, and their families, it is vital that we offer effective treatment for those women who are affected. The effects of maternal depression during pregnancy on women and their families have been well documented. However, less is known about the efficacy of treatment designed to alleviate the effects of depression during pregnancy. Unfortunately, detection and treatment rates for women who reported depression during pregnancy are lower compared with their nonpregnant counterparts (Geier, Hills, Gonzales, Tum, & Finley, 2015; Vesga-López et al., 2008). In a nationally representative sample of women who were either pregnant or nonpregnant in the past 12 months, only 14.3% of pregnant women received treatment for a 12-month *DSM-IV* mood disorder compared to 15.0% of postpartum women and 25.5% of nonpregnant women (Vesga-López et al., 2008). Possible reasons for the lower depression treatment rates among pregnant women include misinterpretation of depression symptoms as normal pregnancy symptoms, the lack of consensus on safe and effective treatments for maternal depression in pregnancy, and reluctance to seek treatment for mental health concerns due to stigma (Battle, Uebelacker, Magee, Sutton, & Miller, 2015; Vesga-López et al., 2008).

A number of treatment interventions for maternal depression during pregnancy are available. Some of these treatment options may pose a risk to women and the fetus, and some treatment interventions are not well studied, making it difficult for women and health professionals to make informed treatment decisions. Given the present limitations in treatment options, how best to treat maternal depression in pregnancy remains a highly debated topic (Meltzer-Brody, 2011).

Psychological Treatment Approaches for Maternal Depression in Pregnancy

The American Psychiatric Association and the ACOG recommend the use of psychological (e.g., psychotherapeutic) approaches without medical therapy as a first-line treatment strategy to treat mild to moderate prenatal depression (Yonkers et al., 2009). Pregnant women often choose psychological treatments for their depression because of their reluctance to use psychopharmacologic approaches that may compromise the safety of the fetus (Goodman, 2009; O'Mahen & Flynn, 2008). In pregnancy, psychotherapeutic interventions, such as interpersonal therapy (IPT) and cognitive behavioral therapy (CBT), have been used both as a treatment option for maternal depression in pregnancy as well as a strategy to prevent the occurrence of postpartum depression (Bittner et al., 2014). Psychotherapeutic approaches have shown efficacy in treating depression in pregnancy (Stuart & Koleva, 2014) and in the treatment of postpartum depression (Sockol, 2015).

Interpersonal Therapy

There exist a small number of controlled studies that examined whether IPT may be an effective strategy for the treatment of major depression or depression symptoms during pregnancy. IPT is designed to treat depression by assisting individuals in addressing one of four interpersonal problem areas (role transition, role dispute, grief, and interpersonal deficits) that may be related to the onset or recurrence of a depressive episode (Grote et al., 2009). Spinelli and Endicott (2003) conducted a 16-week bilingual controlled clinical trial that tested the efficacy of IPT (originally designed for depression during the postpartum period and adapted for prenatal depression) versus a parenting education control program for 38 pregnant women with unipolar major depression. Women in the control group met with a therapist for 45-minute-long weekly sessions to discuss their symptoms and functioning. Study participants receiving IPT reported a significant reduction in depressed mood compared to the control group on the EPDS, BDI, and the Hamilton Depression Rating Scale. The treatment group also had substantially higher rates of recovery according to Clinical Global Impression scores. In an extension of their previous work, Spinelli and colleagues (2013) conducted a second controlled clinical trial that tested the efficacy of IPT among a bilingual sample of 142 pregnant women with unipolar major depression. Women in both groups received either 12 weekly sessions of IPT or a parent education program. Similar to the earlier study, women in the IPT group showed significant improvement in depressed mood based on clinician-rated and self-reported instruments. However, women who received the parenting education program also showed improvement in their mood and functioning by the end of the 12-week program, suggesting that this program may also be an alternative treatment that requires further study.

Two open-pilot trials examined a 12-week course of IPT adapted for pregnant adolescents using a group format (Miller, Gur, Shanok, & Weissman, 2008). The main focus of the modified IPT was promotion of self-advocacy skills among the adolescents to advocate for their needs with adults (Mufson, Weissman, Moreau, & Garfinkel, 1999). The first study tested the adapted IPT for management of depression symptoms among 14 respondents and was delivered during a health class; in the second study, the adapted IPT was tested for its efficacy in the treatment of depression symptoms among 11 respondents, delivered after school on a self-nominating basis. At 12-week termination, the level of depressive symptoms had decreased by 50% and 40%, respectively, with treatment effects maintained at 20 weeks postpartum (Miller et al., 2008).

Grote and colleagues (2009) implemented a randomized controlled trial of brief and enhanced IPT among a low-income sample of 53 pregnant women with elevated depression symptoms on the EDPS. IPT was modified to be culturally relevant to socioeconomically disadvantaged women. The treatment group received one engagement session, eight IPT sessions during their pregnancy, and bi-weekly or monthly maintenance sessions were provided for up to six months postpartum. The control group received enhanced usual care, including psychoeducational materials, and was encouraged to seek treatment for their depression at a local behavioral health clinic or community mental health clinic. Compared with women who received usual care (n = 28), women who received the enhanced IPT (n = 25) reported significantly higher rates of treatment engagement and retention as well as reduced depression diagnoses and depression symptoms before childbirth and at six months postpartum.

Thomas, Komiti, and Judd (2014) conducted a pilot study to investigate a group intervention designed to reduce the severity of depression and anxiety symptoms among pregnant women with current or past depression and anxiety symptoms. The intervention was group based and consisted of six sessions, and participants' partners were invited to attend two of the sessions. The intervention had four components, including behavioral self-care strategies, psychoeducation, IPT, and the parent-infant relationship. Pre- and posttreatment depression and anxiety symptom scores, assessed by the CES-D, EPDS, and the State-Trait Anxiety Inventory (STAI), demonstrated significant reductions in maternal depression in pregnancy.

IPT has also been delivered during pregnancy as an intervention strategy to prevent postpartum depression. In general, prevention interventions for postpartum depression target women who are at risk for maternal depression during pregnancy based on a history of depression or other risk factors previously shown to be associated with major depression or elevated depression symptoms. Zlotnick, Miller, Pearlstein, Howard, and Sweeney (2006) examined whether a brief IPT-based group intervention (four sessions during pregnancy and a booster session after childbirth) reduced the incidence of postpartum depression among depressed pregnant women who received public assistance. In the randomized controlled trial, 53 women were assigned to the IPT-based group intervention and 46 were provided standard prenatal care. At three months postpartum, two women from the intervention group developed postpartum major depressive disorder compared to eight women who received the standard prenatal care group.

Cognitive Behavioral Therapy

CBT is a widely studied treatment for perinatal depression. In brief, CBT targets problematic thinking patterns or behaviors that are linked to individuals' depression through strategies designed to change maladaptive thinking, increase mood-enhancing activities, and solve life problems (Dimidjian & Goodman, 2009). CBT is a validated and effective modality for the treatment of depression in as few as three to six sessions (Richards et al., 2003, Scott, Tacchi, Jones, & Scott, 1997). Numerous randomized control trials of both individual and group-based CBT interventions in pregnancy designed to prevent postpartum depression have been implemented (Austin et al., 2008; Le, Perry, & Stuart, 2011; Leung et al., 2013; O'Mahen, Himle, Fedock, Henshaw, & Flynn, 2013). In general, randomized control trials of CBT group-based interventions have been found to reduce the severity of postpartum depression among treatment groups compared to control groups (Goodman & Santangelo, 2011). Several controlled trials of CBT have been conducted that look to treat depression during pregnancy.

Milgrom and colleagues (2015) implemented a feasibility study and a pilot randomized controlled trial on the efficacy of a brief CBT treatment intervention designed to reduce depression and anxiety symptoms among pregnant women. The brief CBT intervention was adapted from a 12-session group postpartum intervention. Given that there were no studies that examined the effects of treatment interventions on offspring outcomes, the authors explored whether the intervention had an impact on several infant outcomes at nine months postpartum. A total of 42 pregnant women were randomized to either the CBT treatment (n = 20) or usual prenatal care (n = 22). Women in the treatment group received eight one-on-one sessions. Women who received the CBT had a significant reduction in the severity of both depression and anxiety symptoms in pregnancy compared to the usual care group as assessed by the Beck Depression Inventory-Revised (BDI-II) and the EPDS. Improvement in depression symptoms was maintained at nine months for those who were in the treatment group. A dose-response between the number of CBT sessions and improvement of depression symptoms was evident. Infant outcomes were assessed via the Ages and Stages Questionnaire (ASQ-3), the Ages and Stages Questionnaire Social Emotional (ASQ-SE), and the Revised Infant Behavioral Questionnaire Short Form. Infants of mothers in the treatment group showed improvements in three domains of child developmental outcomes, including problem-solving, self-regulation, and stress reactivity, after controlling for postpartum depression and anxiety symptoms.

Bittner and colleagues (2014) conducted a randomized controlled trial to assess the efficacy of an eight-session, group-based CBT with elevated depression and anxiety symptoms (also included were psychoeducation and relaxation techniques) delivered to 36 depressed pregnant women (control group consisted of 57 women). The modified CBT was delivered by trained clinical therapists. It was adapted for pregnancy based on an established program for adolescents and young adults. Women in both groups experienced a decline in depression and anxiety symptoms as measured by the BDI, EPDS, and the STAI. Additionally, three months after childbirth, intervention effects were present for women with high depression symptoms prior to the intervention.

Burns and colleagues (2013) conducted a pilot randomized controlled trial of CBT aimed at successfully treating major depression before the end of pregnancy. The CBT intervention was modified to include the role of maternal beliefs, constraints related to behavioral activation, and principles and strategies to improve communication and social support. Randomization resulted in 18 women in the treatment group and 18 in the control group. The intervention, consisting of up to 12 individual sessions of CBT, was delivered at women's homes by CBT therapists. Findings suggest that by the end of pregnancy (15 weeks postrandomization), 68.7% of women in the intervention group no longer met ICD-10 criteria for depression compared to 38.5% of women who received usual prenatal care.

McGregor, Coghlan, and Dennis (2014) examined the effectiveness of a pilot quasi-experimental trial to treat maternal depression in pregnancy. The CBT intervention was delivered in six sessions by individual obstetricians who provided prenatal care to women in the study. Forty-two women participated in the pilot trial. Women assigned to the intervention group (n = 21) received the CBT intervention, while the control group (n = 21) received standard prenatal care. Although, small sample size prevented detection of group differences, mean depression symptoms (as measured by the EPDS) for women in the intervention group were lower compared to women in the control group.

It is clear that IPT and CBT modalities may be effective therapies in treating maternal depression in pregnancy. However, larger controlled studies are needed to provide consistent and reliable evidence for their application in the treatment of depression in pregnancy.

Antidepressants to Treat Maternal Depression in Pregnancy

The American Psychiatric Association (2010) recommended medical therapy treatment alone or combined with psychotherapeutic approaches when patients experience severe acute depression, or persistent depression symptoms. During the prenatal period, antidepressant medications remain a primary treatment strategy for treating maternal depression (Battle, Salisbury, Schofield, & Ortiz-Hernandez, 2013). In the United States, the proportion of women seeking prenatal care who received a prescription for antidepressant medication increased threefold (0.7%–2.1%) between 2002 and 2010. Over this same period, the proportion of prescriptions for selective serotonin reuptake inhibitors (SSRIs), the most frequently used antidepressant among pregnant women, declined from 87% to 66% (Meunier, Bennett, & Coco, 2013).

The decision whether to use antidepressants at times during pregnancy remains a complicated one. This leaves pregnant women with a history of depression or current depression symptoms and health professionals with many issues to consider (Richards & Payne, 2013). For example, due to ethical issues, the efficacy of SSRIs in pregnant women has not been determined in large randomized control trials (Weisskopf et al., 2015). Rather, the findings from smaller studies provide some evidence of the utility of antidepressant medication in the treatment of depression during pregnancy. Yonkers and colleagues (2011b) conducted a randomized controlled study of 778 pregnant women with a history of any depressive disorder and found that the risk of a major depressive episode during pregnancy was not statistically different for women who took their antidepressant medication from those who discontinued their medication. Cohen and colleagues (2006) investigated the time to relapse among a sample of depressed pregnant women and reported that those who discontinued their antidepressant medication were more likely to experience frequent relapses compared with women who continued their medication (68% vs. 26%). Wisner and colleagues (2009) studied 238 pregnant women and categorized them into three mutually exclusive exposure groups: (1) no major depression or SSRI exposure, (2) major depression with SSRI exposure (either continuous or partial use during pregnancy), and (3) major depression (either the presence of major depression throughout the entire pregnancy or at some point during pregnancy) with no SSRI exposure. Women with continuous major depression and no SSRI treatment had significantly higher depression symptoms compared with women in all other groups. Although findings from these studies suggest antidepressant use may be a treatment option during pregnancy, not all pregnant women will experience this benefit.

Second, the decision to use antidepressants during pregnancy is complicated by the need for women and their clinicians to balance the potential benefits versus the risks of antidepressant medications, as well as to consider that exposure to untreated maternal depression poses risks for both a woman and her fetus. Unfortunately, many of the risks associated with either antidepressant use during pregnancy or exposure to untreated depression during pregnancy are presumably unknown. For example, the effects of fetal exposure to untreated maternal depression are difficult to determine from those of fetal exposure to antidepressant medication (Richards & Payne, 2013). Ethical considerations prohibit the availability of controlled studies among pregnant women to determine the risks to infants associated with exposure to untreated depression or antidepressant exposure in utero. As a result, women and their clinicians must base the decision to use antidepressant medications during pregnancy on naturalistic studies of infant outcomes among depressed pregnant women who either use or do not use antidepressant medication during pregnancy (Suri, Lin, Cohen, & Altshuler, 2014).

The effect of maternal depression during pregnancy and of antidepressants on adverse pregnancy outcomes and neonatal complications has been extensively studied (Accortt, Cheadle, & Dunkel Schetter, 2015; Grote et al., 2009; Yonkers, Blackwell, Glover, & Forray, 2014; Yonkers et al., 2009); however, several limitations must be considered when interpreting this literature. First, many studies that examined the association between antidepressant medication use in pregnancy and adverse birth outcomes excluded data on maternal comorbid psychiatric illness. Second, few studies assessed depressive disorders by using diagnostic criteria or included detailed information regarding length of exposure and dosage levels for antidepressant medications. Third, although more than 80% of women take at least one dose of medication (excluding vitamins) during pregnancy (Headley, Northstone, Simmons, Golding, & ALSPAC Study Team, 2004), most studies failed to account for the frequent use of multiple medications in pregnancy and the impact on obstetric outcomes. Finally, comorbid health behaviors that influence birth outcomes, such as poor prenatal care and prenatal substance use, were not consistently controlled (Richards & Payne, 2013; Yonkers et al., 2009). Despite these limitations, we present a brief review of the primary findings of the available data.

Malformations

There have been conflicting findings for an association between antidepressant medication use in pregnancy and a range of major congenital malformations from the eight meta-analyses that have examined the association. Overall, four of these studies found no association between antidepressant exposure and any major malformation (Addis & Koren, 2000; Einarson & Einarson, 2005; Grigoriadis et al., 2013b; Rahimi, Nikfar, & Abdollahi, 2006), three studies reported an association between antidepressant treatment and cardiac malformation (Bar-Oz et al., 2007; Myles, Newall, Ward, & Large, 2013; Wurst, Poole, Ephross, & Olshan, 2010), and one study found no elevated risk for cardiac malformation (O'Brien, Einarson, Sarkar, Einarson, & Koren, 2008). A Danish population-based cohort study reported an association between major congenital malformations (specifically cardiac malformations) and antidepressant treatment among women with first trimester exposure and paused exposure during the second and third trimesters (Jimenez-Solem et al., 2012). More recently, Huybrechts and colleagues (2014a) investigated whether antidepressant exposure was associated with an increased risk of cardiac malformation among a population-based sample of Medicaid eligible pregnant women. Results suggested there was no substantial increase in the risk of cardiac malformations.

Neonatal Behavioral Syndrome

Exposure to antidepressants during late pregnancy has been linked to infant irritability, abnormal crying, tremors, lethargy, hypoactivity, decreased feeding, tachypnea, and respiratory distress (Byatt, Deligiannidis, & Freeman, 2013). Collectively, these symptoms are referred to as poor (or postnatal) neonatal adaptation syndrome (PNAS). Symptoms usually develop after birth and are time-limited and resolve within days or weeks of delivery with supportive care (Moses-Kolko et al., 2005). Mechanisms for PNAS are not clearly understood, yet serotonin toxicity (Oberlander et al., 2004), withdrawal or discontinuation syndrome (Levinson-Castiel, Merlob, Linder, Sirota, & Klinger, 2006), or infant genotype (Knoppert, Nimkar, Principi, & Yuen, 2006) may be possible explanations. There have been inconsistent findings with regard to a statistically significant association between prenatal antidepressant use and increased risk of PNAS. Warburton, Hertzman, and Oberlander (2010), in a population-based study of 119,547 birth records, examined the risk of adverse neonatal outcomes among infants who were exposed in utero to antidepressants during the last 14 days of pregnancy. Results suggest there was no difference in the risk of developing clinical symptoms of PNAS between infants exposed to antidepressants in late pregnancy compared to infants who had gestational exposure other than during the last 14 days of pregnancy. Findings from a recent meta-analysis revealed a significant association for two specific clinical symptoms of PNAS, respiratory distress and tremors, in infants who were exposed to antidepressants in utero (Grigoriadis et al., 2013a). Ewing, Tatarchuk, Appleby, Schwartz, and Kim (2015) conducted a review that explored whether there are patterns of placental transfer of antidepressants into the fetal environment and increased risk of PNAS. The authors found no consistent pattern between antidepressants with the highest transfer percentages of placental permeability (e.g., fluoxetine, venlafaxine) and increased risk of PNAS.

Adverse Birth Outcomes

Adverse birth outcomes, such as low birth weight (weighing less than 2500g at birth) and preterm birth (less than 37 weeks of completed gestation), are leading causes of infant morbidity and mortality in the United States (Martin et al., 2012). Although previous studies have produced mixed results regarding the effect of antidepressant use during pregnancy on the risk of low birth weight and preterm birth (Chambers, Johnson, Dick, Felix, & Jones, 1996; Källén, 2004; Malm, Klaukka, & Neuvonen, 2005; Marroun et al., 2012; Oberlander, Warburton, Misri, Aghajanian, & Hertzman, 2006;

Wen et al., 2006; Wisner et al., 2013), findings from three recent meta-analyses suggested a small increased risk of both low birth weight and preterm birth among infants exposed in utero to antidepressant medications. Ross and colleagues (2013) reported that gestational age and preterm birth were significantly associated with antidepressant exposure during pregnancy. The authors also found a decrease in birth weight of 74 grams for infants exposed to antidepressants in utero compared to those infants not exposed. However, sensitivity analysis limited to studies that included control groups of depressed mothers who did not use antidepressant medications resulted in differences in birth weight between the two groups that were no longer significant. Huang, Coleman, Bridge, Yonkers, and Katon (2014) observed that both low birth weight and preterm birth were significantly associated with antidepressant use during pregnancy. The association did not differ significantly based on medication type (SSRI vs. other antidepressant, or mixed), study design (prospective vs. retrospective), or control group (depressed mothers without antidepressants vs. mixed or nondepressed). Finally, Huybrechts, Sanghani, Avorn, and Urato (2014b) also found a statistically significant association between antidepressant medication use during pregnancy and preterm birth among infants who were exposed during the second and third trimesters of pregnancy. Notably, the association remained after adjusting for depression diagnosis. Despite the findings of the meta-analyses, there is concern that many of the reviewed articles failed to adequately address confounding associated with the depression illness and its severity. Moreover, this line of inquiry is bolstered by the results of a meta-analysis that revealed that maternal depression during pregnancy was associated with increased risk of low birth weight and preterm birth (Grote et al., 2010). It has been posited that pregnant women with a diagnosis of depression who continue their antidepressant medication do so for reasons that differ from pregnant women who discontinue their medications. If this is the case, then it is likely that the underlying depressive disorder has a role in the increased risk of low birth weight and preterm birth rather than the antidepressant medication alone (Huybrechts et al., 2014b).

Spontaneous Abortion

Spontaneous abortion, or miscarriage, refers to the loss of a fetus before the 20th week of gestation in the absence of outside intervention (Epstein, Moore, & Bobo, 2014). There have been inconsistent findings regarding the link between spontaneous abortion and the use of antidepressants during pregnancy. Some studies establish a link (Chun-Fai-Chan et al., 2005; Einarson, Choi, Einarson, & Koren, 2009; Hemels, Einarson, Koren, Lanctôt, & Einarson, 2005; Klieger-Grossmann et al., 2012; Nakhai-Pour, Broy, & Bérard, 2010), while other studies were negative (Einarson et al., 2003; Kulin et al., 1998). A recent meta-analysis found no support for an association between spontaneous abortion and antidepressant exposure during pregnancy (Ross et al., 2013), which is inconsistent with the findings of two previous meta-analyses (Hemels et al.,

2005; Rahimi et al., 2006). Not included in the previous meta-analyses was a study that used population-based data from the Danish Medical Birth Registry and the Danish National Hospital Registry to generate a sample of 1,005,319 pregnancies in Denmark between February 1997 to December 2008. The authors reported a small increase of spontaneous abortion associated with antidepressant exposure during pregnancy. However, when the sample was restricted to women with a diagnosis of depression, the association was no longer statistically significant (Kjaersgaard et al., 2013).

Neurodevelopmental Outcomes among Offspring Exposed to Antidepressants

There is a growing concern that exposure to antidepressant medications during pregnancy may pose a risk to the developing fetus as well as later infant motor, psychological, and cognitive outcomes. To determine the reproductive safety of antidepressants, studies must separate the effects of maternal depression in pregnancy from the effects of exposure to antidepressants (Nulman et al., 2012). Only a few controlled studies have investigated the neurodevelopmental outcomes of children exposed to antidepressant medication during pregnancy, and these studies report mixed findings. Nulman and colleagues (1997, 2002) reported no difference between young children (aged 1–7) exposed to antidepressant medications during pregnancy and comparison groups on global IQ, language development, or behavior. In their most recent study, Nulman and colleagues (2012) again showed there was no effect of antidepressant exposure in pregnancy on children's IQ or behavioral outcomes. In comparison, Casper and colleagues (2003) suggested that children (aged 6–40 months) exposed to antidepressants during pregnancy experienced subtle problems with motor development and control, as well as lower APGAR scores compared with children of depressed mothers who were not treated with antidepressants. Similar to Casper and colleagues (2003), Galbally, Lewis, & Buist (2011) reported subtle motor development effects among children exposed to antidepressants during pregnancy, yet these findings failed to meet the clinical criteria for developmental delay. Pedersen, Henriksen, and Olsen (2010) found a small developmental delay in gross motor function in children exposed to antidepressants during the second and third trimesters of pregnancy compared to children of depressed mothers who did not use antidepressants during pregnancy. The effect was present at 6 months of age, but no difference in gross motor function was present at 19 months of age.

Persistent Pulmonary Hypertension

Persistent pulmonary hypertension of the newborn (PPHN) is a rare but potentially adverse neonatal outcome that occurs in 1–2 per 1,000 infants and is caused by a failure to transition to newborn circulatory functioning during delivery (Epstein et al., 2014). In 2006, Chambers and colleagues first reported an association between in utero exposure to SSRIs after the 20th week of pregnancy and increased risk of PPHN in a nested case-control study of more than 1,200 women. In that same year, the FDA issued a warning that there is an increased risk of PPHN with SSRI use after the 20th week of pregnancy. This resulted in warning labels outlining the risk of PPHN. Since this article by Chambers and colleagues was published, subsequent studies have found an association in both early pregnancy exposure as well as late pregnancy exposure to antidepressants and increased risk of PPHN (Grigoriadis et al., 2014; Källén & Olausson, 2008; Kieler et al., 2012; Reis & Källén, 2010). However, other studies have suggested no association between antidepressant exposure in utero and increased risk of PPHN (Andrade et al., 2009; Wichman et al., 2009; Wilson et al., 2011). In December 2011, the FDA amended its earlier advisory, which stated that available data is conflicting, and there is insufficient evidence to conclude that antidepressant exposure during pregnancy causes an increased risk of PPHN (US Food and Drug Administration, 2011).

Other Treatment Approaches for Maternal Depression in Pregnancy

Physical Exercise

In 2002, the ACOG recommended that pregnant women without medical or obstetric complications follow the recommendations from the American College of Sports Medicine and Centers for Disease Control and Prevention for physical exercise by engaging in 30 minutes or more of moderate exercise a day (ACOG, 2002). Pregnancy is considered a unique opportunity for women to engage in positive health behaviors, such as physical exercise (Artal & O'Toole, 2003). Given that the physical risks associated with exercise for both women and fetus are rare, physical exercise during pregnancy may result in health benefits across a woman's subsequent life course (Nascimento, Surita, & Cecatti, 2012). A systematic review examined the effectiveness of exercise as an intervention to treat maternal depression in pregnancy as well as to prevent depression during the postpartum period. Six randomized controlled trials were included in the review, and preliminary findings suggest that exercise may be an effective treatment for reducing depression symptoms during pregnancy. There is less evidence that exercise prevented maternal depression during pregnancy (Daley et al., 2015). More recently, an open trial was implemented to investigate the feasibility of a gentle prenatal yoga intervention as an approach to treat prenatal depression. Battle and colleagues (2015) delivered a 10-week prenatal yoga program to 34 depressed pregnant women recruited from prenatal care settings. Results suggested that the intervention was feasible to administer was acceptable to participants, and significant improvements were evident in depression severity. Although prenatal exercise may hold some promise as an effective treatment for maternal depression in pregnancy, existing studies are limited by small sample size, the small number of trials, lack of evidence on what type of exercise might be most effective to treat depression during pregnancy, and mechanisms that, in part, explain the role of exercise in reducing prenatal depression (Field, Diego, Delgado, & Medina, 2013a, 2013b; Robledo-Colonia, Sandoval-

Restrepo, Mosquera-Valderrama, Escobar-Hurtado, & Ramírez-Vélez, 2012). As a result, large-scale controlled studies are needed to determine whether reductions in depression symptoms during pregnancy are attributable to prenatal exercise (Epstein et al., 2014).

Light Therapy

Bright light therapy is effective in the treatment of seasonal and nonseasonal depression (Even, Schröder, Friedman, & Rouillon, 2008) and may be a promising treatment for prenatal depression symptoms. Oren and colleagues (2002) conducted an open trial of 16 pregnant women with prenatal depression in which the participants received 10,000 lux bright light therapy for 60 minutes per day for three weeks. Findings suggest a significant reduction (by 49%) of depression among all participants and a decrease of 59% for seven participants who continued treatment for five weeks.

Epperson and colleagues (2004) conducted a randomized controlled trial in which five women were randomized to the treatment group and received 7,000 lux bright light therapy for 60 minutes per day for five weeks, while women in the placebo group (n = 5) received 500 lux light. Results suggest depression was reduced similarly in both conditions.

Wirz-Justice and colleagues (2011) randomized 16 women to a treatment group that received 7,000 lux bright light therapy for 60 minutes per day for five weeks, while women in the placebo group (n = 11) received 500 lux light. Compared to the placebo group, participants who received the treatment showed improvement in depression symptoms during pregnancy, as measured by the Hamilton Depression Rating Scale and the Structured Interview Guide for the Hamilton Depression Rating Scale with Atypical Depression Supplement (SIGH-ADS).

Despite being limited by small sample sizes, results from existing controlled studies suggest the potential use of bright light therapy as an effective therapy for maternal depression. However, large-scale controlled studies are needed to ascertain the antidepressive effect of bright light therapy in the treatment for maternal depression in pregnancy (Crowley & Youngstedt, 2012).

Acupuncture

Acupuncture, due to its minimal and transient side effects, may be an effective strategy to treat maternal depression in pregnancy. Manber and colleagues (2009) investigated a randomized controlled trial of acupuncture for the treatment of depressed pregnant women. A total of 150 participants were randomized to the treatment group (n = 52), which consisted of acupuncture specific for depression treatment. The remaining participants were randomized into two control groups, including acupuncture not specific for depression (n = 49) or prenatal massage (n = 49). Treatment was delivered in 12 sessions over an eight-week period. The treatment group participants reported a greater rate of decrease in depression symptom severity compared to the control acupuncture alone or the two control groups combined.

Conclusion

In this chapter, we presented some of the important issues surrounding maternal depression during pregnancy, including the ways it is measured as well as its prevalence, risk factors, and treatment alternatives. Given the tremendous burdens that untreated depression during pregnancy pose for women and their children, clinical recommendations underscore the need for universal screening for depression during the prenatal period as well as the implementation of effective treatment options. Although our understanding of maternal depression during pregnancy has improved, unanswered questions remain. Lines of inquiry include: (1) distinguishing the risks associated with the pregnant woman's underlying depressive disorder from those associated with antidepressant medication treatment, (2) the impact of maternal depression during pregnancy on offspring development across the life span, and (3) the effective implementation of treatment strategies that safeguard the short- and long-term health outcomes of mothers and their children.

References

Accortt, E. E., Cheadle, A. C. D., & Dunkel Schetter, C. (2015). Prenatal depression and adverse birth outcomes: An updated systematic review. *Maternal and Child Health Journal, 19*(6), 1306–1337.

Addis, A., & Koren, G. (2000). Safety of fluoxetine during the first trimester of pregnancy: A meta-analytical review of epidemiological studies. *Psychological Medicine, 30*(1), 89–94.

American College of Obstetricians and Gynecologists Committee on Obstetric Practice. (2002). *Committee opinion no. 267: Exercise during pregnancy and the postpartum period.* Retrieved from http://www.acog.org/Resources-And-Publications/Committee-Opinions /Committee-on-Obstetric-Practice/Exercise-During-Pregnancy-and-the-Postpartum-Period

American College of Obstetricians and Gynecologists Committee on Obstetric Practice. (2010). Committee opinion no. 453. Screening for depression during and after pregnancy. *Obstetrics and Gynecology, 115*(2), 394–395.

American College of Obstetricians and Gynecologists Committee on Obstetric Practice. (2015). Committee opinion no. 630. Screening for perinatal depression. *Obstetrics and Gynecology, 125*(5), 1268–1271.

American Psychiatric Association. (2010). *Practice guideline for the treatment of patients with major depressive disorder, 3rd edition.* Washington, DC: American Psychiatric Association.

Andrade, S. E., McPhillips, H., Loren, D., Raebel, M. A., Lane, K., Livingston, J., & Platt, R. (2009). Antidepressant medication use and risk of persistent pulmonary hypertension of the newborn. *Pharmacoepidemiology and Drug Safety, 18*(3), 246–252.

Armstrong, D. S. (2004). Impact of prior perinatal loss on subsequent pregnancies. *Journal of Obstetric, Gynecologic, and Neonatal Nursing, 33*(6), 765–773.

Artal, R., & O'Toole, M. (2003). Guidelines of the American College of Obstetricians and Gynecologists for exercise during pregnancy and the postpartum period. *British Journal of Sports Medicine, 37*(1), 6–12.

Austin, M.-P., Frilingos, M., Lumley, J., Hadzi-Pavlovic, D., Roncolato, W., Acland, S., & Parker, G. (2008). Brief antenatal cognitive behaviour therapy group intervention for the prevention of postnatal depression and anxiety: A randomised controlled trial. *Journal of Affective Disorders, 105*(1–3), 35–44.

Bansil, P., Kuklina, E. V., Meikle, S. F., Posner, S. F., Kourtis, A. P., Ellington, S. R., & Jamieson, D. J. (2010). Maternal and fetal outcomes among women with depression. *Journal of Women's Health, 19*(2), 329–334.

Barker, E. D., Jaffee, S. R., Uher, R., & Maughan, B. (2011). The contribution of prenatal and postnatal maternal anxiety and depression to child maladjustment. *Depression and Anxiety, 28*(8), 696–702.

Bar-Oz, B., Einarson, T., Einarson, A., Boskovic, R., O'Brien, L., Malm, H., & Koren, G. (2007). Paroxetine and congenital malformations: Meta-analysis and consideration of potential confounding factors. *Clinical Therapeutics, 29*(5), 918–926.

Baskin, R., Hill, B., Jacka, F. N., O'Neil, A., & Skouteris, H. (2015). The association between diet quality and mental health during the perinatal period: A systematic review. *Appetite, 91*, 41–47.

Battle, C. L., Salisbury, A. L., Schofield, C. A., & Ortiz-Hernandez, S. (2013). Perinatal antidepressant use: Understanding women's preferences and concerns. *Journal of Psychiatric Practice, 19*(6), 443–453.

Battle, C. L., Uebelacker, L. A., Magee, S. R., Sutton, K. A., & Miller, I. W. (2015). Potential for prenatal yoga to serve as an intervention to treat depression during pregnancy. *Women's Health Issues, 25*(2), 134–141.

Beck, A. T., Ward, C. H., Mendelson, M., Mock, J., & Erbaugh, J. (1961). An inventory for measuring depression. *Archives of General Psychiatry, 4*, 561–571.

Bennett, H. A., Einarson, A., Taddio, A., Koren, G., & Einarson, T. R. (2004). Prevalence of depression during pregnancy: Systematic review. *Obstetrics and Gynecology, 103*(4), 698–709.

Bennett, I. M., Culhane, J. F., McCollum, K. F., Mathew, L., & Elo, I. T. (2007). Literacy and depressive symptomatology among pregnant Latinas with limited English proficiency. *American Journal of Orthopsychiatry, 77*(2), 243–248.

Betts, K. S., Williams, G. M., Najman, J. M., & Alati, R. (2014). Maternal depressive, anxious, and stress symptoms during pregnancy predict internalizing problems in adolescence. *Depression and Anxiety, 31*(1), 9–18.

Betts, K. S., Williams, G. M., Najman, J. M., & Alati, R. (2015). The relationship between maternal depressive, anxious, and stress symptoms during pregnancy and adult offspring behavioral and emotional problems. *Depression and Anxiety, 32*(2), 82–90.

Bittner, A., Peukert, J., Zimmermann, C., Junge-Hoffmeister, J., Parker, L. S., Stöbel-Richter, Y., & Weidner, K. (2014). Early intervention in pregnant women with elevated anxiety and depressive symptoms: Efficacy of a cognitive-behavioral group program. *Journal of Perinatal and Neonatal Nursing, 28*(3), 185–195.

Bixo, M., Sundström-Poromaa, I., Björn, I., & Åström, M. (2001). Patients with psychiatric disorders in gynecologic practice. *American Journal of Obstetrics and Gynecology, 185*(2), 396–402.

Bodnar, L. M., Wisner, K. L., Moses-Kolko, E., Sit, D. K. Y., & Hanusa, B. H. (2009). Pre-pregnancy body mass index, gestational weight gain, and the likelihood of major depressive disorder during pregnancy. *Journal of Clinical Psychiatry, 70*(9), 1290–1296.

Borri, C., Mauri, M., Oppo, A., Banti, S., Rambelli, C., Ramacciotti, D., & Cassano, G. B. (2008). Axis I psychopathology and functional impairment at the third month of pregnancy: Results from the Perinatal Depression-Research and Screening Unit (PND-ReScU) study. *Journal of Clinical Psychiatry, 69*(10), 1617–1624.

Boyce, P., Galbally, M., Snellen, M., & Buist, A. (2014). Pharmacological management of major depression in pregnancy. In M. Galbally, M. Snellen, & A. Lewis (Eds.), *Psychopharmacology and pregnancy: Treatment efficacy, risks, and guidelines* (pp. 67–85). Berlin Heidelberg: Springer-Verlag.

Bunevicius, A., Kusminskas, L., Pop, V. J., Pedersen, C. A., & Bunevicius, R. (2009). Screening for antenatal depression with the Edinburgh Depression Scale. *Journal of Psychosomatic Obstetrics and Gynaecology, 30*(4), 238–243.

Burns, A., O'Mahen, H., Baxter, H., Bennert, K., Wiles, N., Ramchandani, P., & Evans, J. (2013). A pilot randomised controlled trial of cognitive behavioural therapy for antenatal depression. *BMC Psychiatry, 13*, 33.

Byatt, N., Deligiannidis, K. M., & Freeman, M. P. (2013). Antidepressant use in pregnancy: A critical review focused on risks and controversies. *Acta Psychiatrica Scandinavica, 127*(2), 94–114.

Campbell, S. B., Brownell, C. A., Hungerford, A., Spieker, S. I., Mohan, R., & Blessing, J. S. (2004). The course of maternal depressive symptoms and maternal sensitivity as predictors of attachment security at 36 months. *Development and Psychopathology, 16*(2), 231–252.

Canady, R. B., Stommel, M., & Holzman, C. (2009). Measurement properties of the centers for epidemiological studies depression scale (CES-D) in a sample of African American and non-Hispanic white pregnant women. *Journal of Nursing Measurement, 17*(2), 91–104.

Casper, R. C., Fleisher, B. E., Lee-Ancajas, J. C., Gilles, A., Gaylor, E., DeBattista, A., & Hoyme, H. E. (2003). Follow-up of children of depressed mothers exposed or not exposed to antidepressant drugs during pregnancy. *Journal of Pediatrics, 142*(4), 402–408.

Castro, E., Couto, T., Martins Brancaglion, M. Y., Nogueira Cardoso, M., Bergo Protzner, A., Duarte Garcia, F., Nicolato, R., & Corrêa, H. (2015). What is the best tool for screening antenatal depression? *Journal of Affective Disorders, 178*, 12–17.

Chambers, C. D., Hernández-Diaz, S., Van Marter, L. J., Werler, M. M., Louik, C., Jones, K. L., & Mitchell, A. A. (2006). Selective serotonin-reuptake inhibitors and risk of persistent pulmonary hypertension of the newborn. *New England Journal of Medicine, 354*(6), 579–587.

Chambers, C. D., Johnson, K. A., Dick, L. M., Felix, R. J., & Jones, K. L. (1996). Birth outcomes in pregnant women taking fluoxetine. *New England Journal of Medicine, 335*(14), 1010–1015.

Chun-Fai-Chan, B., Koren, G., Fayez, I., Kalra, S., Voyer-Lavigne, S., Boshier, A., & Einarson, A. (2005). Pregnancy outcome of women exposed to bupropion during pregnancy: A prospective comparative study. *American Journal of Obstetrics and Gynecology, 192*(3), 932–936.

Cohen, L. S., Altshuler, L. L., Harlow, B. L., Nonacs, R., Newport, D. J., Viguera, A. C., & Stowe, Z. N. (2006). Relapse of major depression during pregnancy in women who maintain or discontinue antidepressant treatment. *JAMA, 295*(5), 499–507.

Cox, J. L., Holden, J. M., & Sagovsky, R. (1987). Detection of postnatal depression: Development of the 10-item Edinburgh Postnatal Depression Scale. *British Journal of Psychiatry, 150*, 782–786.

Crowley, S. K., & Youngstedt, S. D. (2012). Efficacy of light therapy for perinatal depression: A review. *Journal of Physiological Anthropology, 31*, 15.

Daley, A., Foster, L., Long, G., Palmer, C., Robinson, O., Walmsley, H., & Ward, R. (2015). The effectiveness of exercise for the prevention and treatment of antenatal depression: Systematic review with meta-analysis. *BJOG: An International Journal of Obstetrics and Gynaecology, 122*(1), 57–62.

Dayan, J., Creveuil, C., Dreyfus, M., Herlicoviez, M., Baleyte, J.-M., & O'Keane, V. (2010). Developmental model of depression applied to prenatal depression: Role of present and past life events, past emotional disorders and pregnancy stress. *PloS One, 5*(9), e12942.

Deave, T., Heron, J., Evans, J., & Emond, A. (2008). The impact of maternal depression in pregnancy on early child development. *BJOG: An International Journal of Obstetrics and Gynaecology, 115*(8), 1043–1051.

Dietz, P. M., Williams, S. B., Callaghan, W. M., Bachman, D. J., Whitlock, E. P., & Hornbrook, M. C. (2007). Clinically identified maternal depression before, during, and after pregnancies ending in live births. *American Journal of Psychiatry, 164*(10), 1515–1520.

Dimidjian, S., & Goodman, S. (2009). Nonpharmacologic intervention and prevention strategies for depression during pregnancy and the postpartum. *Clinical Obstetrics and Gynecology, 52*(3), 498–515.

Einarson, A., Bonari, L., Voyer-Lavigne, S., Addis, A., Matsui, D., Johnson, Y., & Koren, G. (2003). A multicenter prospective controlled study to determine the safety of Trazodone and Nefazodone use during pregnancy. *Canadian Journal of Psychiatry, 48*(2), 106–110.

Einarson, A., Choi, J., Einarson, T. R, & Koren, G. (2009). Rates of spontaneous and therapeutic abortions following use of antidepressants in pregnancy: Results from a large prospective database. *Journal of Obstetrics and Gynaecology Canada, 31*(5), 452–456.

Einarson, T. R., & Einarson, A. (2005). Newer antidepressants in pregnancy and rates of major malformations: A meta-analysis of prospective comparative studies. *Pharmacoepidemiology and Drug Safety, 14*(12), 823–827.

Epperson, C. N., Terman, M., Terman, J. S., Hanusa, B. H., Oren, D. A., Peindl, K. S., & Wisner, K. L. (2004). Randomized clinical trial of bright light therapy for antepartum depression: Preliminary findings. *Journal of Clinical Psychiatry, 65*(3), 421–425.

Epstein, R. A., Moore, K. M., & Bobo, W. V. (2014). Treatment of nonpsychotic major depression during pregnancy: Patient safety and challenges. *Drug, Healthcare and Patient Safety, 6*, 109–129.

Ertel, K. A., James-Todd, T., Kleinman, K., Krieger, N., Gillman, M., Wright, R., & Rich-Edwards, J. (2012). Racial discrimination, response to unfair treatment, and depressive symptoms among pregnant black and African American women in the United States. *Annals of Epidemiology, 22*(12), 840–846.

Even, C., Schröder, C. M., Friedman, S., & Rouillon, F. (2008). Efficacy of light therapy in nonseasonal depression: A systematic review. *Journal of Affective Disorders, 108*(1–2), 11–23.

Ewing, G., Tatarchuk, Y., Appleby, D., Schwartz, N., & Kim, D. (2015). Placental transfer of antidepressant medications: Implications for postnatal adaptation syndrome. *Clinical Pharmacokinetics, 54*(4), 359–370.

Fellenzer, J. L., & Cibula, D. A. (2014). Intendedness of pregnancy and other predictive factors for symptoms of prenatal depression in a population-based study. *Maternal and Child Health Journal, 18*(10), 2426–2436.

Field, T., Diego, M., Delgado, J., & Medina, L. (2013a). Tai chi / yoga reduces prenatal depression, anxiety and sleep disturbances. *Complementary Therapies in Clinical Practice, 19*(1), 6–10.

Field, T., Diego, M., Delgado, J., & Medina, L. (2013b). Yoga and social support reduce prenatal depression, anxiety and cortisol. *Journal of Bodywork and Movement Therapies, 17*(4), 397–403.

Flynn, H. A. (2010). Depression and postpartum disorders. In B. L. Levin & M. A. Becker (Eds.), *A Public Health Perspective of Women's Mental Health* (pp. 109–120). New York, NY: Springer.

Flynn, H. A., Davis, J., Marcus, S. M., Cunningham, R., Blow, F. C. (2004). Rates of maternal depression in pediatric emergency and relationship to child service utilization. *General Hospital Psychiatry, 26*(4), 316–322.

Galbally, M., Lewis, A. J., & Buist, A. (2011). Developmental outcomes of children exposed to antidepressants in pregnancy. *Australian and New Zealand Journal of Psychiatry, 45*(5), 393–399.

Gavin, A. R., Melville, J. L., Rue, T., Guo, Y., Dina, K. T., & Katon, W. J. (2011). Racial differences in the prevalence of antenatal depression. *General Hospital Psychiatry, 33*(2), 87–93.

Gavin, N. I., Gaynes, B. N., Lohr, K. N., Meltzer-Brody, S., Gartlehner, G., & Swinson, T. (2005). Perinatal depression: A systematic review of prevalence and incidence. *Obstetrics and Gynecology, 106*(5 Pt 1), 1071–1083.

Gaynes, B. N., Gavin, N., Meltzer-Brody, S., Lohr, K. N., Swinson, T., Gartlehner, G., & Miller, W. C. (2005). Perinatal depression: Prevalence, screening accuracy, and screening outcomes: Summary. *AHRQ evidence report summaries*. Rockville, MD: Agency for Healthcare Research and Quality. Retrieved from http://www.ncbi.nlm.nih.gov/books/NBK11838/

Geier, M. L., Hills, N., Gonzales, M., Tum, K., & Finley, P. R. (2015). Detection and treatment rates for perinatal depression in a state Medicaid population. *CNS Spectrums, 20*(1), 11–19.

Giallo, R., Woolhouse, H., Gartland, D., Hiscock, H., & Brown, S. (2015). The emotional-behavioural functioning of children exposed to maternal depressive symptoms across pregnancy and early childhood: A prospective Australian pregnancy cohort study. *European Child and Adolescent Psychiatry, 24*(10), 1233–1244.

Goodman, J. H. (2009). Women's attitudes, preferences, and perceived barriers to treatment for perinatal depression. *Birth, 36*(1), 60–69.

Goodman, J. H., & Santangelo, G. (2011). Group treatment for postpartum depression: A systematic review. *Archives of Women's Mental Health, 14*(4), 277–293.

Grigoriadis, S., VonderPorten, E. H., Mamisashvili, L., Eady, A., Tomlinson, G., Dennis, C.-L., & Ross, L. E. (2013a). The effect of prenatal antidepressant exposure on neonatal adaptation: A systematic review and meta-analysis. *Journal of Clinical Psychiatry, 74*(4), e309-e320.

Grigoriadis, S., VonderPorten, E. H., Mamisashvili, L., Roerecke, M., Rehm, J., Dennis, C.-L., & Ross, L. E. (2013b). Antidepressant exposure during pregnancy and congenital malformations: Is there an association? A systematic review and meta-analysis of the best evidence. *Journal of Clinical Psychiatry, 74*(4), e293-e308.

Grigoriadis, S., VonderPorten, E. H., Mamisashvili, L., Tomlinson, G., Dennis, C.-L., Koren, G., . . . Ross, L. E. (2013c). The impact of maternal depression during pregnancy on perinatal outcomes: A systematic review and meta-analysis. *Journal of Clinical Psychiatry, 74*(4), e321-e341.

Grigoriadis, S., Vonderporten, E. H., Mamisashvili, L., Tomlinson, G., Dennis, C.-L., Koren, G., & Ross, L. E. (2014). Prenatal exposure to antidepressants and persistent pulmonary hypertension of the newborn: Systematic review and meta-analysis. *BMJ, 348*, f6932.

Grote, N. K., Bridge, J. A., Gavin, A. R., Melville, J. L., Iyengar, S., & Katon, W. J. (2010). A meta-analysis of depression during pregnancy and the risk of preterm birth, low birth weight, and intrauterine growth restriction. *Archives of General Psychiatry, 67*(10), 1012–1024.

Grote, N. K., Swartz, H. A., Geibel, S. L., Zuckoff, A., Houck, P. R., & Frank, E. (2009). A randomized controlled trial of culturally relevant, brief interpersonal psychotherapy for perinatal depression. *Psychiatric Services, 60*(3), 313–321.

Hay, D. F., Pawlby, S., Waters, C. S., Perra, O., & Sharp, D. (2010). Mothers' antenatal depression and their children's antisocial outcomes. *Child Development, 81*(1), 149–165.

Headley, J., Northstone, K., Simmons, H., Golding, J., & ALSPAC Study Team. (2004). Medication use during pregnancy: Data from the Avon Longitudinal Study of Parents and Children. *European Journal of Clinical Pharmacology, 60*(5), 355–361.

Hemels, M. E. H., Einarson, A., Koren, G., Lanctôt, K. L., & Einarson, T. R. (2005). Antidepressant use during pregnancy and the rates of spontaneous abortions: A meta-analysis. *Annals of Pharmacotherapy, 39*(5), 803–809.

Hobfoll, S. E., Ritter, C., Lavin, J., Hulsizer, M. R., & Cameron, R. P. (1995). Depression prevalence and incidence among inner-city pregnant and postpartum women. *Journal of Consulting and Clinical Psychology, 63*(3), 445–453.

Holcomb, W. L., Stone, L. S., Lustman, P. J., Gavard, J. A., & Mostello, D. J. (1996). Screening for depression in pregnancy: Characteristics of the Beck Depression Inventory. *Obstetrics and Gynecology, 88*(6), 1021–1025.

Holzman, C., Eyster, J., Tiedje, L. B., Roman, L. A., Seagull, E., & Rahbar, M. H. (2006). A life course perspective on depressive symptoms in mid-pregnancy. *Maternal and Child Health Journal, 10*(2), 127–138.

Huang, H., Coleman, S., Bridge, J. A., Yonkers, K., & Katon, W. (2014). A meta-analysis of the relationship between antidepressant use in pregnancy and the risk of preterm birth and low birth weight. *General Hospital Psychiatry, 36*(1), 13–18.

Huybrechts, K. F., Palmsten, K., Avorn, J., Cohen, L. S., Holmes, L. B., Franklin, J. M., & Hernández-Díaz, S. (2014a). Antidepressant use in pregnancy and the risk of cardiac defects. *New England Journal of Medicine, 370*(25), 2397–2407.

Huybrechts, K. F., Sanghani, R. S., Avorn, J., & Urato, A. C. (2014b). Preterm birth and antidepressant medication use during pregnancy: A systematic review and meta-analysis. *PloS One, 9*(3), e92778.

Ji, S., Long, Q., Newport, D. J., Na, H., Knight, B., Zach, E. B., & Stowe, Z. N. (2011). Validity of depression rating scales during pregnancy and the postpartum period: Impact of trimester and parity. *Journal of Psychiatric Research, 45*(2), 213–219.

Jimenez-Solem, E., Andersen, J. T., Petersen, M., Broedbaek, K., Jensen, J. K., Afzal, S., & Poulsen, H. E. (2012). Exposure to selective serotonin reuptake inhibitors and the risk of congenital malformations: A nationwide cohort study. *BMJ Open, 2*(3), e001148. Retrieved from http://doi.org/10.1136/bmjopen-2012-001148

Källén, B. (2004). Neonate characteristics after maternal use of antidepressants in late pregnancy. *Archives of Pediatrics and Adolescent Medicine, 158*(4), 312–316.

Källén, B., & Olausson, P. O. (2008). Maternal use of selective serotonin re-uptake inhibitors and persistent pulmonary hypertension of the newborn. *Pharmacoepidemiology and Drug Safety, 17*(8), 801–806.

Kessler, R. C. (2003). Epidemiology of women and depression. *Journal of Affective Disorders, 74*(1), 5–13.

Kieler, H., Artama, M., Engeland, A., Ericsson, O., Furu, K., Gissler, M., & Haglund, B. (2012). Selective serotonin reuptake inhibitors during pregnancy and risk of persistent pulmonary hypertension in the newborn: Population based cohort study from the five Nordic countries. *BMJ, 344*, d8012.

Kjaersgaard, M., Parner, E., Vestergaard, M., Sørensen, M., Olsen, J., Christensen, J., & Pedersen, L. (2013). Prenatal antidepressant exposure and risk of spontaneous abortion - A population-based study. *PLoS One, 8*(8). Retrieved from http://doi.org/10.1371/journal.pone .0072095

Klieger-Grossmann, C., Weitzner, B., Panchaud, A., Pistelli, A., Einarson, T., Koren, G., & Einarson, A. (2012). Pregnancy outcomes following use of escitalopram: A prospective comparative cohort study. *Journal of Clinical Pharmacology, 52*(5), 766–770.

Knoppert, D. C., Nimkar, R., Principi, T., & Yuen, D. (2006). Paroxetine toxicity in a newborn after in utero exposure: Clinical symptoms correlate with serum levels. *Therapeutic Drug Monitoring, 28*(1), 5–7.

Ko, J. Y., Farr, S. L., Dietz, P. M., & Robbins, C. L. (2012). Depression and treatment among US pregnant and nonpregnant women of reproductive age, 2005–2009. *Journal of Women's Health, 21*(8), 830–836.

Kozinszky, Z., & Dudas, R. B. (2015). Validation studies of the Edinburgh Postnatal Depression Scale for the antenatal period. *Journal of Affective Disorders, 176*, 95–105.

Kroenke, K., Spitzer, R. L., & Williams, J. B. (2001). The PHQ-9: Validity of a brief depression severity measure. *Journal of General Internal Medicine, 16*(9), 606–613.

Kulin, N. A., Pastuszak, A., Sage S. R., Schick-Boschetto, B., Spivey, G., Feldkamp, M., . . . Koren, G. (1998). Pregnancy outcome following maternal use of new selective serotonin reuptake inhibitors: A prospective controlled multicenter study. *JAMA, 279*(8), 609–610.

Lancaster, C. A., Gold, K. J., Flynn, H. A., Yoo, H., Marcus, S. M., & Davis, M. M. (2010). Risk factors for depressive symptoms during pregnancy: A systematic review. *American Journal of Obstetrics and Gynecology, 202*(1), 5–14.

Le, H.-N., Perry, D. F., & Stuart, E. A. (2011). Randomized controlled trial of a preventive intervention for perinatal depression in high-risk Latinas. *Journal of Consulting and Clinical Psychology, 79*(2), 135–141.

Leigh, B., & Milgrom, J. (2008). Risk factors for antenatal depression, postnatal depression and parenting stress. *BMC Psychiatry, 8*, 24. Retrieved from https://www.ncbi.nlm.nih.gov/pmc /articles/PMC2375874/pdf/1471-244X-8-24.pdf

Leis, J. A., Heron, J., Stuart, E. A., & Mendelson, T. (2014). Associations between maternal mental health and child emotional and behavioral problems: Does prenatal mental health matter? *Journal of Abnormal Child Psychology, 42*(1), 161–171.

Leung, S. S. K., Lee, A. M., Chiang, V. C. L., Lam, S. K., Kuen, Y. W., & Wong, D. F. K. (2013). Culturally sensitive, preventive antenatal group cognitive-behavioural therapy for Chinese women with depression. *International Journal of Nursing Practice, 19*(Suppl 1), 28–37.

Levinson-Castiel, R., Merlob, P., Linder, N., Sirota, L., & Klinger, G. (2006). Neonatal abstinence syndrome after in utero exposure to selective serotonin reuptake inhibitors in term infants. *Archives of Pediatrics and Adolescent Medicine, 160*(2), 173–176.

Malm, H., Klaukka, T., & Neuvonen, P. J. (2005). Risks associated with selective serotonin reuptake inhibitors in pregnancy. *Obstetrics and Gynecology, 106*(6), 1289–1296.

Malmenström, M., Bixo, M., Björn, I., Åström, M., & Poromaa, I. S. (2006). Patients with psychiatric disorders in gynecologic practice—a three year follow-up. *Journal of Psychosomatic Obstetrics and Gynaecology, 27*(1), 17–22.

Manber, R., Schnyer, R., Chambers, A., Lyell, D., Caughey, A., Carlyle, E., & Allen, J. (2009). Acupuncture for depression during pregnancy. *American Journal of Obstetrics and Gynecology, 201*(6 Suppl), S19.

Marcus, S. M., Flynn, H. A., Blow, F. C., & Barry, K. L. (2003). Depressive symptoms among pregnant women screened in obstetrics settings. *Journal of Women's Health, 12*(4), 373–380.

Marroun, H. El, Jaddoe, V. W. V., Hudziak, J. J., Roza, S. J., Steegers, E. A. P., Hofman, A., & Tiemeier, H. (2012). Maternal use of selective serotonin reuptake inhibitors, fetal growth, and risk of adverse birth outcomes. *Archives of General Psychiatry, 69*(7), 706–714.

Martin, J. A., Hamilton, B. E., Ventura, S. J., Osterman, M. J. K., Wilson, E. C., & Mathews, T. J. (2012). Births: Final data for 2010. *National Vital Statistics Reports: From the Centers for Disease Control and Prevention, National Center for Health Statistics, National Vital Statistics System, 61*(1), 1–72.

McGregor, M., Coghlan, M., & Dennis, C.-L. (2014). The effect of physician-based cognitive behavioural therapy among pregnant women with depressive symptomatology: A pilot quasi-experimental trial. *Early Intervention in Psychiatry, 8*(4), 348–357.

Mei-Dan, E., Ray, J. G., & Vigod, S. N. (2015). Perinatal outcomes among women with bipolar disorder: A population-based cohort study. *American Journal of Obstetrics and Gynecology, 212*(3), 367.e1–8.

Meltzer-Brody, S. (2011). New insights into perinatal depression: Pathogenesis and treatment during pregnancy and postpartum. *Dialogues in Clinical Neuroscience, 13*(1), 89–100.

Melville, J. L., Gavin, A., Guo, Y., Fan, M.-Y., & Katon, W. J. (2010). Depressive disorders during pregnancy: Prevalence and risk factors in a large urban sample. *Obstetrics and Gynecology, 116*(5), 1064–1070.

Meunier, M. R., Bennett, I. M., & Coco, A. S. (2013). Use of antidepressant medication in the United States during pregnancy, 2002–2010. *Psychiatric Services, 64*(11), 1157–1160.

Milgrom, J., & Gemmill, A. W. (2014). Screening for perinatal depression. *Best Practice and Research: Clinical Obstetrics and Gynaecology, 28*(1), 13–23.

Milgrom, J., Holt, C., Holt, C. J., Ross, J., Ericksen, J., & Gemmill, A. W. (2015). Feasibility study and pilot randomised trial of an antenatal depression treatment with infant follow-up. *Archives of Women's Mental Health, 18*(5), 717–730.

Miller, L., Gur, M., Shanok, A., & Weissman, M. (2008). Interpersonal psychotherapy with pregnant adolescents: Two pilot studies. *Journal of Child Psychology and Psychiatry, 49*(7), 733–742.

Mora, P. A., Bennett, I. M., Elo, I. T., Mathew, L., Coyne, J. C., & Culhane, J. F. (2009). Distinct trajectories of perinatal depressive symptomatology: Evidence from growth mixture modeling. *American Journal of Epidemiology, 169*(1), 24–32.

Moses-Kolko, E. L., Bogen, D., Perel, J., Bregar, A., Uhl, K., Levin, B., & Wisner, K. L. (2005). Neonatal signs after late in utero exposure to serotonin reuptake inhibitors: Literature review and implications for clinical applications. *JAMA, 293*(19), 2372–2383.

Mufson, L., Weissman, M. M., Moreau, D., & Garfinkel, R. (1999). Efficacy of interpersonal psychotherapy for depressed adolescents. *Archives of General Psychiatry, 56*(6), 573–579.

Myles, N., Newall, H., Ward, H., & Large, M. (2013). Systematic meta-analysis of individual selective serotonin reuptake inhibitor medications and congenital malformations. *Australian and New Zealand Journal of Psychiatry, 47*(11), 1002–1012.

Nakhai-Pour, H. R., Broy, P., & Bérard, A. (2010). Use of antidepressants during pregnancy and the risk of spontaneous abortion. *Canadian Medical Association Journal, 182*(10), 1031–1037.

Nascimento, S. L., Surita, F. G., & Cecatti, J. G. (2012). Physical exercise during pregnancy: A systematic review. *Current Opinion in Obstetrics and Gynecology, 24*(6), 387–394.

NICHD Early Child Care Research Network. (1999). Chronicity of maternal depressive symptoms, maternal sensitivity, and child functioning at 36 months. *Developmental Psychology, 35*(5), 1297–1310.

Nulman, I., Koren, G., Rovet, J., Barrera, M., Pulver, A., Streiner, D., & Feldman, B. (2012). Neurodevelopment of children following prenatal exposure to venlafaxine, selective serotonin reuptake inhibitors, or untreated maternal depression. *American Journal of Psychiatry, 169*(11), 1165–1174.

Nulman, I., Rovet, J., Stewart, D. E., Wolpin, J., Gardner, H. A., Theis, J. G., & Koren, G. (1997). Neurodevelopment of children exposed in utero to antidepressant drugs. *New England Journal of Medicine, 336*(4), 258–262.

Nulman, I., Rovet, J., Stewart, D. E., Wolpin, J., Pace-Asciak, P., Shuhaiber, S., & Koren, G. (2002). Child development following exposure to tricyclic antidepressants or fluoxetine throughout fetal life: A prospective, controlled study. *American Journal of Psychiatry, 159*(11), 1889–1895.

Oates, M. (2003). Suicide: The leading cause of maternal death. *British Journal of Psychiatry, 183*(4), 279–281.

Oberlander, T. F., Misri, S., Fitzgerald, C. E., Kostaras, X., Rurak, D., & Riggs, W. (2004). Pharmacologic factors associated with transient neonatal symptoms following prenatal psychotropic medication exposure. *Journal of Clinical Psychiatry, 65*(2), 230–237.

Oberlander, T. F., Warburton, W., Misri, S., Aghajanian, J., & Hertzman, C. (2006). Neonatal outcomes after prenatal exposure to selective serotonin reuptake inhibitor antidepressants and maternal depression using population-based linked health data. *Archives of General Psychiatry, 63*(8), 898–906.

O'Brien, L., Einarson, T. R., Sarkar, M., Einarson, A., & Koren, G. (2008). Does paroxetine cause cardiac malformations? *Journal of Obstetrics and Gynaecology Canada, 30*(8), 696–701.

O'Hara, M. W., & Swain, A. M. (1996). Rates and risk of postpartum depression: A meta-analysis. *International Review of Psychiatry, 8*(1), 37–54.

O'Hara, M. W., & Wisner, K. L. (2014). Perinatal mental illness: Definition, description and aetiology. *Best Practice and Research: Clinical Obstetrics and Gynaecology, 28*(1), 3–12.

O'Mahen, H. A., & Flynn, H. A. (2008). Preferences and perceived barriers to treatment for depression during the perinatal period. *Journal of Women's Health, 17*(8), 1301–1309.

O'Mahen, H., Himle, J. A., Fedock, G., Henshaw, E., & Flynn, H. (2013). A pilot randomized controlled trial of cognitive behavioral therapy for perinatal depression adapted for women with low incomes. *Depression and Anxiety, 30*(7), 679–687.

Oren, D. A., Wisner, K. L., Spinelli, M., Epperson, C. N., Peindl, K. S., Terman, J. S., & Terman, M. (2002). An open trial of morning light therapy for treatment of antepartum depression. *American Journal of Psychiatry, 159*(4), 666–669.

Orr, S. T., Blazer, D. G., James, S. A., & Reiter, J. P. (2007). Depressive symptoms and indicators of maternal health status during pregnancy. *Journal of Women's Health, 16*(4), 535–542.

Paschetta, E., Berrisford, G., Coccia, F., Whitmore, J., Wood, A. G., Pretlove, S., & Ismail, K. M. K. (2014). Perinatal psychiatric disorders: An overview. *American Journal of Obstetrics and Gynecology, 210*(6), 501–509.e6.

Paulson, J. F., Dauber, S., & Leiferman, J. A. (2006). Individual and combined effects of postpartum depression in mothers and fathers on parenting behavior. *Pediatrics, 118*(2), 659–668.

Pawlby, S., Hay, D. F., Sharp, D., Waters, C. S., & O'Keane, V. (2009). Antenatal depression predicts depression in adolescent offspring: Prospective longitudinal community-based study. *Journal of Affective Disorders, 113*(3), 236–243.

Payne, J. L. (2012). Depression: Is pregnancy protective? *Journal of Women's Health, 21*(8), 809–810.

Pearson, R. M., Evans, J., Kounali, D., Lewis, G., Heron, J., Ramchandani, P. G., & Stein, A. (2013). Maternal depression during pregnancy and the postnatal period: Risks and possible mechanisms for offspring depression at age 18 years. *JAMA Psychiatry, 70*(12), 1312–1319.

Pedersen, L. H., Henriksen, T. B., & Olsen, J. (2010). Fetal exposure to antidepressants and normal milestone development at 6 and 19 months of age. *Pediatrics, 125*(3), e600-e608.

Pereira, A. T., Soares, M. J., Bos, S., Marques, M., Maia, B., Valente, J., & Macedo, A. (2014). Why should we screen for perinatal depression? Ten reasons to do it. *International Journal of Clinical Neurosciences and Mental Health, 1*, 1–7.

Pina-Camacho, L., Jensen, S. K., Gaysina, D., & Barker, E. D. (2015). Maternal depression symptoms, unhealthy diet and child emotional-behavioural dysregulation. *Psychological Medicine, 45*(9), 1851–1860.

Plant, D. T., Pariante, C. M., Sharp, D., & Pawlby, S. (2015). Maternal depression during pregnancy and offspring depression in adulthood: Role of child maltreatment. *British Journal of Psychiatry, 207*(3), 213–220.

Radloff, L. S. (1977). The CES-D scale: A self-report depression scale for research in the general population. *Applied Psychological Measurement, 1*(3), 385–401.

Rahimi, R., Nikfar, S., & Abdollahi, M. (2006). Pregnancy outcomes following exposure to serotonin reuptake inhibitors: A meta-analysis of clinical trials. *Reproductive Toxicology, 22*(4), 571–575.

Räisänen, S., Lehto, S. M., Nielsen, H. S., Gissler, M., Kramer, M. R., & Heinonen, S. (2014). Risk factors for and perinatal outcomes of major depression during pregnancy: A population-based analysis during 2002–2010 in Finland. *BMJ Open, 4*(11), e004883. Retrieved from http://doi.org/10.1136/bmjopen-2014-004883

Reis, M., & Källén, B. (2010). Delivery outcome after maternal use of antidepressant drugs in pregnancy: An update using Swedish data. *Psychological Medicine, 40*(10), 1723–1733.

Richards, A., Barkham, M., Cahill, J., Richards, D., Williams, C., & Heywood, P. (2003). PHASE: A randomised, controlled trial of supervised self-help cognitive behavioural therapy in primary care. *British Journal of General Practice, 53*(495), 764–770.

Richards, E. M., & Payne, J. L. (2013). The management of mood disorders in pregnancy: Alternatives to antidepressants. *CNS Spectrums, 18*(5), 261–271.

Robertson, E., Grace, S., Wallington, T., & Stewart, D. E. (2004). Antenatal risk factors for postpartum depression: A synthesis of recent literature. *General Hospital Psychiatry, 26*(4), 289–295.

Robledo-Colonia, A. F., Sandoval-Restrepo, N., Mosquera-Valderrama, Y. F., Escobar-Hurtado, C., & Ramírez-Vélez, R. (2012). Aerobic exercise training during pregnancy reduces depressive symptoms in nulliparous women: A randomised trial. *Journal of Physiotherapy, 58*(1), 9–15.

Ross, L. E., Grigoriadis, S., Mamisashvili, L., Vonderporten, E. H., Roerecke, M., Rehm, J., & Cheung, A. (2013). Selected pregnancy and delivery outcomes after exposure to antidepressant medication: A systematic review and meta-analysis. *JAMA Psychiatry, 70*(4), 436–443.

Scott, C., Tacchi, M. J., Jones, R., & Scott, J. (1997). Acute and one-year outcome of a randomised controlled trial of brief cognitive therapy for major depressive disorder in primary care. *British Journal of Psychiatry, 171*, 131–134.

Sidebottom, A. C., Harrison, P. A., Godecker, A., & Kim, H. (2012). Validation of the Patient Health Questionnaire (PHQ)-9 for prenatal depression screening. *Archives of Women's Mental Health, 15*(5), 367–374.

Sockol, L. E. (2015). A systematic review of the efficacy of cognitive behavioral therapy for treating and preventing perinatal depression. *Journal of Affective Disorders, 177*, 7–21.

Spinelli, M. G. (1998). Antepartum and postpartum depression. *Journal of Gender-Specific Medicine, 1*(2), 33–36.

Spinelli, M. G., & Endicott, J. (2003). Controlled clinical trial of interpersonal psychotherapy versus parenting education program for depressed pregnant women. *American Journal of Psychiatry, 160*(3), 555–562.

Spinelli, M. G., Endicott, J., Leon, A. C., Goetz, R. R., Kalish, R. B., Brustman, L. E., & Schulick, J. L. (2013). A controlled clinical treatment trial of interpersonal psychotherapy for depressed pregnant women at 3 New York City sites. *Journal of Clinical Psychiatry, 74*(4), 393–399.

Spitzer, R. L., Williams, J. B., Gibbon, M., & First, M. B. (1992). The Structured Clinical Interview for *DSM-III-R* (SCID). I: History, rationale, and description. *Archives of General Psychiatry, 49*(8), 624–629.

Spitzer, R. L., Williams, J. B., Kroenke, K., Hornyak, R., & McMurray, J. (2000). Validity and utility of the PRIME-MD patient health questionnaire in assessment of 3000 obstetric-gynecologic patients: The PRIME-MD Patient Health Questionnaire Obstetrics-Gynecology Study. *American Journal of Obstetrics and Gynecology, 183*(3), 759–769.

Spitzer, R. L., Williams, J. B., Kroenke, K., Linzer, M., deGruy, F. V., Hahn, S. R., & Johnson, J. G. (1994). Utility of a new procedure for diagnosing mental disorders in primary care: The PRIME-MD 1000 study. *JAMA, 272*(22), 1749–1756.

Stuart, S., & Koleva, H. (2014). Psychological treatments for perinatal depression. *Best Practice and Research: Clinical Obstetrics and Gynaecology, 28*(1), 61–70.

Suri, R., Lin, A. S., Cohen, L. S., & Altshuler, L. L. (2014). Acute and long-term behavioral outcome of infants and children exposed in utero to either maternal depression or antidepressants: A review of the literature. *Journal of Clinical Psychiatry, 75*(10), e1142-e1152.

Thomas, N., Komiti, A., & Judd, F. (2014). Pilot early intervention antenatal group program for pregnant women with anxiety and depression. *Archives of Women's Mental Health, 17*(6), 503–509.

Thoppil, J., Riutcel, T. L., & Nalesnik, S. W. (2005). Early intervention for perinatal depression. *American Journal of Obstetrics and Gynecology, 192*(5), 1446–1468.

US Food and Drug Administration. (2011). *Selective Serotonin Reuptake Inhibitor (SSRI) Antidepressants: Drug Safety Communication—Use During Pregnancy and Potential Risk of Persistent Pulmonary Hypertension of the Newborn*. Retrieved from http://www.fda.gov/Safety /MedWatch/SafetyInformation/SafetyAlertsforHumanMedicalProducts/ucm283696.htm

Vesga-López, O., Blanco, C., Keyes, K., Olfson, M., Grant, B. F., & Hasin, D. S. (2008). Psychiatric disorders in pregnant and postpartum women in the United States. *Archives of General Psychiatry, 65*(7), 805–815.

Warburton, W., Hertzman, C., & Oberlander, T. F. (2010). A register study of the impact of stopping third trimester selective serotonin reuptake inhibitor exposure on neonatal health. *Acta Psychiatrica Scandinavica, 121*(6), 471–479.

Waters, C. S., Hay, D. F., Simmonds, J. R., & van Goozen, S. H. M. (2014). Antenatal depression and children's developmental outcomes: Potential mechanisms and treatment options. *European Child and Adolescent Psychiatry, 23*(10), 957–971.

Weisskopf, E., Fischer, C. J., Bickle Graz, M., Morisod Harari, M., Tolsa, J.-F., Claris, O., & Panchaud, A. (2015). Risk-benefit balance assessment of SSRI antidepressant use during pregnancy and lactation based on best available evidence. *Expert Opinion on Drug Safety, 14*(3), 413–427.

Wen, S. W., Yang, Q., Garner, P., Fraser, W., Olatunbosun, O., Nimrod, C., & Walker, M. (2006). Selective serotonin reuptake inhibitors and adverse pregnancy outcomes. *American Journal of Obstetrics and Gynecology, 194*(4), 961–966.

Westdahl, C., Milan, S., Magriples, U., Kershaw, T. S., Rising, S. S., & Ickovics, J. R. (2007). Social support and social conflict as predictors of prenatal depression. *Obstetrics and Gynecology, 110*(1), 134–140.

Wichman, C. L., Moore, K. M., Lang, T. R., St. Sauver, J. L., Heise, R. H., & Watson, W. J. (2009). Congenital heart disease associated with selective serotonin reuptake inhibitor use during pregnancy. *Mayo Clinic Proceedings, 84*(1), 23–27.

Wilson, K. L., Zelig, C. M., Harvey, J. P., Cunningham, B. S., Dolinsky, B. M., & Napolitano, P. G. (2011). Persistent pulmonary hypertension of the newborn is associated with mode of delivery and not with maternal use of selective serotonin reuptake inhibitors. *American Journal of Perinatology, 28*(1), 19–24.

Wilusz, M. J., Peters, R. M., & Cassidy-Bushrow, A. E. (2014). Course of depressive symptoms across pregnancy in African American women. *Journal of Midwifery and Women's Health, 59*(4), 411–416.

Winkel, S., Einsle, F., Pieper, L., Höfler, M., Wittchen, H.-U., & Martini, J. (2015). Associations of anxiety disorders, depressive disorders and body weight with hypertension during pregnancy. *Archives of Women's Mental Health, 18*(3), 473–483.

Wirz-Justice, A., Bader, A., Frisch, U., Stieglitz, R.-D., Alder, J., Bitzer, J., & Riecher-Rössler, A. (2011). A randomized, double-blind, placebo-controlled study of light therapy for antepartum depression. *Journal of Clinical Psychiatry, 72*(7), 986–993.

Wisner, K. L., Bogen, D. L., Sit, D., McShea, M., Hughes, C., Rizzo, D., & Wisniewski, S. W. (2013). Does fetal exposure to SSRIs or maternal depression impact infant growth? *American Journal of Psychiatry, 170*(5), 485–493.

Wisner, K. L., Sit, D. K. Y., Hanusa, B. H., Moses-Kolko, E. L., Bogen, D. L., Hunker, D. F., & Singer, L. T. (2009). Major depression and antidepressant treatment: Impact on pregnancy and neonatal outcomes. *American Journal of Psychiatry, 166*(5), 557–566.

World Health Organization. (2000). *Women's mental health: An evidence based review*. Retrieved from http://www.who.int/mental_health/publications/women_mh_evidence_review/en/

Wurst, K. E., Poole, C., Ephross, S. A., & Olshan, A. F. (2010). First trimester paroxetine use and the prevalence of congenital, specifically cardiac, defects: A meta-analysis of epidemiological studies. *Birth Defects Research: Part A, Clinical and Molecular Teratology, 88*(3), 159–170.

Yonkers, K. A., Blackwell, K. A., Glover, J., & Forray, A. (2014). Antidepressant use in pregnant and postpartum women. *Annual Review of Clinical Psychology, 10*, 369–392.

Yonkers, K. A., Gotman, N., Smith, M. V., Forray, A., Belanger, K., Brunetto, W. L., . . . Lockwood, C. J. (2011b). Does antidepressant use attenuate the risk of a major depressive episodes in pregnancy? *Epidemiology, 22*(6), 848–854.

Yonkers, K. A., Vigod, S., & Ross, L. E. (2011a). Diagnosis, pathophysiology, and management of mood disorders in pregnant and postpartum women. *Obstetrics and Gynecology, 117*(4), 961–977.

Yonkers, K. A., Wisner, K. L., Stewart, D. E., Oberlander, T. F., Dell, D. L., Stotland, N., & Lockwood, C. (2009). The management of depression during pregnancy: A report from the American Psychiatric Association and the American College of Obstetricians and Gynecologists. *General Hospital Psychiatry, 31*(5), 403–413.

Zlotnick, C., Miller, I. W., Pearlstein, T., Howard, M., & Sweeney, P. (2006). A preventive intervention for pregnant women on public assistance at risk for postpartum depression. *American Journal of Psychiatry, 163*(8), 1443–1445.

CHAPTER 14

Racial and Ethnic Disparities in Depressive Illness and Clinical Care

Challenges and Solutions toward Equality in Care

Alfiee M. Breland-Noble, PhD, MHSc
Jeanne Miranda, PhD

Mental disorders, such as depression with its early age of onset and recurrent nature, are the leading causes of years lived with disability worldwide, and 40.5% of this burden is uniquely attributable to major depression (World Health Organization, 2011). This chapter reviews the evidence about racial and ethnic disparities in depressive illness and care. First, we discuss rates of depression among racially diverse Americans as compared with white Americans. Second, we discuss differential rates of depression among subgroups of people of color, such as immigrants compared with those US-born people of color. Third, we discuss mental health care use by people of color as compared with white Americans, examining factors that are related to disparities. Finally, we discuss what is known about overcoming mental health care disparities, including suggesting some innovative models.

Rates of Depression among People of Color
African Americans

To ensure the most inclusive description of people of African descent living in the United States, we define the African American population as any person with familial roots in Africa currently residing in the United States. This definition includes persons of multiple generations descended from the Transatlantic Slave Trade to the United States and more recent black immigrants from the Caribbean and continental Africa (Caldwell, Assari, & Breland-Noble, 2016).

Youth

Research on African American youth indicates that depression prevalence for this population does not differ significantly from that of white youth. Angold and colleagues

(2002) examined depression prevalence among underresourced, racially diverse youth (9–17 years of age) in rural North Carolina and found that 1.7% of African American youth in the sample met criteria for depression. Doi and colleagues (2001) found a depression prevalence rate of 13.4% for a small sample (n = 636) of African American youth aged 12–15 in Texas using the Diagnostic Interview Schedule for Children. In 2013, Byck and colleagues (2013) also measured depression in underresourced African American youth in Alabama using the Diagnostic Interview Schedule for Children (n = 592) and found a 3.8% prevalence rate. The largest study to date, the National Comorbidity Survey-Adolescent Supplement, conducted face-to-face surveys of 10,123 adolescents aged 13–18 in the continental United States. In this study, rates of depression did not differ between African American and white youth (Avenevoli, Swendsen, He, Burstein, & Merikangas, 2015).

Adults

Four studies funded by the National Institute of Mental Health Consortium on Psychiatric Epidemiology Studies (NIMH-CPES) fielded common questions and unified sampling weights to permit comparisons across white, black (African American and Caribbean descent), Hispanic (Puerto Rican, Cuban, Mexican, and other descent), and Asian (Chinese, Filipino, Vietnamese, and other descent) ethnic groups (Heeringa et al., 2004). Given the disproportionately higher rates of poverty and poor health among US people of color compared with whites, and the fact that poverty and poor health are positively related to mental disorders, one would anticipate that people of color, particularly African Americans and Latinos, would also report higher rates of mental disorders. However, in this large, nationally representative study, whites demonstrated higher depression lifetime prevalence than African Americans and Caribbean blacks. Nonetheless, research indicates that African American adults consistently present for care later in the course of illness with more severe symptoms (Williams et al., 2007).

Older Adults

Rates of depression in older African American populations were studied in early epidemiological surveys. In that earlier data, African American elders were found to have lower rates of depression than their white counterparts (Robins & Regier, 1991; Somervell, Leaf, Weissman, Blazer, & Bruce, 1989).

Latinos

Hispanic Americans, or Latino Americans, are Americans descending from the countries of Latin America. Latinos form an ethnicity sharing a language (Spanish) and cultural heritage, rather than a race. American Latinos are predominantly of Mexican and, to a lesser extent, Puerto Rican, Cuban, Salvadoran, Dominican, Guatemalan, Colombian, and other Latino ancestry.

Youth

As is true of African American youth, rates of depression in Latino youth are similar to those of white youth. The National Comorbidity Survey-Adolescent Supplement did not find differences in rates of depression between white and Latino youth (Avenevoli et al., 2015).

Adult

Latinos of Puerto Rican, Cuban, Mexican, and other decent were studied in the NIMH-CPES (Heeringa et al., 2004). With the exception of Puerto Ricans, all of the subgroups of Latinos reported lower rates of lifetime depression than white Americans reported. Similar advantages existed for the presence of depression in the past year, although Latino rates were relatively close to that of whites.

Older Adults

Rates of depression in older Latinos have been studied in two small community samples. First, rates were studied in Mexican Americans in Sacramento, California (González, Haan, & Hinton, 2001), and Hispanics in Massachusetts (Falcón & Tucker, 2000). In both cases, older Latinos were found to have higher rates of depression than older white Americans. However, these results should be interpreted cautiously, as both studies involved symptom measures of depression rather than clinical diagnoses.

Asian Americans

Asian Americans are persons having origins in any of the original peoples of the Far East, Southeast Asia, or the Indian subcontinent. It includes Indian, Chinese, Filipino, Korean, Japanese, and Vietnamese, among others.

Youth

To our knowledge, no large-scale epidemiological studies of depression among Asian youth exist.

Adults

Asians of Chinese, Filipino, Vietnamese, and other descent were studied in the NIMH-CPES (Heeringa et al., 2004). Additionally, recent reviews of this population have yielded additional estimates of depression prevalence. Prevalence rates varied significantly, ranging from 4.5% to 11.3%, but were all considerably lower than their white counterparts. Interestingly, Korean and Filipino Americans were found to demonstrate higher depression prevalence rates than those of their Chinese counterparts (33%–34% vs. 15%, respectively) (Jackson et al., 2011; Kim, Park, Storr, Tran, & Juon, 2015).

Older Adults

Similar to Hispanic Americans, a number of studies have looked at depressive symptoms in older Asian American populations. Although the studies vary by particular group, the prevalence rates are estimated to be higher than those of community-dwelling older adults in general (Kuo, Chong, & Joseph, 2008).

American Indians / Alaskan Natives

American Indians and Alaskan natives are people having origins in any of the original peoples of North and South America (including Central America), and who maintain tribal affiliation or community attachment. The American Indian and Alaskan Native population includes Navajo, Blackfeet, Inupiat, Yup'ik, and Choctaw, as well as Central American Indian groups and South American Indian groups.

Youth

One of the few psychiatric epidemiological studies that sought to address the mental health status of American Indian youth is the Great Smoky Mountains Study, led by Costello and colleagues (1996). While the primary focus of the study was a racially diverse sample of African American, white, Latino, and Native American youth in underresourced rural areas, the study included a sample of more than 300 Native American youth, all of whom have been followed over time since preadolesence (Costello, Angold, Burns, Erkanli, et al., 1996; Costello, Angold, Burns, Stangl, et al., 1996). Findings from this study indicate that 4.3%–6.4% of these youth (who entered the study as pre/early adolescents and were late adolescents and emerging adults when last studied) met criteria for depressive and anxiety disorders for the three-month period prior to study evaluation (Costello, Erkanli, Copeland, & Angold, 2010; Gone & Trimble, 2012). These findings indicate that depression might be at least as prevalent among American Indian youth as it is among people of other racial ethnic groups.

Adults

Although not part of the NIMH-CPES, mental disorders have been studied in two adult American Indian reservation populations. The single largest attempt to quantify psychiatric epidemiology estimates for a representative sample of Native Americans / American Indians was the American Indian Service Utilization, Psychiatric Epidemiology, Risk and Protective Factors Project (Beals, Manson, Mitchell, Spicer, & Team, 2003; Gone & Trimble, 2012). The prevalence of major psychiatric disorders among Native Americans was collected from a representative sample of persons from two tribes (n = 3,084, with tribes from the Northern Plains and the Southwest). Results from this large-scale study indicated that 7.8%–10.9% of persons surveyed met criteria for a major depressive episode in the recent past. These rates are lower than white comparison samples in the United States.

Older Adults

Data on prevalence of depression in older Native populations is extremely limited. In one study of urban Indians in Los Angeles, rates of depression were 11%, lower than those of older white Americans (Weibel-Orlando & Kramer, 1989).

Summary

Overall, youth of color and white youth are reported to have similar rates of mental disorders. Contrary to what one would expect, given disproportionately higher rates of poverty among people of color as compared with white Americans, racially diverse adults have lower rates of depression than do their white counterparts. The one exception is Puerto Ricans, who have rates of depression similar to those of whites in the US population. Among older people of color, rates have not been established in large studies with diagnostic instruments.

Rates of Disorders by Immigrant Status

Both Latinos and Asian Americans have substantial immigrant populations in the United States. In fact, the foreign-born population from Latin America accounts for more than half (53%) of all foreign-born persons in the United States. By comparison, 28% of foreign-born persons were born in Asia.

Early research found that among Mexican Americans in Los Angeles, immigrants reported lower rates of depression than did their US-born counterparts (Burnam, Hough, Karno, Escobar, & Telles, 1987). In a later investigation, Vega and colleagues (1998) found similar results in Fresno, California. The question of nativity was also examined in the NIMH-CPES. Among Latinos, increased rates of psychiatric disorders, including depression, were observed among US-born, English-language-proficient, and third-generation Latinos (Alegria et al., 2007). Among Asians, immigration-related factors and mental disorders were different for women than men. Among women, nativity was strongly associated with lifetime disorders, with immigrant women having lower rates of most disorders compared with US-born women. Conversely, English proficiency was associated with mental disorders for Asian men. Asian men who spoke English proficiently generally had lower rates of lifetime and 12-month disorders compared with nonproficient speakers (Takeuchi et al., 2007).

Two studies have looked at rates of depression among African Americans compared with white Americans and black Caribbean immigrants. White Americans had the highest rates of depression, with black Caribbean immigrants next, and US-born African Americans with the lowest rates (Williams et al., 2007). Rates of depression among Caribbean African, African, and US-born African American young women who were screened in county entitlement programs were examined. Rates of depression were higher among US-born women as compared with the two immigrant groups (Miranda, Siddique, Belin, & Kohn-Wood, 2005).

In summary, rates of depression appear to be generally lower in immigrant populations as compared with US-born minorities. This appears to be a more consistent finding for women than male immigrants.

Use of Mental Health Services
Evidence on Access, Use, and Spending

Most research comparing mental health care across groups finds evidence of disparities in access and use. As documented in the US Surgeon General's report on mental health and its supplement, people of color have less access to mental health services than whites (due largely to differences in rates of insurance), are less likely to receive needed care, and are more likely to receive poor-quality care when treated (US Department of Health and Human Services, 1999, 2001). Additionally, people of color are reportedly less likely to seek care and more likely to delay seeking care than whites in the United States (Kessler et al., 1996). Furthermore, after entering care, racially diverse patients are less likely than whites to receive the best available treatments for depression (Wang, Berglund, & Kessler, 2000). We also note research indicating that African Americans have a greater propensity than whites to terminate depression treatment and other forms of mental health care prematurely (Arnow et al., 2007; Lester, Resick, Young-Xu, & Artz, 2010; Sue, Zane, & Young, 1994).

Among adults with a diagnosis-based need for mental health or substance abuse care, 37.6% of whites receive care compared with only 22.4% of Latinos and 25.0% of African Americans (K. Wells, Klap, Koike, & Sherbourne, 2001). Among adults of various Asian ethnicities in the United States, only 8.6% had sought any type of mental health care in the prior 12 months (Abe-Kim et al., 2007). Although large-scale studies of Native American populations are not available, in one study of two reservation populations, less than 30% of those who met criteria for a diagnosis talked to or received services from specialty providers, and fewer sought help from other medical providers (Beals et al., 2005). McGuire and colleagues (2006) implemented the Institute of Medicine (IOM) definition of disparities in outpatient mental health care and found that overall spending for blacks and Latinos on outpatient mental health care is about 60% and 75% of spending rates for whites, respectively, after taking into account need for care (McGuire, Alegria, Cook, Wells, & Zaslavsky, 2006).

Trends in Mental Health Care Disparities

Some studies have begun to track trends in mental health care disparities. Three use the IOM definition of disparities. Using a national data set, the Medical Expenditure Panel Survey, Cook, McGuire, and Miranda (2007) found that black-white and Hispanic-white disparities in rates of any mental health care use worsened from 2000–2001 to 2003–2004. Using another nationally representative sample of those with access to services, the National Ambulatory Medical Care Survey, no evidence was found for progress against disparities in depression care in primary care settings over the past decade (Stockdale, Lagomasino, Siddique, McGuire, & Miranda, 2008). In a national sample of English-speaking people, overall rates of treatment for psychiatric disorders increased between 1990 and 2003, but in both years blacks were only 50% as likely to receive psychiatric treatment as whites were for diseases of similar severity (Kessler et al., 2005).

Predictors of Disparities

Research has consistently demonstrated that multiple factors contribute to the lower rates of mental health care utilization among racially diverse youth and adults. Among the strongest predictors of failure to get needed care are instrumental barriers, such as health insurance, transportation, and obtaining time off from work for childcare (Nadeem et al., 2007). Heightened stigma related to mental illness is also related to lower service use among people of color (Breland-Noble, 2012; Nadeem et al., 2007), as are socioeconomic factors such as educational attainment (Broman, 2012) and negative prior experiences with medical and mental health systems (Barksdale, Kenyon, Graves, & Jacobs, 2014; Smith et al., 2014). Individual factors such as implicit bias and other types of bias on the part of providers are also related (Breland-Noble, Bell, & Nicolas, 2006; Sabin & Greenwald, 2012; Smedley, Stith, & Nelson, 2003), as is general lack of access to quality care (Alegria et al., 2002).

Overcoming Mental Health Care Disparities
Effectiveness of Evidence-Based Depression Care for People of Color

Because both antidepressants and brief psychotherapies (specifically cognitive behavioral therapy and interpersonal therapy) have demonstrated utility for depression among underresourced African Americans and Latinos (Breland-Noble, Childers, & Boyce, in press; Miranda et al., 2005; Mufson, Weissman, Moreau, & Garfinkel, 1999; Zhou et al., 2015), with emerging evidence for Asian Americans of varied socioeconomic backgrounds (Hwang et al., 2015; Ratzliff, Ni, Chan, Park, & Unützer, 2013), reducing mental health care disparities might best be approached by creating novel interventions to increase access to treatments and engage underutilizers of treatment in current systems designed to meet their needs in culturally relevant ways.

Collaborative Care

The most promising line of research for overcoming mental health care disparities is through collaborative care, or providing care in primary health care settings where minorities are most likely to receive care. Collaborative care approaches to depression treatment (Archer et al., 2012) have been shown to be effective, with more than 79 randomized controlled research trials establishing a robust evidence base for integrating care for depressive disorders into primary care settings. Collaborative care is highly effective among diverse patient populations, including in safety-net settings, for low-income people of color, and in Spanish-speaking patients (Areán et al., 2005; Areán, Gum, Tang, & Unützer, 2007; Ell, Aranda, Xie, Lee, & Chou, 2010; Ell et al., 2009). To date, collaborative care interventions are the only strategies that have documented decreases in mental health care disparities. Two trials have documented the positive impact on disparities of high-quality collaborative care, achieved through quality improvement interventions in primary health care settings. In a large trial of quality improvement of depression care in managed health care settings, African Americans and Latinos had lower rates of care and higher rates of depression at baseline but enjoyed larger increases in rates receiving appropriate care and improvements in depression than did white participants, resulting in decreased disparities in receiving and benefitting from quality care (Miranda et al., 2003). In five- and nine-year follow-ups of this study (Wells et al., 2004, 2007), improvements in disparities were maintained. Similarly, findings for quality improvement interventions for depression care among adolescent youth demonstrated decreases in disparities for African American and Latino youth (Ngo et al., 2009).

Collaborative care is provided by a primary care–based team (Katon & Unützer, 2006), including (1) the primary care provider; (2) a care manager (e.g., nurse, clinical social worker, counselor) who supports treatment initiated by the primary care provider and provides evidence-based, brief, structured psychotherapy (e.g., CBT or IPT); and (3) a psychiatric consultant, who advises the primary care team by developing treatment plans and suggesting changes to treatment for patients who are not improving. Care managers work closely with primary care providers, who retain primary responsibility for patients' treatment. Care manager duties include: (1) a structured comprehensive mental health assessment; (2) patient engagement and education; (3) proactive follow-up on treatment adherence, effectiveness, and side effects; (4) brief, structured counseling with evidence-based techniques such as motivational interviewing, behavioral activation, and problem-solving treatment; (5) regular (i.e., weekly) review of patients who are not improving with a psychiatric consultant; (6) facilitation of communication among treatment team members; and (7) facilitation of referrals and coordination with community-based agencies.

Collaborative care is patient-centered, involving a shared, evidence-based plan of care while accounting for patient preferences. Patients are tracked in a registry, which facilitates outreach to patients who are not improving or who are not well engaged. Collaborative care is measurement-based, using standardized instruments appropriate for depression. Established tools available in multiple languages are used for screening and to track outcomes, such as the PHQ-9, a nine-item depression scale derived from the Patient Health Questionnaire (Kroenke, Spitzer, & Williams, 2001). Clinical outcomes and progress toward patients' personal goals are used to guide treatment decisions. When patients are not improving as expected, treatments are adjusted, avoiding clinical inertia that accounts for many treatment failures in usual care. This approach is called "stepped care" because treatment is intensified step-by-step until a patient achieves significant improvement.

Settings wishing to implement collaborative care for depression typically receive individualized implementation planning, allowing them to customize the program to the needs of the site and the patients served (Unützer, Katon, et al., 2002; Unützer, Schoenbaum, Druss, & Katon, 2006). One of the leaders in this approach to collaborative care is the Advancing Integrated Mental Health Solutions (AIMS) Center at the University of Washington, whose model includes an initial six-month planning and team-building phase using a systematic process, a training phase, and a 12-month phase of posttraining implementation support that is based on tracking real-time outcomes (i.e., patients engaged and retained in collaborative care) and the clinical outcomes of collaborative care as implemented at each clinic (Gilbody, Bower, Fletcher, Richards, & Sutton, 2006). The AIMS model requires substantial practice change from primary care and mental health providers as well as system-of-care changes, such as the use of registries to track patient outcomes and facilitate consultation along with changes that focus on adjusting treatments to better attain outcome targets (i.e., "treatment to target") if patients are not improving as expected. Emerging evidence suggests that the AIMS model is a promising approach for implementation on a large scale, as in the DIAMOND program in Minnesota (Korsen & Pietruszewski, 2009), the Mental Health Integration program in the state of Washington (Unützer et al., 2012), or the RESPECT-MIL program in the US Army (Engel, 2008). Training includes skills for team members (primary care providers, care managers, psychiatric consultants) such as medication management, brief evidence-based psychotherapies for depression, and support for practices to develop effective workflows and processes that support engagement of patients and provision of evidence-based treatments (Unützer, Choi, Cook, & Oishi, 2002). The model involves tracking patient enrollment, care processes, and clinical outcomes using a web-based registry.

Unfortunately, collaborative care is not yet widely implemented in most safety-net practices, where disparities are greatest (Druss & Goldman, 2003; Miranda, McGuire, Williams, & Wang, 2008; US Department of Health and Human Services, 2001, 2003), and we lack knowledge on how to best implement, scale up, and sustain this positive intervention. To overcome mental health care disparities, engaging depressed people of color into care is critical. The collaborative care model is somewhat successful in that minorities are much more likely to present to primary health care settings than to psychiatric settings, and some have trusting relationships with their primary health care providers. However, people of color have less access to health care (Miranda et al., 2008) (which may improve with expanding Medicaid enrollment through the Affordable Care Act) and report less favorable relationships with primary health care providers (Campbell, Ramsay, & Green, 2001). To address these issues, researchers have evaluated mechanisms used to help bring and keep people in clinical care (Breland-Noble, 2012), such as interventions focused on behavioral activation of patients (Alegria et al., 2014), novel interventions focused on nontraditional settings such as faith communities (Breland-Noble, 2012; Hankerson & Weissman, 2012), and engaging diverse community agencies in implementing depression interventions (Wells et al., 2013).

Community-based participatory partnerships and faith-based depression programs are newer approaches with promise for reducing mental health disparities in access to and outcomes for depression care through engaging trusted settings in implementing depression interventions. Implementation of depression care in underresourced communities requires effective strategies responsive to local culture and context, which engage vulnerable communities to participate in implementation (Smedley, Syme, & Institute of Medicine Committee, 2001).

Overall, underresourced people of color are more likely than their white counterparts to be without a usual care provider and thus are not likely to receive services under collaborative care. Likewise, mental health care providers often are not linguistically and culturally aligned with the racially diverse communities they serve. As such, these communities are far less trustful of providers and services compared to majority culture people. Community engagement, recommended by the National Institutes of Health, the IOM, and disparities scholars to eliminate racial and ethnic disparities in health care, offers an approach to engaging communities in identifying, educating, and increasing use of care to those in need by extending services into trusted agencies with linguistically and culturally aligned staff (Agency for Toxic Substances and Disease Registry, 2011; Breland-Noble, Al-Mateen, & Singh, 2016; Institute of Medicine, 2013; Smedley et al., 2001).

Community engagement has been defined as "the process of working collaboratively with and through groups of people affiliated by geographic proximity, special interest, or similar situations to address issues affecting the well-being of those people" (Centers for Disease Control and Prevention, 1997, p. 9). Recent studies have explored the application of community engagement to mental health care for underresourced persons (Dobransky-Fasiska et al., 2010; Kneipp et al., 2011; Shellman & Mokel, 2010), focusing on broadening engagement of stakeholders to faith-based and other agencies to overcome stigma concerns and distrust of providers (Breland-Noble, Wong, Childers, Hankerson, & Sotomayor, 2015), as well as extending the small pool of racially diverse providers through task shifting to community agencies. Wells and colleagues (2013) tested the added value of community engagement in multiagency networks, such as churches and social service agencies, to implement collaborative care for depression, over and above technical assistance, plus community outreach to individual agencies for clients drawn from health care and community-based agencies in underresourced communities of color in Los Angeles in the Community Partners in Care study. Community engagement was superior to technical assistance after six months on mental health quality of life, physical activity, and reduced behavioral health hospitalizations and risk factors for homelessness among low-income urban, primarily Latino and African American patients. These findings suggest community engagement as a promising approach to implementing collaborative care across health care and social service agencies.

To overcome mental health care disparities, community engagement can supplement implementation of the collaborative care model by joint planning, implementation, and monitoring and adaptations across primary care, integrated care, and social and human service settings within the same community, to build an integrated community approach. Community-based agencies serve a range of complementary roles, including: (1) education and outreach to increase community knowledge and decrease social stigma (e.g., radio shows, faith-based programs) to promote uptake of local depression and anxiety services; (2) task shifting of some collaborative care behavioral management tasks to community-based settings to expand network capacity to deliver collaborative care components while potentially increasing diversity of the overall network workforce, and (3) task enhancement or increasing skills in managing depression and anxiety of social services providers to improve their ability to deliver needed social services (e.g., food, housing) to persons with depression.

In order to engage community agencies in underresourced, minority serving areas into depression interventions, a community participatory model is likely essential. Based on principles of equity, equality, and respect, a primary council may be commissioned, representing health care and community agencies and supporting workgroups on key aspects of care, such as components of collaborative care or technology and payment strategies. Each coalition is charged with implementing an egalitarian, partnered planning process to develop and monitor a culturally and community-relevant implementation strategy for collaborative care training while developing culturally congruent community networks to deliver services. The primary council is designed to promote capacity development among stakeholders, along with community understanding of and competency in collaborative care goals and tasks. Community engagement is built on the principle of trust-building through a two-way knowledge exchange integrating community knowledge, expertise, and passion to improve outcomes with collaborative care expertise (Chung, Dixon, Miranda, Wells, & Jones, 2010). The model generates a shared understanding and reinterpretation of collaborative care within a "co-owned" implementation plan involving joint training and network agreements for services. Goals of this community-engaged collaborative care are to: (1) promote capacity-building and partnership between primary care, mental health, and community agencies around the mental health needs of ethnic minorities; (2) increase awareness of and reduce mental health stigma to increase treatment acceptability; (3) increase adoption and penetration of collaborative care for depression and anxiety across the network; and (4) enhance the of capacity of non–health care agencies to address sociocultural needs of vulnerable clients.

This planning process involves regular meetings at start-up to develop the network and shared training plan, followed by a longer-term period of regular meetings to support the implementation of the intervention training across the network, followed by oversight of the programs as they implement the community's plan for collaborative care. All components are derived from evidence-based collaborative care components (Wennerstrom et al., 2011).

Despite the positive outcomes from the Community Partners in Care projects (Wells et al., 2013), depression outcomes and use of formal depression treatments were similar between conditions, suggesting a need to strengthen the collaborative care intervention within the community-engaged practice. This would suggest maintaining the community engagement but strengthening the collaborative care treatment to ensure quality outcomes in depression.

Technology

An additional innovation for eliminating mental health care disparities is the incorporation of technology support, which has the potential to address disparities in access and effectiveness through increasing the reach of interventions by telephone, internet, and social media, tailored to individual preferences and needs for support. Notwithstanding the disproportionate burden of poverty borne by people of color in the United States, racially diverse Americans are reported to have substantial access to advanced technology, such as smartphones with internet access (Gibbons, 2011). For example, internet interventions have been successful in increasing smoking cessation among Spanish-speaking individuals (Munoz et al., 2006, 2009). Clearly, innovative technology could provide part of the solution to decreasing or eliminating mental health care disparities.

Financing

A community-engaged collaborative care model could be well positioned for widespread implementation under health care reform developments such as patient-centered medical homes and accountable care organizations. Although collaborative care was developed and tested before the development of patient-centered medical homes, payment models would need to be developed to support the community agency participation in this type of care.

Conclusions

Rates of mental disorders are generally not higher among ethnic minorities as compared with their more affluent white counterparts. In part, this is due to generally lower rates of depression among immigrants as compared with US-born populations. Nonetheless, minorities have poorer access to care and are less likely to obtain quality care when they do access care. Evidence suggests that collaborative care programs, or implementing depression care within primary health care settings, offer promise for eliminating mental health care disparities. In order to reach ethnic minorities, we propose a community-engaged approach to care that brings in trusted community agencies to participate in collaborative care depression treatment. We believe that incorporating innovative technology interventions within this type of care would enhance the ability to get and keep generally underserved minorities in care. Finally, we believe that developing strategies through patient-centered health homes could help to finance this model.

References

Abe-Kim, J., Takeuchi, D. T., Hong, S., Zane, N., Sue, S., Spencer, M. S., . . . Alegria, M. (2007). Use of mental health–related services among immigrant and US-born Asian Americans: Results from the National Latino and Asian American Study. *American Journal of Public Health, 97*(1), 91–98.

Agency for Toxic Substances and Disease Registry. (2011). *CTSA community engagement key function committee task force on the principals of community engagement (second edition).* Retrieved from http://www.atsdr.cdc.gov/communityengagement/pce_ctsa.html

Alegria, M., Canino, G., Rios, R., Vera, M., Calderon, J., Rusch, D., & Ortega, A. N. (2002). Inequalities in use of specialty mental health services among Latinos, African Americans, and non-Latino whites. *Psychiatric Services, 53*(12), 1547–1555.

Alegria, M., Carson, N., Flores, M., Xinliang, L., Shi, P., Sophia, A., . . . Shrout, P. E. (2014). Activation, self-management, engagement, and retention in behavioral health care: A randomized clinical trial of the DECIDE intervention. *JAMA Psychiatry, 71*(5), 557–565.

Alegria, M., Shrout, P. E., Woo, M., Guarnaccia, P., Sribney, W., Vila, D., . . . Canino, G. (2007). Understanding differences in past year psychiatric disorders for Latinos living in the US. *Social Science & Medicine, 65*(2), 214–230.

Angold, A., Erkanli, A., Farmer, E. M., Fairbank, J. A., Burns, B. J., Keeler, G., & Costello, E. J. (2002). Psychiatric disorder, impairment, and service use in rural African American and white youth. *Archives of General Psychiatry, 59*(10), 893–901.

Archer, J., Bower, P., Gilbody, S., Lovell, K., Richards, D., Gask, L., . . . Coventry, P. (2012). Collaborative care for depression and anxiety problems. *Cochrane Database of Systematic Reviews, 10*, CD006525. doi:10.1002/14651858.CD006525.pub2

Areán, P. A., Ayalon, L., Hunkeler, E., Lin, E., Tang, L., Harpole, L., . . . Unützer, J. (2005). Improving depression care for older, minority patients in primary care. *Medical Care, 43*(4), 381–390.

Areán, P. A., Gum, A. M., Tang, L., & Unützer, J. (2007). Service use and outcomes among elderly persons with low incomes being treated for depression. *Psychiatric Services, 58*(8), 1057–1064.

Arnow, B. A., Blasey, C., Manber, R., Constantino, M. J., Markowitz, J. C., Klein, D. N., . . . Rush, A. J. (2007). Dropouts versus completers among chronically depressed outpatients. *Journal of Affective Disorders, 97*(1), 197–202.

Avenevoli, S., Swendsen, J., He, J. P., Burstein, M., & Merikangas, K. R. (2015). Major depression in the National Comorbidity Survey-Adolescent Supplement: Prevalence, correlates, and treatment. *Journal of the American Academy of Child and Adolescent Psychiatry, 54*(1), 37–44.

Barksdale, C. L., Kenyon, J., Graves, D. L., & Jacobs, C. G. (2014). Addressing disparities in mental health agencies: Strategies to implement the national clas standards in mental health. *Psychological Services, 11*(4), 369–376.

Beals, J., Manson, S. M., Mitchell, C. M., Spicer, P., & Team, A. S. (2003). Cultural specificity and comparison in psychiatric epidemiology: Walking the tightrope in American Indian research. *Culture Medicine and Psychiatry, 27*(3), 259–289.

Beals, J., Novins, D. K., Whitesell, N. R., Spicer, P., Mitchell, C. M., & Manson, S. M. (2005). Prevalence of mental disorders and utilization of mental health services in two American Indian reservation populations: Mental health disparities in a national context. *American Journal of Psychiatry, 162*(9), 1723–1732.

Breland-Noble, A. M. (2012). Community and treatment engagement for depressed African American youth: The AAKOMA FLOA pilot. *Journal of Clinical Psychology in Medical Settings, 19*(1), 41–48.

Breland-Noble, A. M., Al-Mateen, C., & Singh, N. (Eds.). (2016). *Handbook of mental health in African American youth.* New York, NY: Springer.

Breland-Noble, A. M., Bell, C., & Nicolas, G. (2006). Family first: The development of an evidence-based family intervention for increasing participation in psychiatric clinical care and research in depressed African American adolescents. *Family Process, 45*(2), 153–169.

Breland-Noble, A. M., Childers, T., & Boyce, C. A. (In Press). The evidence for CBT in the treatment of mental illness in African Americans. In F. T. L. Leong, G. Bernal, & N. Buchanan (Eds.), *Clinical psychology of ethnic minorities: Integrating research and practice.* Washington, DC: American Psychological Association.

Breland-Noble, A. M., Wong, M., Childers, T., Hankerson, S., & Sotomayor, J. (2015). Spirituality and religious coping in African American youth with depressive illness. *Culture, Mental Health and Religion, 18*(5), 330–341.

Broman, C. L. (2012). Race differences in the receipt of mental health services among young adults. *Psychological Services, 9*(1), 38–48.

Burnam, M. A., Hough, R. L., Karno, M., Escobar, J. I., & Telles, C. A. (1987). Acculturation and lifetime prevalence of psychiatric disorders among Mexican Americans in Los Angeles. *Journal of Health and Social Behavior, 28*(1), 89–102.

Byck, G. R., Bolland, J., Dick, D., Ashbeck, A. W., & Mustanski, B. S. (2013). Prevalence of mental health disorders among low-income African American adolescents. *Social Psychiatry and Psychiatric Epidemiology, 48*(10), 1555–1567.

Caldwell, C., Assari, S., & Breland-Noble, A. M. (2016). The epidemiology of mental disorders in African American children and adolescents. In A. M. Breland-Noble, C. Al-Mateen, & N. Singh (Eds.), *Handbook of mental health in African American youth.* New York, NY: Springer.

Campbell, J., Ramsay, J., & Green, J. (2001). Age, gender, socioeconomic, and ethnic differences in patients' assessments of primary health care. *Quality in Health Care, 10*(2), 90–95.

Centers for Disease Control and Prevention. (1997). *Principles of community engagement* (1st ed.). Atlanta, GA: US Government Printing Office.

Chung, B., Dixon, E. L., Miranda, J., Wells, K., & Jones, L. (2010). Using a community partnered participatory research approach to implement a randomized controlled trial:

Planning community partners in care. *Journal of Health Care for the Poor and Underserved, 21*(3), 780–795.

Cook, B. L., McGuire, T., & Miranda, J. (2007). Measuring trends in mental health care disparities, 2000–2004. *Psychiatric Services, 58*(12), 1533–1540.

Costello, E. J., Angold, A., Burns, B. J., Erkanli, A., Stangl, D. K., & Tweed, D. L. (1996). The Great Smoky Mountains Study of Youth: Functional impairment and serious emotional disturbance. *Archives of General Psychiatry, 53*(12), 1137–1143.

Costello, E. J., Angold, A., Burns, B. J., Stangl, D. K., Tweed, D. L., Erkanli, A., & Worthman, C. M. (1996). The Great Smoky Mountains Study of Youth: Goals, design, methods, and the prevalence of *DSM-III-R* disorders. *Archives of General Psychiatry, 53*(12), 1129–1136.

Costello, E., Erkanli, A., Copeland, W., & Angold, A. (2010). Association of family income supplements in adolescence with development of psychiatric and substance use disorders in adulthood among an American Indian population. *JAMA, 303*(19), 1954–1960.

Dobransky-Fasiska, D., Nowalk, M., Pincus, H., Castillo, E., Lee, B., Walnoha, A., . . . Brown, C. (2010). Public-academic partnerships: Improving depression care for disadvantaged adults by partnering with non-mental health agencies. *Psychiatric Services, 61*(2), 110–112.

Doi, Y., Roberts, R. E., Takeuchi, K., & Suzuki, S. (2001). Multiethnic comparison of adolescent major depression based on the *DSM-IV* criteria in a US–Japan study. *Journal of the American Academy of Child and Adolescent Psychiatry, 40*(11), 1308–1315.

Druss, B. G., & Goldman, H. H. (2003). New Freedom Commission Report: Introduction to the special section on the president's New Freedom Commission Report. *Psychiatric Services, 54*(11), 1465–1466.

Ell, K., Aranda, M. P., Xie, B., Lee, P.-J., & Chou, C.-P. (2010). Collaborative depression treatment in older and younger adults with physical illness: Pooled comparative analysis of three randomized clinical trials. *American Journal of Geriatric Psychiatry, 18*(6), 520–530.

Ell, K., Katon, W., Cabassa, L. J., Xie, B. I. N., Lee, P.-J., Kapetanovic, S., & Guterman, J. (2009). Depression and diabetes among low-income hispanics: Design elements of a socio-culturally adapted collaborative care model randomized controlled trial. *International Journal of Psychiatry in Medicine, 39*(2), 113–132.

Engel, C. C., Oxman, T., Yamamoto, C., Gould, D., Barry, S., Stewart, P., . . . Dietrich, A. J. (2008). RESPECT-Mil: Feasibility of a systems-level collaborative care approach to depression and post-traumatic stress disorder in military primary care. *Military Medicine, 173*(10), 935–940.

Falcón, L. M., & Tucker, K. L. (2000). Prevalence and correlates of depressive symptoms among Hispanic elders in Massachusetts. *The Journals of Gerontology Series B: Psychological Sciences and Social Sciences, 55*(2), S108-S116.

Gibbons, M. C. (2011). Use of health information technology among racial and ethnic underserved communities. *Perspectives in Health Information Management, 8*(Winter), 1f. Retrieved from http://www.ncbi.nlm.nih.gov/pmc/articles/PMC3035830/

Gilbody, S., Bower, P., Fletcher, J., Richards, D., & Sutton, A. J. (2006). Collaborative care for depression: A cumulative meta-analysis and review of longer-term outcomes. *Archives of Internal Medicine, 166*(21), 2314–2321.

Gone, J. P., & Trimble, J. E. (2012). American Indian and Alaska Native mental health: Diverse perspectives on enduring disparities. *Annual Review of Clinical Psychology, 8*(1), 131–160.

González, H. M., Haan, M. N., & Hinton, L. (2001). Acculturation and the prevalence of depression in older Mexican Americans: Baseline results of the Sacramento Area Latino Study on Aging. *Journal of the American Geriatrics Society, 49*(7), 948–953.

Hankerson, S. H., & Weissman, M. M. (2012). Church-based health programs for mental disorders among African Americans: A review. *Psychiatric Services, 63*(3), 243–249.

Heeringa, S. G., Wagner, J., Torres, M., Duan, N., Adams, T., & Berglund, P. A. (2004). Sample designs and sampling methods for the Collaborative Psychiatric Epidemiology Studies (CPES). *International Journal of Methods in Psychiatric Research, 13*(4), 221–240.

Hwang, W.-C., Myers, H. F., Chiu, E., Mak, E., Butner, J. E., Fujimoto, K., Wood, J. J., Miranda, J. (2015). Culturally adapted cognitive-behavioral therapy for Chinese Americans with depression: A randomized controlled trial. *Psychiatric Services, 66*(10), 1035–1042. doi:10.1176/appi.ps.201400358

Institute of Medicine. Committee to Review the Clinical and Translational Science Awards Program at the National Center for Advancing Translational Sciences. (2013). *The CTSA program at NIH: Opportunities for advancing clinical and translational research.* Washington, DC: National Academies Press.

Jackson, J., Abelson, J., Berglund, P., Mezuk, B., Torres, M., & Zhang, R. (2011). Ethnicity, immigration, and cultural influences on the nature and distribution of mental disorders: An examination of major depression. In D. Regier, W. Narrow, E. Kuhl, & D. Kupfer (Eds.), *Conceptual evolution of DSM 5* (Vol. 5, pp. 267–285). Arlington, VA: American Psychiatric Publishing.

Katon, W., & Unützer, J. (2006). Collaborative care models for depression: Time to move from evidence to practice. *Archives of Internal Medicine, 166*(21), 2304–2306.

Kessler, R. C., Demler, O., Frank, R. G., Olfson, M., Pincus, H. A., Walters, E. E., . . . Zaslavsky, A. M. (2005). Prevalence and treatment of mental disorders, 1990 to 2003. *New England Journal of Medicine, 352*(24), 2515–2523.

Kessler, R. C., Nelson, C. B., McGonagle, K. A., Liu, J., Swartz, M., & Blazer, D.G. (1996). Comorbidity of *DSM-III-R* major depressive disorder in the general population: Results from the US National Comorbidity Survey. *British Journal of Psychiatry Supplement, Jun*(30), 17–30.

Kim, H. J., Park, E., Storr, C. L., Tran, K., & Juon, H. S. (2015). Depression among Asian-American adults in the community: Systematic review and meta-analysis. *PLoS ONE, 10*(6), e0127760.

Kneipp, S. M., Kairalla, J. A., Lutz, B. J., Pereira, D., Hall, A. G., Flocks, J., . . . Schwartz, T. (2011). Public health nursing case management for women receiving temporary assistance for needy families: A randomized controlled trial using community-based participatory research. *American Journal of Public Health, 101*(9), 1769–1775.

Korsen, N., & Pietruszewski, P. (2009). Translating evidence to practice: Two stories from the field. *Journal of Clinical Psychology in Medical Settings, 16*(1), 47–57.

Kroenke, K., Spitzer, R. L., & Williams, J. B. (2001). The PHQ-9. *Journal of General Internal Medicine, 16*(9), 606–613.

Kuo, B. C., Chong, V., & Joseph, J. (2008). Depression and its psychosocial correlates among older Asian immigrants in North America: A critical review of two decades' research. *Journal of Aging and Health, 20*(6), 615–652.

Lester, K., Resick, P. A., Young-Xu, Y., & Artz, C. (2010). Impact of race on early treatment termination and outcomes in posttraumatic stress disorder treatment. *Journal of Consulting and Clinical Psychology, 78*(4), 480–489.

McGuire, T. G., Alegria, M., Cook, B. L., Wells, K. B., & Zaslavsky, A. M. (2006). Implementing the Institute of Medicine definition of disparities: An application to mental health care. *Health Services Research, 41*, 1979–2005.

Miranda, J., Bernal, G., Lau, A., Kohn, L., Hwang, W., & LaFromboise, T. (2005). State of the science on psychosocial interventions for ethnic minorities. *Annual Review of Clinical Psychology, 1*, 113–142.

Miranda, J., Duan, N., Sherbourne, C., Schoenbaum, M., Lagomasino, I., Jackson-Triche, M., & Wells, K. B. (2003). Improving care for minorities: Can quality improvement interventions improve care and outcomes for depressed minorities? Results of a randomized, controlled trial. *Health Services Research, 38*(2), 613–630.

Miranda, J., McGuire, T. G., Williams, D. R., & Wang, P. (2008). Mental health in the context of health disparities. *American Journal of Psychiatry, 165*(9), 1102–1108.

Miranda, J., Siddique, J., Belin, T. R., & Kohn-Wood, L. P. (2005). Depression prevalence in disadvantaged young black women. *Social Psychiatry and Psychiatric Epidemiology, 40*(4), 253–258.

Mufson, L., Weissman, M. M., Moreau, D., & Garfinkel, R. (1999). Efficacy of interpersonal psychotherapy for depressed adolescents. *Archives of General Psychiatry, 56*(6), 573–579.

Munoz, R. F., Barrera, A. Z., Delucchi, K., Penilla, C., Torres, L. D., & Perez-Stable, E. J. (2009). International Spanish/English internet smoking cessation trial yields 20% abstinence rates at 1 year. *Nicotine and Tobacco Research, 11*(9), 1025–1034.

Munoz, R. F., Lenert, L. L., Delucchi, K., Stoddard, J., Perez, J. E., Penilla, C., & Perez-Stable, E. J. (2006). Toward evidence-based internet interventions: A Spanish/English website for international smoking cessation trials. *Nicotine and Tobacco Research, 8*(1), 77–87.

Nadeem, E., Lange, J. M., Edge, D., Fongwa, M., Belin, T., & Miranda, J. (2007). Does stigma keep poor young immigrant and US-born black and Latina women from seeking mental health care? *Psychiatric Services, 58*(12), 1547–1554.

Ngo, V. K., Asarnow, J. R., Lange, J., Jaycox, L. H., Rea, M. M., Landon, C., . . . Miranda, J. (2009). Outcomes for youths from racial-ethnic minority groups in a quality improvement intervention for depression treatment. *Psychiatric Services, 60*(10), 1357–1364.

Ratzliff, A., Ni, K., Chan, Y., Park, M., & Unützer, J. (2013). A collaborative care approach to depression treatment for Asian Americans. *Psychiatric Services, 64*(5), 487–490.

Robins, L. N., & Regier, D. A. (1991). *Psychiatric disorders in America: The Epidemiologic Catchment Area study*: New York, NY: Free Press.

Sabin, J. A., & Greenwald, A. G. (2012). The influence of implicit bias on treatment recommendations for 4 common pediatric conditions: Pain, urinary tract infection, attention deficit hyperactivity disorder, and asthma. *American Journal of Public Health, 102*(5), 988–995.

Shellman, J., & Mokel, M. (2010). Overcoming barriers to conducting an intervention study of depression in an older African American population. *Journal of Transcultural Nursing, 21*(4), 361–369.

Smedley, B. D., Stith, A. Y., & Nelson, A. R. (Eds.). (2003). *Unequal treatment: Confronting racial and ethnic disparities in health care*. Washington, DC: Institute of Medicine.

Smedley, B. D., Syme, S. L., & Institute of Medicine Committee on Capitalizing on Social Science Behavioral Research to Improve the Public's Health. (2001). Promoting health: Intervention strategies from social and behavioral research. *American Journal of Health Promotion, 15*(3), 149–166.

Smith, M. E., Lindsey, M. A., Williams, C. D., Medoff, D. R., Lucksted, A., Fang, L. J., . . . Dixon, L. B. (2014). Race-related differences in the experiences of family members of persons with mental illness participating in the NAMI Family to Family Education Program. *American Journal of Community Psychology, 54*(3–4), 316–327.

Somervell, P. D., Leaf, P. J., Weissman, M. M., Blazer, D. G., & Bruce, M. L. (1989). The prevalence of major depression in black and white adults in five United States communities. *American Journal of Epidemiology, 130*(4), 725–735.

Stockdale, S. E., Lagomasino, I. T., Siddique, J., McGuire, T., & Miranda, J. (2008). Racial and ethnic disparities in detection and treatment of depression and anxiety among psychiatric and primary health care visits, 1995–2005. *Medical Care, 46*(7), 668–677.

Sue, S., Zane, N., & Young, K. (1994). Research on psychotherapy with culturally diverse populations. In A. E. Bergin & S. L. Garfield (Eds.), *Handbook of psychotherapy and behavior change* (4th ed., pp. 783–817). Oxford, England: John Wiley & Sons.

Takeuchi, D. T., Zane, N., Hong, S., Chae, D. H., Gong, F., Gee, G. C., . . . Alegría, M. (2007). Immigration-related factors and mental disorders among Asian Americans. *American Journal of Public Health, 97*(1), 84–90.

Unützer, J., Chan, Y. F., Hafer, E., Knaster, J., Shields, A., Powers, D., & Veith, R. C. (2012). Quality improvement with pay-for-performance incentives in integrated behavioral health care. *American Journal of Public Health, 102*(6), e33-e40.

Unützer, J., Choi, Y., Cook, I. A., & Oishi, S. (2002). Clinical computing: A web-based data management system to improve care for depression in a multicenter clinical trial. *Psychiatric Services, 53*(6), 671–678.

Unützer, J., Katon, W., Callahan, C. M., Williams Jr., J. W., Hunkeler, E., Harpole, L., . . . Lin, E. H. B. (2002). Collaborative care management of late-life depression in the primary care setting. *JAMA: The Journal of the American Medical Association, 288*(22), 2836–2845.

Unützer, J., Schoenbaum, M., Druss, B. G., & Katon, W. J. (2006). Transforming mental health care at the interface with general medicine: Report for the President's Commission. *Psychiatric Services, 57*(1), 37–47.

US Department of Health and Human Services. (1999). *Mental health: A report of the surgeon general.* Washington, DC: US Government Printing Office.

US Department of Health and Human Services. (2001). *Mental health: Culture, race, and ethnicity—A supplement to mental health: A report of the surgeon general.* Washington, DC: US Government Printing Office.

US Department of Health and Human Services. (2003). *New freedom commission on mental health: Achieving the promise: Transforming mental health in America. Final report.* (SMA-03–3832). Rockville, MD: US Government Printing Office.

Vega, W. A., Kolody, B., Aguilar-Gaxiola, S., Alderete, E., Catalano, R., & Caraveo-Anduaga, J. (1998). Lifetime prevalence of *DSM-III-R* psychiatric disorders among urban and rural Mexican Americans in California. *Archives of General Psychiatry, 55*(9), 771–778.

Wang, P. S., Berglund, P., & Kessler, R. C. (2000). Recent care of common mental disorders in the United States. *Journal of General Internal Medicine, 15*(5), 284–292.

Weibel-Orlando, J., & Kramer, B. (1989). *The Urban American Indian Elders Outreach Project: Final report for the Administration of Aging, Grant# 90 AMO273.* Los Angeles, CA: County of Los Angeles.

Wells, K. B., Jones, L., Chung, B., Dixon, E. L., Tang, L. Q., Gilmore, J., . . . Miranda, J. (2013). Community-partnered cluster-randomized comparative effectiveness trial of community engagement and planning or resources for services to address depression disparities. *Journal of General Internal Medicine, 28*(10), 1268–1278.

Wells, K., Klap, R., Koike, A., & Sherbourne, C. (2001). Ethnic disparities in unmet need for alcoholism, drug abuse, and mental health care. *American Journal of Psychiatry, 158*(12), 2027–2032.

Wells, K. B., Sherbourne, C. D., Miranda, J., Tang, L., Benjamin, B., & Duan, N. (2007). The cumulative effects of quality improvement for depression on outcome disparities over 9 years: Results from a randomized, controlled group-level trial. *Medical Care, 45*(11), 1052–1059.

Wells, K., Sherbourne, C., Schoenbaum, M., Ettner, S., Duan, N., Miranda, J., . . . Rubenstein, L. (2004). Five-year impact of quality improvement for depression: Results of a group-level randomized controlled trial. *Archives of General Psychiatry, 61*(4), 378–386.

Wennerstrom, A., Vannoy, S. D., Allen, C. E., Meyers, D., O'Toole, E., Wells, K. B., & Springgate, B. F. (2011). Community-based participatory development of a community health worker mental health outreach role to extend collaborative care in post-Katrina New Orleans. *Ethnicity and Disease, 21*(3 Suppl 1), S1-45-51.

Williams, D. R., Gonzalez, H. M., Neighbors, H., Nesse, R., Abelson, J. M., Sweetman, J., & Jackson, J. S. (2007). Prevalence and distribution of major depressive disorder in African Americans, Caribbean blacks, and non-Hispanic whites—Results from the National Survey of American Life. *Archives of General Psychiatry, 64*(3), 305–315.

World Health Organization. (2011). *Depression.* Retrieved from http://www.who.int/mental _health/management/depression/definition/en/index.html

Zhou, X. Y., Hetrick, S. E., Cuijpers, P., Qin, B., Barth, J., Whittington, C. J., . . . Xie, P. (2015). Comparative efficacy and acceptability of psychotherapies for depression in children and adolescents: A systematic review and network meta-analysis. *World Psychiatry, 14*(2), 207–222.

CHAPTER 15

Public Health Perspectives on Depression in Primary Care

Trina Chang, MD, MPH
Albert Yeung, MD, ScD

The Burden of Major Depression in Primary Care

The majority of depression care in the United States is delivered not by mental health specialists but by primary care providers (PCPs). Depression accounts for nearly 10% of all primary care office visits (Frank, Huskamp, & Pincus, 2003; Stafford, Ausiello, Misra, & Saglam, 2000), and in 2006–2007, close to 60% of all antidepressant prescriptions in the United States were written by PCPs (general practitioners, pediatricians, and obstetrician-gynecologists) (Mark, Levit, & Buck, 2009).

One reason for the greater utilization of PCPs for drug treatment is the availability of selective serotonin reuptake inhibitors and other second-generation antidepressants that are simpler and safer to treat depression than in the past. Until the mid- to late 1980s, the main medication options for depression were tricyclic antidepressants, with their side effects and risks in overdose, and monoamine oxidase inhibitors, with their many food-drug interactions and risk of hypertensive crisis. By contrast, bupropion, selective serotonin reuptake inhibitors, and other newer antidepressants are safer in overdose, better tolerated, and less subject to life-threatening interactions (Gartlehner et al., 2011).

Another reason is the growing difficulty in receiving specialty medication management services for mental health conditions. Psychiatry was one of only five specialties to experience a decline in the number of practicing physicians (by 2%) from 2000 to 2010 (Association of American Medical Colleges, 2012). The Health Resources and Services Administration (2015) estimated that another 2,800 psychiatrists would be needed to adequately cover the federally designated mental health shortage areas. And the gap may only grow bigger. Currently, 59% of psychiatrists in active practice are aged 55 or older, making psychiatry the third-oldest specialty. At the same time, the number of psychiatry residency graduates has been falling, going from 1,142 in

2000 to 985 in 2008 (Insel, 2011). While advanced practice nurses can prescribe medications, only about 300 join the field each year (Hartley, Hart, Hanrahan, & Loux, 2004); whether psychologists may prescribe medications remains highly controversial.

In addition, many patients prefer to receive mental health treatment from their primary care doctors rather than a specialist. For some people, it may stem from practical concerns such as wanting to see someone who already knows them, not needing to travel to multiple appointments, and avoiding specialty copays. For others, stigma may be the deterrent (Corrigan, Druss, & Perlick, 2014). A review of 144 studies found that mental health–related stigma exerted a small- to moderate-sized deterrent effect on help-seeking (Clement et al., 2015); stigma also leads patients to drop out of mental health treatment prematurely (Sirey et al., 2001). As a result, fewer patients engage in mental health care in referral models than in primary care–based models.

Yet the importance of depression management in achieving good health outcomes is becoming increasingly recognized. Compared to nondepressed patients with a chronic medical illness, those with a chronic medical illness plus comorbid depression make more frequent visits to primary care, specialty care, and emergency departments; incur higher inpatient pharmacy costs; and have more diagnostic tests (e.g., Druss & Rosenheck, 1999; Katon, Lin, Russo, & Unützer, 2003; Yoon et al., 2012). They are also three times as likely to be nonadherent to recommended medical treatment as patients without depression (DiMatteo, Lepper, & Croghan, 2000).

As a result, the health care system has begun to pay more attention to the identification and management of depression in primary care settings. The US Preventive Services Task Force (2016) is now recommending screening for the general adult population. The National Committee for Quality Assurance (2014) requires some level of attention to behavioral health conditions in order for primary care practices to receive recognition as patient-centered medical homes. The American College of Physicians has formally declared its support for behavioral health integration into primary care settings and has offered specific recommendations to promote integration, such as payment reform, workforce training, and stigma reduction programs (Crowley & Kirschner, 2015).

Challenges of Depression Management in Primary Care

Nevertheless, many challenges exist regarding the identification and treatment of depression in the primary care setting: lack of expertise and knowledge, competing demands, the emotional burden of managing psychiatric patients, patient factors, financing problems, and fragmentation of the mental health system, among others (e.g., Fuchs et al., 2015; Henke, Chou, Chanin, Zides, & Scholle, 2008; Whitebird et al., 2013).

One problem is that primary care doctors frequently feel undertrained to manage psychiatric issues. In a qualitative study by Loeb and colleagues (2012), PCPs reported feeling that they lack the medical knowledge, behavioral skills, and sometimes interest to manage patients with challenging mental health issues such as treatment-resistant depression with serious medical illness. In a survey of 54 primary care or internal medicine residency directors, 63% felt that more training in psychiatry was needed (Chin, Guillermo, Prakken, & Eisendrath, 2000). Meanwhile, lacking trust in their primary care doctors' knowledge about depression management, patients may be less likely to seek help from them (Kravitz et al., 2011). While the medical training system is starting to place more value on behavioral sciences (Association of American Medical Colleges, 2011; Mann, 2012; Smith et al., 2014), it will take time for the effects of these changes to trickle down through the profession into practice.

Another major limitation is time. In the absence of quick physiological measures or blood tests that can diagnose depression, health care providers must diagnose depression through a clinical interview—something that may be too time-consuming for the typical primary care visit. Adding to the pressure is PCPs' reluctance to discuss sensitive emotional issues with the same rapid approach they might take toward physical illnesses (Henke et al., 2008). Østbye and colleagues (2005) estimated that following patient care guidelines for just ten chronic illnesses, including depression, would require 10.6 hours per day. When comorbidities enter the mix, the problem is magnified; the more physical comorbidity the patient has, the less likely it is that a possible diagnosis of depression is considered, and the more new medical problems a depressed patient manifests, the less likely the physician is to discuss depression treatment changes (Rost et al., 2000). While some have proposed developing quick questionnaires or screeners to substitute for diagnostic interviews, it takes time and effort to free up staff members to process and respond to those results. For example, in one study, just 5% of patients who scored positive on a two-question depression screener were given the full Nine-Item Patient Health Questionnaire to follow up on the screen (Nutting et al., 2002).

The emotional burden of depression management often goes unrecognized but nevertheless affects practice as well. The physicians interviewed by Loeb and colleagues (2012) identified difficulty managing emotional responses to patients as another barrier to managing mental health. Additionally, PCPs must contend with patients who seemingly reject their recommendations—that is, patients who may not believe in or agree with a diagnosis of depression or the provider's treatment recommendations and who may decline or drop out of treatment.

Within-patient factors may also interfere. Some patients with a need for depression treatment who are presenting in primary care instead of specialty mental health settings are there because they do not think—or do not know—that they might need or want depression treatment. This group may include people who have little knowledge about depression and who may not know to report their symptoms to their providers, or who may use different language to describe their symptoms. Some may subscribe to the belief that depression is a temporary reaction to an event and that they can "snap out of it" if they try. Some may come from cultures that do not use the Western concept of depression. They may emphasize somatic symptoms such as poor sleep, weight changes, and low energy rather than psychological symptoms such as feelings of worthlessness. Or they may describe culturally specific syndromes that their providers may not recognize as signs of depression. Primary care doctors who have not been trained to use different vocabulary to describe depression may therefore struggle to discuss diagnoses and negotiate treatment plans with these patients.

Systemic factors represent a third potential set of barriers. Fragmentation in the US health care system has long been problematic (Elhauge, 2010), and when it comes to mental health care, the situation is worse. Patients may be referred for mental health treatment from separate organizations or providers in private practice, raising the risk of communication breakdowns between their health providers. Referral processes may be complicated and slow compared to referrals for other specialty services—for example, if patients must see a therapist before receiving medication management referrals (Henke et al., 2008). Within the mental health system, there are so many possible levels of treatment and services (e.g., different psychotherapy modalities, intensive outpatient treatment, community support services) that nonspecialists may feel lost and uncertain where to send their patients. In addition, many providers and health care leaders point to quirks of the health care financing system as disincentives for providing mental health care in primary care settings. One major issue has been the existence of "carve-outs" for behavioral health services, wherein payers contract with specialty companies to administer (and often bear the financial risk for) mental health and substance use services. With time, some unintended consequences have become apparent. Examining behavioral health integration efforts and barriers, Pincus and colleagues (2005) wrote:

> The existence of a risk-bearing managed behavioral health care organization (MBHO), in conjunction with another health plan's capitation for primary care services only, establishes a potent motivation for primary care doctors to refer behavioral patients to the MBHO. MBHOs do not share any rewards or risks for more efficient management of depression in the primary care setting, nor do they receive any benefit from the reduced costs associated with improved pharmacy or medical/surgical use by members seeking treatment for their mental condition in the primary care setting. (p. 272)

The advent of the Affordable Care Act and accountable care organizations (ACOs), which reward quality improvement and cost reduction, has raised hopes that this split can be corrected (Bartels, Gill & Naslund, 2015). O'Donnell and colleagues (2013) argued that "due to the high financial and health costs of poorly treated chronic mental and physical health conditions, it is unlikely that ACOs will be able to meet quality measures, and benefit from shared savings, without adequately addressing mental health" (p. 181). However, as of January 2015, less than 10% of the US population was covered through ACOs (Muhlestein, 2015).

Currently, providers must contend with what may seem to be arcane and arbitrary rules pertaining to payment and billing. In interviews with primary care leaders, Kathol and colleagues (2010) identified these common barriers to integrating behavioral health into primary care: (1) problems with coding for mental health services in nonpsychiatric settings, (2) confusion about whether to bill medical or behavioral health payers, (3) regulations barring payment for physical and mental condition encounters on the same day, (4) lack of reimbursement for care managers, and (5) low reimbursement rates for mental health services provided in medical settings.

Consequences for Depression Management in Primary Care

The results of these challenges are missed diagnoses and inadequate treatment. In a study using screening and structured clinical interviews in primary care, Simon and Von Korff (1995) found that 64% of the patients who met criteria for current major depression were recognized as being depressed by their PCPs. In another study, only 56% of primary care patients with major depression were recognized as having depression at some point over the next five years (Jackson, Passamonti & Kroenke, 2007). Patients who present with somatic symptoms—approximately two-thirds of primary care patients with depression—or somatic comorbidities may be especially subject to missed diagnoses (Nuyen et al., 2005; Tylee & Gandhi, 2005).

Reaching a diagnosis is no guarantee that the disorder or symptoms will be addressed. Mischoulon and colleagues (2001) found that when they screened community-based primary care patients for major depression using a structured clinical interview and informed their PCPs of diagnoses, only half received any depression treatment or referral during the next three months. Overall, 50.6% of primary care patients with moderately severe or severe depression receive no antidepressant or psychotherapy treatment whatsoever (Shim, Baltrus, Ye, & Rust, 2011).

Conversely, providers sometimes offer depression treatment without having made a formal diagnosis of a depressive disorder. Simon and colleagues (2014) found that 27% of patients filling antidepressant prescriptions in 2010 did not carry an appropriate psychiatric diagnosis, even after they corrected for the use of medications for indications such as pain or tobacco cessation.

Once the patient and provider have agreed on how to manage the patient's depression symptoms, achieving high-quality treatment is the next hurdle. Analyses of the 1996 Midlife Development in the United States survey showed that only 16.9% of patients with major depression received guideline-concordant care (Wang, Berglund, & Kessler, 2000). More recently, Henke and colleagues (2009) found significant "clinical inertia" in the treatment of depression in primary care settings. In cases in which depression had not fully resolved with treatment, further adjustments to the treatment occurred only one-third of the time. Similarly, Chang and colleagues (2012) found that among primary care patients who had been diagnosed with depression and had not improved at least 50% as of three months later, only about 15% had any change in their depression treatment over the subsequent three months.

Finally, whether due to patient or systemic factors, retaining patients in treatment remains challenging. Patients who are started on an antidepressant by a primary care physician show higher rates of immediate nonadherence, as measured by never filling an antidepressant prescription (18% for PCPs vs. 13% for psychiatrists), and six-month nonadherence, as measured by obtaining refills, than those started on an antidepressant by a psychiatrist (53% for PCPs vs. 49% for psychiatrists) (Bambauer, Soumerai, Adams, Zhang, & Ross-Degnan, 2007). Additionally, these patients are less likely to have three or more visits during the first 90 days after the initiation of the medication (generally considered to be guideline-concordant care for depression) than are those started on antidepressants by a psychiatrist (Chen et al., 2010; Simon, Von Korff, Rutter, & Peterson, 2001).

Interventions to Improve Primary Care Management of Depression

A number of interventions have been tested to address these barriers. Single-component interventions have included efforts to enhance screening rates, educate providers, and improve the quality of depression treatment delivered in primary care.

Promoting depression screening in primary care is one of the most popular interventions for improving primary care management of depression. In 2015, the US Preventive Services Task Force proposed expanding its primary care depression screening recommendations to include the general adult population, as opposed to just those treated in settings where adequate systems for diagnosis, treatment, and follow-up were available (US Preventive Services Task Force, 2015). However, some investigators have questioned the quality of the evidence for depression screening and have highlighted the risks and costs of overtreatment (Thombs, Ziegelstein, Roseman, Kloda, & Ioannidis, 2014). Additionally, screening alone is no guarantee of diagnosis or treatment, as discussed earlier.

Another common approach is to offer more training in depression management to PCPs. Unfortunately, this approach has mixed evidence of effectiveness (Lin et al., 1997; Thompson et al., 2000). For example, one study of a training that included multiple educational interventions, didactics, discussion, and role-playing in group or one-on-one formats, followed by opportunities for case discussion and consultation, found no significant change in practice in terms of diagnosing depression or initiating pharmacotherapy. The authors concluded that educating physicians is a "necessary but insufficient strategy" (Lin, Simon, Katzelnick, & Pearson, 2001).

Similarly, providing decision support alone may not suffice. In one study, researchers used the electronic medical record to send PCPs patient-specific treatment advisory messages based on federal depression treatment guidelines and to remind providers to schedule follow-up visits; however, this intervention did not lead to improvements in process or outcome measures compared to simply reminding PCPs of the depression diagnosis and providing a link to more information (Rollman et al., 2002). When five VA primary care clinics added a depression decision support team consisting of a psychiatrist and a nurse to provide patient education, monitoring, and feedback to primary care clinicians, they found improvements in process but not in depression outcomes (Dobscha et al., 2006).

Interventions using a care team member to provide support and medication monitoring have been more successful. For example, when trained nurses provided two medication education sessions averaging no more than 15 minutes each to patients starting a tricyclic antidepressant for depression, medication adherence improved (Peveler, George, Kinmonth, Campbell, & Thompson, 1999). Better yet, when primary care patients starting antidepressants were paired with nurse telehealth managers who made ten six-minute calls over four months to offer emotional support and focused behavioral interventions, both depression symptom severity and response rates improved significantly at six months (Hunkeler et al., 2000). However, similar interventions by pharmacists have shown mixed results in terms of medication adherence and depression outcomes (Adler et al., 2004; Bosmans et al., 2007; Bungay et al., 2004; Capoccia et al., 2004; Finley et al., 2003).

Overall, the limitations of single-component interventions for depression have led many to conclude that multicomponent interventions are more promising (Gilbody, Whitty, Grimshaw, & Thomas, 2003). These interventions generally draw on successes in the management of chronic medical issues in ambulatory care, situating depression management in a well-established framework of care redesign efforts in primary care. In the 1990s, the idea of chronic care models (CCMs) for chronic medical illnesses such as cardiovascular disease (CVD) and diabetes began to take hold (Von Korff, Gruman, Schaefer, Curry, & Wagner, 1997; Wagner, Austin, & Von Korff, 1996). These models aimed to change ambulatory care practice to facilitate long-term disease management, catching problems before they could cause severe complications or emergency room visits and hospitalizations. Themes of CCMs included coordination of care delivery, clinical decision support tools and information systems, patient self-management, an organizational environment that systematically supports chronic illness management, and linkage to community resources (Wagner et al., 2001). On the whole, the evidence suggests that such models are associated with improved process and outcome measures for a variety of disorders and that interventions that utilize multiple CCM elements are associated with better quality of care (Coleman, Austin, Brach, & Wagner, 2009).

Translating these models for use with depressed patients made sense, given that depression can be a lifelong illness whose management requires multiple health care visits, treatment adjustments, and behavior changes (Haddad & Tylee, 2011). Katon and colleagues (1995) studied the effect of a collaborative intervention in which depressed patients had two visits each with their primary care doctor and a psychiatrist during the first four to six weeks of treatment, received additional education on depression, and were monitored for medication refills. The authors tested a similar intervention in which patients also worked with a psychologist for brief counseling around medication adherence and cognitive behavioral strategies to manage depression (Katon et al., 1996). Both interventions were associated with improvements in medication adherence and depression severity in patients with major depression.

Other models emphasized some form of care management. In one study, while providing monitoring and feedback to physicians made no difference in treatment or patient outcomes, adding a care manager who provided telephone follow-up, treatment recommendations, and practice support *did* improve outcomes for an added $80 per patient (Simon, Von Korff, Rutter, & Wagner, 2000). In another study that provided education for physicians and training and role redefinition to enable nurses to provide education about treatment options, promote engagement in treatment, and assess depressive symptoms, the intervention was associated with increased odds of patients with a new depressive episode receiving guideline-concordant pharmacotherapy and/or psychotherapy, as well as with an improvement in depressive symptoms (Rost, Nutting, Smith, Werner, & Duan, 2001).

These efforts evolved into a set of contemporaneous but independent trials of models of depression care integration in primary care for depressed elders: Improving Mood-Promoting Access to Collaborative Treatment (IMPACT), Primary Care Research in Substance Abuse and Mental Health for Elderly (PRISM-E), and Prevention of Suicide in Primary Care Elderly: Collaborative Trial (PROSPECT). Each of these large-scale trials combined broad-based screening for case identification with multiple elements of CCMs, whether care management, algorithm-based treatment, or closer relationships between mental health and PCPs (Alexopoulos et al., 2009; Krahn et al., 2006; Unützer et al., 2002).

Perhaps the best-known of these trials was IMPACT, which was tested in a geriatric population. In this model, the PCP retains responsibility for managing depression but is supported by a team that includes a care manager and a consulting psychiatrist. The care manager is responsible for contacting the patient frequently to monitor treatment adherence, side effects, and response; carry out behavioral interventions such as behavioral activation; review cases with the consulting psychiatrist; and act as a liaison between team members. The consulting psychiatrist may never "lay eyes" on the patient but rather will discuss cases with the care manager in order to provide input on treatment. Other key elements include the use of standardized symptom measurement scales, stepped care, and registries.

The evidence for the IMPACT model is extensive and well documented. In the clinical trial, which spanned 18 sites in five states and enrolled 1801 patients, nearly half of intervention subjects experienced at least a 50% improvement in depression symptoms after 12 months, compared to 19% in the control arm (Unützer et al., 2002). A cost-effectiveness analysis found that compared to usual care, the IMPACT intervention led to lower total health care costs (including outpatient and inpatient costs for medical and mental health care as well as intervention costs) over four years—$29,422 in the intervention arm compared to $32,785 in the usual care arm (Unützer et al., 2008). Furthermore, its benefits may last long after the intervention. A study of participants at one site found that eight years after the intervention ended, intervention patients without baseline CVD experienced a 48% lower risk of hard cardiovascular events (i.e., myocardial infarction or stroke) than did controls without baseline CVD (Stewart, Perkins, & Callahan, 2014).

These findings accorded well with the findings of the PRISM-E and PROSPECT trials. Like IMPACT, these trials found that their approaches to behavioral health integration led to better depression outcomes. In addition, PROSPECT found lower mortality in intervention patients in a follow-up study seven years later (Gallo et al., 2013), and the PRISM-E intervention led to better patient engagement in treatment (Bartels et al., 2004).

Collaborative Care

"Collaborative care" is the most promising chronic care model-based strategy for improving care of depression. While the make-up of collaborative care interventions for treatment of depression vary, they typically include a multi-professional approach to patient care, structured management, scheduled patient follow-ups, and enhanced inter-professional communication. (Coventry et al., 2014, p. 2)

With time, many of these models have converged into the comprehensive systems commonly categorized as collaborative care for depression in primary care. Multiple large reviews and meta-analyses (e.g., Archer et al., 2012; Thota et al., 2012; Woltmann et al., 2012) have concluded that collaborative care is effective at improving depression outcomes such as symptom severity, response and remission rates, quality of life, and treatment satisfaction in the general adult population. It also may improve medication use, mental health quality of life, and patient satisfaction. In addition, a review of 30 studies on economic outcomes of collaborative care found evidence of economic benefit in multiple areas. Five of six cost-utility studies found that collaborative care was cost-effective, and of the seven that measured economic benefits in terms of averted health care or productivity loss, four of seven found benefits due to collaborative care (Jacob et al., 2012).

The success of these collaborative care models has led to numerous adaptations targeting different patient populations and disorders, which we discuss in the following sections.

Adolescents

In the Youth Partners in Care intervention for adolescents aged 13–21, primary care practices received training and access to a psychotherapist care manager who could follow up with patients, coordinate care with the primary care clinician, assist with patient management, and provide manualized cognitive behavioral therapy (CBT) components. Rates of care and depression severity both improved significantly more in the intervention group by the end of six months (Asarnow et al., 2005). In a similar intervention based on IMPACT that targeted adolescents aged 13–17, the Reaching Out to Adolescents in Distress (ROAD) intervention (Richardson et al., 2014), primary care clinics had access to master's-level care managers who could provide education, monitoring and brief CBT, consulting psychiatrists, and stepped-care treatment algorithms. This intervention was associated with significantly greater improvements in depression severity, response, and remission.

Medically Ill Populations

A particularly important area for expanded screening and treatment focus is the comorbidity of depression with other medical disorders. There appears to be a bidirectional relationship between depression and several chronic medical illnesses, wherein the risk of depression appears to be higher in some medically ill populations and vice versa (Patten et al., 2008). Furthermore, depression is associated with poor treatment adherence and medical outcomes, such as higher all-cause mortality in patients with comorbid depression at 5 (Lin et al., 2009), 8 (Egede, Nietert, & Zheng, 2005), and 10 years (Coleman, Katon, Lin, & Von Korff, 2013).

Not surprisingly, a number of collaborative care models have been adapted to target patients with depression and another illness—for example, diabetes, heart disease, and cancer. A meta-analysis of 24 articles based on 12 separate studies of collaborative care suggests that these interventions can improve depression in patients with comorbid medical illnesses, though their effect on medical outcomes requires more study (Watson et al., 2013).

DEPRESSION, DIABETES, AND CARDIOVASCULAR HEALTH

Researchers from the University of Washington who had developed one of the original depression collaborative care models first investigated what would happen if patients with comorbid depression and diabetes received an IMPACT-type intervention. The Pathways case management intervention, which provided collaborative care management for depression in patients with comorbid depression and diabetes, found an improvement in depression outcomes and adequate antidepressant treatment but not in A1C outcomes in intervention compared to usual care (Katon et al., 2004). They then tested a collaborative treatment that included not only a depression treatment phase but also a subsequent phase focused on controlling disease targets such as blood sugar, cholesterol, or blood pressure, and then a phase devoted to promoting healthy habits such as exercise and tobacco cessation. It used a nurse care manager, who met weekly for case review with the PCP and a psychiatrist, and monthly with a psychologist for supervision in behavioral interventions.

This intervention, the TEAMcare model, was tested in a 12-month randomized controlled trial in patients with depression and comorbid diabetes or cardiovascular heart disease. Compared to enhanced usual care, the intervention was associated with greater improvements in depression scores, glycated hemoglobin, systolic blood pressure, and LDL cholesterol at the end of the first year (Katon et al., 2010), though only the depression improvements were sustained 6 and 12 months after the intervention ended (Katon et al., 2012). Intervention patients experienced higher rates of medication initiation and adjustment rates for antidepressants, insulin, and antihypertensive agents; monitored their blood pressure and glucose more frequently; and reported more days of healthy eating and of getting at least 30 minutes of activity (Lin et al., 2012; Rosenberg, Lin, Peterson, Ludman, Von Korff, & Katon, 2014). Medication adherence rates did not differ, though the authors thought this might be due to high baseline adherence rates. Two-year cost-effectiveness analyses showed that the intervention was associated with an estimated decrease of $594 in total outpatient costs compared to usual care and an increase of .335 quality-adjusted life years, an index that is intended to reflect both the quality (morbidity) and the quantity (mortality) of life and that is commonly used in analyses of health care interventions. This decrease translated into an estimated cost of $3297 per quality-adjusted life year, well within the range for interventions that are recommended for rapid dissemination (Katon et al., 2012).

IMPACT and the TEAMCare intervention have been combined with screening, brief intervention, referral, and treatment for substance use disorders into an intervention called COMPASS (Care of Mental, Physical and Substance Use Syndromes) for patients with depression and comorbid diabetes and/or CVD. COMPASS is a three-year, $18 million project that was funded by the federal Centers for Medicaid and Medicare Services and carried out by a consortium of health care delivery organizations and implementation/quality improvement centers nationwide. More than 4,000 patients in seven states were enrolled over the course of the project, and results are promising (2017).

DEPRESSION AND CANCER

A number of trials have tackled the problem of depression in cancer patients, which affects 8%–24% of people with cancer (Krebber et al., 2014). Subgroup analyses of patients in the IMPACT trial previously had suggested that the intervention was effective in elderly patients with cancer (Fann, Fan, & Unützer, 2009). In the United Kingdom, researchers with the Symptom Management Research Trials group (SMaRT2) carried out a series of studies of a collaborative care intervention known as Depression Care for People with Cancer (Walker & Sharpe, 2014). Patients in the intervention arm were offered up to 10 individual sessions (in person or by telephone) with a nurse who could provide education on depression, problem-solving treatment, and coordination with the patient's oncologist and primary care physician, supplemented by advice from a study psychiatrist. The intervention was associated with greater improvements in depression, anxiety, and fatigue (Sharpe et al., 2014; Strong et al., 2008; Walker et al., 2014), and showed evidence of cost-effectiveness (Walker, Cassidy, & Sharpe, 2009).

Racial or Ethnic Minorities

Treating minority patients with depression poses a special challenge, as illustrated by reports that have found continued racial and ethnic disparities in the management of mental health issues (e.g., Agyemang, Mezuk, Perrin, & Rybarczyk, 2014; Hankerson et al., 2011; Lagomasino et al., 2005) such as lower rates of receipt of mental health care (Hahm, Cook, Ault-Brutus, & Alegría, 2015), lower likelihood of receiving guideline-concordant treatment (González et al., 2010), and lower retention in treatment (Fortuna, Alegría, & Gao, 2010; Kales et al., 2013). Issues such as different concepts of psychological symptoms and an emphasis on somatic symptoms may contribute to lower rates of recognizing and diagnosing depression in certain minority populations. Socioeconomic barriers and stigma may keep those who need treatment by mental health specialists from accessing it (Interian, Ang, Gara, Rodriguez, & Vega, 2011; Sirey, Franklin, McKenzie, Ghosh, & Raue, 2014). For these reasons, primary care settings are especially important for diagnosing and treating racial or ethnic minorities with depression.

Research indicates that collaborative care may be particularly useful for minority patients. Subgroup analyses of the depression collaborative care interventions described earlier have shown effectiveness for participants who belonged to minority groups. For example, the IMPACT collaborative care model was as effective for black and Latino elders as it was for non-Latino white elders (Areán et al., 2005). Adaptations of collaborative care models for specific minority groups also have demonstrated success. In a study comparing standard collaborative care and patient-centered collaborative care models for African American patients (Cooper et al., 2013), both models were associated with improvements in depression outcomes comparable to the results of previous collaborative care interventions. Yeung and colleagues (2011) created a culturally sensitive collaborative treatment model for Chinese Americans in primary care, featuring bilingual care managers and a diagnostic interview protocol adaptable for members of different cultural groups. The care management group showed higher rates of treatment engagement, though no difference in treatment outcomes, perhaps because all depressed patients in this study received treatment from a psychiatrist (Yeung et al., 2010). A subsequent adaptation using telepsychiatry found improved depression response and remission rates as well as greater decrease in depressive symptoms (Yeung et al., 2016).

Overall, in a review of depression interventions for older racial and ethnic minority patients in the United States, Fuentes and Aranda (2012) concluded that while the effectiveness of depression care in general has mixed evidence, "collaborative or integrated care shows promise for African Americans and Latinos" (p. 915). Among interventions that focused on treatment engagement of underserved racial and ethnic minorities, a review by Interian, Lewis-Fernández, and Dixon (2013) specifically singled out collaborative care interventions for depression as being effective.

Furthermore, several studies have demonstrated that a quality improvement (QI) intervention for depression treatment has the potential to improve treatment in minority as well as majority groups (Angstman et al., 2015; Miranda et al., 2003; Wells et al., 2004). In fact, perhaps because of existing disparities, minorities actually stood to gain more from a QI intervention in the Partners in Care studies, meaning that QI efforts had the potential to reduce racial or ethnic mental health disparities (Wells et al., 2007).

Dissemination and Implementation

At this point, the evidence base for these models of depression management in primary care is sufficiently well accepted, so their adoption is snowballing across the country. Large health systems, health plans, and even state governments (e.g., Schuffman, Druss & Parks, 2009) have begun to adopt some form of integration of behavioral health care in primary care. The VA has mandated that all of its practice adopt one of three models for depression care improvement in primary care (VHA Handbook, 2008), while the US Army has widely implemented a collaborative care program for posttraumatic stress disorder and depression (Department of Defense Deployment Health Clinical Center, n.d.). Insurers have begun developing their own care management programs for behavioral health conditions (e.g., Boston Medical Center HealthNet Plan, n.d.; Health Care Service Corporation, n.d.). In Minnesota, employers and insurers banded together with the Institute for Clinical Systems Improvement to fund a depression collaborative care service based on the IMPACT model, a program known as Depression Improvement Across Minnesota, Offering a New Direction (DIAMOND) (Institute for Clinical Systems Improvement, 2014).

With this transition from research to practice, the field has turned its attention to questions of dissemination and implementation. For example, can research-based models be implemented with relative fidelity and success in real-world settings? Which elements are necessary for success, and what other variations or expansions could increase their effectiveness? What conditions facilitate success of depression care transformation?

Fidelity and Replication

Both the team behind the IMPACT model and researchers studying the VA models have provided guidance on key steps or practices needed to implement their models with high fidelity (Fortney et al., 2009; University of Washington, 2010). The DIAMOND project reported a high degree of implementation fidelity that was sustained over two years across 75 practices (Solberg et al., 2013). However, whether this translated into improved outcomes was unclear. An analysis funded by the National Institute of Mental Health of some DIAMOND sites did not find significantly better results compared to usual care (Institute for Clinical Systems Improvement, n.d.), but a less rigorous analysis of other sites did show an improvement (Shippee et al., 2013). Conversely, a study of the implementation of TEAMcare at four Canadian clinics showed suboptimal fidelity but nevertheless was associated with improved outcomes (Wozniak et al., 2015). A study of three VA centers and 11 of their affiliated community-based outpatient clinics found both "excellent" fidelity and good clinical outcomes, comparable to those achieved in randomized controlled trials (e.g., 41% depression response rates) (Fortney et al., 2012).

In any case, fidelity is not the sole goal. "There is a natural tension between fidelity to a particular model and blending or transforming models to respond to local needs and preferences," wrote Pomerantz and Sayers (2010, p. 81) about the VA experience implementing behavioral health integration. "Within a short time after funding these programs, it became apparent that the most effective approaches to integrated care were those that blended the models together and now, after only 3 years, most programs blend models in a way that assures adaptation to local culture, resources and patient care needs."

Key Components and Variations

Complementing efforts to study treatment fidelity are investigations asking which intervention components are the most important to retain. A 2006 meta-analysis examining 37 trials of collaborative care for depression across the United States and Europe identified active care management, support of medication management in primary care, and psychiatric consultation as key elements of successful programs (Gilbody, Bower, Fletcher, Richards, & Sutton, 2006). A metaregression of 62 studies found that some of the variables most strongly associated with improvement in depressive symptoms were subject recruitment via systematic case identification, use of care managers with a background in mental health, and the provision of regular supervision for care managers (Bower, Gilbody, Richards, Fletcher, & Sutton, 2006). A subsequent metaregression of 79 studies suggested that increased antidepressant use was seen with systematic case identification and studies including patients with a chronic physical condition; it also identified psychological treatment as an element associated with greater depression improvement (Coventry et al., 2014).

Other studies are focusing on variations of ways to deliver collaborative care to increase its utility, such as workforce questions. IMPACT's original studies showed cost-effectiveness using psychologists and nurses as care managers; many other studies successfully utilized social workers. The DIAMOND project in Minnesota found no difference in outcomes whether the care managers were registered nurses, licensed practical nurses, or certified medical assistants (Pietruszewski, Mundt, Hadzic, & Brown, 2015). It did, however, note a trend toward better enrollment and outcomes with dedicated care managers, rather than with care managers who filled multiple clinic roles.

Ideal caseload is another unknown. The original IMPACT trial had an average caseload of 100 to 120 patients per care manager, including both patients in active management and those being monitored to establish stability before being discharged from active management. The VA estimated that its telephone care managers in one study were carrying a maximum caseload of 143 to 165 patients apiece (Liu et al., 2007), but caring for more psychiatrically ill or complicated patients may require lower patient-to–care manager ratios.

Telemedicine offers another promising way to extend the reach of depression collaborative care. Telephonic care management and psychotherapy appear to enhance depression outcomes for a modest cost compared to usual care (Simon, Ludman, & Rutter, 2009), and current collaborative care programs frequently rely on telephone calls from care managers to supplement or replace in-person visits. A study at rural federally qualified health centers found that telemedicine-based collaborative care yielded better depression outcomes than practice-based collaborative care at its sites, perhaps due to greater treatment fidelity on the part of the centrally based care managers (Fortney et al., 2013); thus, while more expensive, it also was more cost-effective (Pyne et al., 2015). Yeung and colleagues (2016) successfully used videoconferencing to enable psychiatric consultants in a collaborative model to evaluate depressed Chinese American primary care patients. Project ECHO (Project Extension for Community Healthcare Outcomes) (Arora et al., 2007) allows physicians in distant locations to discuss cases in telemedicine "clinics" with specialists at an academic center, increasing their knowledge and enhancing patient care; it is being used to improve access to treatment for addiction and mental illnesses in New Mexico (Project ECHO, n.d.).

Another potential use of technology involves software or applications to support components of depression care integration. For example, a software platform that supports assessment, treatment, and QI is a central component of the Behavioral Health Laboratory (BHL), one of three integrated care models used by the VA (Tew, Klaus, & Oslin, 2010). BHL's software can be used to record responses to validated symptom questionnaires, generate clinical notes, carry out patient tracking functions, and facilitate other quality management functions. The software is programmed with a number of different evidence-based treatment pathways that can be customized to the specific needs of the clinic—for example, recommending specialty referral for patients with subsyndromal illness in one clinic that is minimally equipped to manage this and allowing for monitoring and management within primary care at another clinic. Modules include "watchful waiting" (p. 136), at-risk drinking, and others.

Implementation Issues

A third question is what is needed to implement collaborative care and similar depression care redesign efforts successfully. Researchers with the DIAMOND project in Minnesota found that "practice leaders' " relative commitment to depression care improvement may be a useful measure of the likelihood that a practice is ready to implement evidence-based depression care changes (Rubenstein et al., 2014). A qualitative and quantitative analysis of the clinics participating in DIAMOND found that practices with strong leadership support, a strong care manager, a well-defined and well-implemented role for the care manager, a care manager who was onsite and accessible, and a strong PCP champion enrolled more patients. Factors linked with improved clinical outcomes were slightly different; better six-month remission rates were associated with practices having an engaged consulting psychiatrist, doing "warm handoffs" (introducing patients to the care manager in person at the time of referral), and not perceiving operating costs as a barrier (Whitebird et al., 2014).

Overall, noting a high degree of adoption of depression practice systems and depression care improvement strategies—albeit with much interpractice variation—the DIAMOND researchers observed: "This study demonstrates that under the right circumstances, primary care clinics that are prepared to implement evidence-based care can do so if financial barriers are reduced, effective training and facilitation are provided, and the new design introduces the specific mental models, new care processes, and workers and expertise that are needed" (Solberg et al., 2013, p. 10).

At the VA, a survey of 225 clinics that had implemented one of the administration's three endorsed models of primary care–mental health integration found that 48% of clinics had implemented co-location, 17% had chosen an IMPACT-like model known as Translating Initiatives in Depression into Effective Solutions (TIDES), and 8% went with the BHL (Chang et al., 2013). The researchers hypothesized that the comparative simplicity of the co-location model explained its seeming popularity. Clinics in a VA regional network that endorsed the TIDES model were more likely to implement TIDES. Those with psychologists or psychiatrists on staff, greater financial sufficiency, or greater spatial sufficiency appeared more likely to implement BHL.

In addition, the VA found that patients whose primary care clinicians were early adopters of the collaborative care model were more likely to complete adequate care manager follow-up. There appeared to be a dose-response pattern for care manager visits, with patients who had four or more care manager visits having significantly better outcomes on the Nine-Item Patient Health Questionnaire at 24 weeks than patients with just baseline and 24-week visits (Chaney et al., 2011).

Financing

Restructuring the payment system to support depression collaborative care and similar integration models is perhaps the biggest challenge currently facing depression care redesign. The DIAMOND project in Minnesota was revolutionary in that it brought together employers and health plans to create a single billing code and a bundle of depression collaborative care services, which the payers would reimburse for a monthly fee (American Psychiatric Association, 2010; Bao et al., 2011). But even if ongoing services are funded, the costs of organizational transformation are significant. The VA estimated that the cost of implementing its depression care QI program at seven primary care clinics in three multistate VA regions over four years totaled $84,438 for clinical leaders from the regional systems, health centers, and individual practices, and $197,787 for the technical expert team providing support for the implementation, with the bulk of the costs being incurred during initial engagement activities and the care model design process (Liu et al., 2009).

As noted earlier, incentives to treat depression in primary care patients are slowly shifting with the Affordable Care Act and the rise of shared risk contracts. In fact, Medicare has recently started paying for collaborative care management of behavioral health conditions. Still, less than half of the nation's economic burden of depression is due to direct health care costs; nearly 50% is due to workplace costs such as lost productivity and disability (Greenberg, Fournier, Sisitsky, Pike, & Kessler, 2015). Thus, greater transformation in payments for depression treatment may yet be needed, whether through partnerships with employers similar to the DIAMOND program or arrangements with Medicare and Medicaid such as the temporary matching Medicaid funding that Missouri received to fund behavioral health consultants and care management (Crowley & Kirschner, 2015).

Conclusion

Depression in primary care settings remains a high public health priority due to both the substantial number of depressed patients who are managed in primary care and the interrelationship between depression and poor medical outcomes. The good news is that a robust evidence base suggests that there are indeed efficacious—and cost-effective—interventions to reduce the burden of depression in primary care patients. The bad news is that the interventions with the broadest evidence base at present are generally complex multicomponent interventions that require a significant investment of time, commitment, and labor up front, as well as changes in current payment systems, to be sustainable in the long run.

Thus, from a public health perspective, organizations must consider how to modify systems to support any extra work required for depression management in primary care, such as the manpower to administer, document, and follow up on screens and the technology to operate population management registries. Payers and policy-makers must grapple with how to structure health care financing to better align payment with the true societal costs of depression and other behavioral health conditions. And there is a pressing need for additional research to understand how to implement such models, such as the most important components to include and possible stepwise approaches to bring about change, as well as for research to optimize current models and treatments—at least until the next paradigm shift in managing depression in primary care takes place.

References

Adler, D. A., Bungay, K. M., Wilson, I. B., Pei, Y., Supran, S., Peckham, E., . . . Rogers, W. H. (2004). The impact of a pharmacist intervention on 6-month outcomes in depressed primary care patients. *General Hospital Psychiatry, 26*(3), 199–209.

Agyemang, A. A., Mezuk, B., Perrin, P., & Rybarczyk, B. (2014). Quality of depression treatment in black Americans with major depression and comorbid medical illness. *General Hospital Psychiatry, 36*(4), 431–436.

Alexopoulos, G. S., Reynolds, C. F., Bruce, M. L., Katz, I. R., Raue, P. J., Mulsant, B. H., . . . the PROSPECT Group. (2009). Reducing suicidal ideation and depression in older primary care patients: 24-month outcomes of the PROSPECT study. *American Journal of Psychiatry, 166*(8), 882–890.

American Psychiatric Association. (2010). A new direction in depression treatment in Minnesota: DIAMOND program, Institute for Clinical Systems Improvement, Blooming-ton, Minnesota. *Psychiatric Services, 61*(10), 1042–1044.

Angstman, K. B., Phelan, S., Myszkowski, M. R., Schak, K. M., DeJesus, R. S., Lineberry, T. W., & van Ryn, M. (2015). Minority primary care patients with depression: Outcome disparities improve with collaborative care management. *Medical Care, 53*(1), 32–37.

Archer, J., Bower, P., Gilbody, S., Lovell, K., Richards, D., Gask, L., . . . Coventry, P. (2012). Collaborative care for depression and anxiety problems. *Cochrane Database of Systematic Reviews, 10*, CD006525.

Areán, P. A., Ayalon, L., Hunkeler, E., Lin, E. H., Tang, L., Harpole, L., . . . Unützer, J. (2005). Improving depression care for older, minority patients in primary care. *Medical Care, 43*(4), 381–390.

Arora, S., Geppert, C. M. A., Kalishman, S., Dion, D., Pullara, F., Bjeletich, B., . . . Scaletti, J. V. (2007). Academic health center management of chronic diseases through knowledge networks: Project ECHO. *Academic Medicine, 82*(2), 154–160.

Asarnow, J. R., Jaycox, L. H., Duan, N., LaBorde, A. P., Rea, M. M., Murray, P., . . . Wells, K. B. (2005). Effectiveness of a quality improvement intervention for adolescent depression in primary care clinics: A randomized controlled trial. *Journal of the American Medical Association, 293*(3), 311–319.

Association of American Medical Colleges. (2012). *2012 Physician Specialty Data Book.* Retrieved from https://www.aamc.org/download/313228/data/2012physicianspecialtydatabook.pdf

Bambauer, K. Z., Soumerai, S. B., Adams, A. S., Zhang, F., & Ross-Degnan, D. (2007). Provider and patient characteristics associated with antidepressant nonadherence: The impact of provider specialty. *Journal of Clinical Psychiatry, 68*(6), 867–873.

Bao, Y., Casalino, L. P., Ettner, S. L., Bruce, M. L., Solberg, L. I., & Unützer, J. (2011). Design-ing payment for collaborative care for depression in primary care. *Health Services Research, 46*(5), 1436–1451.

Bartels, S. J., Coakley, E. H., Zubritsky, C., Ware, J. H., Miles, K. M., Areán, P. A., . . . Levkoff, S. E. (2004). Improving access to geriatric mental health services: A randomized trial comparing treatment engagement with integrated versus enhanced referral care for depression, anxiety, and at-risk alcohol use. *American Journal of Psychiatry, 161*(8), 1455–1462.

Bartels, S. J., Gill, L., & Naslund, J. A. (2015). The Affordable Care Act, accountable care organizations, and mental health care for older adults: Implications and opportunities. *Harvard Review of Psychiatry, 23*(5), 304–319.

Bosmans, J. E., Brook, O. H., van Hout, H. P., de Bruijne, M. C., Nieuwenhuyse, H., Bouter, L. M., . . . van Tulder, M. W. (2007). Cost effectiveness of a pharmacy-based coaching programme to improve adherence to antidepressants. *Pharmacoeconomics, 25*(1), 25–37.

Boston Medical Center HealthNet Plan. (n.d.). Mental health or substance abuse. Retrieved from http://www.bmchp.org/members/care-management-program/behavioral-health

Bower, P., Gilbody, S., Richards, D., Fletcher, J., & Sutton, A. (2006). Collaborative care for depression in primary care. Making sense of a complex intervention: Systematic review and meta-regression. *British Journal of Psychiatry, 189*(6), 484–493.

Bungay, K. M., Adler, D. A., Rogers, W. H., McCoy, C., Kaszuba, M., Supran, S., . . . Wilson, I. B. (2004). Description of a clinical pharmacist intervention administered to primary care patients with depression. *General Hospital Psychiatry, 26*(3), 210–218.

Capoccia, K. L., Boudreau, D. M., Blough, D. K., Ellsworth, A. J., Clark, D. R., Stevens, N. G., . . . Sullivan, S. D. (2004). Randomized trial of pharmacist interventions to improve depression care and outcomes in primary care. *American Journal of Health-System Pharmacy, 61*(4), 364–372.

Chaney, E. F., Rubenstein, L. V., Liu, C.-F., Yano, E. M., Bolkan, C., Lee, M., . . . Uman, J. (2011). Implementing collaborative care for depression treatment in primary care: A cluster randomized evaluation of a quality improvement practice redesign. *Implementation Science, 6*, 121. Retrieved from http://doi.org/10.1186/1748-5908-6-121

Chang, E. T., Rose, D. E., Yano, E. M., Wells, K. B., Metzger, M. E., Post, E. P., . . . Rubenstein, L. V. (2013). Determinants of readiness for primary care-mental health integration (PC-MHI) in the VA health care system. *Journal of General Internal Medicine, 28*(3), 353–362.

Chang, T. E., Jing, Y., Yeung, A. S., Brenneman, S. K., Kalsekar, I., Hebden, T., . . . Fava, M. (2012). Effect of communicating depression severity on physician prescribing patterns: Findings from the Clinical Outcomes in Measurement-based Treatment (COMET) trial. *General Hospital Psychiatry, 34*(2), 105–112.

Chen, S. Y., Hansen, R. A., Farley, J. F., Gaynes, B. N., Morrissey, J. P., & Maciejewski, M. L. (2010). Follow-up visits by provider specialty for patients with major depressive disorder initiating antidepressant treatment. *Psychiatric Services, 61*(1), 81–85.

Chin, H. P., Guillermo, G., Prakken, S., & Eisendrath, S. (2000). Psychiatric training in primary care medicine residency programs: A national survey. *Psychosomatics, 41*(5), 412–417.

Clement, S., Schauman, O., Graham, T., Maggioni, F., Evans-Lacko, S., Bezborodovs, N., . . . Thornicroft, G. (2015). What is the impact of mental health–related stigma on help-seeking? A systematic review of quantitative and qualitative studies. *Psychological Medicine, 45*(1), 11–27.

Coleman, K., Austin, B. T., Brach, C., & Wagner, E. H. (2009). Evidence on the chronic care model in the new millennium. *Health Affairs, 28*(1), 75–85.

Coleman, S. M., Katon, W., Lin, E., & Von Korff, M. (2013). Depression and death in diabetes: 10-year follow up of all cause and cause specific mortality in a diabetic cohort. *Psychosomatics, 54*(5), 428–436.

Cooper, L. A., Ghods Dinoso, B. K., Ford, D. E., Roter, D. L., Primm, A. B., Larson, S. M., . . . Wang, N. Y. (2013). Comparative effectiveness of standard versus patient-centered collaborative care interventions for depression among African Americans in primary care settings: The BRIDGE Study. *Health Services Research, 48*(1), 150–174.

Corrigan, P. W., Druss, B. G., & Perlick, D. A. (2014). The impact of mental illness stigma on seeking and participating in mental health care. *Psychological Science in the Public Interest, 15*(2), 37–70.

Coventry, P. A., Hudson, J. L., Kontopantelis, E., Archer, J., Richards, D. A., Gilbody, S., . . . Bower, P. (2014). Characteristics of effective collaborative care for treatment of depression: A systematic review and meta-regression of 74 randomised controlled trials. *PLoS ONE, 9*(9), e108114.

Crowley, R. A., & Kirschner, N. (2015). The integration of care for mental health, substance abuse, and other behavioral health conditions into primary care: Executive summary of an American College of Physicians position paper. *Annals of Internal Medicine, 163*(4), 298–299.

Department of Defense Deployment Health Clinical Center. (n.d.). *RESPECT-Mil*. Retrieved from http://www.pdhealth.mil/respect-mil/index1.asp

DiMatteo, M. R., Lepper, H. S., & Croghan, T. W. (2000). Depression is a risk factor for noncompliance with medical treatment: Meta-analysis of the effects of anxiety and depression on patient adherence. *Archives of Internal Medicine, 160*(14), 2101–2107.

Dobscha, S. K., Corson, K., Hickam, D. H., Perrin, N. A., Kraemer, D. F., & Gerrity, M. S. (2006). Depression decision support in primary care: A cluster randomized trial. *Annals of Internal Medicine, 145*(7), 477–487.

Druss, B. G., & Rosenheck, R. A. (1999). Patterns of health care costs associated with depression and substance abuse in a national sample. *Psychiatric Services, 50*(2), 214–218.

Egede, L. E., Nietert, P. J., & Zheng, D. (2005). Depression and all-cause and coronary heart disease mortality among adults with and without diabetes. *Diabetes Care, 28*(6), 1339–1345.

Elhauge, E. (2010). *The fragmentation of US health care: Causes and solutions.* New York, NY: Oxford University Press.

Fann, J. R., Fan, M. Y., & Unützer, J. (2009). Improving primary care for older adults with cancer and depression. *Journal of General Internal Medicine, 24*(Suppl. 2), S417–424.

Finley, P. R., Rens, H. R., Pont, J. T., Gess, S. L., Louie, C., Bull, S. A., . . . Bero, L. A. (2003). Impact of a collaborative care model on depression in a primary care setting: A randomized controlled trial. *Pharmacotherapy, 23*(9), 1175–1185.

Fortney, J., Enderle, M., McDougall, S., Clothier, J., Otero, J., Altman, L., & Curran, G. (2012). Implementation outcomes of evidence-based quality improvement for depression in VA community based outpatient clinics. *Implementation Science, 7*, 30. Retrieved from http://doi.org/10.1186/1748-5908-7-30

Fortney, J. C., Pyne, J. M., Mouden, S. B., Mittal, D., Hudson, T. J., Schroeder, G. W., . . . Rost, K. M. (2013). Practice based versus telemedicine based collaborative care for depression in rural federally qualified health centers: A pragmatic randomized comparative effectiveness trial. *American Journal of Psychiatry, 170*(4), 414–425.

Fortney, J. C., Pyne, J. M., Smith, J. L., Curran, G. M., Otero, J. M., Enderle, M. A., & McDougall, S. (2009). Steps for implementing collaborative care programs for depression. *Population Health Management, 12*(2), 69–79.

Fortuna, L. R., Alegría, M., & Gao, S. (2010). Retention in depression treatment among ethnic and racial minority groups in the United States. *Depression and Anxiety, 27*(5), 485–494.

Frank, R. G., Huskamp, H. A., & Pincus, H. A. (2003). Aligning incentives in the treatment of depression in primary care with evidence-based practice. *Psychiatric Services, 54*(5), 682–687.

Fuchs, C. H., Haradhvala, N., Hubley, S., Nash, J. M., Keller, M. B., Ashley, D., . . . Uebe-lacker, L. A. (2015). Physician actions following a positive PHQ-2: Implications for the implementation of depression screening in family medicine practice. *Families, Systems and Health, 33*(1), 18–27.

Fuentes, D., & Aranda, M. P. (2012). Depression interventions among racial and ethnic minority older adults: A systematic review across 20 years. *American Journal of Geriatric Psychiatry, 20*(11), 915–931.

Gallo, J. J., Morales, K. H., Bogner, H. R., Raue, P. J., Zee, J., Bruce, M. L., & Reynolds, C. F. (2013). Long term effect of depression care management on mortality in older adults: Follow-up of cluster randomized clinical trial in primary care. *British Medical Journal, 346*, f2570. Retrieved from http://doi.org/10.1136/bmj.f2570

Gartlehner, G., Hansen, R. A., Reichenpfader, U., Kaminski, A., Kien, C., Strobelberger, M., . . . Gaynes, B. (Eds.). (2011). Drug class review. Second-generation antidepressants: Final update 5 report. Portland, OR: Oregon Health and Science University. Retrieved from http://www.healthandwelfare.idaho.gov/Portals/0/Medical/MedicaidCHIP /AntidepressantsFinalReport.pdf

Gilbody, S., Bower, P., Fletcher, J., Richards, D., & Sutton, A. J. (2006). Collaborative care for depression: A cumulative meta-analysis and review of longer-term outcomes. *Archives of Internal Medicine, 166*(21), 2314–2321.

Gilbody, S., Whitty, P., Grimshaw, J., & Thomas, R. (2003). Improving the detection and management of depression in primary care. *Quality and Safety in Health Care, 12*(2), 149–155.

González, H. M., Vega, W. A., Williams, D. R., Tarraf, W., West, B. T., & Neighbors, H. W. (2010). Depression care in the United States: Too little for too few. *Archives of General Psychiatry, 67*(1), 37–46.

Greenberg, P. E., Fournier, A. A., Sisitsky, T., Pike, C. T., & Kessler, R. C. (2015). The economic burden of adults with major depressive disorder in the United States (2005 and 2010). *Journal of Clinical Psychiatry, 76*(2), 155–162.

Haddad, M., & Tylee, A. (2011). The chronic disease management model for depression in primary care. *Clinical Neuropsychiatry, 8*(4), 252–259.

Hahm, H. C., Cook, B. L., Ault-Brutus, A., & Alegría, M. (2015). Intersection of race-ethnicity and gender in depression care: Screening, access, and minimally adequate treatment. *Psychiatric Services, 66*(3), 258–264.

Hankerson, S. H., Fenton, M. C., Geier, T. J., Keyes, K. M., Weissman, M. M., & Hasin, D. S. (2011). Racial differences in symptoms, comorbidity, and treatment for major depressive disorder among black and white adults. *Journal of the National Medical Association, 103*(7), 576–584.

Hartley, D., Hart, V., Hanrahan, N., & Loux, S. (2004). Are advanced practice psychiatric nurses a solution to rural mental health workforce shortages? Working paper #31. Portland, ME: University of Southern Maine. Retrieved from https://muskie.usm.maine.edu /Publications/rural/wp31.pdf

Health Care Service Corporation. (n.d.). *Behavioral health care management program*. Retrieved from http://www.bcbsil.com/provider/clinical/behavioral_health.html

Health Resources and Services Administration. (2015). Shortage designation: Health professional shortage areas and medically underserved areas/populations. Retrieved from http://www.hrsa.gov/shortage/

Henke, R. M., Chou, A. F., Chanin, J. C., Zides, A. B., & Scholle, S. H. (2008). Physician attitude toward depression care interventions: Implications for implementation of quality improvement initiatives. *Implementation Science, 3*, 40. Retrieved from http://doi.org/10 .1186/1748-5908-3-40

Henke, R. M., Zaslavsky, A. M., McGuire, T. G., Ayanian, J. Z., & Rubenstein, L.V. (2009). Clinical inertia in depression treatment. *Medical Care, 47*(9), 959–967.

Hunkeler, E. M., Meresman, J. F., Hargreaves, W. A., Fireman, B., Berman, W. H., Kirsch, A. J., . . . Salzer, M. (2000). Efficacy of nurse telehealth care and peer support in augmenting treatment of depression in primary care. *Archives of Family Medicine, 9*(8), 700–708.

Insel, T. (2011, June 3). Psychiatry: Where are we going? [Web log entry]. Retrieved from http://www.nimh.nih.gov/about/director/2011/psychiatry-where-are-we-going.shtml

Institute for Clinical Systems Improvement. (n.d.). DIAMOND study findings. Retrieved from https://www.icsi.org/_asset/nn7ofc/ICSI-DIAMOND-Study-Finding-6-4-14.pdf

Institute for Clinical Systems Improvement. (2014, June). *The DIAMOND program: Treatment for patients with depression in primary care.* White paper. Retrieved from https://www.icsi .org/_asset/rs2qfi/DIAMONDWP0614.pdf

Interian, A., Ang, A., Gara, M. A., Rodriguez, M. A., & Vega, W. A. (2011). The long-term trajectory of depression among Latinos in primary care and its relationship to depression care disparities. *General Hospital Psychiatry, 33*(2), 94–101.

Interian, A., Lewis-Fernández, R., & Dixon, L. B. (2013). Improving treatment engagement of underserved US racial-ethnic groups: A review of recent interventions. *Psychiatric Services, 64*(3), 212–222.

Jackson, J. L., Passamonti, M., & Kroenke, K. (2007). Outcome and impact of mental disorders in primary care at 5 years. *Psychosomatic Medicine, 69*(3), 270–276.

Jacob, V., Chattopadhyay, S. K., Sipe, T. A., Thota, A. B., Byard, G. J., & Chapman, D. P., . . . Community Preventive Services Task Force. (2012). Economics of collaborative care for management of depressive disorders: A community guide systematic review. *American Journal of Preventive Medicine, 42*(5), 539–549.

Kales, H. C., Nease, D., Sirey, J. A., Zivin, K., Kim, H. M., Kavanagh, J., . . . Blow, F. C. (2013). Racial differences in adherence to antidepressant treatment in later life. *American Journal of Geriatric Psychiatry, 21*(10). Retrieved from http://doi.org/10.1016/j.jagp.2013.01.046

Kathol, R. G., Butler, M., McAlpine, D. D., & Kane, R. L. (2010). Barriers to physical and mental condition integrated service delivery. *Psychosomatic Medicine, 72*(6), 511–518.

Katon, W. J., Lin, E., Russo, J., & Unützer, J. (2003). Increased medical costs of a population-based sample of depressed elderly patients. *Archives of General Psychiatry, 60*(9), 897–903.

Katon, W. J., Lin, E. H. B., Von Korff, M., Ciechanowski, P., Ludman, E., Young, B., . . . McGregor, M. (2010). Integrating depression and chronic disease care among patients with diabetes and/or coronary heart disease: The design of the TEAMcare study. *Contemporary Clinical Trials, 31*(4), 312–322.

Katon, W., Robinson, P., Von Korff, M., Lin, E., Bush, T., Ludman, E., . . . Walker, E. (1996). A multifaceted intervention to improve treatment of depression in primary care. *Archives of General Psychiatry, 53*(10), 924–932.

Katon, W., Russo, J., Lin, E. H. B., Schmittdiel, J., Ciechanowski, P., Ludman, E., . . . Von Korff, M. (2012). Cost-effectiveness of a multicondition collaborative care intervention: A randomized controlled trial. *Archives of General Psychiatry, 69*(5), 506–515.

Katon, W. J., Von Korff, M., Lin, E. H., Simon, G., Ludman, E., Russo, J., . . . Bush, T. (2004). The Pathways Study: A randomized trial of collaborative care in patients with diabetes and depression. *Archives of General Psychiatry, 61*(10), 1042–1049.

Katon, W., Von Korff, M., Lin, E., Walker, E., Simon, G. E., Bush, T., . . . Russo, J. (1995). Collaborative management to achieve treatment guidelines: Impact on depression in primary care. *Journal of the American Medical Association, 273*(13), 1026–1031.

Krahn, D. D., Bartels, S. J., Coakley, E., Oslin, D. W., Chen, H., McIntyre, J., . . . Levkoff, S. E. (2006). PRISM-E: Comparison of integrated care and enhanced specialty referral models in depression outcomes. *Psychiatric Services, 57*(7), 946–953.

Kravitz, R. L., Paterniti, D. A., Epstein, R. M., Rochlen, A. B., Bell, R. A., Cipri, C., . . . Duberstein, P. (2011). Relational barriers to depression help-seeking in primary care. *Patient Education and Counseling, 82*(2), 207–213.

Krebber, A. M. H., Buffart, L. M., Kleijn, G., Riepma, I. C., de Bree, R., Leemans, C. R., . . . Verdonck-de Leeuw, I. M. (2014). Prevalence of depression in cancer patients: A meta-analysis of diagnostic interviews and self-report instruments. *Psycho-Oncology, 23*(2), 121–130.

Lagomasino, I. T., Dwight-Johnson, M., Miranda, J., Zhang, L., Liao, D., Duan, N., & Wells, K. B. (2005). Disparities in depression treatment for Latinos and site of care. *Psychiatric Services, 56*(12), 1517–1523.

Lin, E. H. B., Heckbert, S. R., Rutter, C. M., Katon, W. J., Ciechanowski, P., Ludman, E. J., . . . Von Korff, M. (2009). Depression and increased mortality in diabetes: Unexpected causes of death. *Annals of Family Medicine, 7*(5), 414–421.

Lin, E. H., Katon, W. J., Simon, G. E., Von Korff, M., Bush, T. M., Rutter, C. M., . . . Walker, E. A. (1997). Achieving guidelines for the treatment of depression in primary care: Is physician education enough? *Medical Care, 35*(8), 831–842.

Lin, E. H. B., Simon, G. E., Katzelnick, D. J., & Pearson, S. D. (2001). Does physician education on depression management improve treatment in primary care? *Journal of General Internal Medicine, 16*(9), 614–619.

Lin, E. H., Von Korff, M., Ciechanowski, P., Peterson, D., Ludman, E. J., Rutter, C. M., . . . Katon, W. J. (2012). Treatment adjustment and medication adherence for complex patients with diabetes, heart disease, and depression: A randomized controlled trial. *Annals of Family Medicine, 10*(1), 6–14.

Liu, C.-F., Fortney, J., Vivell, S., Vollen, K., Raney, W. N., Revay, B., . . . Chaney, E. (2007). Time allocation and caseload capacity in telephone depression care management. *American Journal of Managed Care, 13*(12), 652–660.

Liu, C.-F., Rubenstein, L. V., Kirchner, J. E., Fortney, J. C., Perkins, M. W., Ober, S. K., . . . Chaney, E. F. (2009). Organizational cost of quality improvement for depression care. *Health Services Research, 44*(1), 225–244.

Loeb, D. F., Bayliss, E. A., Binswanger, I. A., Candrian, C., & deGruy, F. V. (2012). Primary care physician perceptions on caring for complex patients with medical and mental illness. *Journal of General Internal Medicine, 27*(8), 945–952.

Mann S. (2012). AAMC approves new MCAT exam with increased focus on social, behavioral sciences. *AAMC Reporter.* Retrieved from https://www.aamc.org/newsroom/reporter /march2012/276588/mcat2015.html

Mark, T. L., Levit, K. R., & Buck, J. A. (2009). Datapoints: Psychotropic drug prescriptions by medical specialty. *Psychiatric Services, 60*(9), 1167.

Miranda, J., Duan, N., Sherbourne, C., Schoenbaum, M., Lagomasino, I., Jackson-Triche, M., & Wells, K. B. (2003). Improving care for minorities: Can quality improvement interventions improve care and outcomes for depressed minorities? Results of a randomized, controlled trial. *Health Services Research, 38*(2), 613–630.

Mischoulon, D., McColl-Vuolo, R., Howarth, S., Lagomasino, I. T., Alpert, J. E., Nierenberg, A. A., & Fava, M. (2001). Management of major depression in the primary care setting. *Psychotherapy and Psychosomatics, 70*(2), 103–107.

Muhlestein, D. (2015, March 31). Health Affairs Blog: Growth and dispersion of accountable care organizations in 2015. [Web log entry]. Retrieved from http://healthaffairs.org/blog /2015/03/31/growth-and-dispersion-of-accountable-care-organizations-in-2015-2/

National Committee for Quality Assurance. (2014, March 24). New NCQA patient-centered medical home standards raise the bar. Retrieved from http://www.ncqa.org/newsroom /news-archive/2014-news-archive/news-release-march-24-2014

Nutting, P. A., Rost, K., Dickinson, M., Werner, J. J., Dickinson, P., Smith, J. L., & Gallovic, B. (2002). Barriers to initiating depression treatment in primary care practice. *Journal of General Internal Medicine, 17*(2), 103–111.

Nuyen, J., Volkers, A. C., Verhaak, P. F., Schellevis, F. G., Groenewegen, P. P., & Van den Bos, G. A. (2005). Accuracy of diagnosing depression in primary care: The impact of chronic somatic and psychiatric co-morbidity. *Psychological Medicine, 35*(8), 1185–1195.

O'Donnell, A. N., Williams, B. C., Eisenberg, D., & Kilbourne, A. M. (2013). Mental health in ACOs: Missed opportunities and low hanging fruit. *American Journal of Managed Care, 19*(3), 180–184.

Østbye, T., Yarnall, K. S. H., Krause, K. M., Pollak, K. I., Gradison, M., & Michener, J. L. (2005). Is there time for management of patients with chronic diseases in primary care? *Annals of Family Medicine, 3*(3), 209–214.

Patten, S. B., Williams, J. V., Lavorato, D. H., Modgill, G., Jetté, N., & Eliasziw, M. (2008). Major depression as a risk factor for chronic disease incidence: Longitudinal analyses in a general population cohort. *General Hospital Psychiatry, 30*(5), 407–413.

Peveler, R., George, C., Kinmonth, A.-L., Campbell, M., & Thompson, C. (1999). Effect of antidepressant drug counselling and information leaflets on adherence to drug treatment in primary care: Randomised controlled trial. *British Medical Journal, 319*(7210), 612–615.

Pietruszewski, P. B., Mundt, M. P., Hadzic, S., & Brown, R. L. (2015). Effects of staffing choices on collaborative care for depression at primary care clinics in Minnesota. *Psychiatric Services, 66*(1), 101–103.

Pincus, H. A., Houtsinger, J. K., Bachman, J., & Keyser, D. (2005). Depression in primary care: Bringing behavioral health care into the mainstream. *Health Affairs, 24*(1), 271–276.

Pomerantz, A. S., & Sayers, S. L. (2010). Primary care–mental health integration in healthcare in the Department of Veterans Affairs. *Family Systems and Health, 28*(2), 78–82.

Project ECHO. (n.d.). Integrated addiction and psychiatry. [Web page]. Retrieved from http://echo.unm.edu/nm-teleecho-clinics/integrated-addiction-and-psychiatry-clinic/

Pyne, J. M., Fortney, J. C., Mouden, S., Lu, L., Hudson, T. J., & Mittal, D. (2015). Cost-effectiveness of on-site versus off-site collaborative care for depression in rural FQHCs. *Psychiatric Services, 66*(5), 491–499.

Report of the Behavioral and Social Science Expert Panel. (2011). Washington, DC: Association of American Medical Colleges. Retrieved from https://www.aamc.org/download/271020/data /behavioralandsocialsciencefoundationsforfuturephysicians.pdf

Richardson, L. P., Ludman, E., McCauley, E., Lindenbaum, J., Larison, C., Zhou, C., . . . Katon, W. (2014). Collaborative care for adolescents with depression in primary care: A randomized clinical trial. *JAMA, 312*(8), 809–816.

Rollman, B. L., Hanusa, B. H., Lowe, H. J., Gilbert, T., Kapoor, W. N., & Schulberg, H. C. (2002). A randomized trial using computerized decision support to improve treatment of major depression in primary care. *Journal of General Internal Medicine, 17*(7), 493–503.

Rosenberg, D., Lin, E., Peterson, D., Ludman, E., Von Korff, M., & Katon, W. (2014). Integrated medical care management and behavioral risk factor reduction for multicondition patients: Behavioral outcomes of the TEAMcare trial. *General Hospital Psychiatry, 36*(2), 129–134.

Rossom, R.C., Solberg, L. I., Magnan, S., Crain, A. L., Beck, A., Coleman, K. J., . . . Unützer, J. (2017). Impact of a national collaborative care initiative for patients with depression and diabetes or cardiovascular disease. *General Hospital Psychiatry, 44*, 77–85.

Rost, K., Nutting, P., Smith, J., Coyne, J. C., Cooper-Patrick, L., & Rubenstein, L. (2000). The role of competing demands in the treatment provided primary care patients with major depression. *Archives of Family Medicine, 9*(2), 150–154.

Rost, K., Nutting, P., Smith, J., Werner, J., & Duan, N. (2001). Improving depression outcomes in community primary care practice: A randomized trial of the QuEST intervention. *Journal of General Internal Medicine, 16*(3), 143–149.

Rubenstein, L. V., Danz, M. S., Crain, A. L., Glasgow, R. E., Whitebird, R. R., & Solberg, L. I. (2014). Assessing organizational readiness for depression care quality improvement: Relative commitment and implementation capability. *Implementation Science, 9*, 173. Retrieved from http://doi: 10.1186/s13012-014-0173-1

Schuffman, D., Druss, B. G., & Parks, J. J. (2009). State mental health policy: Mending Missouri's safety net: Transforming systems of care by integrating primary and behavioral health care. *Psychiatric Services, 60*(5), 585–588.

Sharpe, M., Walker, J., Holm Hansen, C., Martin, P., Symeonides, S., Gourley, C., . . . Murray, G. (2014). Integrated collaborative care for comorbid major depression in patients with cancer (SMaRT Oncology-2): A multicentre randomised controlled effectiveness trial. *The Lancet, 384*(9948), 1099–1108.

Shim, R. S., Baltrus, P., Ye, J., & Rust, G. (2011). Prevalence, treatment, and control of depressive symptoms in the United States: Results from the National Health and Nutrition Examination Survey (NHANES), 2005–2008. *Journal of the American Board of Family Medicine, 24*(1), 33–38.

Shippee, N. D., Shah, N. D., Angstman, K. B., DeJesus, R. S., Wilkinson, J. M., Bruce, S. M., & Williams, M. D. (2013). Impact of collaborative care for depression on clinical, functional, and work outcomes: A practice-based evaluation. *Journal of Ambulatory Care Management, 36*(1), 13–23.

Simon, G. E., Ludman, E. J., & Rutter, C. M. (2009). Incremental benefit and cost of telephone care management and telephone psychotherapy for depression in primary care. *Archives of General Psychiatry, 66*(10), 1081–1089.

Simon, G. E., Stewart, C., Beck, A., Ahmedani, B., Coleman, K. J., Whitebird, R., . . . Hunkeler, E. M. (2014). National prevalence of receipt of antidepressant prescriptions by persons without a psychiatric diagnosis. *Psychiatric Services, 65*(7), 944–946.

Simon, G. E., & Von Korff, M. (1995). Recognition, management, and outcomes of depression in primary care. *Archives of Family Medicine, 4*(2), 99–105.

Simon, G. E., Von Korff, M., Rutter, C. M., & Peterson, D. A. (2001). Treatment process and outcomes for managed care patients receiving new antidepressant prescriptions from psychiatrists and primary care physicians. *Archives of General Psychiatry, 58*(4), 395–401.

Simon, G. E., Von Korff, M., Rutter, C., Wagner, E. (2000). Randomised trial of monitoring, feedback, and management of care by telephone to improve treatment of depression in primary care. *British Medical Journal, 320*(7234), 550–554.

Sirey, J. A., Bruce, M. L., Alexopoulos, G. S., Perlick, D. A., Friedman, S. J., & Meyers, B. S. (2001). Stigma as a barrier to recovery: Perceived stigma and patient-rated severity of illness as predictors of antidepressant drug adherence. *Psychiatric Services, 52*(12), 1615–1620.

Sirey, J. A., Franklin, A. J., McKenzie, S., Ghosh, S., & Raue, P. (2014). Race, stigma and mental health recommendations among depressed older persons in aging services. *Psychiatric Services, 65*(4), 537–540.

Siu, A. L., US Preventive Services Task Force, Bibbins-Domingo, K., Grossman, D. C., Baumann, L. C., Davidson, K. W., . . . Pignone, M. P. (2016). Screening for depression in adults: US Preventive Services Task Force recommendation statement. *JAMA, 315*(4):380–387.

Smith, R. C., Laird-Fick, H., D'Mello, D., Dwamena, F. C., Romain, A., Olson, J., . . . Frankel, R. (2014). Addressing mental health issues in primary care: An initial curriculum for medical residents. *Patient Education and Counseling, 94*(1), 33–42.

Solberg, L. I., Crain, A. L., Jaeckels, N., Ohnsorg, K. A., Margolis, K. L., Beck, A., . . . Van de Ven, A. H. (2013, November 16). The DIAMOND initiative: Implementing collaborative care for depression in 75 primary care clinics. *Implementation Science, 8*, 135. Retrieved from http://doi: 10.1186/1748-5908-8-135

Stafford, R. S., Ausiello, J. C., Misra, B., & Saglam, D. (2000). National patterns of depression treatment in primary care. *Primary Care Companion to the Journal of Clinical Psychiatry, 2*(6), 211–216.

Stewart, J. C., Perkins, A. J., & Callahan, C. M. (2014). Effect of collaborative care for depression on risk of cardiovascular events: Data from the IMPACT randomized controlled trial. *Psychosomatic Medicine, 76*(1), 29–37.

Strong, V., Waters, R., Hibberd, C., Murray, G., Wall, L., Walker, J., . . . Sharpe, M. (2008). Management of depression for people with cancer (SMaRT Oncology 1): A randomised trial. *Lancet, 372*(9632), 40–48.

Tew, J., Klaus, J., & Oslin, D. W. (2010). The behavioral health laboratory: Building a stronger foundation for the patient-centered medical home. *Families, Systems and Health, 28*(2), 130–145.

Thombs, B. D., Ziegelstein, R. C., Roseman, M., Kloda, L. A., & Ioannidis, J. P. (2014). There are no randomized controlled trials that support the United States Preventive Services Task

Force guideline on screening for depression in primary care: A systematic review. *BMC Medicine, 12*, 13. Retrieved from http://doi.org/10.1186/1741-7015-12-13

Thompson, C., Kinmonth, A. L., Stevens, L., Peveler, R. C., Stevens, A., Ostler, K. J., . . . Campbell, M. J. (2000). Effects of a clinical-practice guideline and practice-based education on detection and outcome of depression in primary care: Hampshire Depression Project randomised controlled trial. *Lancet, 355*(9199), 185–191.

Thota, A. B., Sipe, T. A., Byard, G. J., Zometa, C. S., Hahn, R. A., McKnight-Eily, L. R., . . . Williams, S. P. (2012). Collaborative care to improve the management of depressive disorders: A community guide systematic review and meta-analysis. *American Journal of Preventive Medicine, 42*(5), 525–538.

Tylee, A., & Gandhi, P. (2005). The importance of somatic symptoms in depression in primary care. *Primary Care Companion to the Journal of Clinical Psychiatry, 7*(4), 167–176.

University of Washington. (2010). *IMPACT fidelity scale.* Retrieved from http://impact-uw.org /files/FidelityScale-Dec2010.pdf

Unützer, J., Katon, W., Callahan, C. M., Williams, J. W. Jr., Hunkeler, E., Harpole, L., . . . Langston, C. (2002). Improving mood-promoting access to collaborative treatment. Collaborative care management of late-life depression in the primary care setting: A randomized controlled trial. *JAMA, 288*(22), 2836–2845.

Unützer, J., Katon, W. J., Fan, M.-Y., Schoenbaum, M. C., Lin, E. H. B., Penna, R. D. D., & Powers, D. (2008). Long-term cost effects of collaborative care for late-life depression. *American Journal of Managed Care, 14*(2), 95–100.

VHA Handbook 1160.01. (2008). *Uniform mental health services in VA medical centers and clinics.* Washington, DC: Department of Veterans Affairs Office of Patient Care Services.

Von Korff, M., Gruman, J., Schaefer, J., Curry, S. J., & Wagner, E. H. (1997). Collaborative management of chronic illness. *Annals of Internal Medicine, 127*(12), 1097–1102.

Wagner, E. H., Austin, B. T., Davis, C., Hindmarsh, M., Schaefer, J., & Bonomi, A. (2001). Improving chronic illness care: Translating evidence into action. *Health Affairs, 20*(6), 64–78.

Wagner, E. H., Austin, B. T., & Von Korff, M. (1996). Organizing care for patients with chronic illness. *Milbank Quarterly, 74*(4), 511–544.

Walker, J., Cassidy, J., & Sharpe, M. (2009). The second Symptom Management Research Trial in Oncology (SMaRT Oncology-2): A randomised trial to determine the effectiveness and cost-effectiveness of adding a complex intervention for major depressive disorder to usual care for cancer patients. *Trials, 10*, 18.

Walker, J., Hansen, C. H., Martin, P., Symeonides, S., Gourley, C., Wall, L., . . . Sharpe, M. (2014). Integrated collaborative care for major depression comorbid with a poor prognosis cancer (SMaRT Oncology-3): A multicentre randomised controlled trial in patients with lung cancer. *The Lancet Oncology, 15*(10), 1168–1176.

Walker, J., & Sharpe, M. (2014). Integrated management of major depression for people with cancer. *International Review of Psychiatry, 26*(6), 657–668.

Wang, P. S., Berglund, P., & Kessler, R. C. (2000). Recent care of common mental disorders in the United States: Prevalence and conformance with evidence-based recommendations. *Journal of General Internal Medicine, 15*(5), 284–292.

Watson, L. C., Amick, H. R., Gaynes, B. N., Brownley, K. A., Thaker, S., Viswanathan, M., & Jonas, D. E. (2013). Practice-based interventions addressing concomitant depression and chronic medical conditions in the primary care setting: A systematic review and meta-analysis. *Journal of Primary Care and Community Health, 4*(4), 294–306.

Wells, K. B., Sherbourne, C. D., Miranda, J., Tang, L., Benjamin, B., & Duan, N. (2007). The cumulative effects of quality improvement for depression on outcome disparities over 9 years: Results from a randomized, controlled group-level trial. *Medical Care, 45*(11), 1052–1059.

Wells, K., Sherbourne, C., Schoenbaum, M., Ettner, S., Duan, N., Miranda, J., . . . Rubenstein, L. (2004). Five-year impact of quality improvement for depression: Results of a group-level randomized controlled trial. *Archives of General Psychiatry, 61*(4), 378–386.

Whitebird, R. R., Solberg, L. I., Jaeckels, N. A., Pietruszewski, P. B., Hadzic, S., Unützer, J., . . . Rubenstein, L. V. (2014). Effective implementation of collaborative care for depression: What is needed? *American Journal of Managed Care, 20*(9), 699–707.

Whitebird, R. R., Solberg, L. I., Margolis, K. L., Asche, S. E., Trangle, M. A., & Wineman, A. P. (2013). Barriers to improving primary care of depression: Perspectives of medical group leaders. *Qualitative Health Research, 23*(6), 805–814.

Woltmann, E., Grogan-Kaylor, A., Perron, B., Georges, H., Kilbourne, A. M., & Bauer, M. S. (2012). Comparative effectiveness of collaborative chronic care models for mental health conditions across primary, specialty, and behavioral health care settings: Systematic review and meta-analysis. *American Journal of Psychiatry, 169*(8), 790–804.

Wozniak, L., Soprovich, A., Rees, S., Al Sayah, F., Majumdar, S. R., & Johnson, J. A. (2015, October). Contextualizing the effectiveness of a collaborative care model for primary care patients with diabetes and depression (TEAMCare): A qualitative assessment using RE-AIM. *Canadian Journal of Diabetes, 39*(Suppl 3), S83-S91.

Yeung, A., Martinson, M. A., Baer, L., Chen, J., Clain, A., Williams, . . . Fava, M. (2016). The effectiveness of telepsychiatry-based culturally sensitive collaborative treatment for depressed Chinese immigrants: A randomized controlled trial. *Journal of Clinical Psychiatry, 77*(8), e996-e1002.

Yeung, A., Shyu, I., Fisher, L., Wu, S., Yang, H., & Fava, M. (2010). Culturally sensitive collaborative treatment for depressed Chinese Americans in primary care. *American Journal of Public Health, 100*(12), 2397–2402.

Yeung, A., Trinh, N.-H. T., Chang, T. E., & Fava, M. (2011). The Engagement Interview Protocol (EIP): Improving the acceptance of mental health treatment among Chinese immigrants. *International Journal of Culture and Mental Health, 4*(2), 91–105.

Yoon, J., Yano, E. M., Altman, L., Cordasco, K. M., Stockdale, S. E., Chow, A., . . . Rubenstein, L. V. (2012). Reducing costs of acute care for ambulatory care-sensitive medical conditions: The central roles of comorbid mental illness. *Medical Care, 50*(8), 705–713.

CHAPTER 16

A Twenty-First-Century Public Health Challenge and Opportunity

Addressing Depressive Disorders in an Aging Population

Neal L. Cohen, MD

Population aging worldwide is a daunting challenge for twenty-first-century public health. Driven by falling fertility rates and expanding life expectancies, we will reach a demographic milestone for the first time by 2020 with adults worldwide aged 65 and older outnumbering children under age 5 (United Nations, 2013). By 2050, the number of people aged 65 or older is projected to triple, from an estimated 524 million in 2010 to nearly 1.5 billion in 2050 (National Institute on Aging, 2011). In the United States, the first of the postwar baby boomers turned 65 in 2011, with projections to nearly double by 2030 to 70 million older adults (US Census Bureau, 2014). This population surge between 2010 and 2030 for the US population of older adults will result in an expected increase from 13% to 20% of the total population.

Along with these demographic changes, the success of public health systems in economically advanced nations in addressing twentieth-century infectious disease threats has led to a new priority focus on the twenty-first-century public health challenges of chronic diseases faced by an aging population. Fueled in part by the heightened focus on chronic health conditions, the past 20 years have seen advances toward a population approach to mental health and greater understanding of the impact of mental disorders on overall population health (Cohen & Galea, 2011). In these past two decades, significant developments in psychiatric epidemiology have advanced our understanding from mainly prevalence and incidence of mental disorders toward greater measurement of impairment and quality of life (Susser & Smith, 2011). The WHO World Mental Health Surveys (Kessler & Üstün, 2008) have greatly expanded our understanding of morbidity attributable to mental illness worldwide and the far-reaching health consequences of mental disorders that make them a core public health challenge. And, although the interrelationship of mental disorders with physical illness is not yet fully understood, the chronic disease burden impacting older adults highlights the importance of addressing population mental health as a central element of the late-life public health paradigm.

With major depressive disorder (MDD) now recognized as the second leading cause of years lived with disability worldwide, exceeded only by lower back pain (Kessler, Bromet, de Jonge, Shahly, & Wilcox, 2017), a focus on depression as a major component of public health for older adults is particularly salient given the aging of the population. The incidence of depression peaks in early adult life, but there is a secondary peak in incidence beginning among people in their 50s, with modest increases in depressive symptoms with further aging (Davey, Halverson, Zonderman, & Costa, 2004). The public health significance for depression in older adults is pronounced with potential life-threatening consequences associated with increased risks of morbidity; physical, social, and cognitive dysfunction; suicide; and increased mortality (Aziz & Steffens, 2013; Conwell et al., 2010; Gleason, Pierce, Walker, & Warnock, 2013). Furthermore, depression in older adults is associated with significant increases in health care costs, with about 50% higher costs compared to nondepressed older adults, even after adjusting for chronic medical illness and mental health treatment (Katon, Lin, Russo, & Unützer, 2003). In a two-year study of 1,740 community-dwelling older adults aged 65 and older (Choi, Hasche, & Nguyen, 2015), additional health care expenditures of $3,855 were incurred in year two by depressed older adults compared to nondepressed older adults at the start of the study, even after controlling for co-occurring health conditions.

Key to the development of potential public health approaches to depression in older adults is an understanding of the unique factors associated with its onset. More than half of cases represent a first onset in later life with distinctive risk factors and presentation than those with earlier adult onset. The former, so called "late-life depression," is commonly associated with risk factors that represent complex interactions among genetic vulnerabilities, cognitive diathesis, age-associated neurobiological changes, and stressful events (Fiske, Wetherell, & Gatz, 2009). Compared to younger adults, the presentation of late-life depression is more likely to display somatic symptoms and cognitive changes, thereby masking the common symptoms of major depression and appearing to be cognitive impairment or an early sign of a neuroendocrine or related chronic disorder.

Estimating the prevalence of depression among older adults is particularly challenging given that late-life depression very often goes undetected or is undertreated (Fahs, Cabin, & Gallo, 2011). Contrary to popular perception, with a prevalence of MDD at any given time in community samples of adults aged 65 and older ranging from 1% to 5%, major depression is less frequent among older adults than at earlier ages (Hasin, Goodwin, Stinson, & Grant, 2005). Among elderly primary care patients, the prevalence of major depression has been estimated at 6.5%–9% (Lyness, Caine, King, Cox, & Yoediono, 1999). Studies of subsyndromal depressive symptomatology indicate that 15%–27% of older adults in the community (Zivin, Wharton, & Rostant,

2013) and up to 37% seen in primary care settings experience significant depressive symptoms (Hybels & Pieper, 2009; Weyerer et al., 2008) that are felt to require clinical intervention. An Institute of Medicine report (2012) on adults 65 years and older reviewed 12-month prevalence rates of major depressive episodes (3.0%–4.3%), dysthymic disorder (0.6%–1.6%), and depressive symptoms (1.1%–11.1%).

Despite not reaching the clinical thresholds for a diagnosis of MDD, the high prevalence of subsyndromal depressive symptomatology among older adults produces a uniquely high burden for late-life depressive illness. For example, in a study of older adults at least 60 years of age receiving usual care across multiple primary care practice settings, Lyness and colleagues (2006) found that those with minor or subsyndromal depression were five and a half times as likely to develop major depression after one year compared to those without depression.

The diagnosis of "dysthymic disorder" was first established in the *Diagnostic and Statistical Manual of Mental Disorders, Third Edition* (American Psychiatric Association, 1980) to describe a depressive syndrome of mild to moderate severity of at least two years' duration that did not meet criteria for MDD. In the *DSM-5* edition (American Psychiatric Association, 2013), the diagnosis of dysthymic disorder was replaced by "persistent depressive disorder," which includes both chronic major depression and dysthymic disorder. The presentation of persistent depressive disorder in older adults frequently occurs at a late age of onset, without other psychiatric disorders, and at a low rate of family history of mood disorders. Associated stressors are commonly loss of social support and bereavement, while some display signs of cerebrovascular or neurodegenerative pathology. Despite subsyndromal symptomatology, persistent depressive disorder is strongly associated with disability and poor medical outcomes (Devanand, 2014).

Neighborhood and Environmental Influences on Depression

Although individual risk factors (e.g., educational status, income, stressful life events) for depressive disorders have long attracted the greatest research attention, a growing body of literature is finding an influence of neighborhood environments on individual health and well-being, including depressed mood in the general population (e.g., Mair, Diez-Roux, & Galea, 2008; Paczkowski & Galea, 2010). In a systematic review of the research literature, Kim (2008) found evidence for harmful effects of neighborhood social disorder and, to a lesser extent, protective effects for higher neighborhood socioeconomic status. Older adults may be particularly vulnerable to the health impacts of neighborhood factors. Julien and colleagues (2012) cited multiple reasons for this vulnerability, including declines in physical and cognitive competencies in older adults that lessen their capacity to cope with environmental stressors; greater reliance on community resources as older adults lose support from friends who may be ill or die, and from family members who live at far distances; and, due to retirement and decreased mobility, older adults may be more restricted to their immediate residential neighborhoods than younger adults. In their review of 19 studies of depressed mood and neighborhood variables among adults aged 65 years or older, Julien and colleagues (2012) found complex but significant multivariate associations that supported their conclusion that "selected neighborhood variables, especially those related to poverty and material deprivation, are associated with worse mental health" (p. 1223).

The findings in most of the literature are limited by studies having a cross-sectional design, which does not allow for inferences about causal mechanisms. More longitudinal and experimental studies are needed to better uncover the processes by which neighborhood factors may influence mental well-being. In a longitudinal design study, Wright, Cummings, Karlamangla, and Aneschensel (2009) examined associations between urban neighborhood sociodemographic characteristics and change over time in late-life depressive symptoms. Using large national survey data from three time periods in the 1990s, the worsening of depressive symptoms varied significantly across urban neighborhoods and was most prominent with neighborhood-level disadvantage; however, those neighborhood factors diminished in significance when underlying individual-level demographic and aging processes were accounted for. The authors posit that neighborhood disadvantage may have the greatest impact where there is cross-level interaction with those older adults who are at greatest personal disadvantage. In another longitudinal design study that examined neighborhood influences on depression in older adults while accounting for individual-level factors, Beard and colleagues (2009) surveyed 808 New York City residents aged 50 years or older in 2005 and 2007. The multivariate model found the cluster of socioeconomic influence to be associated both with protection from depression symptoms (neighborhood affluence) and subsequent risk of depression (neighborhood disadvantage).

Although the research literature on the relationship between neighborhood characteristics and depression has been mixed and limited by methodologic issues, further study of mental health and broader neighborhood health effects remains indicated as an important public health focus. Our efforts to improve health and mental well-being among an aging US population will need to consider the role of residential context and those structural interventions at the community level that can best promote public health.

Social Capital and Mental Well-Being

Recognizing the limitations of individual targeted health care interventions, the public health literature has focused attention to concepts of "social capital" to better understand the influences of social relationships and the social environment on population health. Social capital theories and various definitions of the concept generally share the perspective that it derives from community activities and not the activities of individuals alone (Nyqvist, Forsman, Giuntoli, & Cattan, 2013). Both the resources that are available to all members of certain communities and the resources that are embedded within an individual's social network comprise assets to contribute to the social capital. Furthermore, a number of studies find that social capital mediates the contextual effect of neighborhood disadvantage, thereby improving individuals' mental well-being with fewer depressive symptoms reported (Haines, Beggs, & Hurlbert, 2011; Kawachi & Berkman, 2001; Poortinga, 2006).

Considerable evidence from the research literature has linked social capital and various indicators of health (Murayama, Fujiwara, & Kawachi, 2012). Increasingly, studies of the link between concepts of social capital and health, including mental well-being, suggest that older adults are particularly vulnerable to suffer poor mental health in association with low-level social capital (Nyqvist et al., 2013). As the senior years are associated with changes in health and losses in social network size as well as quality of network participation, the broader concept of social capital can be regarded either as a relevant risk or as a protective factor in the mental well-being of older adults.

Social capital can be examined at individual, family, and community levels, each of which can be a focus of intervention to promote mental well-being and to prevent ill health. In their review of the public health literature on the influences of social capital, Szreter and Woolcock (2004) found the social support aspect of social capital to be empirically linked to numerous health-related outcomes, including improved child development, adolescent well-being, lower violent crime rates and youth delinquency, increased mental health, and lower mortality. At the individual level of intervention, psychosocial therapies for depression with older adults frequently focus on mobilizing the person's social resources to strengthen the sense of connectedness and civic engagement. In a meta-analysis of 69 depression prevention studies, Jané-Llopis, Hosman, Jenkins, and Anderson (2003) found social support interventions (e.g., network-building, fostering socialization) to be most effective among older adults. Forsman and colleagues' (2013) study of social capital in later life found that family and close friendship ties were the key factor in promoting mental well-being, by providing social support, mutual trust, and sense of security. In this digital age, there are numerous technological ways to allow older adults to remain connected and interactive with their social networks despite the challenges of physical separation and distancing. At a community level, social capital is particularly connected to the neighborhood of residence for older adults since the familiarity and comfort level of their surroundings function as a stable foundation for everyday routines. As a result, the physical characteristics of neighborhoods (e.g., walkability, green spaces, access to public transportation) can provide community assets to better maintain the social networks and connectedness of older adults. Consequently, public policies, whether they are aimed at strengthening family support, existing networks, or the built environment of neighborhoods, are important strategies to promote active and healthy aging.

Suicide

The World Health Organization (2014) described suicide in later life as a global public health problem, with completed suicide rates higher than in any of the younger age groups in most countries reporting suicide statistics. In the United States in 2010, adults aged 65 and older comprised 13% of the total population but accounted for 20.9% of individuals who died by suicide between 2000–2010 (Ahmedani et al., 2014). Addressing the suicidal behavior in older adults is particularly daunting given multiple challenges. In the United States, among those older adults who commit their first suicidal act, nearly 75% of older adults die as a consequence (Conwell, Rotenberg, & Caine, 1990), which may be explained by deliberate planning, physical frailty, and method lethality (Fassberg et al., 2012).

Despite the lower rates of major depression among older age populations, Alexopoulos and colleagues (1999) found that depression severity was the most important determinant of contemporaneous suicidal ideation and suicidal intent. In response to their suicidal ideation, older adults are more likely than younger age groups to complete a suicide. While the ratio of attempted to completed suicide among adolescents is estimated to be 200:1, and for the overall population from 8:1 to 33:1, among adults aged 65 and older there are as few as two to four attempts for each completed suicide (Conwell, 2014). While worldwide suicide rates are generally higher for both men and women in older age groups, in the United States the highest rates of suicide are committed by older white men, increasing with age and peaking for the oldest age group (i.e., > 85 years old; Centers for Disease Control and Surveillance [CDC], 2013).

In the largest longitudinal study to date, collecting data on nearly 6,000 individuals who died by suicide between 2000 and 2010, Ahmedani and colleagues (2014) found that 67% of adults aged 65 and older had made a visit to a health care provider within four weeks of death, the majority of whom did not have a mental health diagnosis. Of those who made any visit to a health care provider, only about one-third had a mental health–related office visit. Psychological autopsy studies of late-life suicide in the United States indicate that 71%–95% of persons aged 65 years and older who completed suicide had a diagnosable major psychiatric disorder, most often major depression, at the time of death (Cavanagh, Carson, Sharpe, & Lawrie, 2003; Conwell & Duberstein, 2005). Consequently, the high percentage of contact with primary care providers by older adults within weeks of their suicides underscores the loss of a significant public health opportunity to improve detection and take action to reduce suicide risk.

Prevention of suicidal behavior in older adults is particularly daunting, with multiple challenges. Given that the suicidality of older adults is strongly associated with major depression but the majority of those who completed suicide did not see a mental health professional in the year prior (Ahmedani et al., 2014), the detection and treatment of depression in the primary care setting constitutes a particularly pivotal suicide prevention strategy for this age group. In 2001, the US Public Health Service issued its report titled *National Strategy for Suicide Prevention: Goals and Objectives for Action* in a public health framework, which recognized primary care physicians' potential role in mitigating suicidality among older adults.

While a large-scale study by Szanto and colleagues (2003) found that suicidality in older adults with late-life depression responded well overall to a course of antidepressant therapy, those patients with higher risk experience a slower and less robust response requiring more persistent therapeutic attention. The task of treating depressed older adults with suicidal ideation in primary care settings therefore may often require greater ability to identify and manage these patients with more frequent and ongoing treatment sessions than generally available from primary care physicians. Consequently, those collaborative care models that provide primary care physicians with supports from depression care managers to monitor symptoms, treatment response, side effects, and enhance communications between physicians and patients are especially important in the office-based management of depressed older adults.

Primary Care Models of Detection and Depression Care

Rates of major depression have been rising markedly over the past two decades (Akincigil et al., 2011; Compton, Conway, Stinson, & Grant, 2006), suggesting that with the aging population we can expect to see increased numbers of older adults who have experienced or are contending with depressive disorders. However, most older adults with clinically significant depressive symptoms do not seek mental health specialty care but do see primary care providers (Gallo & Coyne, 2000). Despite the availability of effective treatment for depression, case finding and adequate treatment in the primary care setting are inadequate (Sonnenberg, Beekman, Deeg, & Van Tilburg, 2003; Tiemens, Ormel, & Simon, 1996). The depressive disorders of older adults presenting in primary care settings are frequently masked by associated impairments in cognition and by psychomotor agitation or retardation (*DSM-5*, American Psychiatric Association, 2013), a symptom presentation that may be regarded by primary care practitioners as related to the older patient's physical health conditions or drug interactions. Older adults are more likely to be seen in primary care with multiple complaints related to a number of chronic health conditions with which they are clinically managed with multiple medications (Drayer et al., 2005). Further complicating reliable detection and treatment of depressive disorders in older adults is the common misconception in the general population (including health care providers) that depression is an expectable and normal response to aging. Furthermore, there is a large body of research that recognizes that depressive illness characteristically complicates the course of many physical illnesses, resulting in poorer health outcomes (see chapter 4, this volume). With high suicide rates and poorer health outcomes, untreated depressive disorders may be seen as a serious threat to the health and survival of older adults (Chapman & Perry, 2008).

The co-occurrence of chronic health conditions with depression is particularly prevalent in the older adult population. The CDC (2013) reported that while one-quarter of all Americans have multiple chronic health conditions, two-thirds of older adults have multiple chronic conditions. Older adults are also disproportionately represented among the almost 2.5 million hospitalizations in the United States with depression as a secondary diagnosis (Russo, Hambrick, & Owens, 2007). Chronic conditions most frequently endured by older adults, including cardiovascular disease, visual impairment, falls, hearing loss, arthritis, and functional disability, are commonly co-occurring with depressive illness (Cabin & Fahs, 2010). Nevertheless, primary care physicians treating multiple chronic health conditions comorbid with depressive illness will generally have difficulty finding adequate time and resources to follow patients closely enough to ensure compliance with adequate trials of antidepressant medications (Callahan, 2001; Unützer et al., 2001).

Although better recognition of depressive illness in primary care settings is clearly a public health goal, the formal screening for depression in primary care has been an issue of debate (Thombs et al., 2012). In 2009, the US Preventive Services Task Force recommended the screening of patients for depression in primary care but only in the context of integrated systems where nonmedical specialists such as case managers are available to provide management and follow-up for those who are found to need treatment. Concerns about screening in primary care are raised about the possible overidentification of patients with milder symptoms of depression for whom antidepressant medication is of much less benefit than those with more severe symptoms (Barbui, Cipriani, Patel, Ayuso-Mateos, & van Ommeren, 2011; Fournier et al., 2010).

During the 1990s, there was significant expansion in the number of Americans receiving treatment for depression in office-based physician practice, with increased emphasis on pharmacologic treatments but less psychotherapy among those receiving care (Olfson et al., 2002). In a study of the treatment of depression in older adult Medicare enrollees from 1992 to 2005, Akincigil and colleagues (2011) found that among those who received a depression diagnosis, antidepressant prescribing increased from 53.7% to 67.1%, whereas the proportion receiving psychotherapy declined from 26.1% to 14.8%. This trend evolved in large measure as a result of the introduction and availability of the serotonin specific reuptake inhibitor (SSRI) antidepressants, with much better safety profiles compared to the earlier classes of antidepressants. With more confidence in drug safety, less patient abuse, and lower suicide risk from overdose, primary care physicians have become the most frequent prescribers of antidepressant medications. Coyne and Katz (2001) pointed to the elevated rates of antidepressant prescribing in primary care as evidence that older adults with minor or subsyndromal depression are being treated even without a clinically diagnosable depression. Furthermore, despite the expansion of depression treatment by primary care physicians, studies suggest that only 20%–30% of patients treated exclusively in a primary care setting receive adequate care and follow-up (Fernandez et al., 2007; Mojtabai & Olfson, 2008). Thus, office-based primary care practice is challenged both by the task of reliable detection of proper candidates for antidepressant medications and the delivery of adequate care for depressed older adults.

Over the last several decades, research studies have detected disparities in access to and quality of health care in the United States, especially for minority populations with a need for mental health care (Aguilar-Gaxiola et al., 2011). Despite overall increases in the diagnosis and treatment rates for depression beginning in the 1990s, some studies find that those increases were not consistent across racial and ethnic subgroups (e.g., Areán & Unützer, 2003), and that disparities in treatment of diagnosed depression among minority elders have been persistent (e.g., Akincigil et al., 2012; Crystal, Sambamoorthi, & Akincigil, 2003). Older minorities are even less likely to use mental health services than nonminority elders (Swartz et al., 1998), as they are challenged by multiple barriers to treatment including limited financial and geographical access to specialty mental health services, lack of culturally competent care, distrust of mental health providers, and stigma (Alegría et al., 2002; Areán et al., 2005).

Importantly, a number of population-based models of depression care have demonstrated greater efficacy in overcoming the barriers to adequate treatment in primary care settings for both minority and nonminority older adults. Developed to address the resource limitations in primary care, these "collaborative care" models utilize care managers to link primary care providers, patients, and mental health specialists. In treating depressed patients, the care manager coordinates services and facilitates patient use of depression interventions. Both Gilbody, Bower, Fletcher, Richards, and Sutton (2006) and Thota and colleagues (2012) carried out cumulative meta-analyses of the research literature, finding collaborative care models to be more effective than standard care in achieving clinically meaningful improvements in depression outcomes and public health benefits across multiple settings and populations. While collaborative care includes a wide range of interventions of varying intensity of treatments and care management, the Improving Mood-Promoting Access to Collaborative Treatment (IMPACT) (Hunkeler et al., 2006; Williams, Unützer, Lee, & Noel, 2009) and the PROSPECT (Alexopoulos et al., 2005, 2009; Bogner, Morales, Post, & Bruce, 2007) models of care have received the most research study and attention to outcomes with older adults.

The IMPACT intervention model involves close collaboration among primary care and specialist practitioners to create a personalized treatment plan that includes patient preferences, proactive follow-up, protocols for stepped care for greater or lesser intensity, and outcomes monitoring by a depression care manager. Hunkeler and colleagues (2006) reported on a randomized clinical trial of 1801 US primary care patients aged 60 and older who received either IMPACT collaborative care or usual care for depression. IMPACT-treated patients fared significantly better than controls in measures of remission of depression, continuation of antidepressant medications, physical functioning, quality of life, self-efficacy, and satisfaction with care at 18 and 24 months. Areán and colleagues (2005) found comparable improvements for IMPACT-treated patients from ethnic minority groups (African Americans and Latinos) as the nonminority older adults.

An analysis of the cost-effectiveness of the IMPACT study (Katon et al., 2005) found that over a two-year period, total outpatient costs were $295 higher than usual care, with 107 more depression-free days experienced by the IMPACT patients than those receiving usual care. The authors conclude that the IMPACT intervention is a worthwhile investment for older adults, as it is associated with high clinical benefits at a low increment in health care costs. Furthermore, in a follow-up study of cost-effectiveness over four years of a subgroup of these IMPACT study older adults, health care costs were found to be statistically lower than usual care patients, suggesting that the initial investment in better depression care results in longer-term total health care cost savings (Unützer et al., 2008).

Another collaborative care model, the Prevention of Suicide in Primary Care Elderly: Collaborative Trial (PROSPECT), was designed specifically to target suicidal ideation and depression in older primary care patients. The intervention consisted of services of trained care managers who offered algorithm-based recommendations to physicians and helped patients with treatment adherence over 18 months. These depression care managers (social workers, nurses, and psychologists) made home visits to patients unable to travel and offered interpersonal therapy to patients who declined medication. Alexopoulos and colleagues (2005, 2009) found that sustained collaborative care with the PROSPECT model promoted higher utilization of depression treatment, reduced suicidal ideation, and improved the outcomes of major depression over a two-year period.

Coronary heart disease and diabetes are among the most common chronic health conditions seen in primary care (Katon et al., 2012), with depression co-occurring in up to 20% of these patients (Ali, Stone, Peters, Davies, & Khunti, 2006; Carney & Freedland, 2008). With both poorer health outcomes (Katon et al., 2004; Ludman et al., 2004) and higher medical costs (Lustman & Clouse, 2005; Unützer et al., 2009) reported among those older adults with depression comorbid with diabetes or coronary heart disease, the potential overall health benefits of collaborative care in the primary care setting are of particular public health interest.

Evidence has mounted over the past few decades for a bidirectional link between depression and medical illness that derives from a complex interaction between physiological and environmental factors (Gleason et al., 2013). Nemeroff and Owens (2009) reviewed findings for the altered functioning of multiple biological systems in depression that place older adults with multiple comorbidities at even greater health risk. In a large population-based study of the association between depression and mortality in adults aged 65 and older, Schulz and colleagues (2000) found significantly higher mortality rates over a six-year period for depressed older adults with cardiovascular disease after controlling for a wide range of sociodemographic risk factors. In a controlled study of patients who suffer from MDD, within a few weeks after an acute coronary syndrome, Glassman, Bigger, and Gaffney (2009) found that mortality more than doubled over 6.7 years of follow-up for those with greater MDD severity or failure of MDD to improve over the first six-month follow-up.

Effective and persistent treatment of depression among those with comorbid chronic health conditions appears to mitigate the likelihood of increased morbidity and mortality. Bogner and colleagues (2007) found that depressed older patients with diabetes were less likely to die from any cause over a five-year period when treated in the PROSPECT care management model than were a comparable group of patients treated with usual care. Similarly, Katon and colleagues (2006) applied an IMPACT model of care management in the primary care setting to depressed older adults with diabetes, resulting in better depression outcomes at no greater cost than usual care. A systematic literature review by Huffman and colleagues (2014) found that those integrated care interventions that targeted both mental health and chronic medical illness are likely to serve an increasingly large role in health care, given its potential to improve the quality of patient care, improve the health of populations, and reduce health care costs.

Late-Life Depression Prevention and Mental Health Promotion

The prevalence and disabling nature of depressive episodes in older adults along with the excess mortality associated with depression underscores the need for a priority public health focus on prevention. Andrews and colleagues (2004) estimated that even with optimal case finding and treatment with evidence-based interventions, only 34% of the overall disease burden associated with depressive disorders could be averted. Additionally, despite the relative safety of the SSRI antidepressant drugs, older adults are at greater risk for adverse drug responses, given the greater prevalence of chronic diseases as aging advances. Consequently, a focus on depression prevention among older adults has the potential to have an even greater beneficial public health impact than treatment strategies alone (Beekman, Smit, Stek, Reynolds III, & Cuijpers, 2010).

Preventive approaches to late-life depression are informed by the launch of a framework for a preventive science approach to mental disorders in 1994 with the publication of a report prepared by the National Institute of Mental Health (NIMH Prevention Research Committee, 1994) and a groundbreaking report by the Institute of Medicine (1994), both from Congressional requests. The NIMH report, *The Prevention of Mental Disorders: A National Research Agenda* (NIMH Prevention Research Committee, 1994), described the components of a prevention science that would undertake risk and protective factor studies, controlled preventive intervention trials, and evidence-based implementation efforts. The Institute of Medicine report, *Reducing Risks for*

Mental Disorders: Frontiers for Preventive Intervention Research (Institute of Medicine, 1994), reaffirmed the distinct parameters of treatment and prevention with a risk and protective factor framework for interventions prior to the onset of illness. The report advanced a typology for the pathways through which prevention-oriented interventions are targeted:

- "Universal" preventive interventions are directed at a population base without specific knowledge of their health and mental well-being;
- "Selective" preventive interventions are directed at those who are deemed to be at elevated risk for mental health problems;
- "Indicated" preventive interventions are directed at individuals already manifesting psychological symptoms suggesting high risk for mental illness.

Given the absence of any evidence-based universal prevention approach for depression, Schoevers and colleagues (2006) underscored the need to target preventive interventions toward groups with a significant a priori risk for incident depression through exposure to multiple risk factors. In their study to find an optimal strategy for prevention of late-life depression in the primary care setting, the researchers found that screening for subsyndromal depression symptoms had the greatest potential benefit in terms of feasibility, costs, and effectiveness. In a focus on both high risk and already-mildly symptomatic older adults, Lyness, Yu, Tang, Tu, and Conwell (2009) found that a combination of risks, including minor or subsyndromal depression, impaired functional status, and a history of major or minor depression, identified a group of older adults seen in primary care at very high risk for incident depression.

With the aim to identify a population at sufficiently high risk to justify the expense and risk of pharmacological or psychological preventive interventions, Robinson and colleagues (2008) targeted older nondepressed stroke victims who are at 30%–40% risk for incident depression contributing to poor recovery and increased mortality following acute stroke. The study demonstrated significant reductions in poststroke depression over a 12-month period for patients receiving either problem-solving therapy or an SSRI antidepressant (escitalopram) compared to placebo control.

The mental health promotion concept in older adults can be defined as encompassing both positive mental health promotion and disorder prevention (Forsman, Nordmyr, & Wahlbeck, 2011). Jané-Llopis and colleagues (2011) defined mental health promotion as an enabling process with and for individuals to achieve positive mental health and to enhance quality of life. In their review of psychosocial interventions for the promotion of mental health, Forsman and colleagues (2011) found that "meaningful social activities tailored to the older individual's abilities, preferences and needs should be considered when aiming to improve mental health among older people" (p. 198). The authors underscore that greater investment in developing an evidence base through the evaluation of measures to promote mental health and prevent depression among older adults is needed to become a far greater research priority.

Looking Ahead

The Institute of Medicine (2012) has labeled the surge in the aging population "the silver tsunami," as it will rapidly increase demand for health services and overwhelm the relatively small health care workforce properly trained in integrated health and mental health care for older adults. Despite decades of mounting evidence for the benefits of integrated mental health care for overall health (Gilbody et al., 2006), there has been insufficient movement to place integrated care into those community health centers that can best reach low-income populations of all ages in disadvantaged neighborhoods and advance public health. However, more recent policies and legislative initiatives have created new opportunities for improved health and mental health care of older adults.

For decades, professional practice organizations and mental health advocates attempted to change the discriminatory mental health benefits coverage that dominated the policies of the health insurance industry and discouraged utilization of mental health services. Despite the prevalence and impact of mental disorders on the overall well-being of older adults, mental health care spending is disproportionately small relative to both population size and Medicare health expenditures (SAMHSA, 2013). The Wellstone and Domenici Mental Health Parity and Addiction Equity Act of 2008 represented a major step toward ending the inequity between mental health / substance use disorders and medical/surgical benefits in commercial plans; however, Medicare was not required to comply with the law. Congress did enact the Medicare Improvements for Patients and Providers Act in 2008, which was to be phased in over five years, allowing for incremental movement toward parity of health-related benefits. Beginning in January 2014, the five-year phase-out of mental health treatment limitations ended, allowing Medicare beneficiaries coverage for outpatient mental health services at full parity with medical and surgical benefits. Furthermore, the passage of the Affordable Care Act (2010) was a watershed in US public health policy that has incentivized expanded health care coverage along with improving health care quality, efficiency, and accountability, such as making primary health care more accessible to medically underserved populations. Medicare beneficiaries are entitled to expanded access to wellness visits, more preventive care, and less costly drugs, with little or no change to their insurance costs. Improving the overall health of older adults improves mental well-being; improving public health through greater focus on preventive and primary health care at younger ages will undoubtedly improve the health of the nation's seniors going forward.

The stimulus for greater access to health services that integrate a public health model of health promotion and disease prevention with improved care for those with complex and chronic conditions will need to be met with new and transformational training models for both public health and clinical practitioners. And importantly, the burgeoning of the older adult populations in the coming decades must also stimulate a research agenda for an integrated health / mental health promotion and prevention framework to identify the public policies and the real-life community practices that will further advance twenty-first-century public health.

The World Health Organization has defined active and healthy aging as "the process of optimizing opportunities for health, participation and security in order to enhance quality of life as people age" (WHO, 2002). Consequently, the public health agenda for healthy aging must be one component of broader public policies of a "preventive gerontology" that recognizes the roles of the social and physical environment, health care delivery, and mental health care as vital.

References

Aguilar-Gaxiola, S., Sribney, W. S., Raingruber, B., Wenzel, N., Fields-Johnson, D., & Loera, G. (2011). Disparities in mental health status and care in the US. In N. L. Cohen & S. Galea (Eds.), *Population mental health: Evidence, policy, and public health practice* (pp. 69–91). New York, NY: Routledge.

Ahmedani, B. K., Simon, G. E., Stewart, C., Beck, A., Waitzfelder, B. E., Rossom, R., . . . Solberg, L. I. (2014). Health care contacts in the year before suicide death. *Journal of General Internal Medicine, 29*(6), 870–874.

Akincigil, A., Olfson, M., Siegel, M. J., Zurlo, K. A., Walkup, J. T., & Crystal, S. (2012). Racial and ethnic disparities in depression care in community-dwelling elderly in the United States. *American Journal of Public Health, 102*(2), 319–328.

Akincigil, A., Olfson, M., Walkup, J. T., Siegel, M. J., Kalay, E., Amin, S., . . . Crystal, S. (2011). Diagnosis and treatment of depression in older community-dwelling adults: 1992–2005. *Journal of the American Geriatrics Society, 59*(6), 1042–1051.

Alegría, M., Canino, G., Rios, R., Vera, M., Calderon, J., Rusch, D., & Ortega, A. N. (2002). Mental health care for Latinos: Inequalities in use of specialty mental health services among Latinos, African Americans, and non-Latino whites. *Psychiatric Services, 53*(12), 1547–1555.

Alexopoulos, G. S., Bruce, M. L., Hull, J., Sirey, J. A., & Kakuma, T. (1999). Clinical determinants of suicidal ideation and behavior in geriatric depression. *Archives of General Psychiatry, 56*, 1048–1053.

Alexopoulos, G. S., Katz, I. R., Bruce, M. L., Hero, M., Have, T. T., Raue, P., & Reynolds III, C. F. (2005). Remission in depressed geriatric primary care patients: A report from the PROSPECT study. *American Journal of Psychiatry, 162*(4), 718–724.

Alexopoulos, G. S., Reynolds III, C. F., Bruce, M. L., Katz, I. R., Raue, P., Mulsant, B. H., . . . Have, T. T. (2009). Reducing suicidal ideation and depression in older primary care patients: 24-month outcomes of the PROSPECT study. *American Journal of Psychiatry, 166*(8), 882–890.

Ali, S., Stone, M. A., Peters, J. L., Davies, M. J., & Khunti, K. (2006). The prevalence of co-morbid depression in adults with type 2 diabetes: A systematic review and meta-analysis. *Diabetes Medicine, 23*(11), 1165–1173.

American Psychiatric Association. (1980). *Diagnostic and statistical manual of mental disorders, 3rd edition*. Arlington, VA: American Psychiatric Publishing, Inc.

American Psychiatric Association. (2013). *Diagnostic and statistical manual of mental disorders, 5th edition.* Arlington, VA: American Psychiatric Publishing, Inc.

Andrews, G., Issakidis, C., Sanderson, K., Corry, J., & Lapsley, H. (2004). Utilising survey data to inform public policy: Comparison of the cost-effectiveness of treatment of ten mental disorders. *British Journal of Psychiatry, 184*(6), 526–533.

Areán, P. A., Ayalon, L., Hunkeler, E., Lin, E. H. B., Tang, L., Harpole, L., . . . Unützer, J. (2005). Improving depression care for older, minority patients in primary care. *Medical Care, 43*(4), 381–390.

Areán, P. A., & Unützer, J. (2003). Inequalities in depression management in low-income, minority, and old-old adults: A matter of access to preferred treatments? *Journal of the American Geriatric Society, 51*(12), 1808–1809.

Aziz, R., & Steffens, D. C. (2013). What are the causes of late-life depression? *Psychiatric Clinics of North America, 36*, 497–516.

Barbui, C., Cipriani, A., Patel, V., Ayuso-Mateos, J. L., & van Ommeren, M. (2011). Efficacy of antidepressants and benzodiazepines in minor depression: Systematic review and meta-analysis. *British Journal of Psychiatry, 198*, 11–16.

Beard, J. R., Cerda, M., Blaney, S., Ahern, J., Vlahov, D., & Galea, S. (2009). Neighborhood characteristics and change in depressive symptoms among older residents of New York City. *American Journal of Public Health, 99*(7), 1308–1314.

Beekman, A. T., Smit, F., Stek, M. L., Reynolds III, C. F., & Cuijpers, P. C. (2010). Preventing depression in high-risk groups. *Current Opinion in Psychiatry, 23*(1), 8–11.

Bogner, H. R., Morales, K. H., Post, E. P., & Bruce, M. L. (2007). Diabetes, depression, and death: A randomized controlled trial of a depression treatment program for older adults based in primary care. *Diabetes Care, 30*(12), 3005–3010.

Cabin, W., & Fahs, M. (2010). Developing a predictive model for depression among seniors attending senior centers in NYC neighborhoods. Unpublished manuscript, Brookdale Center for Healthy Aging and Longevity, Hunter College, New York, NY.

Callahan, C. M. (2001). Quality improvement research on late life depression in primary care. *Medical Care, 39*(8), 772–784.

Carney, R. M., & Freedland, K. E. (2008). Depression in patients with coronary heart disease. *American Journal of Medicine, 121*(11 Suppl. 2), S20–S27.

Cavanagh, J. T. O., Carson, A. J., Sharpe, M., & Lawrie, S. M. (2003). Psychological autopsy studies of suicide: A systematic review. *Psychological Medicine, 33*(3), 395–405.

Centers for Disease Control and Surveillance. (2013). *The state of aging and health in America 2013.* Atlanta, GA: US Department of Health and Human Services. Retrieved from http://www.cdc.gov/aging/pdf/state-aging-health-in-america-2013.pdf

Chapman, D. P., & Perry, G. S. (2008). Depression as a major component of public health for older adults. *Prevention of Chronic Disease, 5*(1). Retrieved from http://www.cdc.gov/pcd/issues/2008/jan/07_0150.htm

Choi, S., Hasche, L., & Nguyen, D. (2015). Effects of depression on the subsequent year's healthcare expenditures among older adults: Two-year panel study. *Psychiatric Quarterly, 86*, 225–241.

Cohen, N., & Galea, S. (Eds.). (2011). *Population mental health: Evidence, policy, and public health practice.* New York, NY: Routledge.

Compton, W. M., Conway, K. P., Stinson, F. S., & Grant, B. F. (2006). Changes in the prevalence of major depression and comorbid substance use disorders in the United States between 1991–1992 and 2001–2002. *American Journal of Psychiatry, 163*(12), 2141–2147.

Conwell, Y. (2014). Suicide later in life: Challenges and priorities for prevention. *American Journal of Preventive Medicine, 47*(3 Suppl. 2), S244–250.

Conwell, Y., & Duberstein, P. (2005). Suicide in older adults: Determinants of risk and opportunities for prevention. In K. Hawton (Ed.), *Prevention and treatment of suicidal behavior: From science to practice* (pp. 221–237). Oxford, England: Oxford University Press.

Conwell, Y., Duberstein, P. R., Hirsch, J. K., Conner, K. R., Eberly, S., & Caine, E. D. (2010). Health status and suicide in the second half of life. *International Journal of Geriatric Psychiatry, 25*, 371–379.

Conwell, Y., Rotenberg, M., & Caine, E. D. (1990). Completed suicide at age 50 and over. *Journal of the American Geriatric Society, 38*, 640–644.

Coyne, J., & Katz, I. R. (2001). Improving the primary care treatment of late life depression: Progress and opportunities. *Medical Care, 39*(8), 756–759.

Crystal, S., Sambamoorthi, U., & Akincigil, A. (2003). Diagnosis and treatment of depression in the elderly Medicare population: Predictors, disparities, and trends. *Journal of the American Geriatric Society, 51*(12), 1718–1728.

Davey, A., Halverson, Jr., C. F., Zonderman, A. B., & Costa, P. T. (2004). Change in depressive symptoms in the Baltimore Longitudinal Study of Aging. *Journals of Gerontology, Series B: Psychological Sciences and Social Sciences, 59B*(6), P270–P277.

Devanand, D. P. (2014). Dysthymic disorder in the elderly population. *International Psychogeriatrics, 26*(1), 39–48.

Drayer, R. A., Mulsant, B. H., Lenze, E. J., Rollman, B. L., Dew, M. A., Kelleher, K., . . . Reynolds III, C. F. (2005). Somatic symptoms of depression in elderly patients with medical comorbidities. *International Journal of Geriatric Psychiatry, 20*(10), 973–982.

Fahs, M. C., Cabin, W., & Gallo, W. T. (2011). Healthy aging and mental health: A public health challenge for the 21st century. In N. Cohen & S. Galea (Eds.), *Population mental health: Evidence, policy, and public health practice* (pp. 248–282). New York, NY: Routledge.

Fassberg, M. M., van Orden, K. A., Duberstein, P., Erlangsen, A., Lapierre, S., Bodner, E., . . . Waern, M. (2012). A systematic review of social factors and suicidal behavior in older adulthood. *International Journal of Environmental and Public Health, 9*, 722–745.

Fernandez, A., Haro, J. M., Martinez-Alonso, M., Demyttenaere, K., Brugha, T. S., Autonell, J., . . . Alonso, J. (2007). Treatment adequacy for anxiety and depressive disorders in six European countries. *British Journal of Psychiatry, 190*, 172–173.

Fiske, A., Wetherell, J. L., & Gatz, M. (2009). Depression in older adults. *Annual Review of Clinical Psychology, 5*, 363–389.

Forsman, A. K., Herberts, C., Nyqvist, F., Wahlbeck, K., & Schierenbeck, I. (2013). Understanding the role of social capital for mental wellbeing among older adults. *Ageing and Society, 33*(5), 804–825.

Forsman, A. K., Nordmyr, J., & Wahlbeck, K. (2011). Psychosocial interventions for the promotion of mental health and the prevention of depression among older adults. *Health Promotion International, 26*(S1), i85–i107.

Fournier, J. C., DeRubeis, R. J., Hollon, S. D., Dimidjian, S., Amsterdam, M. D., Shelton, R. C., & Fawcett, J. (2010). Antidepressant drug effects and depression severity: A patient-level meta-analysis. *Journal of the American Medical Association, 303*, 47–53.

Gallo, J. J., & Coyne, J. C. (2000). The challenge of depression in late life: Bridging science and service in primary care. *JAMA, 284*, 1570–1572.

Gilbody, S., Bower, P., Fletcher, J., Richards, D., & Sutton, A. J. (2006). Collaborative care for depression: A cumulative meta-analysis and review of longer-term outcomes. *Archives of Internal Medicine, 166*(2), 2314–2321.

Glassman, A. H., Bigger, J. T., & Gaffney, M. (2009). Psychiatric characteristics associated with long-term mortality among 361 patients having an acute coronary syndrome and major depression. *Archives of General Psychiatry, 66*(9), 1022–1029.

Gleason, O. C., Pierce, A. M., Walker, A. E., & Warnock, J. K. (2013). The two-way relationship between medical illness and late-life depression. *Psychiatric Clinics of North America, 36*, 533–544.

Haines, V. A., Beggs, J. J., & Hurlbert, J. S. (2011). Neighborhood disadvantage, network social capital, and depressive symptoms. *Journal of Health and Social Behavior, 52*(1), 58–73.

Hasin, D. S., Goodwin, R. D., Stinson, F. S., & Grant, B. F. (2005). Epidemiology of major depressive disorder: Results from the National Epidemiologic Survey on Alcoholism and Related Conditions. *Archives of General Psychiatry, 62*, 1097–1106.

Huffman, J. C., Niazi, S. K., Rundell, J. R., Sharpe, M., & Katon, W. J. (2014). Essential articles on collaborative care models for the treatment of psychiatric disorders in medical settings: A publication by the Academy of Psychosomatic Medicine research and evidence-based practice committee. *Psychosomatics, 55*, 109–122.

Hunkeler, E. M., Katon, W., Tang, L., Williams Jr., J. W., Kroenke, K., Lin, E. H. B., . . . Unützer, J. (2006). Long term outcomes from the IMPACT randomized trial for depressed elderly patients in primary care. *British Medical Journal, 332*, 259–262.

Hybels, C. F., & Pieper, C. F. (2009). Epidemiology and geriatric psychiatry. *American Journal of Geriatric Psychiatry, 17*(8), 627–631.

Institute of Medicine. (1994). *Reducing risks for mental disorders: Frontiers for preventive intervention research.* Washington, DC: The National Academies Press.

Institute of Medicine. (2012). *The mental health and substance use workforce for older adults: In whose hands?* Washington, DC: The National Academies Press.

Jané-Llopis, E., Hosman, C., Jenkins, R., & Anderson, P. (2003). Predictors of efficacy in depression programmes. *British Journal of Psychiatry, 183*, 384–397.

Jané-Llopis, E., Katschnig, H., McDaid, D., & Wahlbeck, K. (2011). Supporting decision-making processes for evidence-based mental health promotion. *Health Promotion International, 26*(S1), i140–i146.

Julien, D., Richard, L., Gauvin, L., & Kestens, Y. (2012). Neighborhood characteristics and depressive mood among older adults: An integrative review. *International Psychogeriatrics, 24*(8), 1207–1225.

Katon, W. J., Lin, E., Russo, J., & Unützer, J. (2003). Increased medical costs of a population-based sample of depressed elderly patients. *Archives of General Psychiatry, 60*(9), 897–903.

Katon, W. J., Lin, E., Russo, J., Von Korff, M., Ciechanowski, P., Simon, G., . . . Young, B. (2004). Cardiac risk factors in patients with diabetes mellitus and major depression. *Journal of General Internal Medicine, 19*, 1192–1199.

Katon, W. J., Russo, J., Lin, E. H. B., Schmittdiel, J., Ciechanowski, P., Ludman, E., . . . Von Korff, M. (2012). Cost-effectiveness of a multicondition collaborative care intervention: A randomized controlled trial. *Archives of General Psychiatry, 69*(5), 506–514.

Katon, W. J., Schoenbaum, M., Fan, M.-Y., Callahan, C. M., Williams Jr., J., Hunkeler, E., . . . Unützer, J. (2005). Cost-effectiveness of improving primary care treatment of late-life depression. *Archives of General Psychiatry, 62*(2), 1313–1320.

Katon, W. J., Unützer, J., Fan, M.-Y., Williams Jr., J. W., Schoenbaum, M., Lin, E. H. B., & Hunkeler, E., (2006). Cost-effectiveness and net benefit of enhanced treatment of depression for older adults with diabetes and depression. *Diabetes Care, 29*(2), 265–270.

Kawachi, I., & Berkman, L. F. (2001). Social ties and mental health. *Journal of Urban Health, 78*, 458–467.

Kessler, R. C., Bromet, E. J., de Jonge, P., Shahly, V., & Wilcox, M. (2016). The burden of depressive illness. In N. Cohen (Ed.), *Public health perspectives on depressive disorders* (pp. 40–66). Baltimore, MD: Johns Hopkins University Press.

Kessler, R. C., & Ustün, T. B. (Eds.). (2008). *The WHO world mental health surveys: Global perspectives on the epidemiology of mental disorders.* New York, NY: Cambridge University Press.

Kim, D. (2008). Blues from the neighborhood? Neighborhood characteristics and depression. *Epidemiologic Reviews, 30*, 101–117.

Ludman, E. J., Katon, W., Russo, J., Von Korff, M., Simon, G., Ciechanowski, P., . . . Young, B. (2004). Depression and diabetes symptom burden. *General Hospital Psychiatry, 26*, 430–436.

Lustman, P. J., & Clouse, R. E. (2005). Depression in diabetic patients: The relationship between mood and glycemic control. *Journal of Diabetes Complications, 19*(2), 113–122.

Lyness, J. M., Caine, E., King, D., Cox, C., & Yoediono, Z. (1999). Psychiatric disorders in older primary care patients. *Journal of General Internal Medicine, 14*, 249–254.

Lyness, J. M., Heo, M., Datto, C. J., Ten Have, T. R., Katz, I. R., Drayer, R., . . . Bruce, M. L. (2006). Outcomes of minor and subsyndromal depression among elderly patients in primary care settings. *Annals of Internal Medicine, 144*(7), 496–504.

Lyness, J. M., Yu, Q., Tang, W., Tu, X., & Conwell, Y. (2009). Risks for depression onset in primary care elderly patients: Potential targets for preventive interventions. *American Journal of Psychiatry, 166*(12), 1375–1393.

Mair, C., Diez-Roux, A. V., & Galea, S. (2008). Are neighbourhood characteristics associated with depressive symptoms? A review of evidence. *Journal of Epidemiology and Community Health, 62*, 940–946.

Mojtabai, R., & Olfson, M. (2008). National patterns in antidepressant treatment by psychiatrists and general medical providers: Results from the National Comorbidity Survey Replication. *Journal of Clinical Psychiatry, 69*, 1064–1074.

Murayama, H., Fujiwara, Y., & Kawachi, I. (2012). Social capital and health: A review of prospective multilevel studies. *Journal of Epidemiology, 22*(3), 179–187.

National Institute on Aging. (2011). *Global health and aging.* Rockville, MD: US Government Printing Office.

Nemeroff, C. B., & Owens, M. J. (2009). The role of serotonin in the pathophysiology of depression: As important as ever. *Clinical Chemistry, 55*, 12578–12579.

NIMH Prevention Research Committee. (1994). *The prevention of mental disorders: A national research agenda.* Washington, DC: US Government Printing Office.

Nyqvist, F., Forsman, A. K., Giuntoli, G., & Cattan, M. (2013). Social capital as a resource for mental well-being in older people: A systematic review. *Aging and Mental Health, 17*(4), 394–410.

Olfson, M., Marcus, S. C., Druss, B., Elinson, L., Tanielian, T., & Pincus, H. A. (2002). National trends in the outpatient treatment of depression. *Journal of the American Medical Association, 287*(2), 203–209.

Paczkowski, M. M., & Galea, S. (2010). Sociodemographic characteristics of the neighborhood and depressive symptoms. *Current Opinion in Psychiatry, 23*, 337–341.

The Patient Protection and Affordable Care Act (PPACA), Public Law No.111-148, 124 Stat. 119 (March 23, 2010).

The Paul Wellstone and Pete Domenici Mental Health Parity and Addiction Parity Act (MHPAEA). (2008). Public Law 110-343.

Poortinga, W. (2006). Social capital: An individual or collective resource for health? *Social Science & Medicine, 62*, 292–302.

Robinson, R. G., Jorge, R. E., Moser, D. J., Acion, L., Solodkin, A., Small, S. L., . . . Arndt, S. (2008). Escitalopram and problem-solving therapy for prevention of poststroke depression: A randomized controlled trial. *JAMA, 299*(2), 2391–2400.

Russo, A., Hambrick, M., & Owens, P. (2007). *Healthcare cost and utilization project (HCUP)* (Statistical Brief No. 40). Rockville, MD: Agency for Healthcare Research and Quality. Retrieved from www.hcup-us.ahrq.gov/reports/statbriefs/sb40.jsp

SAMHSA. (2013). *National expenditures for mental health services and substance abuse treatment, 1986–2009.* (DHHS Publication No. SMA-13-4740). Rockville, MD: US Government Printing Office.

Schoevers, R. A., Smit, F., Deeg, D. J. H., Cuijpers, P., Dekker, J., Van Tilburg, W., & Beekman, A. T. F. (2006). Prevention of late-life depression in primary care: Do we know where to begin? *American Journal of Psychiatry, 163*(9), 1611–1621.

Schulz, R., Beach, S. R., Ives, D. G., Maartire, L. M., Ariyo, A. A., & Kop, W. J. (2000). Association between depression and mortality in older adults: The cardiovascular health study. *Archives of Internal Medicine, 160*(12), 1761–1768.

Sonnenberg, C. M., Beekman, A. T., Deeg, D. J., & Van Tilburg, W. (2003). Drug treatment in depressed elderly on the Dutch community. *International Journal of Geriatric Psychiatry, 18*, 99–104.

Susser, E., & Smith, R. P. (2011). Epidemiology in public mental health. In N. L. Cohen, & S. Galea (Eds.), *Population mental health: Evidence, policy, and public health practice* (pp. 38–50). New York, NY: Routledge.

Swartz, M. S., Wagner, H. R., Swanson, J. W., Burns, B. J., George, L. K., & Padgett, D. K. (1998). Comparing use of public and private mental health services: The enduring barriers of race and age. *Community Mental Health Journal, 34*, 133–144.

Szanto, K., Mulsant, B. H., Houck, P., Dew, M. A., & Reynolds III, C. F. (2003). Occurrence and course of suicidality during short-term treatment of late-life depression. *Archives of General Psychiatry, 60*, 610–617.

Szreter, S., & Woolcock, M. (2004). Health by association? Social capital, social theory, and the political economy of public health. *International Journal of Epidemiology, 33*, 650–667.

Thombs, B. D., Coyne, J. C., Cuijpers, P., de Jonge, P., Gilbody, S., Ioannidis, J. P., . . . Ziegelstein, R. C. (2012). Rethinking recommendations for screening for depression in primary care. *Canadian Medical Association Journal, 184*(4), 413–417.

Thota, A. B., Sipe, T. A., Byard, G. J., Zometa, C. S., Hahn, R. A., McKight-Eily, L. R., . . . Williams, S. P. (2012). Collaborative care to improve the management of depressive disorders: A community guide systematic review and meta-analysis. *American Journal of Preventive Medicine, 42*(5), 525–538.

Tiemens, B. G., Ormel, J., & Simon, G. E. (1996). Occurrence, recognition, and outcome of psychological disorders in primary care. *American Journal of Psychiatry, 153*(5), 636–644.

United Nations. (2013). *World population prospects: The 2012 revision.* Retrieved from http://esa.un.org/unpd/wpp

Unützer, J., Katon, W. J., Fan, M., Schoenbaum, M. C., Elizabeth, H. B., Della Penna, R. D., & Powers, D. (2008). Long-term cost effects of collaborative care for late-life depression. *American Journal of Managing Care, 13*(2), 95–100.

Unützer, J., Katon, W., Williams, J. W., Callahan, C. M., Harpole, L., Hunkeler, E. M., . . . Langston, C. A. (2001). Improving primary care for depression in late life. *Medical Care, 39*(8), 785–799.

Unützer, J., Schoenbaum, M., Katon, W. J., Fan, M. Y., Pincus, H. A., Hogan, D., & Taylor, J. (2009). Healthcare costs associated with depression in medically ill fee-for-service Medicare participants. *Journal of the American Geriatric Society, 57*(3), 506–510.

US Census Bureau. (2014). *An aging nation: The older population in the United States.* Retrieved from http://www.census.gov/prod/2014pubs/p25-1140.pdf

US Department of Health and Human Services, Public Health Service. (2001). *National strategy for suicide prevention: Goals and objectives for action.* (DHHS Publication No. SMA 01-3517). Rockville, MD: US Government Printing Office.

US Preventive Services Task Force. (2009). Screening for depression in adults: US Preventive Services Task Force recommendation statement. *Annals of Internal Medicine, 161*, 784–792.

Weyerer, S., Eiflaender-Gorfer, S., Kohler, L., Jessen, F., Maier, W., Fuchs, A., . . . Bickel, H. (2008). Prevalence and risk factors for depression in non-demented primary care attenders aged 75 years and older. *Journal of Affective Disorders, 111*, 153–163.

Williams, E. V., Unitzer, J., Lee, S., & Noel, H. (2009). Collaborative care for depression: A systematic review and cumulative meta-analysis. *American Journal of Geriatric Psychiatry, 17*, 1040–1049.

World Health Organization. (2002). *Active ageing: A policy framework.* Geneva, Switzerland: World Health Organization.

World Health Organization. (2014). *Preventing suicide: A global imperative.* Geneva, Switzerland: World Health Organization. Retrieved from http://apps.who.int/iris/bitstream/10665/67215/1/WHO_NMH_NPH_02.8.pdf

Wright, R. G., Cummings, J. R., Karlamangla, A. S., & Aneschensel, C. S. (2009). Urban neighborhood context and changes in depressive symptoms in late life. *Journals of Gerontology, Series B: Psychological Sciences and Social Sciences, 64B*(2), 247–251.

Zivin, K., Wharton, T., & Rostant, O. (2013). The economic, public health, and caregiver burden of late-life depression. *Psychiatric Clinics of North America, 36*(4), 631–649.

CHAPTER 17

The Digital Revolution and Its Potential Impact on Detection and Treatment of Depressive Disorders

Charles Platkin, PhD, MPH

Alissa R. Link, MPH

Amy Kwan, MPH

The digital revolution over the past 25 years has transformed the way we communicate, educate, conduct business, and obtain information (e.g., Harlow & Guo, 2014; Helbing, 2014; Purcell, Heaps, Buchanan, & Friedrich, 2013; Samson, Mehta, & Chandani, 2014; Toumache, Rouaski, Talbi, & Djelloul, 2014). This is evidenced by the increasingly wide reach of digital technologies: in 2015, 92% of adults in the United States had a mobile phone, 68% had a smartphone, 84% used the internet, and 65% used social media or social networking sites (Duggan, Ellison, Lampe, Lenhart, & Madden, 2015; Perrin, 2015; Perrin & Duggan, 2015), and as of September 2016 there were more than 1.8 billion active daily users on Facebook, 400 million monthly users on Instagram, 313 million monthly active users on Twitter, and billions of daily views on YouTube (Facebook, 2016; Instagram, 2016a; Twitter, 2016; YouTube, 2016). Globally, 32% of the population has a mobile phone (ICT Data and Statistics Division, 2014) and 46% uses the internet (ICT Data and Statistics Division, 2015). Of particular promise is the use of smartphones by underresourced individuals and the expansion of mobile phone and smartphone use in developing countries (Anderson, 2015; Anderson & Perrin, 2015; Pew Research Center, 2014).

Technology has enhanced efficiency and quality of service in most industries, yet health care has been slower to adopt certain technological advances (Herzlinger, 2006; Hwang & Christensen, 2008). However, nearly three-quarters (72%) of internet users and more than half (52%) of smartphone users have gone online or used their phones to seek health or medical information (Pew Research Center, 2015). Thus, there exists great potential for "disruptive innovation" (Hwang & Christensen, 2008; Klein, Hostetter, & McCarthy, 2014) that broadly changes health care practice. This chapter begins with an overview of different types of health technology and the applications already being developed to improve depression care. We then examine the advantages and challenges of social media surveillance, followed by examples and applications of health technology for depression screening, treatment, and suicide prevention.

History and Overview

The first wave of health technology began in the 1960s-1980s with innovations such as the electronic health or medical record (EHR or EMR) and telemedicine, offering new tools that facilitate health care delivery for providers, patients, and systems at large (Atherton, 2011; Chan, Parish, & Yellowlees, 2015). While the EHRs of the 1980s (with the Veterans Health Administration's VISTA serving as an early model) bear little resemblance to those today, adoption of these systems has increased dramatically during the early 2000s, with just 18% of physicians' offices using an EHR system in 2001 and 78% using one in 2013 (Hsiao & Hing, 2014). The second wave of health technology developed from strong consumer demand and the expansion of mobile and internet technologies, and a wide range of tools, resources, and interventions that can be accessed directly by patients and the public (Atkinson, Saperstein, & Pleis, 2009; Becker et al., 2014; Donker et al., 2013). The following are examples of the different delivery methods; however, it should be noted that there is significant overlap between the following categories and the ways they can be used to monitor and improve health (Klein et al., 2014).

- **EHRs** may include physician notes, electronic test and imaging results, and computerized provider-order entry, plus more advanced functions, such as clinical decision support. Through decision support, such as risk calculation, review of test result history, and reminders for preventive care, the burden on health care utilization can decrease by up to 24% (Chaudhry et al., 2006). An important and related function of health information technology is the capacity for health information exchange, the ability for separate organizations to communicate electronically and exchange patient data. The EHR and health information technology also present an unprecedented opportunity to amass large data sets ("big data") that can be powerful research tools for epidemiologists and clinicians (Angus, 2015; Paul et al., 2015). But while many health care providers are currently using EHRs, these records are not communicating across health care systems and are poorly designed from a user perspective, making it difficult for health care providers to find what they need to know about a patient when they need to know it (Cifuentes et al., 2015).
- **Telemedicine**, broadly defined, is the use of digital communication to exchange medical information with the goal of improving health (American Telemedicine Association, 2015). This is commonly in the form of two-way video but also includes communication by email, text messaging, smartphones, and other mechanisms. Some of the earliest applications of telemedicine have been in rural

areas to alleviate the shortage of health care providers, as well as in fields such as radiology, where in-person contact is not always essential (Chan et al., 2015).

- **Mobile Health (mHealth)** involves the use of mobile communication devices to promote health and deliver health care services. In its most basic form, text messaging, or Short Message Service (SMS), has multiple health applications (e.g., appointment reminders, health behavior promotion, disaster management alerts) (US Department of Health and Human Services, 2014). mHealth includes health-related smartphone software applications (apps) that can serve as tools for education, self-management, and intervention delivery (Donker et al., 2013). mHealth also includes wearables and sensors that can track physical activity, heart rate, skin conductivity, and so forth (Intille, 2007). In a 2015 US-based online survey, 58% of adults had downloaded a health-related app and 65% of those opened health apps daily (Krebs & Duncan, 2015).
- **Internet-based applications** to health care are wide reaching and can include web-based interventions, educational resources, social networking sites, or social media, as well as gaming/gamification. Websites can be used to disseminate health information, screen and monitor for symptoms and diseases, and deliver evidence-based interventions. Social media are websites and apps that facilitate the creation and sharing of content, including social networking sites (e.g., Facebook and Twitter), message boards or forums (e.g., PatientsLikeMe), and socially curated information sources (e.g., Wikipedia and Reddit, https://www.reddit.com/r/depression/). Social media has broad implications for health through its ability to engender peer-to-peer information exchange and social support. Computer-based gaming technology has recently been applied to the realm of health care to create interventions that are interactive and engaging (Cheek et al., 2015; Coyle, Doherty, & Sharry, 2009; Knox et al., 2011).

Health Technology Approaches to Depressive Disorders

Health technologies provide a number of unique and innovative opportunities for the prevention and treatment of depression. First, technology can help to meet the demands associated with the shortage of psychiatric and mental health resources in the United States, whereby 55% of counties in the United States have no practicing mental health providers and only 27% of community hospitals have operating inpatient psychiatry units, with many state and county psychiatric hospitals closing due to budget cuts (American Hospital Association, 2012). Second, technology can be used to identify those at risk for depression by expanding the reach and accessibility to treatment, as some people may neglect to mention symptoms or concerns to their primary care doctor (Cape & McCulloch, 1999) but may search for information about depression online (Leykin, Munoz, & Contreras, 2012; Pew Research Center, 2015). Third, technology can be used for real-time monitoring of symptoms, both where and when they occur in the natural environment (Juengst et al., 2015; Saeb et al., 2015; Tomita, Kandolo, Susser, & Burns, 2015). Given that most mental health interactions take place in a health care setting, providers may not be able to address fluctuations in mood or symptoms that are context- or time-dependent. Fourth, health technology can provide access to resources and interventions at times of greatest need—for example, at 3 a.m. when a depressed individual is unable to sleep or is having thoughts of self-harm. Fifth, technology can help to overcome barriers in access to care, such as reducing the stigma associated with seeking help by doing so in a private and anonymous online environment (Barak & Gluck-Ofri, 2007; Burns, Durkin, & Nicholas, 2009; Corrigan, Druss, & Perlick, 2014). Finally, technologies provide a unique opportunity for leveraging social support that can improve health outcomes (Morris, Schueller, & Picard, 2015; Shepherd, Sanders, Doyle, & Shaw, 2015).

There are also disadvantages, including lack of an in-person connection between patients and providers, which can come across as disconnected and not as personal (Rogers, Griffin, Wykle, & Fitzpatrick, 2009); distrust in the use of technology in a health care context (Charman, Harms, & Myles-Pallister, 2010); and data security and potential confidentiality concerns (Elhai & Frueh, 2015). In a qualitative study exploring telemedicine in the treatment of depression in rural settings, both patients and providers felt that it was an acceptable solution but expressed reservations about interference with the development of a productive provider-patient relationship (Swinton, Robinson, & Bischoff, 2009). Thus, extra attention can be allocated to relationship-building activities (e.g., ensuring that the patient knows he or she has the provider's undivided attention, maintaining eye contact, using a community health worker to facilitate the visit, or having one in-person visit prior to the telepsychiatry follow-up) to promote a therapeutic relationship despite the lack of in-person contact (Swinton et al., 2009). It is also likely that opinions on this aspect of health technology will evolve as the population becomes increasingly comfortable with the use of technologies, and as two-way video technologies, such as Skype, Google Hangouts, and Apple's FaceTime, become increasingly ubiquitous (Lenhart, 2015; Rivera & van der Meulen, 2014). Indeed, attitudes toward the use of digital technology to communicate with providers are already shifting, with half of US adults in a nationally representative panel indicating that they are willing to communicate with their doctor through email and 20% indicating interest in engaging with providers through social media (Jenssen, Mitra, Shah, Wan, & Grande, 2015).

Social Media Surveillance

Social media platforms, such as Facebook, Instagram, Twitter, YouTube, and Google, are increasingly popular and contain an unprecedented volume of data about people's everyday lives, thoughts, opinions, and behaviors. These mammoth websites process, store, and analyze data on personal characteristics, usage behaviors, communication patterns, and social networks. Social media enables interpersonal surveillance, in which peers can "watch over" one another without necessarily communicating directly, parents can monitor children, and employers can make judgments about future or current employees based on prior behaviors that are provided from online writings, postings, and photographs (Trottier, 2012). Companies and marketers use social media to track consumer behavior, deliver targeted advertising, and use the power of peer influence to help sell their products (Trottier, 2013). Additionally, law enforcement and investigative agencies use social media to track potential terrorist suspects and collect information on criminal activities (with or without warrants or subpoenas) (Bartlett & Reynolds, 2015).

While people who maintain public profiles knowingly post information that can be seen by anyone, other users selectively post information privately among their networks, and the use of social media data for surveillance or other research raises ethical questions. For instance, researchers at Cornell University collaborated with Facebook to conduct a one-week experiment in which they manipulated the content on users' news feeds (the Facebook homepage on which you can see all the recent posts of others in your network) (Kramer, Guillory, & Hancock, 2014). They selectively filtered the content viewed by 689,003 Facebook users such that half had reduced exposure to positive emotional expressions (e.g., "15 Photos That Restore Our Faith in Humanity") and half had reduced exposure to negative emotional expressions (e.g., status updates about a friend losing their job). Those who were exposed to more positive content posted more positive content themselves, and those with more negative content exposure posted more negative content, demonstrating the power of large-scale emotional contagion (Kramer et al., 2014). After the results were released, many Facebook users felt manipulated and upset by the fact that research could be done on them without their explicit consent, or felt that their privacy had been violated. Cornell University's ethics committee waived review of the study, citing the research methodology as the responsibility of Facebook, since Facebook receives agreement to this sort of research when members create a user account (Hill, 2014). Many, if not most, individuals do not carefully read the data use policies of these sites or apps, so should their agreement to such a policy as mandated to create an account be considered "informed consent"? How do we deal with issues of privacy when information that is shared "in confidence" among friends or family members could be used to solve a crime or prevent someone from harm? As social media data become increasingly ubiquitous, so does the power to harness these data toward the common good, and these questions must be addressed.

Indeed, social media and other digital surveillance have broad applications within public health. In many cases, the wide availability of data can result in innovative approaches to care. Hospital claims data have been used to identify "hot spots" for certain diseases, zip codes, or persons with high numbers of hospital readmissions. For example, an outreach team in Camden, New Jersey, targeted the sickest patients and those generating the highest health care costs for home visits with consultations on lifestyle and other health behaviors (e.g., medication adherence), resulting in a 40%–50% reduction in hospital and emergency room visits and costs (Gawande & Brenner, 2011). In New York City, public health officials at the Department of Health and Mental Hygiene launched a surveillance system in the wake of 9/11 using emergency department data and pharmacy medication sales to track early warning signs of respiratory distress or other disease outbreaks (Farley & Weisfuse, 2011). Patwardhan and Bilkovski (2012) also used pharmacy sales data extracted from a national pharmacy chain's enterprise data warehouse to model trends of influenza infection and found the data highly correlated with both Google Flu trend and CDC data. Google Flu trends used online search data (e.g., "flu symptoms," "what to do if I have the flu") tagged by geographic location to predict the spread of influenza. Until very recently, these data were publicly available and easy to mine (Patwardhan & Bilkovski, 2012); however, as of 2015, Google no longer builds their own models of flu trends and instead provides these data directly to researchers at Columbia University's Mailman School of Public Health, Boston Children's Hospital, and the CDC's Influenza Center (Google Research Blog, 2015).

Twitter has also been used to successfully model the spread and locations of influenza infections at the local and national level, identifying trends at least a week faster and at a lower cost than traditional surveillance methods (Broniatowski, Paul, & Dredze, 2013; Paul, Dredze, & Broniatowski, 2014). Paul and colleagues (2014) used an algorithm that applies logistic regression classifiers in three steps: (1) is the tweet about health? (2) is it about influenza? and (3) is it about an influenza infection (vs. general comments about flu season)? While the CDC provides weekly reports of the previous week's health activity, Twitter and Google have the advantage of "nowcasting" and measuring changes in real time. Twitter has since implemented a Data Grants program, which makes its volumes of public and historical data available to researchers. This sort of work is encompassed in the emerging field of "infodemiology," which applies electronic information typically obtained via the internet to epidemiology (understanding the distribution and determinants of health and disease at the population level) with the goal of informing public health and policy (Eysenbach, 2009).

With respect to mental health and surveillance, there are a number of implications for the use of social media, particularly given the common practice of using social media to share one's moods and emotions. Cavazos-Rehg and colleagues (2016) conducted a content analysis of 2,000 depression-related tweets from the United States and Canada over three weeks in 2014 by working with a social media analytics company to collect tweets containing the key words "(#)depressed" and "(#)depression" and remove tweets unrelated to mental health (e.g., "Great Depression," economics, real estate). Of the tweets they analyzed, 32% disclosed symptoms of depression and 40% offered support and help, while only 6% of overall tweets were generated by health or government organizations and 3% from clinicians or therapists. They used a software package called DemographicsPro, which applies algorithms based on Twitter usage and behavior, to extrapolate demographic characteristics and estimated that the majority of users (94%) who tweeted about "feeling depressed" were aged 25 or younger, and 77% were female (see Box 17.1 for sample tweets).

Box 17.1. Depression on Twitter

Sample depression-disclosing tweets:
- "Why am I depressed and sad 24/7 #Done"
- "All my frendz hate me :/ #depressed #emo"
- "I keep reading that working out helps with depression, I literally work out everyday and everyday I still want to stop existing so now what."

Sample supportive tweets:
- "Depressed? We can Help! [URL] #depression #mentalhealth #therapy"
- "Exercise has been scientifically proven to treat depression just as well as taking medication would and it's much more natural!" (Cavazos-Rehg et al., 2016)

Other researchers have sought to validate social media content about depression by comparing it to valid and reliable depression scales. Moreno and colleagues (2012) evaluated 224 public Facebook profiles at two universities and found that one-third displayed references to depressive symptoms. They used the *DSM-IV* symptom criteria and related synonyms to generate keywords that defined relevant content, such as feeling hopeless ("I feel like giving up"), loss of interest or pleasure in doing things, changes in eating behavior, trouble sleeping, and so forth. Qualifying posts also had to relate to the profile owner, rather than describe a friend's symptoms ("Joe looked so sad in class today"), and were not situational ("I'm having a bummer of a day") (Moreno et al., 2011). They then invited these users to complete an online Patient Health Questionnaire (PHQ-9) and found that these Facebook references were positively associated with scores for mild, moderate, or severe depression, although not statistically significant ($p = 0.056$; Moreno et al., 2012). Other studies have also shown associations between online behavior (e.g., number of friends and posted location tags, such as visiting restaurants, parks, concerts) and known measures of depressive symptoms and behaviors (Park, Lee, Kwak, Cha, & Jeong, 2013). These cross-sectional studies mirror work that is being done on a larger scale and can be used to monitor depression at the population level.

Computer scientists are able to use artificial intelligence and linguistics strategies to automate social media surveillance (e.g., De Choudhury, Gamon, Counts, & Horvitz, 2013; Karmen, Hsiung, & Wetter, 2015; Yin, Fabbri, Rosenbloom, & Malin, 2015). A group of researchers at Microsoft has done considerable work in this area and developed a model that uses Twitter to predict the risk of developing depression. The researchers used crowdsourcing to identify internet users with a self-reported clinical diagnosis of major depressive disorder (MDD), and then administered two screening tests, the Center for Epidemiologic Studies Depression Scale (CES-D) and the Beck Depression Inventory (BDI). The authors compared Twitter content (e.g., emotion, linguistic style, language) and usage behavior (e.g., replies, retweets, time of posting) from the year leading up to the first depressive episode. Findings showed that tweets of depressed individuals included late night posts, decreases in posting frequency, self-centricity, words about symptoms, concerns about medications, emotional disclosures, and reduced social activity. Their resulting model predicted depression onset with an average accuracy of 70% and high precision (74%) (De Choudhury et al., 2013). Using similar methodology, the same group of researchers created a social media depression index that they applied to a 30% random sample of all US tweets over a one-year period (De Choudhury, Counts, & Horvitz, 2013). They were able to observe population-level trends in depression patterns across seasons, time of day, gender, and cities that mirror CDC data on depression (De Choudhury et al., 2013). Taking this work further, Coppersmith, Dredze, and Harman (2014) used natural language processing (NLP) methods to automate data collection and classify tweets relevant to depression, bipolar disorder, posttraumatic stress disorder, and seasonal affective disorder with predictable validity. NLP breaks contextual information into grammatical units, and then detects words that are predefined, in this case as indicators of depression or its symptoms, as well as frequency of those symptoms (e.g., never, sometimes, often, always). Karmen and colleagues (2015) merged lists of symptoms from the *DSM-IV* and ICD-10 as well as the most frequently used depression scales (CES-D, BDI, GDS, HAM-D, MADRS, SDS, WHO-5), and then translated jargon into colloquial language. They calculated a score that included weighted sums based on frequency and severity of symptoms, and simple weights based on detection of pronouns (e.g., self vs. other) and negation. NLP methods were able to detect depressive symptoms and their frequency on an internet forum with good precision. These and other studies (e.g., Coppersmith, 2015; Yin et al., 2015) represent considerable progress toward a scalable public health approach to depression surveillance.

Social media surveillance is particularly valuable given the potential for efficiently analyzing data and the capacity for rapid or automated responses (Foldy, 2004; Patwardhan & Bilkovski, 2012). Strong surveillance systems must consider confidentiality and the sensitivity and specificity of given screening methods (Buehler, 2004; Patwardhan & Bilkovski, 2012). By understanding demographic, geographic, and time trends, social media surveillance can help health care systems and government officials determine where to allocate resources for depression prevention, screening, and treatment. These trends can be used to target preventive strategies for at-risk populations; for example, mental health–related organizations could use Twitter to send tailored tweets that match the ages and interests of individuals disclosing depressive symptoms (Cavazos-Rehg et al., 2016) (see box 17.1 for examples of supportive tweets and Table 17.1 for sample hashtags that can be used to target depressed social media users).

Table 17.1. *Using hashtags to target depressed social media users*

Hashtag	No. of images posted on Instagram[a]
#depression	9,622,808
#depressed	8,886,132
#emo	9,915,572
#suicide	5,614,989
#selfharmmm[b]	1,802,331
#selfhate	1,322,276

Note. Hashtags are metadata tags used on Facebook, Twitter, and Instagram that allow users to find messages relating to a specific theme.
[a] Data as of November 11, 2016.
[b] Instagram's policy prevents hashtags that promote self-harm from being searchable, so people use misspellings to circumvent this (Instagram, 2016b).

Despite the popularity of social media, these surveillance methods do not reach certain at-risk populations who do not frequently use social media, such as: older adults (35% of those aged 65 and older use social media vs. 90% of those aged 18–29), rural residents (58% of rural residents use social media vs. 68% of suburban and 64% of urban residents), those of lower education (56% of those with high school or less use social media vs. 70% of those with some college or an associate's degree and 76% of college graduates), and those of lower socioeconomic status (56% of those earning less than $30K annually vs. 78% of those earning $75K or more) (Perrin, 2015). However, there is still significant reach within these subgroups, and use of social media continues to increase over time.

Other applications of social media include promoting mental health and depression awareness. Reality TV celebrity Kim Kardashian recently produced a documentary called *#RedFlag*, which is about how social media can be used as a tool to help identify and assist young adults with mental illness. Indeed, the reach and sway of celebrities and other influencers through social media can be a powerful mechanism for promoting awareness and reducing stigma of mental health issues such as depression.

Health Technology and Screening for Depression

While social media represents an almost "naturalistic" approach to depression surveillance, internet and mobile technologies can extend the reach of current screening methods. An early application of this was tested in 1999 using an online CES-D screen placed on a large online health information portal. More than 24,000 screens were completed during an eight-month period, of which 58% screened positive for depression, 47% of whom had never been treated for depression (Houston et al., 2001). A more recent study recruited more than 50,000 users over one year to a "Free Online Depression Screener" using a worldwide Google AdWords campaign that was designed to target individuals who were searching for depression-related keywords (e.g., "depression symptoms," "sad mood," or "am I depressed"). While many more people clicked on the link than actually engaged with the website, nearly 25,000 provided enough data for evaluation based on the major depressive episode (MDE) screener; two-thirds screened positive for an MDE, with 44% indicating some degree of suicidality and 8% reporting a suicide attempt in the past two weeks (Leykin et al., 2012). However, these screening tools were utilized by people who searched for information about depression or mental health and thus cannot be used to estimate population prevalence of depression. Indeed, compared to the 6.8% of US adults reporting moderate-to-severe depression according to the CDC's Behavioral Risk Factor Surveillance System (Reeves et al., 2011), the percentage of users screening positive for depression with these online screening tools could be viewed as inflated. While online screening methods show promise for detecting incidence of depression and suicidality, only 5% of participants agreed to monthly rescreening (Leykin et al., 2012), thus future research should explore factors that promote adherence, as well as innovative ways to incentivize ongoing monitoring and follow-up (e.g., rewards, social support or community-building, gamification).

There is also a plethora of publicly available depression screening mobile apps (e.g., What's My M3, Depression Screening, Hamilton Depression Scale Lite, CESD-Depression Test). BinDhim and colleagues (2015) developed a free "Depression Monitor" app that they released on the global Apple App Store in late 2012; 8,241 participants from 66 countries downloaded the app during a four-month span, with 74% completing the PHQ-9 questionnaire within the app. One-quarter had a prior depression diagnosis, and those with prior diagnoses were more likely to have higher education levels or have other comorbid conditions; of those without a prior depression diagnosis, 83% were at high risk of depression (PHQ-9 ≥ 11) (BinDhim et al., 2015). These studies are limited by the fact that users were searching for depression-related information online or in the app store; however, given the high prevalence of health-related searches online (Atkinson et al., 2009), these are feasible methods to reach a wide audience of at-risk individuals.

In addition to mobile apps, depression screening can be delivered via SMS (e.g., "On a scale of 1 to 10, what was your average mood today?"), extending its reach in populations with lower health literacy, in low-resource settings, and among populations who are known to be at risk for depression (US Department of Health and Human Services, 2014). Tomita and colleagues (2015) used SMS to assess depressive symptoms among refugees in South Africa, recruited by nurse clinicians who delivered services to refugees. The SMS assessment was based on the Quick Inventory of Depressive Symptomatology and found high rates of depression symptoms, with 26% reporting mild symptoms and 52% reporting moderate or severe symptoms. SMS represented a feasible, reliable, and acceptable means of communicating with and screening this population—99% of the participants owned a mobile phone and every participant responded to all SMS questions on depression; notably, only 43% owned a computer and one-third used the internet (including on their phones), demonstrating the more limited reach of other screening methods and intervention tools.

The combination of push notifications and mobile apps has also been shown to be effective for measuring and assessing depression. Ecological momentary assessment (EMA) involves short, repeated assessments of emotional and physical symptoms, mood/affect, behavior, or thoughts that are measured in real time and in the natural environment. Juengst and colleagues (2015) used a smartphone app to push daily EMAs of depression (PHQ-2 and -9) and anxiety scales (GAD-7) to adults with traumatic brain injuries, with 73% compliance and high satisfaction. EMA can include items taken directly from validated questionnaires or novel ways to deliver validated scales that are optimized for a mobile phone and are thus more engaging for the user, such as the Photographic Affect Meter (PAM; Pollak, Adams, & Gay, 2011). PAM sends an alert that prompts the user to "touch the image that best captures how you feel right now" and is validated as a proxy for the Positive and Negative Affect Scale (Pollak et al., 2011). EMA represents a way to monitor symptoms and behaviors over time and in real-world settings, as the prompts can be sent at varying times of the day, capturing mood fluctuations and reducing recall bias.

Novel screening methods can also apply mobile phone sensor data, such as GPS and phone usage, to monitor at-risk populations for depression. Saeb and colleagues (2015) used an Android app called Purple Robot to gather GPS and phone usage sensor data and correlated these data with PHQ-9 scores in a small sample of adults. They found that individuals with PHQ-9 $\geq$ 5 visited fewer locations with less variety, moved less through geographic space, had increased home stays, and had greater phone usage duration and frequency than those with lower PHQ-9 scores. While these results are very preliminary, the methodology represents a screening mechanism that is unobtrusive and very low effort. As mobile phones become increasingly ubiquitous and technology advances, there is great potential for passive screening methods to monitor at-risk populations.

The combined use of mobile sensor data, social media surveillance, and EMA represents a very important and exciting new frontier in health technology. EMA methods can be used to specifically target an individual's behavior during high-risk key moments in time. If mobile sensor data and social media surveillance can be used to identify patterns of behavior that are associated with depression, suicidal ideation, and so forth, EMA-style alerts or mini-interventions could be pushed to that user and potentially reach an at-risk individual at the time of greatest need.

Health Technology and Depression Treatment

In addition to using technology for screening previously undiagnosed cases of depression, health technology also offers useful tools for monitoring, assessing, and engaging currently depressed individuals. Specifically, technology can be used to augment or replace existing evidence-based depression treatments, deliver novel interventions, and support behavior change. The mode of intervention delivery ranges from use of SMS and phone calls as telemedicine in its most basic form (van den Berg, Grabe, Baumeister, Freyberger, & Hoffmann, 2015) to complex and interactive mobile or web-based applications (e.g., Renton et al., 2014; Rice et al., 2014; Shen et al., 2015). SMS-based mood ratings and single-item responses have been demonstrated as a clinically useful proxy for the PHQ-9 (Aguilera, Schueller, & Leykin, 2015; Keding, Bohnke, Croudace, Richmond, & MacPherson, 2015). Another example is the T2 Mood Tracker, developed by the Department of Defense, which is a smartphone app designed to monitor emotional health in an easy and accurate manner, with the original intention of tracking and recording military service members' behavior and moods, especially after combat deployments. It was downloaded more than 100,000 times between 2010 and 2012 (Jimenez, 2013). Users rate their moods according to six categories (e.g., Anxiety, Depression, General Well-Being [see table 17.1]) and use sliding scales to self-monitor symptoms. The app contains graphs to visualize changes over time, as well as the capability to report experiences to providers. T2 Mood Tracker was tested by a small group of veterans who were receptive to the app and would recommend it to other veterans (Bush, Ouellette, & Kinn, 2014). In the following section, we provide an overview of additional treatment methods for depression, within the context of health technology.

Telepsychiatry

While telepsychiatry has traditionally been used to expand the reach of the health care system in rural areas, it has become more popular over time, with demonstrated clinical efficacy in a range of populations (adult, pediatric, geriatric, ethnic) and in varied settings (emergency room, rural, home health) (Chan et al., 2015; Hilty et al., 2013). The Veterans Health Administration has been a frequent user of telepsychiatry, with more than 3.3 million rural veterans served through community-based outpatient clinics equipped with videoconferencing technology. It grew its telepsychiatry programs dramatically (140%–218% growth) between 2006 and 2010, primarily in the areas of psychotherapy with or without medication management, group psychotherapy, and diagnostic assessment (Deen, Godleski, & Fortney, 2012). Over that time period, hospitalizations decreased by an average of 25% (Godleski, Darkins, & Peters, 2012).

A new method used in telepsychiatry mirrors the "store and forward" methods used in teledermatology and teleradiology, in which a recording of a clinician-patient interview is forwarded for later review by a psychiatrist, who makes an assessment and treatment recommendations, with evidence of feasibility plus clinical efficacy (Chan et al., 2015; Yellowlees et al., 2011). Given ample patient volume, this model is more cost-effective than in-person psychiatric consultations (Butler & Yellowlees, 2012).

Specific to depression, a number of telehealth interventions have been shown to be effective (Hilty et al., 2013). One intervention provided a treatment arm with access to a nurse care manager, pharmacist, psychologist, and psychiatrist via video conferencing and compared it to usual care comprised only of an in-person nurse care manager–based depression treatment. Both groups also had access to an in-person primary care provider. The video conferencing group had greater reductions in depressive symptom severity and higher remission sustained over 18 months, and no increased visits to the primary care physician. The authors hypothesize that these improvements were related to better self-management activities as a result of increased contact with the depression care manager instead of increased access to psychotherapy (Fortney et al., 2013). Patients in a telemedicine-based collaborative care model also reported fewer antidepressant-related side effects compared with those in a low-intensity model (Hudson, Fortney, Pyne, Lu, & Mittal, 2015).

Web and Mobile Applications

Renton and colleagues (2014) conducted a "scoping review" of existing web-based programs for the interactive treatment of depression and found that only 12 of 32 available programs had a published randomized controlled trial (RCT) evaluating efficacy. Another review and content analysis of the depression app marketplace found 243 mobile apps on depression, two-thirds of which had the goal of therapeutic treatment. However, most did not report organizational affiliation or content source, thereby limiting credibility (Shen et al., 2015). These findings are reflective of the broader mHealth field in general—while there are many websites and applications created by well-intending developers, many of them do not utilize theory or evidence-based approaches, nor are they vetted by trusted sources; as the market continues to grow, it may become increasingly difficult for patients to identify reliable and credible apps (Donker et al., 2013).

For those apps that are evidence based, one particular advantage of utilizing web or mobile applications is the ability to track exactly how people engage with the intervention, in order to determine which aspects are most popular or effective. This can allow for iterative improvements to the design that can evolve to meet the needs of users. For example, myCompass (https://www.mycompass.org.au/) is a mobile and web-based program that is fully automated and designed to treat mild or moderate symptoms of depression, anxiety, and stress. It contains 12 modules (see table 17.2), each made up of three sections that take 5–10 minutes to complete, plus a homework exercise; users are asked to complete one module per week. myCompass also has features such as symptom tracking and a diary to record insights and "snippets" (brief tips) that the user could sign up for to receive via SMS or email. The snippets were the most used feature, and those who signed up for such alerts were more likely to see a reduction in symptoms (controlling for severity of baseline symptoms). The most popular modules were those on managing stress, communication, and problem solving. The authors speculate that the snippets were popular and effective because they required little effort in terms of behavior change or time commitments and were supportive, normalizing, and hope instilling (Whitton et al., 2015).

Other companies have taken an educational approach, using technology as the method of delivery. For example, Kognito (www.kognito.com) develops web-based interactive trainings and role-play simulations using computerized animations for health care providers, educators, parents, and caregivers that help people to identify, approach, and refer to mental health support services for those with psychological distress or those who are at risk for suicide. Their interventions are listed under the US Substance Abuse and Mental Health Services Administration's National Registry of Evidence-Based Programs and Practices.

Cognitive Behavioral Therapy

Technology has been applied to both augment the standard delivery of cognitive behavioral therapy (CBT), one of the most widely used and effective therapies for depression, and to "replace" face-to-face CBT. Computerized CBT (cCBT) can refer to a variety of methods of CBT delivery, ranging from interactive voice response systems to websites (internet-based CBT) to mobile apps that have a number of interactive modules covering techniques such as thought recording, attributional style, cognitive restructuring, goal setting, assertiveness training, and so forth (Kaltenthaler & Cavanagh, 2010). Some of the more popular and well-studied cCBT programs include MoodGYM (https://moodgym.anu.edu.au/welcome) and Beating the Blues (http://www.beatingtheblues.co.uk/), both of which are available online. There have been several systematic reviews and meta-analyses establishing that computerized or internet-based CBT is as effective as therapist-led CBT and more effective than usual care in depression treatment (e.g., Andersson & Cuijpers, 2009; Andrews, Cuijpers, Craske, McEvoy, & Titov, 2010; Foroushani, Schneider, & Assareh, 2011; Kaltenthaler et al., 2006; Spek et al., 2007). Internet-based CBT (iCBT) interventions that included therapist support had a larger combined effect size than those without support in meta-analyses (Andersson & Cuijpers, 2009; Spek et al., 2007). Andrews and colleagues (2010) noted that cCBT/iCBT interventions are well accepted and have good adherence while requiring minimal clinician or tech time (approximately 10 minutes per patient per week) but underscore that many of the studies have been done with participants who are self-selected.

There is a range of other evidence-based psychological therapies used to treat depression, such as psychotherapy, problem-solving therapy (PST), acceptance and commitment therapy (ACT), interpersonal therapy (IPT), psychodynamic therapy (PDT), and mindfulness-based cognitive therapy (MBCT). Andersson and Cuijpers (2009) included three studies of non-CBT computerized interventions in their review, two of PST and one of psychoeducation, and found them to be on par with the CBT-based interventions. For the most part, research on computerized or internet-based adaptations of these therapies is still emerging and is limited to protocol papers (Krieger et al., 2014) or case-reports (Felder, Dimidjian, Beck, Boggs, & Segal, 2014).

Promoting Medication Adherence

Several reviews show that SMS reminders and mobile apps in general can be effective at promoting medication adherence across several health conditions (Choi, Lovett, Kang, Lee, & Choi, 2015; Vervloet et al., 2012). Examples of medication adherence–oriented mobile apps (that were available in the Apple, Android, and Black-Berry app marketplaces during August and September 2012) include MyMedSchedule, MyMeds, and RxmindMe; however, these have not yet been supported by any clinical trials (Dayer, Heldenbrand, Anderson, Gubbins, & Martin, 2013). Health technology thus has the potential to further support traditional depression treatment by promoting antidepressant adherence. For example, a recent study assessed antidepressant adherence among 40 undergraduates, 20 of whom were randomized to use a smartphone app. Those using the app were three and a half times more likely to be adherent (measured by pill counts and defined as taking 80%–100% of their prescribed medications), although this did not reach statistical significance (p = 0.057) (Hammonds et al., 2015).

Exercise and Lifestyle Interventions

There is a significant body of literature, including a number of systematic reviews and meta-analyses, demonstrating the efficacy of exercise on improving depressive symptoms in all age groups, particularly for those with mild and moderate depression (e.g., Brown, Pearson, Braithwaite, Brown, & Biddle, 2013; Josefsson, Lindwall, & Archer, 2014; Rhyner & Watts, 2015; Rosenbaum, Tiedemann, Sherrington, Curtis, & Ward, 2014; Silveira et al., 2013; Stanton & Reaburn, 2014). There is additional evidence supporting the use of mHealth interventions such as mobile sensors (accelerometers, pedometers), goal setting, real-time feedback, and social support networking to promote increases in physical activity (e.g., Bort-Roig, Gilson, Puig-Ribera, Contreras, & Trost, 2014; Muntaner, Vidal-Conti, & Palou, 2015). We are not aware of any published studies that have evaluated mHealth interventions to promote physical activity as a component of depression treatment; however, there are a number of blogs and anecdotal reports of using devices such as Fitbits to combat depression (e.g., Brennan, 2014), and some fitness trackers, such as the Jawbone Up24, allow users to record their mood by selecting one of several cartoon faces (Shu, 2014).

One comprehensive depression self-management app, MoodHacker (http://www .orcasinc.com/products/moodhacker/), combines CBT and positive psychology with healthy habit promotion and syncs with fitness trackers to promote physical activity and improved sleep (see table 17.2) (Birney, Gunn, Russell, & Ary, 2016). In an RCT testing MoodHacker versus an email with links to helpful resources about depression (e.g., Mayo Clinic, NIMH), mild to moderately depressed adults who used the app had significantly greater reductions in depression symptoms and negative thoughts as well as significant improvements in behavioral activation and knowledge. Birney and colleagues (2016) tested the app among employees, some of whom had access to an employee assistance program (EAP), and found that MoodHacker users had increased work productivity as well as decreased absenteeism and work distress, and that the app was more effective for those with access to an EAP. Integrating a depression self-management app into workplaces via an EAP or other benefits program can have a wide reach and appeal to employers with increased productivity benefits supporting employer goals.

Social Support Interventions

More novel technology-based interventions for depression have capitalized on the unique characteristics of online social networks. In a RCT with 60 Portuguese adults who had not previously used Facebook, using the site for at least one hour per day was associated with decreased scores on the HAMD-17 and BDI-II over three months, with even stronger improvements for those in the treatment group with the psychiatrist as a "Facebook friend." While only 3 of 20 participants assigned to the "psychiatrist as a friend" condition actually used Facebook chat to communicate with the psychiatrist, the author postulates that knowing the support was there if needed provided some degree of comfort and assurance (Mota Pereira, 2014). In another study of social networks, Morris, Schueller, and Picard (2015) randomized 217 individuals to use (for 25 minutes per week for three weeks) either an "expressive writing" control condition or Panoply, a peer-to-peer support app that allows users to post content, respond to others, and get notifications about new interactions. The control condition and Panoply were visually identical; however, Panoply used briefly trained, crowd-sourced respondents (from Amazon's Mechanical Turk service) to provide feedback in the form of cognitive reappraisal (based on CBT) and socioaffective support. While there was not a significant difference between posttest depression levels among the two groups, Panoply users demonstrated twice as much activity on the site compared with control users and reported significantly higher levels of reappraisal. Individuals with higher baseline depression scores ended with significantly less depression.

Treatments for Youth

The majority of studies have focused on treatment of depression in adults; however, there is enormous potential in using health technology to reach adolescents and young adults. Depression most often has its onset prior to age 26 (Kessler et al., 2012), and given the high risk of relapse and associated worsening of symptoms over time (Keller et al., 1984; Kennard, Emslie, Mayes, & Hughes, 2006), a population approach to depression must prevent and treat early symptoms of depression in children, adolescents, and young adults.

Given the extremely high rates of youth adoption of smartphones, social media, internet- and app-based communication, and online games, health technology represents an important way to engage youth in mental health treatment. A systematic review of the literature found that both online- and social networking–based interventions are effective in treating youth depression. The authors caution, however, that social networking–based interventions can have mixed effects and should be carefully designed with considerations such as ensuring that the social networking site highlights positive interactions, feelings of inclusion, supportive relationships, self-esteem, and learning (Rice et al., 2014).

CBT interventions that incorporate health technology are also being adapted for youth, comprised of online therapist training, in-session tablet use for learning CBT skills and concepts, and between-session SMS homework reminders and self-monitoring prompts. This pilot study demonstrated that the tablet and SMS-enhanced CBT was at least as good as usual care (both the treatment as usual group and the tablet CBT group experienced significant reductions in depression), and 95% of adolescents found the SMS component helpful with high general satisfaction among both patients and providers (Kobak, Mundt, & Kennard, 2015). Indeed, many of the effective tools used within adult populations can be successful among youth but may require adaptation for literacy levels, content complexity, and increased engagement.

Gamification

Game-based interventions have generally been targeted to youth. Ninety-seven percent of US youth aged 12–17 play video games, and half of respondents had played a game the day prior to the survey (Lenhart et al., 2008). Teenagers in the United States spend an average of 6.3 hours per week playing video games (Nielson, 2014), and 81% of them use game consoles (e.g., PlayStation, Xbox, Wii) (Lenhart, 2015), so delivering an intervention in the format of a game can be an acceptable and engaging treatment option. Indeed, computer games have been used in the context of adolescent therapy, where the therapist and adolescent sit together and play the game (Coyle et al., 2009). For example, a computer-based CBT game designed to treat anxiety in children aged 7–13 called Camp Cope-A-Lot (table 17.2) has been shown to have similar outcomes to in-person CBT (Khanna & Kendall, 2010).

Another example is SPARX (Smart, Positive, Active, Realistic, X-factor thoughts), a free online interactive fantasy game based on CBT that is designed to help young people with mild to moderate depression, anxiety, or stress, with seven modules delivered over a four-to-seven-week period (Cheek et al., 2015; Merry et al., 2012) (table 17.2). In developing and refining the game, Cheek and colleagues (2015) conducted a series of focus groups and individual interviews to map user perceptions to

Table 17.2. Technology-based tools and interventions for depression

Program/app	Reference	Goal	Features	Modules, content, or other details
Depression Monitor	(BinDhim et al., 2015)	Screening	PHQ-9; high scores prompt recommendation to share results with a health care provider, plus links to informational websites; weekly reminders via push notifications	Other measures include: demographics, Charlson comorbidity index, single-item anxiety
myCompass	(Whitton et al., 2015)	CBT, IPP, PST	Educational modules; symptom and behavior tracking; "snippets" containing brief mental health tips, motivational content, or facts; diary for recording notes on insights or situational factors that are linked to symptoms	Managing stress and overload, communicating clearly, problem-solving, tackling unhelpful thinking, fear and anxiety, happiness, sleep, relaxation, taking charge of worry, increasing pleasurable activities, smart goals, managing loss
T2 Mood Tracker	(Bush, Ouellette, & Kinn, 2014; Jimenez, 2013)	Symptom monitoring	Symptom and mood tracking, visual feedback and changes over time, provider reports (see http://t2health.dcoe.mil /apps/t2-mood-tracker for screenshots)	Anxiety, depression, general well-being, head injury, posttraumatic stress, stress
MoodGYM	(Calear, Christensen, Mackinnon, Griffiths, & O'Kearney, 2009)	iCBT, prevention	Interactive web program to prevent depression, 5 modules, interactive game, anxiety and depression assessments, relaxation audio download, workbook, feedback assessment	Relationship between thoughts and emotions, dealing with stress, relationship breakups, relaxation and meditation techniques
SPARX	(Cheek et al., 2015; Merry et al., 2012)	CBT	Avatar-based gaming intervention platform via CD-ROM; modules introduce users to therapeutic content via a virtual therapist/guide, then transition to fantasy setting to apply/practice skills, with the goal of "restoring balance" to the fantasy world; reflect on how tasks can be applied in their own life	Level 1: finding hope (cave province), Level 2: being active (ice province), Level 3: dealing with emotions (volcano province), Level 4: overcoming problems (mountain province), Level 5: recognizing unhelpful thoughts (swamp province), Level 6: challenging unhelpful thoughts (bridgeland province). Level 7: bringing it all together (canyon province). Based on self-determination theory, supplemental paper guide

(continued)

Program/app	Reference	Goal	Features	Modules, content, or other details
Depression Quest	http://www .depressionquest .com/	Self-management	Interactive fiction game as a character living with depression, 40,000 interactive words, 150 unique encounters that fluctuate with character's depression level, 5 endings, reactive audio/visual	Characters undergo and complete everyday life events, such as managing a job, relationships, their illness, and treatment
MoodHacker	(Birney, Gunn, Russell, & Ary, 2016)	CBT, positive psychology	Mobile-web app based on the Coping with Depression CBT skills-training program, mood tracking, trigger journaling, goal-setting, daily emails, in-app messaging, video content, syncs with fitness and sleep trackers	Goals are to improve mood self-management, promote positive behaviors, decrease negative and increase positive thinking; incorporates mindfulness and positive psychology; tracker emphasizes connection between positive activities (e.g., social, exercise) and mood over time
Interactive Screening Program	(Garlow et al., 2008); American Foundation for Suicide Prevention	Screening	Brief, confidential screening via PHQ-9, plus a measure of past suicide attempts; written follow-up by counseling service through university, college, or employer; user can converse through the program or schedule to meet via phone or in person	Other measures: anger, anxiety, alcohol and drug abuse, eating disorder symptoms; 35 questions, <10 minutes to complete. Self-assigned user ID protects anonymity

the theoretical model (self-determination theory) that guided the design. Shepherd and colleagues (2015) conducted focus groups to further refine aspects of the game and to ensure that it was seen as effective and appealing among Maori adolescents, an ethnic minority group in New Zealand. SPARX was tested in a RCT among 187 adolescents (aged 12–19), and remission rates were significantly higher in the SPARX arm (44% vs. 26%, p = 0.03) (Merry et al., 2012). Most of the games that have been tested through RCTs are not yet available to the public (Cheek et al., 2015).

Another approach to incorporating gaming into existing treatments is using game activities in conjunction with biofeedback. A small group of children aged 9–17 wore three skin electrodes that monitored heart rate variability and skin conductivity to measure stress. The game used imagery and sounds to help promote relaxation and the biological stress measures determined success within the game; those who played the game had decreased symptoms of anxiety and depression (Knox et al., 2011).

Health Technology and Suicide Prevention

There is particular interest in the application of health technology tools in screening for and preventing suicide. Given that many people who attempt suicide do not seek help first, nor do they remain connected to health services afterward, health technology provides a novel way of screening those at risk, delivering proactive interventions and offering help (Christensen, Batterham, & O'Dea, 2014). The American Foundation for Suicide Prevention has an online screening tool, combining the PHQ-9 with a measure of past suicide attempts, that has been effective in identifying university students at risk for suicide, although only 10%–20% of those students agreed to service referral and even fewer actually engaged with services (Garlow et al., 2008; Haas et al., 2008; Moutier et al., 2012). While there is evidence that web-based screening programs can identify people at risk for suicide, these studies lack a control or nonscreened comparison group, so it is unclear whether online screening leads to increased mental health care utilization among those at risk. Several internet depression programs (e.g., cCBT, SPARX) have demonstrated reductions in suicidal ideation (or proxies thereof) in response to depression-oriented interventions (Christensen et al., 2014).

There are not many examples of online self-help interventions specifically designed to reduce suicidal thoughts. However, in one program, participants were recruited to the site through websites, newspapers, and Google AdWords, and completed the Beck Scale for Suicide Ideation and the BDI to determine eligibility; users with severe depression were not eligible for the online intervention and were referred to other mental health services. The unguided online intervention employed CBT as well as elements of dialectical behavior therapy, PST, and MBCT. Participants were asked to complete one of six modules each week and spend 30 minutes on the site each day. Findings showed that those randomized to the intervention (vs. an educational website) had a significantly greater improvement in and reduction of suicidal thoughts (effect size = 0.28) that appeared to sustain over 12 weeks, with greater improvements among those with a history of repeated suicide attempts (van Spijker, van Straten, & Kerkhof, 2014).

Social media can also be a vehicle to address suicidality in a number of ways, ranging from individuals posting suicide notes online (Ahuja, Biesaga, Sudak, Draper, & Womble, 2014) to suicide prevention social networks, blogs, or Twitter accounts (Christensen et al., 2014; Luxton, June, & Fairall, 2012). Facebook, for example, has a "Report Suicidal Content" feature and connects users with the National Suicide Prevention Lifeline in response (Ahuja et al., 2014). As such, social media, and particularly Twitter, can be useful for monitoring and identifying suicidal or self-harm risk factors (Cavazos-Rehg et al., 2016; Jashinsky et al., 2014; Sueki, 2015). Based on their content analysis of depression-related tweets, Cavazos-Rehg and colleagues (2016) extrapolated that there could be approximately 700 tweets each day related to self-harm or suicide. Sueki (2015) found significant associations between suicide-related tweets and risk factors for suicide. Given that half of suicide attempters announce their plans to family or friends (Beck, Steer, & Ranieri, 1988), future interventions could employ social media data to alert family, friends, or mental health providers when an individual is particularly vulnerable.

Conclusion

With more than 25 years of advances toward a population-level approach to mental health, "mainstream" public health agenda and policy-makers are increasingly recognizing mental health as critical to its twenty-first-century agenda and goals (Cohen & Galea, 2011). With its high prevalence and significant long-term effects, both personal and societal, depressive disorders are a leading cause of disease burden worldwide. Like most mental disorders, major depression goes underdetected, undertreated, and stigmatized by public opinion. However, with burgeoning advances in digital technology, both population mental health (e.g., surveillance, health promotion, illness prevention) and clinical care (e.g., improved treatment outcomes) are particularly good targets for innovative applications of health technology.

Social media provides unique capability for destigmatizing public attitudes toward mental health and improving both health and mental health literacy. The "real-time" expression of dysphoric mood and depression symptoms that do not meet thresholds for *DSM*-based clinical diagnosis offer opportunities for community-level interventions (e.g., supportive peers and family) that may interrupt progression toward MDD. Additionally, more professionally structured treatment can be delivered outside traditional office-based treatment settings. While there is a need for evidence-based mobile applications, the dearth of tested and validated apps compared to the wide availability of commercial apps necessitates greater public education, development, and research (Donker et al., 2013).

The application of digital technologies to health care must also be accompanied by attention to information security and federal HIPAA (Health Insurance Portability and Accountability Act, 1996) laws that protect personal health information. Additionally, the potential adverse mental health consequences of an online health ecosystem include cyberbullying (Hamm et al., 2015; Selkie, Fales, & Moreno, 2015), emotional contagion (Kramer et al., 2014), and pathological internet use (Hanprathet, Manwong, Khumsri, Yingyeun, & Phanasathit, 2015). Although phenomena such as cyberbullying represent novel exposures that can be widespread, there is no evidence of a direct relationship between depression and social media at the population level (Davila et al., 2012; Jelenchick, Eickhoff, & Moreno, 2013). The economic benefits of expanding health technology resources presents an enormous cost-saving potential by increasing efficiency in care delivery and reducing clinician and staff time involved in direct treatment. Online and mobile applications may have relatively high start-up costs, but they can be used by large numbers of people at an extremely low marginal cost per user (American Hospital Association, 2012). While larger efficacy and effectiveness trials are mostly lacking in this area, several efforts have demonstrated cost-effectiveness (e.g., Choi Yoo, Nyman, Cheville, & Kroenke, 2014; van Spijker, Majo, Smit, van Straten, & Kerkhof, 2012). One perceived barrier to the use of technology-based tools is the lack of a reimbursement model to cover a mental health care provider's time when engaged in therapeutic activities beyond the traditional office visit. However, recent policy changes are enhancing reimbursement for telehealth and digital communication between providers and patients. The Centers for Medicare and Medicaid have recently expanded coverage for telehealth with new treatment codes (Centers for Medicare and Medicaid Services, 2015) and increased reimbursement payments (Wicklund, 2014).

Going forward, the use and integration of digital health technologies for mental health practice, at both the individual and population levels, offer potentially much wider access to preventive and therapeutic interventions than through traditional office-based care, providing much-needed opportunities to reduce the heavy burden of mental disorders worldwide.

References

Aguilera, A., Schueller, S. M., & Leykin, Y. (2015). Daily mood ratings via text message as a proxy for clinic based depression assessment. *Journal of Affective Disorders, 175,* 471–474.

Ahuja, A. K., Biesaga, K., Sudak, D. M., Draper, J., & Womble, A. (2014). Suicide on Facebook. *Journal of Psychiatric Practice, 20*(2), 141–146.

American Hospital Association. (2012). *Trendwatch: Bringing behavioral health into the care continuum: Opportunities to improve quality, costs and outcomes.* Washington, DC: American Hospital Association.

American Telemedicine Association. (2015). *What is telemedicine?* Retrieved from http://www .americantelemed.org/about/about-telemedicine

Anderson, M. (2015). *Technology device ownership: 2015*. Washington, DC: Pew Research Center.

Anderson, M., & Perrin, A. (2015). *15% of Americans don't use the internet. Who are they?* Washington, DC: Pew Research Center.

Andersson, G., & Cuijpers, P. (2009). Internet-based and other computerized psychological treatments for adult depression: A meta-analysis. *Cognitive Behaviour Therapy, 38*(4), 196–205.

Andrews, G., Cuijpers, P., Craske, M. G., McEvoy, P., & Titov, N. (2010). Computer therapy for the anxiety and depressive disorders is effective, acceptable and practical health care: A meta-analysis. *PloS One, 5*(10), e13196.

Angus, D. C. (2015). Fusing randomized trials with big data: The key to self-learning health care systems? *JAMA, 314*(8), 767–768.

Atherton, J. (2011). Development of the electronic health record. *AMA Journal of Ethics, 13*(3), 186–189.

Atkinson, N. L., Saperstein, S. L., & Pleis, J. (2009). Using the internet for health-related activities: Findings from a national probability sample. *Journal of Medical Internet Research, 11*, e4.

Barak, A., & Gluck-Ofri, O. (2007). Degree and reciprocity of self-disclosure in online forums. *Cyberpsychology and Behavior, 10*(3), 407–417.

Bartlett, J., & Reynolds, L. (2015). *The state of the art 2015: A literature review of social media intelligence capabilities for counterterrorism*. London, England: Demos.

Beck, A. T., Steer, R. A., & Ranieri, W. F. (1988). Scale for suicide ideation: Psychometric properties of a self-report version. *Journal of Clinical Psychology, 44*(4), 499–505.

Becker, S., Miron-Shatz, T., Schumacher, N., Krocza, J., Diamantidis, C., & Albrecht, U. V. (2014). mHealth 2.0: Experiences, possibilities, and perspectives. *JMIR mHealth and uHealth, 2*(2), e24.

BinDhim, N. F., Shaman, A. M., Trevena, L., Basyouni, M. H., Pont, L. G., & Alhawassi, T. M. (2015). Depression screening via a smartphone app: Cross-country user characteristics and feasibility. *Journal of the American Medical Informatics Association: JAMIA, 22*(1), 29–34.

Birney, A. J., Gunn, R., Russell, J. K., & Ary, D. V. (2016). MoodHacker mobile web app with email for adults to self-manage mild-to-moderate depression: Randomized controlled trial. *JMIR Mhealth Uhealth, 4*(1), e8. doi:10.2196/mhealth.4231

Bort-Roig, J., Gilson, N. D., Puig-Ribera, A., Contreras, R. S., & Trost, S. G. (2014). Measuring and influencing physical activity with smartphone technology: A systematic review. *Sports Medicine (Auckland, N.Z.), 44*(5), 671–686.

Broniatowski, D. A., Paul, M. J., & Dredze, M. (2013). National and local influenza surveillance through Twitter: An analysis of the 2012–2013 influenza epidemic. *PloS One, 8*(12), e83672.

Brown, H. E., Pearson, N., Braithwaite, R. E., Brown, W. J., & Biddle, S. J. (2013). Physical activity interventions and depression in children and adolescents: A systematic review and meta-analysis. *Sports Medicine (Auckland, N.Z.), 43*(3), 195–206.

Buehler, J. W. (2004). Review of the 2003 National Syndromic Surveillance conference: Lessons learned and questions to be answered. *Centers for Disease Control and Prevention: Morbidity and Mortality Weekly Report, 53 Suppl*, 18–22.

Burns, J. M., Durkin, L. A., & Nicholas, J. (2009). Mental health of young people in the United States: What role can the internet play in reducing stigma and promoting help seeking? *Journal of Adolescent Health, 45*(1), 95–97.

Bush, N. E., Ouellette, G., & Kinn, J. (2014). Utility of the T2 mood tracker mobile application among army warrior transition unit service members. *Military Medicine, 179*(12), 1453–1457.

Butler, T. N., & Yellowlees, P. (2012). Cost analysis of store-and-forward telepsychiatry as a consultation model for primary care. *Telemedicine Journal and E-Health, 18*(1), 74–77.

Cape, J., & McCulloch, Y. (1999). Patients' reasons for not presenting emotional problems in general practice consultations. *British Journal of General Practice, 49*(448), 875–879.

Cavazos-Rehg, P. A., Krauss, M. J., Sowles, S., Connolly, S., Rosas, C., Bharadwaj, M., & Bierut, L. J. (2016). A content analysis of depression-related tweets. *Computers in Human Behavior, 54*, 351–357.

Centers for Medicare and Medicaid Services. (2015). *Telemedicine*. Retrieved from http://www.medicaid.gov/Medicaid-CHIP-Program-Information/By-Topics/Delivery-Systems/Telemedicine.html

Chan, S., Parish, M., & Yellowlees, P. (2015). Telepsychiatry today. *Current Psychiatry Reports, 17*(11), 89.

Charman, D., Harms, C., & Myles-Pallister, J. (2010). Help and e-help: Young people's perspectives of mental healthcare. *Australian Family Physician, 39*(9), 663–665.

Chaudhry, B., Wang, J., Wu, S., Maglione, M., Mojica, W., Roth, E., . . . Shekelle, P. G. (2006). Systematic review: Impact of health information technology on quality, efficiency, and costs of medical care. *Annals of Internal Medicine, 144*(10), 742–752.

Cheek, C., Fleming, T., Lucassen, M. F., Bridgman, H., Stasiak, K., Shepherd, M., & Orpin, P. (2015). Integrating health behavior theory and design elements in serious games. *JMIR Mental Health, 2*(2), e11.

Choi, A., Lovett, A. W., Kang, J., Lee, K., & Choi, L. (2015). Mobile applications to improve medication adherence: Existing apps, quality of life and future directions. *Advances in Pharmacology and Pharmacy, 3*(3), 64–74.

Choi Yoo, S. J., Nyman, J. A., Cheville, A. L., & Kroenke, K. (2014). Cost effectiveness of telecare management for pain and depression in patients with cancer: Results from a randomized trial. *General Hospital Psychiatry, 36*(6), 599–606.

Christensen, H., Batterham, P. J., & O'Dea, B. (2014). E-health interventions for suicide prevention. *International Journal of Environmental Research and Public Health, 11*(8), 8193–8212.

Cifuentes, M., Davis, M., Fernald, D., Gunn, R., Dickinson, P., & Cohen, D. J. (2015). Electronic health record challenges, workarounds, and solutions observed in practices integrating behavioral health and primary care. *Journal of the American Board of Family Medicine, 28 Suppl 1*, S63–S72.

Cohen, N., & Galea, S. (Eds.). (2011). *Population mental health: Evidence, policy, and public health practice*. New York, NY: Routledge.

Coppersmith, G. (2015). *[Un]shared task: Computational linguistics and clinical psychology 2015*. Baltimore, MD: Human Language Technology Center of Excellence.

Coppersmith, G., Dredze, M., & Harman, C. (2014). Quantifying mental health signals in Twitter. *Association for Computational Linguistics Workshop on Computational Linguistics and Clinical Psychology [ACL2014]*. Cambridge, MA.

Corrigan, P. W., Druss, B. G., & Perlick, D. A. (2014). The impact of mental illness stigma on seeking and participating in mental health care. *Psychological Science in the Public Interest, 15*(2), 37–70.

Coyle, D., Doherty, G., & Sharry, J. (2009). An evaluation of a solution focused computer game in adolescent interventions. *Clinical Child Psychology and Psychiatry, 14*(3), 345–360.

Davila, J., Hershenberg, R., Feinstein, B. A., Gorman, K., Bhatia, V., & Starr, L. R. (2012). Frequency and quality of social networking among young adults: Associations with depressive symptoms, rumination, and corumination. *Psychology of Popular Media Culture, 1*(2), 72–86.

Dayer, L., Heldenbrand, S., Anderson, P., Gubbins, P. O., & Martin, B. C. (2013). Smartphone medication adherence apps: Potential benefits to patients and providers. *Journal of the American Pharmacists Association, 53*(2), 172–181.

De Choudhury, M., Counts, S., & Horvitz, E. (2013). Social media as a measurement tool of depression in populations. *WebSci '13. Proceedings of the 5th Annual ACM Web Science Conference.* New York, NY. 47–56.

De Choudhury, M., Gamon, M., Counts, S., & Horvitz, E. (2013). Predicting depression via social media. *International Conference on Web an Social Media, Association for the Advancement of Artificial Intelligence.* Cambridge, MA.

Deen, T. L., Godleski, L., & Fortney, J. C. (2012). A description of telemental health services provided by the Veterans Health Administration in 2006–2010. *Psychiatric Services, 63*(11), 1131–1133.

Donker, T., Petrie, K., Proudfoot, J., Clarke, J., Birch, M. R., & Christensen, H. (2013). Smartphones for smarter delivery of mental health programs: A systematic review. *Journal of Medical Internet Research, 15*(11), e247.

Duggan, M., Ellison, N., Lampe, C., Lenhart, A., & Madden, M. (2015, January 9). *Frequency of media use.* Washington, DC: Pew Internet and American Life Project. http://www.pewinternet.org/2015/01/09/frequency-of-social-media-use-2/

Elhai, J. D., & Frueh, B. C. (2015). Security of electronic mental health communication and record-keeping in the digital age. *Journal of Clinical Psychiatry, 77*(2), 262–268.

Eysenbach, G. (2009). Infodemiology and infoveillance: Framework for an emerging set of public health informatics methods to analyze search, communication and publication behavior on the internet. *Journal of Medical Internet Research, 11*(1), e11.

Facebook. (2016). *Company info.* Retrieved from http://newsroom.fb.com/company-info/

Farley, T. A., & Weisfuse, I. (2011). Redefining of public health preparedness after 9/11. *The Lancet, 378*(9794), 957–959.

Felder, J., Dimidjian, S., Beck, A., Boggs, J. M., & Segal, Z. (2014). Mindful mood balance: A case report of web-based treatment of residual depressive symptoms. *The Permanente Journal, 18*(4), 58–62.

Foldy, S. L. (2004). Linking better surveillance to better outcomes. *MMWR: Morbidity and Mortality Weekly Report, 53 Suppl*, 12–17.

Foroushani, P. S., Schneider, J., & Assareh, N. (2011). Meta-review of the effectiveness of computerised CBT in treating depression. *BMC Psychiatry, 11*, 131.

Fortney, J. C., Pyne, J. M., Mouden, S. B., Mittal, D., Hudson, T. J., Schroeder, G. W., . . . Rost, K. M. (2013). Practice-based versus telemedicine-based collaborative care for depression in rural federally qualified health centers: A pragmatic randomized comparative effectiveness trial. *American Journal of Psychiatry, 170*(4), 414–425.

Garlow, S. J., Rosenberg, J., Moore, J. D., Haas, A. P., Koestner, B., Hendin, H., & Nemeroff, C. B. (2008). Depression, desperation, and suicidal ideation in college students: Results from the American Foundation for Suicide Prevention college screening project at Emory University. *Depression and Anxiety, 25*(6), 482–488.

Gawande, A., & Brenner, J. (2011). Doctor hotspot. Retrieved from http://www.pbs.org/wgbh /pages/frontline/doctor-hotspot/#4

Godleski, L., Darkins, A., & Peters, J. (2012). Outcomes of 98,609 US Department of Veterans Affairs patients enrolled in telemental health services, 2006–2010. *Psychiatric Services, 63*(4), 383–385.

Google Research Blog. (2015). *The next chapter for flu trends.* Retrieved from http:// googleresearch.blogspot.com/2015/08/the-next-chapter-for-flu-trends.html

Haas, A., Koestner, B., Rosenberg, J., Moore, D., Garlow, S. J., Sedway, J., . . . Nemeroff, C. B. (2008). An interactive web-based method of outreach to college students at risk for suicide. *Journal of American College Health, 57*(1), 15–22.

Hamm, M. P., Newton, A. S., Chisholm, A., Shulhan, J., Milne, A., Sundar, P., . . . Hartling, L. (2015). Prevalence and effect of cyberbullying on children and young people: A scoping review of social media studies. *JAMA Pediatrics, 169*(8), 770–777.

Hammonds, T., Rickert, K., Goldstein, C., Gathright, E., Gilmore, S., Derflinger, B., . . . Hughes, J. W. (2015). Adherence to antidepressant medications: A randomized controlled trial of medication reminding in college students. *Journal of American College Health, 63*(3), 204–208.

Hanprathet, N., Manwong, M., Khumsri, J., Yingyeun, R., & Phanasathit, M. (2015). Facebook addiction and its relationship with mental health among Thai high school students. *Journal of the Medical Association of Thailand = Chotmaihet Thangphaet, 98*(Suppl 3), S81–S90.

Harlow, S., & Guo, L. (2014). Will the revolution be tweeted or Facebooked? Using digital communication tools in immigrant activism. *Journal of Computer-Mediated Communication, 19*, 463–478.

Health Insurance Portability and Accountability Act of 1996, Pub. L. No. 104-191.

Helbing, D. (2014). *What the digital revolution means for us.* Retrieved from http://www .sciencebusiness.net/news/76591/What-the-digital-revolution-means-for-us

Herzlinger, R. E. (2006). Why innovation in health care is so hard. *Harvard Business Review.* Retrieved from https://hbr.org/2006/05/why-innovation-in-health-care-is-so-hard

Hill, K. (2014). Facebook manipulated 689,003 users' emotions for science. *Forbes.* Retrieved from http://www.forbes.com/sites/kashmirhill/2014/06/28/facebook-manipulated-689003 -users-emotions-for-science/

Hilty, D. M., Ferrer, D. C., Parish, M. B., Johnston, B., Callahan, E. J., & Yellowlees, P. M. (2013). The effectiveness of telemental health: A 2013 review. *Telemedicine Journal and E-Health, 19*(6), 444–454.

Houston, T. K., Cooper, L. A., Vu, H. T., Kahn, J., Toser, J., & Ford, D. E. (2001). Screening the public for depression through the internet. *Psychiatric Services, 52*(3), 362–367.

Hsiao, C., & Hing, E. (2014). *Use and characteristics of electronic health record systems among office-based physician practices: United Sates, 2001–2013* (NCHS Data Brief No. 143). Atlanta, GA: US Department of Health and Human Services, Centers for Disease Control and Prevention.

Hudson, T. J., Fortney, J. C., Pyne, J. M., Lu, L., & Mittal, D. (2015). Reduction of patient-reported antidepressant side effects, by type of collaborative care. *Psychiatric Services, 66*(3), 272–278.

Hwang, J., & Christensen, C. M. (2008). Disruptive innovation in health care delivery: A framework for business-model innovation. *Health Affairs, 27*(5), 1329–1335.

ICT Data and Statistics Division. (2014). *The world in 2014: ICT facts and figures.* Geneva, Switzerland: International Telecommunication Union.

ICT Data and Statistics Division. (2015). *The world in 2015: ICT facts and figures.* Geneva, Switzerland: International Telecommunication Union.

Instagram. (2016a). *Statistics.* Retrieved from https://www.instagram.com/press/?hl=en

Instagram. (2016b). *Instagram, LLC (version 9.7)* [Mobile application software]. Retrieved from http://itunes.apple.com

Intille, S. S. (2007). Technological innovations enabling automatic, context sensitive ecological momentary assessment. In A. Stone, S. Shiffinan, A. Atienza, & L. Nebeling (Eds.), *The science of real-time data capture: Self-reports in health research* (pp. 308–337). Oxford: Oxford University Press.

Jashinsky, J., Burton, S. H., Hanson, C. L., West, J., Giraud-Carrier, C., Barnes, M. D., & Argyle, T. (2014). Tracking suicide risk factors through Twitter in the US. *Crisis, 35*(1), 51–59.

Jelenchick, L. A., Eickhoff, J. C., & Moreno, M. A. (2013). "Facebook depression?" Social networking site use and depression in older adolescents. *Journal of Adolescent Health, 52*(1), 128–130.

Jenssen, B. P., Mitra, N., Shah, A., Wan, F., & Grande, D. (2015, September). Using digital technology to engage and communicate with patients: A survey of patient attitudes. *Journal of General Internal Medicine, 31*(1), 85–92.

Jimenez, J. (2013). *T2Mood tracker mobile app adds new features* (Press Release). Joint Base Lewis-McChord. Washington, DC: National Center for Telehealth and Technology.

Josefsson, T., Lindwall, M., & Archer, T. (2014). Physical exercise intervention in depressive disorders: Meta-analysis and systematic review. *Scandinavian Journal of Medicine and Science in Sports, 24*(2), 259–272.

Juengst, S. B., Graham, K. M., Pulantara, I. W., McCue, M., Whyte, E. M., Dicianno, B. E., . . . Wagner, A. K. (2015). Pilot feasibility of an mHealth system for conducting ecological momentary assessment of mood-related symptoms following traumatic brain injury. *Brain Injury, 29*(11), 1351–1361.

Kaltenthaler, E., Brazier, J., De Nigris, E., Tumur, I., Ferriter, M., Beverley, C., . . . Sutcliffe, P. (2006). Computerised cognitive behaviour therapy for depression and anxiety update: A systematic review and economic evaluation. *Health Technology Assessment, 10*(33), iii, xi–xiv, 1–168.

Kaltenthaler, E., & Cavanagh, K. (2010). Computerised cognitive behavioural therapy and its uses. *Progress in Neurology and Psychiatry, 14*(3), 22–29.

Karmen, C., Hsiung, R. C., & Wetter, T. (2015). Screening internet forum participants for depression symptoms by assembling and enhancing multiple NLP methods. *Computer Methods and Programs in Biomedicine, 120*(1), 27–36.

Keding, A., Bohnke, J. R., Croudace, T. J., Richmond, S. J., & MacPherson, H. (2015). Validity of single item responses to short message service texts to monitor depression: An mHealth sub-study of the UK ACUDep trial. *BMC Medical Research Methodology, 15*, 56.

Keller, M. B., Klerman, G. L., Lavori, P. W., Coryell, W., Endicott, J., & Taylor, J. (1984). Long-term outcome of episodes of major depression: Clinical and public health significance. *JAMA, 252*(6), 788–792.

Kennard, B. D., Emslie, G. J., Mayes, T. L., & Hughes, J. L. (2006). Relapse and recurrence in pediatric depression. *Child and Adolescent Psychiatric Clinics of North America, 15*(4), 1057–1079, xi.

Kessler, R. C., Avenevoli, S., Costello, E. J., Georgiades, K., Green, J. G., Gruber, M. J., . . . Merikangas, K. R. (2012). Prevalence, persistence, and sociodemographic correlates of *DSM-IV* disorders in the National Comorbidity Survey Replication Adolescent Supplement. *Archives of General Psychiatry, 69*(4), 372–380.

Khanna, M. S., & Kendall, P. C. (2010). Computer-assisted cognitive behavioral therapy for child anxiety: Results of a randomized clinical trial. *Journal of Consulting and Clinical Psychology, 78*(5), 737–745.

Klein, S., Hostetter, M., & McCarthy, D. (2014). *A vision for using digital health technologies to empower consumers and transform the US health care system*. Washington, DC: The Commonwealth Fund.

Knox, M., Lentini, J., Cummings, T., McGrady, A., Whearty, K., & Sancrant, L. (2011). Game-based biofeedback for paediatric anxiety and depression. *Mental Health in Family Medicine, 8*(3), 195–203.

Kobak, K. A., Mundt, J. C., & Kennard, B. (2015). Integrating technology into cognitive behavior therapy for adolescent depression: A pilot study. *Annals of General Psychiatry, 14*, 37-015-0077-8.

Kramer, A. D., Guillory, J. E., & Hancock, J. T. (2014). Experimental evidence of massive-scale emotional contagion through social networks. *Proceedings of the National Academy of Sciences of the United States of America, 111*(24), 8788–8790.

Krebs, P., & Duncan, D. T. (2015). Health app use among US mobile phone owners: A national survey. *JMIR mHealth and uHealth, 3*(4), e101.

Krieger, T., Meyer, B., Sude, K., Urech, A., Maercker, A., & Berger, T. (2014). Evaluating an e-mental health program ("deprexis") as adjunctive treatment tool in psychotherapy for depression: Design of a pragmatic randomized controlled trial. *BMC Psychiatry, 14*, 285.

Lenhart, A. (2015). *Teens, social media and technology overview 2015*. Washington, DC: Pew Research Center.

Lenhart, A., Kahne, J., Middaugh, E., Macgil, A., Evans, C., & Vitak, J. (2008). *Teens, video games and civics*. Washington, DC: Pew Research Center.

Leykin, Y., Munoz, R. F., & Contreras, O. (2012). Are consumers of internet health information "cyberchondriacs"? Characteristics of 24,965 users of a depression screening site. *Depression and Anxiety, 29*(1), 71–77.

Luxton, D. D., June, J. D., & Fairall, J. M. (2012). Social media and suicide: A public health perspective. *American Journal of Public Health, 102*(Suppl 2), S195–S200.

Merry, S. N., Stasiak, K., Shepherd, M., Frampton, C., Fleming, T., & Lucassen, M. F. (2012). The effectiveness of SPARX, a computerised self help intervention for adolescents seeking help for depression: Randomised controlled non-inferiority trial. *BMJ (Clinical Research Ed.), 344*, e2598.

Moreno, M. A., Christakis, D. A., Egan, K. G., Jelenchick, L. A., Cox, E., Young, H., . . . Becker, T. (2012). A pilot evaluation of associations between displayed depression references on Facebook and self-reported depression using a clinical scale. *Journal of Behavioral Health Services and Research, 39*(3), 295–304.

Moreno, M. A., Jelenchick, L. A., Egan, K. G., Cox, E., Young, H., Gannon, K. E., & Becker, T. (2011). Feeling bad on Facebook: Depression disclosures by college students on a social networking site. *Depression and Anxiety, 28*(6), 447–455.

Morris, R. R., Schueller, S. M., & Picard, R. W. (2015). Efficacy of a web-based, crowdsourced peer-to-peer cognitive reappraisal platform for depression: Randomized controlled trial. *Journal of Medical Internet Research, 17*(3), e72.

Mota Pereira, J. (2014). Facebook enhances antidepressant pharmacotherapy effects. *Scientific World Journal, 2014*, 892048. Retrieved from https://www.hindawi.com/journals/tswj/2014/892048/

Moutier, C., Norcross, W., Jong, P., Norman, M., Kirby, B., McGuire, T., & Zisook, S. (2012). The suicide prevention and depression awareness program at the University of California, San Diego School of Medicine. *Academic Medicine, 87*(3), 320–326.

Muntaner, A., Vidal-Conti, J., & Palou, P. (2015, February 3). Increasing physical activity through mobile device interventions: A systematic review. *Health Informatics Journal*. pii:1460458214567004.

Nielson. (2014). *Multi-platform gaming: For the win!* New York, NY: The Nielsen Company.

Park, S., Lee, S. W., Kwak, J., Cha, M., & Jeong, B. (2013). Activities on Facebook reveal the depressive state of users. *Journal of Medical Internet Research, 15*(10), e217.

Patwardhan, A., & Bilkovski, R. (2012). Comparison: Flu prescription sales data from a retail pharmacy in the US with Google flu trends and US ILINet (CDC) data as flu activity indicator. *PloS One, 7*(8), e43611.

Paul, M. J., Dredze, M., & Broniatowski, D. (2014). Twitter improves influenza forecasting. *PLoS Currents, 6*, 10.1371.

Paul, M. M., Greene, C. M., Newton-Dame, R., Thorpe, L. E., Perlman, S. E., McVeigh, K. H., & Gourevitch, M. N. (2015). The state of population health surveillance using electronic health records: A narrative review. *Population Health Management, 18*(3), 209–216.

Perrin, A. (2015). *Social media usage: 2005–2015*. Washington, DC: Pew Research Center.

Perrin, A., & Duggan, M. (2015). *Americans' internet access: 2000–2015*. Washington, DC: Pew Research Center.

Pew Research Center. (2014). *Emerging nations embrace internet, mobile technology*. Washington, DC: Pew Research Center.

Pew Research Center. (2015). *Health fact sheet*. (Fact Sheet). Washington, DC: Pew Research Center.

Pollak, J. P., Adams, P., & Gay, G. (2011). PAM: A photographic affect meter for frequent, in situ measurement of affect. *Proceedings of CHI 2011*, 725–734.

Purcell, K., Heaps, A., Buchanan, J., & Friedrich, L. (2013). *How teachers are using technology at home and in their classrooms*. Washington, DC: Pew Research Center.

Reeves, W. C., Strine, T. W., Pratt, L. A., Thompson, W., Ahluwalia, I., Dhingra, S. S., . . . Safran, M. A. (2011). *Mental illness surveillance among adults in the United States*. (Morbidity and Mortality Weekly Report No. 60). Atlanta, GA: Centers for Disease Control and Prevention.

Renton, T., Tang, H., Ennis, N., Cusimano, M. D., Bhalerao, S., Schweizer, T. A., & Topolovec-Vranic, J. (2014). Web-based intervention programs for depression: A scoping review and evaluation. *Journal of Medical Internet Research, 16*, e209.

Rhyner, K. T., & Watts, A. (2015, September 15). Exercise and depressive symptoms in older adults: A systematic meta-analytic review. *Journal of Aging and Physical Activity, 24*(2). doi:10.1123/japa.2015-0146

Rice, S. M., Goodall, J., Hetrick, S. E., Parker, A. G., Gilbertson, T., Amminger, G. P., . . . Alvarez-Jimenez, M. (2014). Online and social networking interventions for the treatment of depression in young people: A systematic review. *Journal of Medical Internet Research, 16*(9), e206.

Rivera, J., & van der Meulen, R. (2014). *Gartner says more than a third of US adult smartphone users use their smartphones for video calling.* (Press Release). Stamford, CT: Gartner, Inc.

Rogers, V. L., Griffin, M. Q., Wykle, M. L., & Fitzpatrick, J. J. (2009). Internet versus face-to-face therapy: Emotional self-disclosure issues for young adults. *Issues in Mental Health Nursing, 30*(10), 596–602.

Rosenbaum, S., Tiedemann, A., Sherrington, C., Curtis, J., & Ward, P. B. (2014). Physical activity interventions for people with mental illness: A systematic review and meta-analysis. *Journal of Clinical Psychiatry, 75*(9), 964–974.

Saeb, S., Zhang, M., Karr, C. J., Schueller, S. M., Corden, M. E., Kording, K. P., & Mohr, D. C. (2015). Mobile phone sensor correlates of depressive symptom severity in daily-life behavior: An exploratory study. *Journal of Medical Internet Research, 17*(7), e175.

Samson, R., Mehta, M., & Chandani, A. (2014). Impact of online digital communication on customer buying decision. *Procedia Economics and Finance, 11*, 872–880.

Selkie, E. M., Fales, J. L., & Moreno, M. A. (2015). Cyberbullying prevalence among US middle and high school–aged adolescents: A systematic review and quality assessment. *Journal of Adolescent Health, 58*(2), 125–133.

Shen, N., Levitan, M. J., Johnson, A., Bender, J. L., Hamilton-Page, M., Jadad, A. A., & Wiljer, D. (2015). Finding a depression app: A review and content analysis of the depression app marketplace. *MJIR Mhealth Uhealth, 3*, e16.

Shepherd, A., Sanders, C., Doyle, M., & Shaw, J. (2015). Using social media for support and feedback by mental health service users: Thematic analysis of a Twitter conversation. *BMC Psychiatry, 15*, 29.

Shu, C. (2014). Every fitness app and wearable should have a mood tracker. Retrieved from http://techcrunch.com/2014/04/27/every-fitness-app-and-wearable-should-have-a-mood -tracker/

Silveira, H., Moraes, H., Oliveira, N., Coutinho, E. S., Laks, J., & Deslandes, A. (2013). Physical exercise and clinically depressed patients: A systematic review and meta-analysis. *Neuropsychobiology, 67*(2), 61–68.

Spek, V., Cuijpers, P., Nyklicek, I., Riper, H., Keyzer, J., & Pop, V. (2007). Internet-based cognitive behaviour therapy for symptoms of depression and anxiety: A meta-analysis. *Psychological Medicine, 37*(3), 319–328.

Stanton, R., & Reaburn, P. (2014). Exercise and the treatment of depression: A review of the exercise program variables. *Journal of Science and Medicine in Sport/Sports Medicine Australia, 17*(2), 177–182.

Sueki, H. (2015). The association of suicide-related Twitter use with suicidal behaviour: A cross-sectional study of young internet users in Japan. *Journal of Affective Disorders, 170*, 155–160.

Swinton, J. J., Robinson, W. D., & Bischoff, R. J. (2009). Telehealth and rural depression: Physician and patient perspectives. *Family System Health, 27*(2), 172–182.

Tomita, A., Kandolo, K. M., Susser, E., & Burns, J. K. (2015, September 24). Use of short messaging services to assess depressive symptoms among refugees in South Africa: Implications for social services providing mental health care in resource-poor settings. *Journal of Telemedicine and Telecare.* doi:10.1177/1357633X15605406.

Toumache, R., Rouaski, K., Talbi, B., & Djelloul, B. (2014). The impact of the information and communication technology (ICT) on economic growth: Statistical econometric approach. *Business and Management Review, 5*(1), 256.

Trottier, D. (2012). Interpersonal surveillance on social media. *Canadian Journal of Communication, 37*(2), 319–332.

Trottier, D. (2013). The business of conversations: Market social media surveillance and visibility. *First Monday, 18*(2). Retrieved from http://journals.uic.edu/ojs/index.php/fm/article/view/3930/3413

Twitter. (2016). Twitter usage / company facts. Retrieved from https://about.twitter.com/company

US Department of Health and Human Services. (2014). *Using health text messages to improve consumer health knowledge, behaviors, and outcomes: An environmental scan.* Rockville, MD: US Department of Health and Human Services.

van den Berg, N., Grabe, H. J., Baumeister, S. E., Freyberger, H. J., & Hoffmann, W. (2015). A telephone- and text message–based telemedicine concept for patients with mental health disorders: Results of a randomized controlled trial. *Psychotherapy and Psychosomatics, 84*(2), 82–89.

van Spijker, B. A., Majo, M. C., Smit, F., van Straten, A., & Kerkhof, A. J. (2012). Reducing suicidal ideation: Cost-effectiveness analysis of a randomized controlled trial of unguided web-based self-help. *Journal of Medical Internet Research, 14*(5), e141.

van Spijker, B. A., van Straten, A., & Kerkhof, A. J. (2014). Effectiveness of online self-help for suicidal thoughts: Results of a randomised controlled trial. *PloS One, 9*(2), e90118.

Vervloet, M., Linn, A. J., van Weert, J. C., de Bakker, D. H., Bouvy, M. L., & van Dijk, L. (2012). The effectiveness of interventions using electronic reminders to improve adherence to chronic medication: A systematic review of the literature. *Journal of the American Medical Informatics Association, 19*(5), 696–704.

Whitton, A. E., Proudfoot, J., Clarke, J., Birch, M. R., Parker, G., Manicavasagar, V., & Hadzi-Pavlovic, D. (2015). Breaking open the black box: Isolating the most potent features of a web- and mobile phone–based intervention for depression, anxiety, and stress. *JMIR Mental Health, 2*(1), e3.

Wicklund, E. (2014). *CMS boosts telehealth in 2015 physician pay schedule.* Retrieved from http://www.mhealthnews.com/news/cms-boosts-telehealth-2015-physician-pay-schedule

Yellowlees, P., Odor, A., Patrice, K., Parish, M. B., Nafiz, N., Iosif, A. M., & Hilty, D. (2011). Disruptive innovation: The future of healthcare? *Telemedicine Journal and E-Health, 17*(3), 231–234.

Yin, Z., Fabbri, D., Rosenbloom, S. T., & Malin, B. (2015). A scalable framework to detect personal health mentions on Twitter. *Journal of Medical Internet Research, 17*(6), e138.

YouTube (2016). *Statistics.* Retrieved from https://www.youtube.com/yt/press/statistics.html

CHAPTER 18

Preventing the Onset of Depressive Disorders
An Overview

Pim Cuijpers, PhD

Preventing the onset of depressive disorders has long been considered to be impossible, because the causes and etiology of these disorders are too complex and not yet well understood. Over the past two decades, however, a growing number of randomized controlled trials have shown that it is in some cases possible to prevent or at least delay the onset of depressive disorders. Psychosocial preventive interventions, typically based on psychological treatments such as cognitive behavioral therapy (CBT) or interpersonal psychotherapy (IPT), have been tested in at-risk populations and in people with subthreshold depression who do not meet diagnostic criteria for a depressive disorder. These interventions appeared in several studies to be effective in reducing the incidence of new cases of depressive disorders at follow-up (Van Zoonen et al., 2014).

In this chapter, I give an overview of the field of prevention of depressive disorders. I first give arguments why prevention of depression is important, describe methods to identify the most optimal target groups for prevention, and then describe the different subfields of preventive interventions, including adolescents, prevention of postpartum depression, prevention of depression in patients with comorbid somatic disorders, and prevention in older adults.

Most researchers and practitioners have defined prevention as those interventions that are conducted before people meet the formal criteria of a depressive disorder according to the *DSM-IV* (Mrazek & Haggerty, 1994; O'Connell, Boat, & Warner, 2009). Acute and maintenance treatment are aimed at people who have established disorders meeting diagnostic criteria. Three types of prevention can be discerned: universal prevention, which is aimed at the general population or parts of the general population, regardless of whether they have a higher-than-average risk of developing a disorder (e.g., school programs or mass media campaigns); selective prevention, which is aimed at high-risk groups who have not yet developed a mental disorder; and indicated prevention, which is aimed at individuals who have some symptoms of a mental disorder but do not meet diagnostic criteria.

Why Is Prevention of Depression Important?

Prevention of depression is important for several reasons. First, depressive disorders are highly prevalent (Alonso et al., 2004; Kessler et al., 1994) and have a high incidence (Waraich, Goldner, Somers, & Hsu, 2004), and they are associated with a substantial loss of quality of life for patients and their relatives (Saarni et al. 2007; Ustün, Ayuso-Mateos, Chatterji, Mathers, & Murray, 2004), increased mortality rates (Cuijpers, Vogelzangs, Twisk, Kleiboer, Li, & Penninx, 2014), high levels of service use, and enormous economic costs (Greenberg & Birnbaum 2005; Smit et al., 2006a). Major depression is currently ranked fourth worldwide in disease burden, and it is expected to rank first in disease burden in high-income countries by the year 2030 (Mathers & Loncar, 2006).

Prevention is also important because current treatments can reduce the disease burden of depression only to a limited extent. A modeling study in Australia estimated that current treatments can reduce the disease burden of depression by only 34%, and that is in optimal conditions with 100% of all depressed patients receiving an evidence-based treatment. When the actual numbers of patients who receive an evidence-based treatment are used in the model, only 16% of the disease burden is reduced. So, although current treatments are usually considered to be effective in treating depressive disorders, it is estimated that these treatments can reduce the disease burden of depression by a maximum of 34% (Andrews, Issakidis, Sanderson, Corry, & Lapsley, 2004). Although these figures are calculated for the current situation in Australia, it is not expected that the situation in other Western countries will differ very much, as is evidenced by yet another modeling study (Chisholm, Sanderson, Ayoso-Mateos, & Saena, 2004). Furthermore, more than 40% of the patients do not respond or only partially respond to treatment and less than 33% of patients completely recover after treatment (Hollon, 2002). In addition, relapse rates are very high, with 29% relapse in one year, 48% in two years, and up to 85% within five years after recovery from an initial episode (Vittengl, Clark, Dunn, & Jarrett, 2007).

Prevention of the incidence of new cases of major depression has been suggested as an alternative for treatment that may reduce a part of the 66% of the disease burden that is not averted by current treatments (Cuijpers, van Straten, Smit, Mihalopoulos, & Beekman, 2008; Smit, Ederveen, Cuijpers, Deeg, & Beekman, 2006b; Van Zoonen et al., 2014).

Is Prevention of Depression Possible?

Over the past few decades, hundreds of controlled studies have examined the effects of mental health programs aimed at preventing mental health problems at school (Durlak & Wells, 1997, 1998), work-related stress (Ruotsalainen, Serra, Marine, & Verbeek, 2008; Tan et al., 2014; Van der Klink, Blonk, & van Dijk, 2001), distress among caregivers for the elderly (Chien et al., 2011), and many other conditions (O'Connell et al., 2009). This considerable body of research has shown that some prevention programs in mental health are capable of strengthening protective factors such as social skills, problem-solving skills, stress-management skills, prosocial behavior, and social support; reducing the consequences of risk factors and psychiatric symptoms; and having positive economic effects. Despite this large body of research, few studies have examined whether these prevention programs are actually capable of reducing the incidence of new cases of major depression or other mental disorders defined according to diagnostic criteria.

In the past 20 years, however, the number of studies examining the effects of preventive interventions on the incidence of new cases of depressive disorders has increased considerably. After the first studies were conducted in the 1990s (Clarke et al., 1995; Muñoz et al., 1995; Seligman, Schulman, DeRubeis, & Hollon, 1999), the number of studies has increased rapidly since 2000. Our meta-analysis of these studies (Van Zoonen et al., 2014) found a total of 32 studies in which subjects with a depressive disorder according to *DSM* criteria at baseline were excluded, and only subjects with no formal depressive disorder were included. In all these studies, it was examined whether the incidence rate of mental disorders was reduced in the recipients of preventive interventions compared to subjects who did not participate in the intervention. The overall incidence rate ratio was 0.79 (95% CI: 0.69~0.91). The incidence rate ratio is the incidence rate of developing a depressive disorder in experimental subjects relative to the incidence rate in control subjects. An incidence rate ratio of 0.79 indicates a reduction of about 21% in the risk of developing a depressive disorder in the next year compared to people in the control groups. This study indicates that prevention of new cases of depressive disorders seems to be possible and may become a realistic strategy to reduce the enormous burden of these disorders, along with treatment of existing depressive disorders.

Preventive interventions have been developed in several settings and include prevention of depression in school settings, maternal care settings, and medical settings. In the next section, I describe these settings and the research conducted in these settings.

Prevention in the School Setting

The school is a suitable setting for conducting prevention research for several reasons. First, depression in children during adolescence is an important problem from a public health perspective. With an estimated prevalence of 2.8% for children under the age of 13 and 5.6% for young people aged 13–18 years (Costello, Erkanli, & Angold, 2006), depression is a frequent condition in underage groups, with high recurrence rates, often poor psychosocial and academic outcomes, and an increased risk for other mental disorders (Birmaher et al., 1996). Furthermore, clinically relevant depressive symptoms that do not meet criteria for major depressive disorder are found in up to 30% of adolescents (Ryan, 2005).

Second, depression rates begin to rise in early adolescence, until they have reached adult levels in late adolescence (Costello et al., 2006). By the age of 19, about one in every four adolescents has had at least one depressive episode (Lewinsohn, Hops, Roberts, Seeley, & Andrews, 1993; Lewinsohn, Rohde, & Seeley, 1998). Most adults with recurrent depression have their initial depressive episodes as teenagers (Pine, Cohen, Gurley, Brook, & Ma, 1988); consequently, a considerable number of people develop their first depressive disorder during adolescence. If prevention is effective during that period, it may prevent the first episode ever as well as a chronic course of depression later in life.

The age of onset for major depressive disorder (MDD) symptoms has been estimated to be 19.1 years for 20% of those ever suffering from MDD and 25.8 years for 50% of those ever suffering from MDD (Mrazek & Haggerty, 1994). The age of first diagnosis, however, has been estimated to be 25.3 years for 20% of those ever suffering MDD and 38.8 years for 50% of those ever suffering MDD. As a result, many people who eventually develop MDD have subthreshold symptoms of depression for several years. During these years (often during adolescence or young adulthood), preventive interventions may be able to reduce the risk of developing depressive disorders.

A third reason is that prevention research at school is relatively easy from a logistic point of view, because all children and adolescents can be screened at schools, at which preventive interventions can be organized relatively easily.

Preventive interventions in the school setting are very diverse. Many interventions are universal (Brunwasser, Gillham, & Kim, 2009; Merry et al., 2011), but there are also indicated interventions aimed at students who already have some symptoms of depression (Van Zoonen et al., 2014). The content of the interventions is also very different, with most interventions being based on principles of CBT (Clarke et al., 1995; Sheffield et al., 2006), but there are also interventions that are based on IPT (Young, Mufson, & Davies, 2006; Young, Mufson, & Gallop, 2010).

A considerable number of studies has examined the possibilities of prevention in the school setting (e.g., Merry et al., 2011; Van Zoonen et al., 2014). However, most of these studies have only examined whether school programs are capable of reducing the overall level of depressive symptoms in students, suggesting that these programs may have a small effect on depressive symptoms (Merry et al., 2011). Although this is interesting in its own right, and positive effects may be indicative of effects on depressive disorders, the results of these studies do not provide clear evidence of a preventive effect of these interventions on depressive disorders.

In a meta-analysis of school-based programs for depression, it was found that 16 trials examined whether students had a depressive disorder (established with a diagnostic interview) at follow-up (Merry et al., 2011). It was found that these programs had a significant effect up to 12 months after the intervention (risk difference at 12 months was RD = -0.06; 95% CI: -0.11~-0.01). In another meta-analysis, only studies in which participants did not have a depressive disorder at baseline were included, and the incidence at follow-up was also established with a diagnostic interview (Van Zoonen et al., 2014). In this meta-analysis, 14 comparisons were found, and the incidence rate ratio (IRR = 0.81; 95% CI: 0.68~0.97) was also significant and reduced the incidence by 19% compared to the "no treatment" control conditions. In both meta-analyses, however, a considerable risk of bias in the included studies was found, so these results should be considered with caution.

Prevention of Postpartum Depression

Another important target group for preventive interventions is women with postpartum depression (PPD). PPD is a depressive disorder with the same characteristics as other depressive disorders, except that it occurs within four weeks postpartum (Elliott et al., 2000). About one in every seven new mothers is affected by PPD (Wisner, Chambers, & Sit, 2006), resulting in an overall prevalence rate of 13% (O'Hara & Swain, 1996). Postpartum mood disorders represent the most frequent form of maternal morbidity following delivery (Stocky & Lynch, 2000).

PPD is an important public health problem (Cuijpers, Brännmark, & van Straten, 2008). Apart from the direct suffering in patients caused by PPD and the increased risk of hospitalization (Dennis, 2004), several areas in the life of a patient can be adversely affected. PPD has been reported to result in an increased risk of marital stress and divorce (Holden, 1991), child abuse and neglect (Buist, 1998), and even maternal suicide and infanticide (Sit, Rothschild, & Wisner, 2006). PPD can also have serious consequences for the children of affected mothers in the short term and in the long term (Murray & Cooper, 2004). The negative effects of maternal depression on children include an increased risk of impaired mental and motor development, impairments in social engagement and emotional regulation, increased negative emotionality, difficult temperament, poor self-regulation, low self-esteem, and long-term behavioral problems (Feldman et al., 2009; Goodman & Gotlib, 1999; Wisner, Chambers, & Sit, 2006). It can also result in insecure attachment (Hipwell, Goossens, Melhuish, & Kumar, 2000; Murray, 1992), difficulties with social interactions (Cummings & Davies, 1994; Dennis, 2004), and a negative influence on cognitive skills (Whiffen & Gotlib, 1989) and expressive language development (Cox, Puckering, Pound, & Mills, 1987).

PPD often goes undetected due to a lack of proper screening and to the shame and loneliness that often make a woman hide it from her surroundings (Murray & Cooper,

1997). Untreated PPD often remits spontaneously after four to six months (O'Hara, 1997) but can in some cases easily last much longer, causing prolonged, serious suffering (Cooper & Murray, 1998). Because it causes considerable distress and disruption to women and their families, prevention is generally considered a priority (Cooper, Murray, Wilson, & Romaniuk, 2003). Research on the prevention of PPD is relatively easy, because all or most new mothers are seen regularly by health professionals during pregnancy.

A considerable number of studies has examined the possibilities of preventing PPD (e.g., Dennis, 2005; Dennis & Creedy, 2007; Sockol, Epperson, & Barber, 2013), but, again, most of these studies have not used diagnostic criteria at pretest and posttest to exclude women who already have a depressive disorder at pretest, and then examine the effects of prevention on the incidence. Most studies have used self-report measures and have only examined whether the level of depressive symptoms has decreased in the prevention groups compared to control groups. Many of these studies have used cognitive behavioral interventions (Brugha et al., 2000; Hagan, Evans, & Pope, 2004; Muñoz et al., 2007), although other studies have used psychoeducational interventions (Elliott et al., 2000), debriefing (Priest, Henderson, Evans, & Hagan, 2003), and IPT (Zlotnick, Johnson, Miller, Pearlstein, & Howard, 2001; Zlotnick, Miller, Pearlstein, Howard, & Sweeney, 2006).

A recent meta-analysis of 37 randomized or quasi-randomized trials on prevention of PPD found that these interventions had a small effect on depressive symptomatology ($g = 0.18$) and reduced the incidence of PPD by 27% at 6 months follow-up (Sockol et al., 2013). In another meta-analysis, only studies in which participants did not have a depressive disorder at baseline were included, and the incidence at follow-up was also established with a diagnostic interview (Van Zoonen et al., 2014). In this meta-analysis, nine comparisons were found for PPD, but the pooled effects were not significant, possibly due to lack of statistical power. Again, in both meta-analyses, a considerable risk of bias in the included studies was found, so all results should be considered with caution.

Prevention of Depressive Disorders in General Medical Disorders

General medical disorders are associated with increased rates of depressive disorders (Cassem, 1995), as found in coronary heart disease (Baune, Adrian, Arolt, & Berger, 2006; Frasure-Smith & Lesperance, 2006), stroke (Brodaty, Withall, Altendorf, & Sachdev, 2007; Robinson, 2003), cancer (Massie, 2004), multiple sclerosis (Rickards, 2006; Wallin, Wilken, Turner, Williams, & Kane, 2006), diabetes (Ali, Stone, Peters, Davies, & Khunti, 2006), rheumatoid arthritis (Dickens, McGowan, Clark-Carter, & Creed, 2002; Isik, Koca, Ozturk, & Mermi, 2007), and many other disorders. Prevention of depression in general medical patients is attractive because, if proven effective, it can be relatively easily integrated into routine care for these patients.

Relatively more research on prevention of depressive disorders has been conducted in stroke patients. It is widely acknowledged that depression is an important complication of stroke that may impede rehabilitation, recovery, quality of life, and caregiver health (Hackett, Anderson, & House, 2005; Hackett & Pickles, 2014). Furthermore, stroke-associated depression is found to have lower recovery rates, reduced survival rates, and increased risks of recurrent vascular events (House, Knapp, Bamford, & Vail, 2001; Morris, Robinson, Andrzejewski, Samuels, & Price, 1993).

In a recent meta-analysis of studies on the prevention of poststroke depression, four small randomized controlled trials of psychological interventions that examined the number of patients meeting criteria for depression at the end of treatment were found (Hackett, Anderson, House, & Halteh, 2008). The pooled results of these four trials indicated a significant reduction in the proportion of participants meeting study criteria for depression at the end of treatment (OR 0.64; 95% CI: 0.42~0.98). But again, the quality of these studies was not optimal. This meta-analysis also examined the effects of pharmacotherapy on the incidence of depression, but found no effects.

Apart from the prevention of depressive disorders in stroke patients, several other groups of general medical patients have been examined, including adolescents with newly diagnosed epilepsy and subthreshold depression (but no MDD) (Martinovic, Simonovic, & Djokic, 2006), diabetes patients (Bot, Pouwer, Ormel, Slaets, & de Jonge, 2010), and older patients with neovascular macular degeneration (Rovner, Casten, Hegel, Leiby, & Tasman, 2007; Rovner et al., 2014). Furthermore, several studies have examined preventive interventions in the care for older adults in nursing homes (Konnert, Dobson, & Stelmach, 2009) and residential homes for the elderly (Dozeman et al., 2012; van Schaik et al., 2014), as well as family caregivers of dementia patients (Joling et al. 2012; Vázquez et al., 2013).

In the meta-analysis we described earlier, in which only prevention trials in which participants did not have a depressive disorder at baseline were included, and the incidence at follow-up was also established with a diagnostic interview (Van Zoonen et al., 2014), 10 trials were found in patients with general medical disorders. The incidence rate ratio for these studies was IRR = 0.69 (95% CI: 0.54~0.89), suggesting that the prevention of depressive disorders may be effective in these target groups.

Prevention in Primary Care

Over the past 20 years, research on the prevention of depressive disorders has been conducted in several other settings. Some studies have examined the possibility of preventing depressive disorders in primary care. For example, in the San Francisco Depression Prevention Research project, an early prevention study, 150 predominantly chronically ill, public sector, and ethnically diverse primary care patients who did not have a depressive disorder in the past six months were randomized to an eight-session cognitive behavioral prevention group or a care-as-usual control group (Muñoz et al.,

1995). No significant difference between the conditions was found, possibly because of low statistical power.

In another study in primary care (Willemse, Smit, Cuijpers, & Tiemens, 2004), 209 patients with subthreshold depression (but no depressive disorder) were randomized to a preventive intervention (guided self-help with telephone support) or a care-as-usual control group. At one-year follow-up, significantly fewer patients in the intervention group developed a depressive disorder. One year after baseline, the incidence of MDD was found to be significantly lower in the psychotherapy group (12%) than in those receiving usual care (18%).

In another trial in primary care, 175 older adults with subthreshold depression were randomized to stepped care or care as usual (Van't Veer-Tazelaar et al., 2009). The stepped-care intervention consisted of watchful waiting, guided self-help, brief problem-solving therapy, and, if required, referral to primary care for medication. The relative risk of developing a depressive or anxiety disorder was $RR = 0.49$ (95% CI: 0.24~0.98). Because the number of studies is so small, it is not possible to pool the results of these trials in a meta-analysis.

Prevention of Depression in Other Settings

Although prevention of depression seems the most feasible in schools, maternal care, and medical settings, several other studies have attempted to identify target groups for preventive interventions and use these in different settings. For example, several studies have recruited adolescents with depressive symptoms (no disorder) through large health maintenance organizations (e.g., Clarke et al., 2001; Gillham, Hamilton, Freres, Patton, & Gallop, 2006). In other studies, adults with subthreshold depression were recruited from the general population through media announcements (Allart-van Dam, Hosman, Hoogduin, & Schaap, 2007; Reynolds et al., 2014). Other studies have focused on the identification of high-risk individuals among college students (Seligman et al., 1999; Seligman, Schulman, & Tryon, 2007).

The internet is potentially a new way to deliver preventive interventions. It is accessible for the majority of people in high-income countries, and it has been shown that psychological interventions for depression can be delivered effectively via the internet (Andersson & Cuijpers, 2009). Preventive interventions aimed at preventing the onset of depressive disorders, however, have not yet been conducted, although one study is ongoing (Ebert et al., 2014).

Problems in Identifying Target Groups for Preventive Interventions

In the preceding paragraphs, we saw that a considerable number of recent studies have examined the effects of preventive interventions on the incidence of depressive disorders, and, when taken together, with considerable success. However, the success of these interventions depends very much on the selection of the right target populations. The first step in every intervention is to select a target population that has an increased risk of developing MDD within a year. In the following paragraphs, we explain why this selection of high-risk groups is very complicated and present some recently developed methods in epidemiology to solve the problems in the selection of target groups.

Over the past few decades, an enormous body of research has shown that many biological, psychological, and psychosocial risk indicators are associated with the onset of depressive disorders. These include genetic factors, characteristics of personality, socioeconomic status, stress and burden, urbanization, loneliness, life events, and somatic factors such as complications during pregnancy, developmental disorders, neuroendocrinological factors, and general medical disorders. (Note that we define these variables as risk indicators, and not as risk factors, as risk factors suggest that these are causally associated with the onset of depressive disorders. Risk indicators only indicate that there is an association between the variable and the onset, while no causal association is assumed.) In principle, these risk indicators can be used to identify target groups for preventive interventions. In the next section of this chapter, we describe several groups of interventions that have focused on such high-risk groups.

Although many risk indicators are known to be associated with the onset of depression, most of them have low specificity. This low specificity implies that most subjects who are exposed to the risk indicator do not develop the disorder, and that one such risk indicator by itself is not sufficient to bring the disorder into being (Cuijpers, 2003; Maclure, 1988). Furthermore, most risk indicators are related to lifetime risk, while target populations for preventive interventions must have an increased shorter-term risk. Suppose, for example, that the risk of developing MDD in the general population is 2.5% in one year (Bijl, De Graaf, Ravelli, Smit, & Vollebergh, 2002; Smit, Beekman, Cuijpers, De Graaf, & Vollebergh, 2004). If a high-risk group has a relative risk of developing a depressive disorder of 4.0, this will be highly significant (if the research population is large enough). But, this means that still only about 10% of the high-risk group will actually develop a depressive disorder, and about 90% will not.

Many epidemiological researchers are satisfied after finding a highly significant relative risk of 4.0, but from the perspective of prevention this is clearly not enough. A high-risk group will probably be difficult to motivate for participation in a preventive program if only 10% will eventually develop the disorder, apart from the question of whether it is ethically acceptable to identify such a population as being "at risk" when most are, in fact, not at risk, or to intervene in such a population when, for the vast majority of participants, the intervention is not needed, and thus the time they spend on it is not needed. Furthermore, such an intervention is probably not very efficient and cost-effective, because the majority will never develop a disorder and the intervention has no preventive effect in this majority.

From the perspective of preventive intervention research, this low specificity is also problematic because very large numbers of subjects are needed to provide sufficient statistical power for these intervention studies (Cuijpers, 2003). Suppose, for example, that we would be able to motivate people from the high-risk group (10% of whom will develop a depressive disorder in the following year) to participate in a preventive intervention. In order to show that such an intervention is capable of reducing the incidence from 10% to 5% (a risk reduction of 50%), we would need about 950 persons in a controlled trial (assuming a statistical power of 0.80; alpha level 0.05; calculations in STATA/SE 8.2). Trials of this size are logistically complex, expensive, and have a high risk of failure.

Toward an Improved Method of Identifying Target Groups for Prevention

Since traditional indicators of the strength between a risk indicator and the incidence of a depressive disorder are not sufficient to identify the best target populations for preventive interventions, improving the selection of target groups can be made by using indices other than odds ratios (ORs), relative risks (RRs), or incidence rate ratios (IRRs) alone, and, in particular, by studying the cumulative effect of joint exposures to several risk indicators rather than the effect of a single risk indicator. The proposed method can be carried out in several steps.

First, a set of significant risk indicators is identified, such that each of them has a statistically significant impact on the likelihood that the disorder will develop. To do this, any of the available measures of association for binary outcomes (OR, RR, or IRR) can be used.

Second, if an OR can be calculated, then it is also possible to say how many people are exposed to that risk indicator. This measure is called exposure rate (ER). For prevention, the ER is important, because it tells us how many people have to be targeted by the preventive intervention. Clearly, smaller groups (smaller ER) are associated with less effort and, hence, lower costs of delivering the intervention.

Third, with the OR and ER in hand, one can calculate the population attributable fraction (AF). The AF indicates by what percentage the current incidence rate of depression in the population could be reduced when the adverse effect of the risk indicator is completely blocked (Miettinen, 1974; Rothman, Lash, & Greenland, 1998; Smit et al., 2006a). This equals the maximum possible health gain of a completely successful preventive intervention.

Fourth, if the OR can be calculated, then it is also possible to obtain the risk difference (e.g., under a linear probability model) and its inverse: the number needed to be treated (NNT). In the context of these analyses, the NNT can be interpreted as the number of people that should be the recipients of a preventive intervention to avoid the onset of the disorder in one person. Again, we have to assume that the preventive intervention is completely successful in containing the adverse effect of the risk factor. This assumption is not realistic, but the NNT may still help create a hierarchy of risk indicators to be targeted in prevention.

Now comes the important part of the method. We want to maximize the health gain (large AF) and minimize the effort to generate this health gain by targeting the smallest possible group (small ER) in the most efficient way (small NNT). Best values overall can be found by looking at combinations of risk indicators. That is, we can see what combinations of exposures (joint exposures) help to minimize and maximize the indices, such that a target group is selected where prevention is most likely to become cost-effective.

There are several ways of finding specific combinations of risk indicators, whether genetic or environmental, that meet the aforementioned criteria, including sophisticated statistical techniques, such as CART analyses (classification and regression trees analysis), and bootstrap aggregation (bagging; Schoevers et al., 2006; Smit et al., 2007). The most straightforward method, which we use here for illustrative purposes, is to select significant predictors of incidence (with standard techniques such as logistic regression) after which all possible combinations of these significant risk indicators are explored in terms of maximizing the OR and AF, and minimizing ER and NNT associated with each of the joint exposures. We used this approach in a population-based sample of older adults (Smit et al., 2006b) and found that subjects with (subclinical) depressive symptoms, functional limitations, a small social network, and female gender comprised only 8% of the total population (ER), while 24.2% of the new incident cases could be attributed to this group (AF). The number of subjects from this population that would have to receive a preventive intervention in order to prevent one incident case (NNT) was four (assuming that the intervention is 100% successful).

There is little doubt that these methods will help to identify the best target groups for preventive interventions in the near future; however, these methods have not yet been applied to intervention studies.

Future Research

Future research in the area of prevention of depressive disorders is certainly warranted. In each of the specific areas of target focus, such as school-based prevention, prevention of PPD, and prevention of depression in general medical disorders, more trials should be conducted in order to increase understanding of the interventions and recruitment methods in these settings.

An issue that has yet to be examined is whether preventive interventions have actually prevented the onset of new disorders or only delayed the onset. Only one of the studies until now has used a follow-up period of more than two years (Seligman et al., 1999). In the meta-analysis of prevention studies, we found a trend indicating that the length of the follow-up period was associated with the increased risk of developing a depressive disorder. This can be seen as an indication of effect decay over time and suggests a delay of onset rather than prevention (Van Zoonen et al., 2014). From a clinical perspective, both preventing and delaying onsets are important. Actual prevention of new cases would, of course, be preferable, as it would result in a reduction of the disease burden of all prevented cases. Delay of onset (i.e., depression-free survival) is also important, because the disease burden of depression is high.

Another question that should be answered by future research is which intervention is the most effective. Many studies have used an adapted version of the "Coping with Depression" course (Lewinsohn, Antonucci, Breckenridge, & Teri, 1984), or another cognitive behavioral intervention. However, a few studies have examined IPT-based interventions, and the effects of these studies were very strong and somewhat more effective than cognitive behavioral interventions (Van Zoonen et al., 2014). It is also necessary to examine the active components of the preventive interventions. All studies up to this point have compared a preventive intervention with a care-as-usual control group. Such studies are very useful for examining the additional effects of preventive interventions in current health care, but they do not give much information about the active components of the interventions. Research on active components may result in interventions with stronger effects than the current interventions.

As indicated earlier, the introduction of internet-based interventions in recent years may be important for the delivery of preventive interventions. Preventive and early interventions for depression are becoming increasingly easy to access online. Internet-based cognitive behavioral interventions appear to be as effective as regular cognitive behavioral interventions (Andersson, Cuijpers, Carlbring, Riper, & Hedman, 2014; Andrews, Cuijpers, Craske, McEvoy, & Titov, 2010) and have several other advantages: they allow participants to (1) work at their own pace, (2) abolish the need to schedule appointments, and (3) save traveling time. Furthermore, internet-based interventions may advance research into the outcome of interventions because every keystroke of users can be recorded for subsequent analysis. Several cognitive behavioral systems aimed at depression are already available, and meta-analyses have shown that these systems are effective in reducing depressive symptoms as much as regular treatments (Andersson & Cuijpers, 2009). Although most of these systems are aimed at the treatment of depression, there is no reason to assume that they cannot be used as (indicated) preventive interventions.

Stronger effects may also be realized when stepped-care approaches are used in indicated preventive interventions. When someone has a subthreshold depression, it seems logical to monitor these symptoms regularly, and when they do not improve, a nonintrusive intervention seems to be the best option. If such an intervention is not sufficiently effective in reducing the symptoms, a more intensive intervention should be used, and when nothing else helps, full pharmacological and psychological treatment can be applied. A trial examining the possibility of stepped care in prevention has very promising outcomes (Van't Veer-Tazelaar et al., 2009).

Future research may also focus on prevention of multiple types of mental disorders, especially anxiety disorders. Although mood and anxiety disorders often co-occur, and CBT often contains common components, only one study up to this point has examined the possibility of preventing both in one trial (Seligman et al., 1999).

Conclusions

Over the past 20 years, considerable progress has been made in the field of depression prevention. Important advances have been made in the epidemiological field, in which more traditional approaches have been improved considerably by other, relatively simple statistics such as the ER, the population AF, and the numbers needed to be treated. These statistical measures can be used to select those high-risk groups that are as small as possible but account for many of the new incident cases. Research on preventive interventions has been conducted in several settings and with several target groups, such as school-based interventions, prevention of PPD in maternal care settings, and prevention of depression in general medical patients.

Although some of these studies found positive effects of preventive interventions on the incidence of depressive disorders, several other studies do not have sufficient statistical power to detect significant effects or did not find any indication of a positive effect. However, a meta-analysis, in which all of these studies were analyzed together, found a clear and significant effect of these interventions (Van Zoonen et al., 2014). Thus, available data indicate that preventive interventions are actually capable of preventing the onset of depressive disorders.

It is encouraging that the prevention of new cases of depressive disorders seems to be feasible and effective. In addition to treatment, prevention may be an important alternative to reduce the enormous burden of depression in the future. The development of evidence-based preventive interventions for MDD and other mental disorders should be an important scientific and public health objective for the twenty-first century.

References

Ali, S., Stone, M. A., Peters, J. L., Davies, M. J., & Khunti, K. (2006). The prevalence of co-morbid depression in adults with type 2 diabetes: A systematic review and meta-analysis. *Diabetes Medicine, 23*(11), 1165–1173.

Allart-van Dam, E., Hosman, C. M., Hoogduin, C. A., & Schaap, C. P. (2007). Prevention of depression in subclinically depressed adults: Follow-up effects on the "Coping with Depression" course. *Journal of Affective Disorders, 97*(1), 219–228.

Alonso, J., Angermeyer, M. C., Bernert, S., Bruffaerts, R., Brugha, T. S., Bryson, H., . . . Vollebergh, W. A. (2004). Prevalence of mental disorders in Europe: Results from the European Study of the Epidemiology of Mental Disorders (ESEMeD) project. *Acta Psychiatrica Scandinavica, Supplement, 109*(s420), 21–27.

Andersson, G., & Cuijpers, P. (2009). Internet-based and other computerized psychological treatments for adult depression: A meta-analysis. *Cognitive Behaviour Therapy, 38*(4), 196–205.

Andersson, G., Cuijpers, P., Carlbring, P., Riper, H., & Hedman, E. (2014). Guided internet-based vs. face-to-face cognitive behaviour therapy for psychiatric and somatic disorders: A systematic review and meta-analysis. *World Psychiatry, 13*(3), 288–295.

Andrews, G., Cuijpers, P., Craske, M. G., McEvoy, P., & Titov, N. (2010). Computer therapy for the anxiety and depressive disorders is effective, acceptable and practical health care: A meta-analysis and pilot implementation. *PLos One, 5*(10), e13196.

Andrews, G., Issakidis, C., Sanderson, K., Corry, J., & Lapsley, H. (2004). Utilising survey data to inform public policy: Comparison of the cost-effectiveness of treatment of ten mental disorders. *British Journal of Psychiatry, 184*(6), 526–533.

Baune, B. T., Adrian, I., Arolt, V., & Berger, K. (2006). Associations between major depression, bipolar disorders, dysthymia and cardiovascular diseases in the general adult population. *Psychotherapy and Psychosomatics, 75*(5), 319–326.

Bijl, R. V., De Graaf, R., Ravelli, A., Smit, F., & Vollebergh, W. A. M. (2002). Gender and age specific first incidence of *DSM-III-R* psychiatric disorders in the general population: Results from the Netherlands Mental Health Survey and Incidence Study (NEMESIS). *Social Psychiatry Psychiatric Epidemiology, 37*(8), 372–379.

Birmaher, B., Ryan, N. D., Williamson, D. E., Brent, D. A., Kaufman, J., Dahl, R. E., . . . Nelson, B. (1996). Childhood and adolescent depression, I: A review of the past 10 years. *Journal of the American Academy of Child Adolescent Psychiatry, 35*(11), 1427–1439.

Bot, M., Pouwer, F., Ormel, J., Slaets, J. P. J., & de Jonge, P. (2010). Education and psychological aspects: Predictors of incident major depression in diabetic outpatients with subthreshold depression. *Diabetic Medicine, 27*(11), 1295–1301.

Brodaty, H., Withall, A., Altendorf, A., & Sachdev, P. S. (2007). Rates of depression at 3 and 15 months poststroke and their relationship with cognitive decline: The Sydney Stroke Study. *American Journal of Geriatric Psychiatry, 15*(6), 477–486.

Brugha, T. S., Wheatly, S., Taub, N. A., Culverwell, A., Freidman, T., Kirwan, P., . . . Shapiro, D. A. (2000). Pragmatic randomized trial of antenatal intervention to prevent post-natal depression by reducing psychosocial risk factors. *Psychological Medicine, 30*(6), 1273–1281.

Brunwasser, S. M., Gillham, J. E., & Kim, E. S. (2009). A meta-analytic review of the Penn Resiliency Program's effect on depressive symptoms. *Journal of Consulting and Clinical Psychology, 77*(6), 1042–1054.

Buist, A. (1998). Childhood abuse, parenting and postpartum depression. *Australian and New Zealand Journal of Psychiatry, 32*(4), 479–487.

Cassem, E. H. (1995). Depressive disorders in the medically ill: An overview. *Psychosomatics, 36*(2), S2–S10.

Chien, L. Y., Chu, H., Guo, J. L., Liao, Y. M., Chang, L. I., Chen, C. H., & Chou, K. R. (2011). Caregiver support groups in patients with dementia: A meta-analysis. *International Journal of Geriatric Psychiatry, 26*(10), 1089–1098.

Chisholm, D., Sanderson, K., Ayoso-Mateos, J. L., & Saena, S. (2004). Reducing the global burden of depression: Population-level analysis of intervention cost-effectiveness in 14 world regions. *British Journal of Psychiatry, 184*(5), 393–403.

Clarke, G. N., Hawkins, W., Murphy, M., Sheeber, L. B., Lewinsohn, P. M., & Seeley, J. R. (1995). Targeted prevention of unipolar depressive disorder in an at-risk sample of high school adolescents: A randomized trial of a group cognitive intervention. *Journal of the American Academy of Child and Adolescent Psychiatry, 34*(3), 312–321.

Clarke, G. N., Hornbrook, M., Lynch, F., Polen, M., Gale, J., Beardslee, . . . Seeley, J. (2001). A randomized trial of a group cognitive intervention for preventing depression in adolescent offspring of depressed parents. *Archives of General Psychiatry, 58*(12), 1127–1134.

Cooper, P. J., & Murray, L. (1998). Fortnightly review: Postnatal depression. *British Medical Journal, 316*(7148), 1884–1886.

Cooper, P. J., Murray, L., Wilson, A., & Romaniuk, H. (2003). Controlled trial of the short- and long-term effect of psychological treatment of post-partum depression; 1. Impact on maternal mood. *British Journal of Psychiatry, 182*(5), 412–419.

Costello, J. E., Erkanli, A., & Angold, A. (2006). Is there an epidemic of child or adolescent depression? *Journal of Child Psychology and Psychiatry, 47*(12), 1263–1271.

Cox, A. D., Puckering, C., Pound, A., & Mills, M. (1987). The impact of maternal depression in young children. *Journal of Child Psychology and Psychiatry, 28*(6), 917–928.

Cuijpers, P. (2003). Examining the effects of prevention programs on the incidence of new cases of mental disorders: The lack of statistical power. *American Journal of Psychiatry, 160*(8), 1385–1391.

Cuijpers, P., Brännmark, J. G., & van Straten, A. (2008). Psychological treatment of postpartum depression: A meta-analysis. *Journal of Clinical Psychology, 64*(1), 103–118.

Cuijpers, P., van Straten, A., Smit, F., Mihalopoulos, C., & Beekman, A. (2008). Preventing the onset of depressive disorders: A meta-analytic review of psychological interventions. *American Journal of Psychiatry, 165*(10), 1272–1280.

Cuijpers, P., Vogelzangs, N., Twisk, J., Kleiboer, A., Li, J., & Penninx, B. (2014). Comprehensive meta-analysis of excess mortality in depression in the general community versus patients with specific illnesses. *American Journal of Psychiatry, 171*(4), 453–462.

Cummings, E. M., & Davies, P. T. (1994). Maternal depression and child development. *Journal of Child Psychology and Psychiatry, 35*(1), 73–112.

Dennis, C. L. (2004). Treatment of postpartum depression, part 2: A critical review of nonbiological interventions. *Journal of Clinical Psychiatry, 65*(9), 1252–1265.

Dennis, C. L. (2005). Psychosocial and psychological interventions for prevention of postnatal depression: Systematic review. *British Medical Journal, 331*(7507), 15.

Dennis, C. L., & Creedy, D. (2007). Psychosocial and psychological interventions for preventing postpartum depression. *Cochrane Database of Systematic Reviews, 4*, Art. No.: CD001134. doi:10.1002/14651858.CD001134.pub2

Dickens, C., McGowan, L., Clark-Carter, D., & Creed, F. (2002). Depression in rheumatoid arthritis: A systematic review of the literature with meta-analysis. *Psychosomatic Medicine, 64*(1), 52–60.

Dozeman, E., van Marwijk, H. W., van Schaik, D. J., Smit, F., Stek, M. L., van der Horst, H. E., . . . Beekman, A. T. (2012). Contradictory effects for prevention of depression and anxiety in residents in homes for the elderly: A pragmatic randomized controlled trial. *International Psychogeriatrics, 24*(8), 1242–1251.

Durlak, J. A., & Wells, A. M. (1997). Primary prevention mental health programs for children and adolescents: A meta-analytic review. *American Journal of Community Psychology, 25*(2), 115–152.

Durlak, J. A., & Wells, A. M. (1998). Evaluation of indicated preventive intervention (secondary prevention) mental health programs for children and adolescents. *American Journal of Community Psychology, 26*(5), 775–802.

Ebert, D. D., Lehr, D., Baumeister, H., Boß, L., Riper, H., Cuijpers, P., . . . Berking, M. (2014). GET.ON Mood Enhancer: Efficacy of internet-based guided self-help compared to psychoeducation for depression: An investigator-blinded randomised controlled trial. *Trials, 15*(1), 39.

Elliott, S. A., Leverton, T. J., Sanjack, M., Turner, H., Cowmeadow, P., Hopkins, J., & Bushnell, D. (2000). Promoting mental health after childbirth: A controlled trial of primary prevention of postnatal depression. *British Journal of Clinical Psychology, 39*(3), 223–241.

Feldman, R., Granat, A., Pariente, C., Kanety, H., Kuint, J., & Gilboa-Schechtman, E. (2009). Maternal depression and anxiety across the postpartum year and infant social engagement, fear regulation, and stress reactivity. *Journal of the American Academy of Child and Adolescent Psychiatry, 48*(9), 919–927.

Frasure-Smith, N., & Lesperance, F. (2006). Recent evidence linking coronary heart disease and depression. *Canadian Journal of Psychiatry, 51*(12), 730–737.

Gillham, J. E., Hamilton, J., Freres, D. R., Patton, K., & Gallop, R. (2006). Preventing depression among early adolescents in the primary care setting: A randomized controlled study of the Penn Resiliency Program. *Journal of Abnormal Child Psychology, 34*(2), 203–219.

Goodman, S. H., & Gotlib, I. H. (1999). Risk for psychopathology in the children of depressed mothers: A developmental model for understanding mechanisms of transmission. *Psychological Review, 106*(3), 458–490.

Greenberg, P. E., & Birnbaum, H. G. (2005). The economic burden of depression in the US: Societal and patient perspectives. *Expert Opinion on Pharmacotherapy, 6*(3), 369–376.

Hackett, M. L., Anderson, C. S., & House, A. O. (2005). Management of depression after stroke: A systematic review of pharmacological therapies. *Stroke, 36*(5), 1092–1097.

Hackett, M. L., Anderson, C. S., House, A., & Halteh, C. (2008). Interventions for preventing depression after stroke. *Cochrane Database of Systematic Reviews, 3*, Art. No.: CD003689.

Hackett, M. L., & Pickles, K. (2014). Part I: Frequency of depression after stroke: An updated systematic review and meta-analysis of observational studies. *International Journal on Stroke, 9*(8), 1017–1025.

Hagan, R., Evans, S. F., & Pope, S. (2004). Preventing postnatal depression in mothers of very preterm infants: A randomised controlled trial. *BJOG, 111*(7), 641–647.

Hipwell, A. E., Goossens, F. A., Melhuish, E. C., & Kumar, R. (2000). Severe maternal psychopathology and infant-mother attachment. *Developmental Psychopathology, 12*(2), 157–175.

Holden, J. M. (1991). Postnatal depression: Its nature, effects, and identification using the Edinburgh Postnatal Depression scale. *Birth, 18*(4), 211–221.

Hollon, S. D. (2002). Psychosocial intervention development for the prevention and treatment of depression: Promoting innovation and increasing access. *Biological Psychiatry, 52*(6), 610–630.

House, A., Knapp, P., Bamford, J., & Vail, A. (2001). Mortality at 12 and 24 months after stroke may be associated with depressive symptoms at 1 month. *Stroke, 32*(3), 696–701.

Isik, A., Koca, S. S., Ozturk, A., & Mermi, O. (2007). Anxiety and depression in patients with rheumatoid arthritis. *Clinical Rheumatology, 26*(6), 872–878.

Joling, K. J., van Marwijk, H. W., Smit, F., van der Horst, H. E., Scheltens, P., van de Ven, P. M., . . . van Hout, H. P. (2012). Does a family meetings intervention prevent depression and anxiety in family caregivers of dementia patients? A randomized trial. *PLoS One, 7*(1), e30936.

Kessler, R. C., McGonagle, K. A., Zhao, S., Nelson, C. B., Hughes, M., Eshleman, S., . . . Kendler, K. S. (1994). Lifetime and 12-month prevalence of *DSM-III-R* psychiatric disorders in the United States: Results from the National Comorbidity Survey. *Archives of General Psychiatry, 51*(1), 8–19.

Konnert, C., Dobson, K., & Stelmach, L. (2009). The prevention of depression in nursing home residents: A randomized clinical trial of cognitive-behavioral therapy. *Aging and Mental Health, 13*(2), 288–299.

Lewinsohn, P. M., Antonucci, D. O., Breckenridge, J. S., & Teri, L. (1984). *The "Coping with Depression" course.* Eugene, OR: Castalia Publishing Company.

Lewinsohn, P. M., Hops, H., Roberts, R. E., Seeley, J. R., & Andrews, J. A. (1993). Adolescent psychopathology, I: Prevalence and incidence of depression and other *DSM-III-R* disorders in high school students. *Journal of Abnormal Psychology, 102*(1), 133–144.

Lewinsohn, P. M., Rohde, P., & Seely, J. R. (1998). Major depressive disorder in older adolescents: Prevalence, risk factors, and clinical implications. *Clinical Psychology Review, 18*(7), 765–794.

Maclure, M. (1988). Refutation in epidemiology: Why else not? In K. J. Rothman (Ed.), *Causal inference* (pp. 131–138). Chestnut Hill, PA: Epidemiology Resources.

Martinovic, Z., Simonovic, P., & Djokic, R. (2006). Preventing depression in adolescents with epilepsy. *Epilepsy and Behavior, 9*(4), 619–624.

Massie, M. J. (2004). Prevalence of depression in patients with cancer. *Journal of the National Cancer Institute Monographs, 32*(1), 57–71.

Mathers, C. D., & Loncar, D. (2006). Projections of global mortality and burden of disease from 2002 to 2030. *PLoS Medicine, 3*(11), e442.

Merry, S. N., Hetrick, S. E., Cox, G. R., Brudevold-Iversen, T., Bir, J. J., & McDowell, H. (2011). Psychological and educational interventions for preventing depression in children and adolescents. *Cochrane Database of Systematic Reviews, 12*, Art. No.: CD003380.

Miettinen, O. S. (1974). Proportion of disease caused or prevented by a given exposure, trait, or intervention. *American Journal of Epidemiology, 99*(5), 325–332.

Morris, P. L., Robinson, R. G., Andrzejewski, P., Samuels, J., & Price, T. R. (1993). Association of depression with 10-year poststroke mortality. *American Journal of Psychiatry, 150*(1), 124–129.

Mrazek, P. J., & Haggerty, R. (1994). *Reducing risks of mental disorder: Frontiers for preventive intervention research.* Washington, DC: National Academy Press.

Muñoz, R. F., Le, H. N., Ippen, C. G., Diaz, M. A., Urizar Jr., G. G., Soto, J., . . . Lieberman, A. F. (2007). Prevention of postpartum depression in low-income women: Development of the Mamas y Bebes / Mothers and Babies course. *Cognitive Behavior Practice, 14*(1), 70–83.

Muñoz, R. F., Ying, Y. W., Bernal, G., Perez-Stable, E. J., Sorensen, J. L., Hargreaves, W. A., . . . Miller, L. S. (1995). Prevention of depression with primary care patients: A randomized controlled trial. *American Journal of Community Psychology, 23*(2), 199–222.

Murray, L. (1992). The impact of postnatal depression on infant development. *Journal of Child Psychology and Psychiatry, 33*(3), 543–561.

Murray, L., & Cooper, P. J. (1997). *Postpartum depression and child development.* New York, NY: Guilford Press.

Murray, L., & Cooper, P. J. (2004). The impact of postpartum depression on child development. In I. Goodyer (Ed.), *Aetiological mechanisms in developmental psychopathology.* Oxford: Oxford University Press.

O'Connell, M. E., Boat, T., & Warner, K. E. (2009). *Preventing mental, emotional, and behavioral disorders among young people: Progress and possibilities.* Washington DC: The National Academies Press.

O'Hara, M. W. (1997). The nature of postpartum depressive disorders. In L. Murray & P. J. Cooper (Eds.), *Postpartum depression and child development* (pp. 3–34). New York, NY: Guilford Press.

O'Hara, M. W., & Swain, A. M. (1996). Rates and risk of postpartum depression: A meta-analysis. *International Review of Psychiatry, 8*(1), 37–54.

Pine, D. S., Cohen, P., Gurley, D., Brook, J., & Ma, Y. (1998). The risk for early-adulthood anxiety and depressive disorders in adolescents with anxiety and depressive disorders. *Archives of General Psychiatry, 55*(1), 56–64.

Priest, S., Henderson, J., Evans, S., & Hagan, R. (2003). Stress debriefing after childbirth: A randomized controlled trial. *Medical Journal of Australia, 178*(11), 542–545.

Reynolds, C. F. III, Thomas, S. B., Morse, J. Q., Anderson, S. J., Albert, S., Dew, M. A., . . . Quinn, S. C. (2014). Early intervention to preempt major depression among older black and white adults. *Psychiatric Services, 65*(6), 765–773.

Rickards, H. (2006). Depression in neurological disorders: An update. *Current Opinions in Psychiatry, 19*(3), 294–298.

Robinson, R. G. (2003). Poststroke depression: Prevalence, diagnosis, treatment, and disease progression. *Biological Psychiatry, 54*(3), 376–387.

Rothman, K. J., Lash, T. L., & Greenland, S. (1998). *Modern Epidemiology* (2nd ed.). Philadelphia, PA: Lippincott-Raven.

Rovner, B. W., Casten, R. J., Hegel, M. T., Leiby, B. E., & Tasman, W. S. (2007). Preventing depression in age-related macular degeneration. *Archives of General Psychiatry, 64*(8), 886–892.

Rovner, B. W., Casten, R. J., Hegel, M. T., Massof, R. W., Leiby, B. E., Ho, A. C., . . . Tasman, W. S. (2014). Low vision depression prevention trial in age-related macular degeneration: A randomized clinical trial. *Ophthalmology, 121*(11), 2204–2211.

Ruotsalainen, J., Serra, C., Marine, A., & Verbeek, J. (2008). Systematic review of interventions for reducing occupational stress in health care workers. *Scandinavian Journal of Work and Environmental Health, 34*(3), 169–178.

Ryan, N. D. (2005). Treatment of depression in children and adolescents. *Lancet, 366*(9489), 933–940.

Saarni, S. I., Suvisaari, J., Sintonen, H., Pirkola, S., Koskinen, S., Aromaa, A., & Lönnqvist, J. (2007). Impact of psychiatric disorders on health-related quality of life: General population survey. *British Journal of Psychiatry, 190*(4), 326–332.

Schoevers, R. A., Smit, F., Deeg, D. J. H., Cuijpers, P., Dekker, J., Van Tilburg, W., & Beekman, A. T. F. (2006). Prevention of late-life depression in primary care: Do we know where to begin? *American Journal of Psychiatry, 163*(9), 1611–1621.

Seligman, M. E. P., Schulman, P., DeRubeis, R. J., & Hollon, S. D. (1999). The prevention of depression and anxiety. *Prevention and Treatment, 2*(1). Retrieved from http://dx.doi.org/10.1037/1522-3736.2.1.28a

Seligman, M. E. P., Schulman, P., & Tryon, A. M. (2007). Group prevention of depression and anxiety symptoms. *Behaviour Research and Therapy, 45*(6), 1111–1126.

Sheffield, J. K., Spence, S. H., Rapee, R. M., Kowalenko, N., Wignall, A., Davis, A., & McLoone, J. (2006). Evaluation of universal, indicated, and combined cognitive-behavioral approaches to the prevention of depression among adolescents. *Journal of Consulting and Clinical Psychology, 74*(1), 66–79.

Sit, D., Rothschild, A. J., & Wisner, K. L. (2006). A review of postpartum psychosis. *Journal of Women's Health, 15*(4), 352–368.

Smit, F., Beekman, A., Cuijpers, P., De Graaf, R., & Vollebergh, W. (2004). Selecting key variables for depression prevention: Results from a population-based prospective epidemiological study. *Journal of Affective Disorders, 81*(3), 241–249.

Smit, F., Comijs, H. C., Schoevers, R., Cuijpers, P., Deeg, D., & Beekman, A. (2007). Target groups for the prevention of late-life anxiety. *British Journal of Psychiatry, 190*(5), 428–434.

Smit, F., Cuijpers, P., Oostenbrink, J., Batelaan, N., de Graaf, R., & Beekman, A. (2006a). Excess costs of common mental disorders: Population-based cohort study. *Journal of Mental Health Policy and Economics, 9*(4), 193–200.

Smit, F., Ederveen, A., Cuijpers, P., Deeg, D., & Beekman, A. (2006b). Opportunities for cost-effective prevention of late-life depression: An epidemiological approach. *Archives of General Psychiatry, 63*(3), 290–296.

Sockol, L. E., Epperson, C. N., & Barber, J. P. (2013). Preventing postpartum depression: A meta-analytic review. *Clinical Psychology Review, 33*(8), 1205–1217.

Stocky, A., & Lynch, J. (2000). Acute psychiatric disturbance in pregnancy and the puerperium. *Bailliere's Best Practice Research in Clinical Obstetric Gynaecology, 14*(1), 73–87.

Tan, L., Wang, M. J., Modini, M., Joyce, S., Mykletun, A., Christensen, H., & Harvey, S. B. (2014). Preventing the development of depression at work: A systematic review and meta-analysis of universal interventions in the workplace. *BMC Medicine, 12*(1), 74. Retrieved from http://www.doi:10.1186/1741-7015-12-74

Ustün, T. B., Ayuso-Mateos, J. L., Chatterji, S., Mathers, C., & Murray, C. J. L. (2004). Global burden of depressive disorders in the year 2000. *British Journal of Psychiatry, 184*(5), 386–392.

Van der Klink, J., Blonk, R., & van Dijk, F. (2001). The benefits of interventions for work-related stress. *American Journal of Public Health, 91*(2), 270–276.

van Schaik, D. J., Dozeman, E., van Marwijk, H. W., Stek, M. L., Smit, F., Beekman, A. T., & van der Horst, H. E. (2014). Preventing depression in homes for older adults: Are effects sustained over 2 years? *International Journal of Geriatric Psychiatry, 29*(2), 191–197.

Van't Veer-Tazelaar, P. J., van Marwijk, H. W., van Oppen, P., van Hout, H. P., van der Horst, H. E., Cuijpers, P., . . . Beekman, A. T. (2009). Stepped-care prevention of anxiety and depression in late life: A randomized controlled trial. *Archives of General Psychiatry, 66*, 297–304.

Van Zoonen, K., Buntrock, C., Ebert, D. D., Smit, F., Reynolds, C. F., Beekman, A. T. F., & Cuijpers, P. (2014). Preventing the onset of major depressive disorder: A meta-analytic review of psychological interventions. *International Journal of Epidemiology, 43*(2), 318–329.

Vázquez, G. F. L, Otero, O. P., Iglesias, T. A., García, H. E., Seoane, B. V., & Fernández, D. O. (2013). A brief problem-solving indicated-prevention intervention for prevention of depression in nonprofessional caregivers. *Psicothema, 25*(1), 87–92.

Vittengl, J. R., Clark, L. A., Dunn, T. W., & Jarrett, R. B. (2007). Reducing relapse and recurrence in unipolar depression: A comparative meta-analysis of cognitive-behavioral therapy's effects. *Journal of Consulting and Clinical Psychology, 75*(3), 475–488.

Wallin, M. T., Wilken, J. A., Turner, A. P., Williams, R. M., & Kane, R. (2006). Depression and multiple sclerosis: Review of a lethal combination. *Journal of Rehabilitation, Research and Development, 43*(1), 45–62.

Waraich, P., Goldner, E. M., Somers, J. M., & Hsu, L. (2004). Prevalence and incidence studies of mood disorders: A systematic review of the literature. *Canadian Journal of Psychiatry, 49*(2), 124–138.

Whiffen, V. E., & Gotlib, I. H. (1989). Infants of postpartum depressed mothers: Temperament and cognitive status. *Journal of Abnormal Psychology, 98*(3), 274–279.

Willemse, G. R., Smit, F., Cuijpers, P., & Tiemens, B. G. (2004). Minimal contact psychotherapy for sub-threshold depression in primary care: A randomised trial. *British Journal of Psychiatry, 185*(5), 416–421.

Wisner, K. L., Chambers, C., & Sit, D. K. Y. (2006). Postpartum depression: A major public health problem. *Journal of the American Medical Association, 296*(21), 2616–2618.

Young, J. F., Mufson, L., & Davies, M. (2006). Efficacy of interpersonal psychotherapy-adolescent skills training: An indicated preventive intervention for depression. *Journal of Child Psychology and Psychiatry, 47*(12), 1254–1262.

Young, J. F., Mufson, L., & Gallop, R. (2010). Preventing depression: A randomized trial of interpersonal psychotherapy-adolescent skill training. *Depression and Anxiety, 27*(5), 426–433.

Zlotnick, C., Johnson, S. L., Miller, I. W., Pearlstein, T., & Howard, M. (2001). Postpartum depression in women receiving public assistance: Pilot study of an interpersonal-therapy-oriented group intervention. *American Journal of Psychiatry, 158*(4), 638–640.

Zlotnick, C., Miller, I. W., Pearlstein, T., Howard, M., & Sweeney, P. (2006). A preventive intervention for pregnant women on public assistance at risk for postpartum depression. *American Journal of Psychiatry, 163*(8), 1443–1445.

INDEX

Page numbers in italics indicate figures.